The Bright Side of Shame

Claude-Hélène Mayer · Elisabeth Vanderheiden
Editors

The Bright Side of Shame

Transforming and Growing Through Practical
Applications in Cultural Contexts

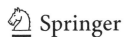 Springer

Editors
Claude-Hélène Mayer
Institut für Therapeutische Kommunikation
und Sprachgebrauch
Europa Universität Viadrina
Frankfurt (Oder), Germany

Department of Management
Rhodes University
Grahamstown, South Africa

Elisabeth Vanderheiden
Katholische Erwachsenenbildung
Rheinland-Pfalz
Mainz, Rheinland-Pfalz, Germany

ISBN 978-3-030-13408-2   ISBN 978-3-030-13409-9   (eBook)
https://doi.org/10.1007/978-3-030-13409-9

Library of Congress Control Number: 2019931533

This Springer imprint is published by the registered company Springer Nature Switzerland AG.
The registered company address is: Gewerbestrasse 11, 6330 Cham, Switzerland

Foreword: From Shame to Wholeness: An Existential Positive Psychology Perspective

> *Then the eyes of both of them were opened, and they realized they were naked; so they sewed fig leaves together and made coverings for themselves.*
>
> (Genesis 3:7, NIV)

Keywords Existential shame, Existential competency, Second wave positive psychology, PP2.0, Human dignity, Compassion

According to this biblical story, shame, guilt, and anxiety are the tragic triangle of existential emotions that have plagued humanity ever since Adam and Eve ate the forbidden fruit and became conscious of their sin and the need to cover themselves from God and each other. Human beings gained their independence and became as wise as God at a heavy cost: our ancestors became conscious of their shame and guilt for the first time after breaking the divine covenant and felt anxious when they faced an uncertain future after expulsion from the Garden of Eden.

The metaphorical truth in this ancient narrative is that shame is a deep-rooted existential emotion which stems from the human condition of being conscious of our own nothingness, aloneness, and insignificance in this vast cosmos as helpless orphans.

Shame is indeed a deep-rooted emotion, hiding behind all kinds of negative emotions (Malik, in this book). "It encompasses the whole of ourselves; it generates a wish to hide, to disappear, or even to die" (Lewis, 1995, p. 2). It is the normal part of the human nature. Shame is also "among the most intense and painful affects" (Andrieux, in this book). Thus, any effective therapy would benefit from an existential positive psychology perspective (Wong, 2009), which both normalises shame and affirms that the greatest potential for growth only comes from the most intense pain.

An Existential Perspective of Shame

The existential perspective of therapy (Wong, 2017a) has at least three advantages. First, it recognises shame as a universal condition of human existence; therefore, all therapies need to address this fundamental existential issue. Second, it recognises the common humanity and human frailty of all human beings; therefore, this consciousness should contribute to our empathy and compassion for all people, regardless of their race, culture, socio-economic status, or physical condition. Third, it also makes us aware of the existential–spiritual core that exists in all individuals; therefore, it behoves us to tap into this spiritual resource to address mental health issues. In other words, all therapists can benefit from existential competency.

The book makes it very clear that shame permeates our entire existence, from the unconscious to the collective; it is experienced in all situations—when we feel out of place, inferior in our social standing, inadequate in our performance, deficient in our body image, or humiliated and rejected by others. Even in places where no one is watching, we can still be haunted by fear that someone may find out our dark secret or have witnessed our shameful act.

Shame is the mother of all negative emotions. We may become angry, when we are humiliated or shamed; depressed and even suicidal, when we are ashamed of our own existence; rude and arrogant, when we want to cover up our inferior feelings; lonely and isolated, when we feel too ashamed of ourselves to reach out; addicted, when we are too ashamed to live with our failure and guilt. Ageing and dying pose further challenges; we feel ashamed of the physical changes that come with advanced age, and our sense of shame becomes even more painful when we become totally dependent on others during the last stage of life. In fact, dignity therapy (Martínez et al., 2017) has been increasingly used to reduce this existential crisis in palliative care. In short, in every stage of development, we cannot achieve wholeness without first finding healing for our existential shame regarding our brokenness and nothingness.

Thus, shame is pervasive in various mental health issues. Our shame can turn into social withdrawal, helplessness, depression, addiction (Baharudin, Sumari, & Hamdani, in this book) or aggression and self-harm—all inadequate attempts to deal with the problem of shame. Therapists need to have the clinical skill to identify the source of shame and treat it as an existential emotion common to all human beings.

External and Collective Shame

Gilbert (in this book) differentiates between external and internal shame. The former refers to our thoughts about other people's perception and opinions about us; the latter refers to self-evaluation and self-criticism. Different intervention strategies are needed for these two kinds of shame. While mindfulness and reframing can reduce both types of pain, external shame also requires challenges to a toxic culture, such as discrimination and stigmatisation.

External shame is often associated with social sanction and collective shame, as shown by Mayer's chapter (in this book) on the German society. Her chapter reminds us of the importance of a historical understanding of collective shame. For example, the best way to understand Chinese sensitivity to slights from the West as well as the current Chinese nationalism is to remember the 100 years of painful humiliation in the hands of foreign invaders starting from the Opium Wars. At a deeper level, collective shame is related to the tribal mentality and territorial instincts with evolutionary roots in the struggle for survival. In other words, collective shame reflects the existential shame of people who exist as social herd animals.

Another example of collective existential shame is Sueda's chapter (in this book) on the repatriation training of Japanese returnees to their homeland. This chapter is relevant to the broader existential need of feeling fully accepted by the country accepted as one's new home. A sense of shame because of one's language and cultural handicap is a big part of acculturation stress, which happens to all people transplanted to a different country, whether as refugees, immigrants, or returnees.

Second Wave Positive Psychology and the Transformation of Shame

This book is a logical next step since Vanderheiden and Mayer's (2017) first book on the nature of shame across cultures. Their shift from pathology to health and well-being is consistent with the perspective of second wave positive psychology (PP 2.0; Wong, 2011). More specifically, I (Wong, 2017b) have pointed out that their first book on the nature of shame recognises that all emotions are dualistic in nature, with both healthy and unhealthy sides. Instead of focusing on the up side of negative emotions, PP 2.0 maintains that well-being is based on how we manage the polarities of each emotion in order to achieve optimal well-being. Moreover, their first book also recognises that there are both intrapsychic and interpersonal dimensions of the dark side of human existence. The intrapsychic dark side may include abuse or a damaged ego due to personal handicaps. The interpersonal dark side of existence includes the accumulated toxic experiences of rejection, bullying, marginalisation, and alienation. Thus, PP 2.0 emphasises the need to embrace the dark side as a necessary gateway to resilience and flourishing.

For the present book by Vanderheiden and Mayer, I also want to mention that, in addition to existential positive psychology (Wong, 2009), PP 2.0 also includes a cross-cultural positive and indigenous psychology (Wong, 2013). PP 2.0 acknowledges that although there is only one human nature, there are many expressions and experiences across different cultures.

This book is encyclopedic in coverage, covering nine major parts involving different contexts, theoretical frameworks, and modalities of shame therapy. To name a few, this book covers the elective approach (Malik, in this book), cognitive-behavioural therapy (Merkin, in this book), motivational interview (Andrieux, in this book), appreciative inquiry (Nel & Govender, in this book), mindfulness (Vanderheiden, in this book), art therapy (Sherwood, in this book), dream work (Mayer, in this book), narrative theory (Nel & Govender, in this book), and failure management (Baumann & Handrock, in this book).

It not only covers "body shame, group shame, empathetic and intimacy shame, traumatic and more shame" (Mayer & Vanderheiden, p. 31, in this book) but also discusses the extensive role culture plays "in the definition, development and experience of shame and how it is addressed, managed, and transformed" (Mayer & Vanderheiden, p. 31, in this book).

It is refreshing to see so many contributors in this book introduce their indigenous ways to treating shame (e.g. Wang & Sang; Kunin; Baharudin, Sumari, & Hamdani; in this book). Seldom does one see a clinical handbook where "researchers as well as practitioners from different countries all over the world have been invited to contribute... and explain how they address shame from within their theoretical stance, their professional practice, and their cultural perspective at various levels" (Mayer & Vanderheiden, p. 30, in this book).

Regardless of their cultures and preferred treatment modality, all contributors bring out different facets and methods of the transformation of shame from a painful experience to resilience, well-being, and personal growth through its remedial function ("I want to change my shameful existence and overcome my feeling of inferiority"), protective function ("I don't want to violate my conscience and normative ethical rules"), and motivational function ("I want to become someone who no longer needs to hide from others").

Conclusion: Existential Competency in Shame Therapy

I want to conclude my forward by returning to the theme of existential positive psychology. The painful ontological aspects of shame indicate that shame is analogous to physical pain, signalling that some injury or deficiency, such as experiences of rejections, imperfections, limitations, and brokenness. As such, it serves as "a survival strategy" (Geldenhuys, in this book). But shame is also "a life-serving signal" (Larsson, in this book), which safeguards our dignity (Boness, in this book) and motivates us to move up from the bottom of the pyramid (Ungerer, in this book). Thus, shame is a double-edged sword in therapy.

Existential competency in therapy deals with both the negative and positive aspects of shame. I can readily distil several basic skills in existential competency from various chapters. These clinical skills include:

- Self-awareness, acceptance, and acknowledgement of one's failures and limitations
- Self-forgiveness and self-compassion
- Self-affirmation through re-authoring and reframing
- Self-affirming the intrinsic value and sacredness of life
- Taking personal responsibility for positive change
- Seeking a support group
- Focusing on the meaning people attach to events
- Seeking deeper meaning and self-transcendence
- Seeking deeper understanding through verbalising one's emotions and dreams.

Most of the above skills are rooted in humanistic–existential psychology and have been incorporated into PP 2.0 (Wong, 2016, 2017c). This book provides further evidence that therapy is more effective when it moves from a pathological focus to an existential positive psychology approach in treating shame.

Toronto, ON, Canada   Paul T. P. Wong
                                        Meaning-Centered Counselling Institute Inc.

References

Lewis, M. (1995). *Shame: The exposed self*. New York, NY: Simon & Schuster.

Martínez, M., Arantzamendi, M., Belar, A., Carrasco, J. M., Carvajal, A., Rullán, M., & Centeno, C. (2017). 'Dignity therapy', a promising intervention in palliative care: A comprehensive systematic literature review. *Palliative Medicine, 31*(6), 492–509. https://doi.org/10.1177/0269216316665562

Vanderheiden, E., & Mayer, C.-H. (Eds.) (2017). *The value of shame: Exploring a health resource in cultural contexts*. Cham, CH: Springer.

Wong, P. T. P. (2009). Existential positive psychology. In S. J. Lopez (Ed.), *Encyclopedia of positive psychology* (Vol. 1, pp. 361–368). Oxford, UK: Wiley Blackwell.

Wong, P. T. P. (2011). Positive psychology 2.0: Towards a balanced interactive model of the good life. *Canadian Psychology, 52*(2), 69–81. https://doi.org/10.1037/a0022511

Wong, P. T. P. (2013). Positive psychology. In K. Keith (Ed.), *Encyclopedia of cross-cultural psychology* (pp. 1021–1026). Oxford, UK: Wiley Blackwell.

Wong, P. T. P. (2016). Self-transcendence: A paradoxical way to become your best. *International Journal of Existential Psychology and Psychotherapy, 6*(1). Retrieved from http://journal.existentialpsychology.org/index.php/ExPsy/article/view/178/141

Wong, P. T. P. (2017a). Existential theoretical framework. In A. Wenzel (Ed.), *The SAGE encyclopedia of abnormal and clinical psychology* (pp. 1375–1378). New York, NY: Sage.

Wong, P. T. P. (2017b). The positive psychology of shame and the theory of PP 2.0 [Review of the book *The value of shame: Exploring a health resource in cultural contexts*, by E. Vanderheiden & C. H. Mayer] *PsycCRITIQUES, 62*(34). https://doi.org/10.1037/a0040971

Wong, P. T. P. (2017c). Meaning-centered approach to research and therapy, second wave positive psychology, and the future of humanistic psychology. *The Humanistic Psychologist, 45*(3), 207–216. https://doi.org/10.1037/hum0000062

Acknowledgements

We would like to thank all the individuals who provided such positive and constructive feedback to our first book, *The Value of Shame. Exploring a Health Resource in Cultural Contexts*, and who encouraged us to take the matter further by exploring shame in cultural contexts with regard to practical perspectives and interventions for transformation.

Further, we would like to thank all of our colleagues and authors for participating in the book project at hand. Special thanks go to Ruth Coetzee who has language edited many of the chapters and thereby contributed strongly to the language quality of this book. We would also like to thank Prof. Paul T. P. Wong who has inspired us with his contributions to the Positive Psychology Wave Two (PP2.0) and who has stimulated us to rethink shame in the context of PP2.0 and meaningfulness. Further thanks go to Prof. Lynette Louw at Rhodes University in Grahamstown, South Africa, who always supports our projects in whichever way possible.

Finally, we would like to thank our publisher Springer International Publishing AG for continuous support and interest in our projects. Especially, we would like to thank Hendrikje Tuerlings, Esther Otten, Ritu Chandwani, and Ram Prasad Chandrasekar for their commitment and engagement with regard to this book project.

Contents

About the Editors

Claude-Hélène Mayer (Dr. habil., PhD, PhD) is a Professor in Industrial and Organisational Psychology at the Department of Industrial Psychology and People Management at the University of Johannesburg, an Adjunct Professor at the Europa Universität Viadrina in Frankfurt (Oder), Germany and a Senior Research Associate in the Department of Management at Rhodes University, Grahamstown, South Africa. She holds a Ph.D. in psychology (University of Pretoria, South Africa), a Ph.D. in management (Rhodes University, South Africa), a Doctorate in political sciences (Georg-August-Universität, Göttingen, Germany), and a Habilitation with a Venia Legendi (Europa Universität Viadrina, Germany) in psychology with focus on work, organizational, and cultural psychology. She has published numerous monographs, edited text books, accredited journal article, and special issues on transcultural mental health, salutogenesis and sense of coherence, shame, transcultural conflict management and mediation, women in leadership in culturally diverse work contexts, constellation work, coaching, and psychobiography.

Elisabeth Vanderheiden (Second state examination) is a Pedagogue, Theologian, Intercultural Mediator, Managing Director of the Catholic Adult Education Rhineland-Palatinate, and Federal Chairwoman of the Catholic Adult Education of Germany. She has published books and articles in the context of vocational qualifications, in particular qualification of teachers and trainers, as well as current topics of general, vocational, and civic education, and intercultural opening processes, mediation, and shame. She lives in Germany and Florida.

Calling on Shame! An Introduction to Transforming Shame

Shame! Since we published our first book on shame (Vanderheiden & Mayer, 2017), we have been drawn deeper into reflections on the question of how shame can be transformed from a toxic into a healthy emotion, which can then be used as a source of individual and collective growth.

This book, *The Bright Side of Shame—Transforming and Growing through Practical Applications in Cultural Contexts*, develops from our previous explorations of how shame is experienced and transformed in different cultural contexts. Here, we focus on how to manage shame from different disciplinary and cultural perspectives, and propose concrete interventions and applications, with examples of how this can be implemented in the respective contexts. The aim of this book is to collect and integrate concepts with theoretical and practical approaches and applications based on research and professional practice, in order to understand, manage, and transform shame from different national, societal, cultural, and organisational stances. Some of the chapters do have practical guidelines for therapy, training, contemplation, and self-reflection, while other chapters do not. Depending on the approach of each author to the topic of shame in cultural contexts, authors chose to either provide questions for reflections, practical guidelines, suggestions for exercises, or cases. As editors we aimed at providing the reader with a variety of approaches to the topic of shame and thereby relate to various learning styles, contexts, and intercultural or culture-specific approaches to transform shame. The aim was therefore not to present a complete set of a certain structured methodological approach, but to present a variety of possible approaches which feed into the academic discourse on positive psychology, culture, and shame as theoretical approaches and therapeutic applications on theoretical and practical levels.

In further exploring cultural perspectives on shame, we present in-depth chapters on the cultural aspects of shame; shame in the context of social-, gender-, and religious-/spiritual-based transformation; shame and organisation in education, in medical contexts, and in therapy; and shame in counselling, and self-development. The underlying purpose is to provide new spaces of discussion and discourse on shame across cultures, disciplines, and individuals, providing a theoretical background and then focusing on the application by responding to the overall questions: How can shame be transformed in different contexts? Which perspectives, theoretical models, methods, and interventions can be used to transform toxic shame into healthy shame?

Researchers as well as practitioners from different countries all over the world have been invited to contribute to this book and explain how they address shame from within their theoretical stance, their professional practice, and their cultural perspective at various levels.

The reader will find that there are a number of parts in this book with regard to cultural perspectives and shame. Obviously, there is a focus on shame in therapeutical contexts; however, the book aims at the same time to open perspectives across disciplines and therefore includes a variety of disciplinary approaches which might not be weighted in terms of a balanced quantity to each of the disciplines explored, but which provides insights into the diverse approaches to shame, thereby promoting diverse cultural, academic, theoretical, and practical approaches.

The reader, no matter from which scientific discipline, will find stimulating approaches across disciplines and see that this book aims at bringing theoretical and practical aspects on shame and culture together from a positive psychology perspective.

Where Do We Stand and Where Do We Go?

In our previous book on shame in cultural contexts (Vanderheiden & Mayer, 2017), we provided the reader with an insight into shame research using transdisciplinary and transcultural perspectives. This shifts the previous focus of shame from psychoanalysis and psychotherapy (Freud, 1961/1933) towards an understanding of shame through transcultural perspectives (Andrieux, 2012), and as a health resource (Wurmser, 2010). In Vanderheiden and Mayer (2017), we have viewed shame within a positive psychology framework, emphasising the importance of moving the view from a pathological concept of shame towards a health-related perspective on shame as an emotion which can have a destructive impact on a person or group members. Wong (2017) responded to Vanderheiden and Mayer (2017) by highlighting that the book has contributed to the theoretical development of PP2.0 (Wong, 2011) which has been described as the second wave of positive psychology (Ivtzan, Lomas, Heffron, & Worth, 2015; Kashdan & Biswas-Diener, 2014). Wong (2017) points out that the book on the value of shame by Vanderheiden and Mayer (2017) contributes in two ways to PP2.0: on the one hand, it shows that all emotions, including shame, are dualistic in nature with healthy and unhealthy sides. On the other hand, the editors and authors emphasise that emotions have both, intrapsychic and interpersonal dark sides. Wong (2017) firstly emphasises that in PP2.0 it is assumed that maintaining well-being is based on how a person manages to deal with the polarities of an emotion, such as shame, which inherently carries positive and negative aspects and which can be contributive to reflect on personal conviction and self-evaluation. Secondly, Wong (2017) points out that emotions, such as shame, have both intrapsychic and interpersonal dark sides which need to be embraced—as what Jung highlights with regard to the shadow—to then build upon the self-recognition and self-knowledge to increase resilience and flourishing.

A question that needs to be explored in future is what values, beliefs, and actions predispose the PP2.0 perspective on shame to discover how positive and negative emotional experiences complement and yield optimal well-being. Practical approaches to recognise, explore, and transform the dark sides of shame into bright sides of shame need to be exercised to develop the individual further into a direction of personal and collective conscious and unconscious growth, well-being, and human flourishing. This is what this book aims at by keeping Lomas (2016) and Parrott (2014) in mind who both point out that in toxics and negative experienced emotions, there is a huge power in exploring their positive aspects after having worked, embraced, and acknowledged the darker sides.

Thereby, we keep in mind Hilgers' (2013) perspective that shame develops early in life and accompanies individuals across their entire lives. Shame can be triggered by different life events and manifests differently depending on age, in various environments and cultures, influencing individual development (Hilgers, 2013). Further, individuals are prone to different categories of shame (Marks, 2011), such as body shame, group shame, empathetic and intimacy shame, traumatic and moral shame. Therefore, it is important that individuals become aware of the proneness to their individual and sociocultural categories of shame, embrace them, and work with them towards developing them as a health resource.

According to the perspective that shame is a highly complex phenomenon that is contextually influenced, there is a need for different methods and interventions to work with shame on individual as well as collective levels. Thereby, culture plays an extraordinary role in the definition, development, and experience of shame and how it is addressed, managed, and transformed (Markus & Kitayama, 1995; Casimir & Schnegg, 2002; Wong & Tsai, 2007), while being a universal emotion (Werden, 2015). An overview of research on shame and culture has already been presented in Vanderheiden and Mayer (2017) and will therefore not be covered here.

We continue to follow the call of previous researchers to explore shame, not only from a Western viewpoint, but also from various culture-specific and transcultural perspectives (Casimir & Schnegg, 2002; Furukawa, Tangney, & Higashibara, 2012; Tracy & Matsumoto, 2008; Wong & Tsai, 2007). In this anthology, we, as editors, also aim at making the invisible shame which Scheff (1988, 2013) has defined for Western cultures, more visible in and for different cultural contexts. Starrin (2016) adds onto Scheff's (1988, 2013) perspective and emphasises that the concept of shame is tabooed in Western cultures, which might be a result of the fact—at least according to Ryan (2017, 6)—that shame includes an aspect of "being out of place". The exploration of this facet and shame needs a culture-specific and culture-relative approach (Röttger-Rössler, 2004, 2010) to come closer to a deeper understanding of shame. Other diverse aspects of shame also need to be considered, such as gender (see Hernandez & Mendoza, 2011; Lewis, 1992; Tangney & Dearing, 2002), age (Brown, 2012; Hilgers, 2013), and religion (Brown, 2012).

An additional point of interest in this book is the focus on the application of theoretical stances to transform shame into a health-orientated, empowering, and resourceful emotion from various sociocultural perspectives, which might impact positively on the individual's and group's self-development.

In the past, the question of how to deal with shame on a practical level has been responded to by other researchers and practitioners, for example Bradshaw (2005) with regard to self-development and healing, and Brown (2004) with specific regard to women, using a narrative approach to overcoming shame. Brown (2004) emphasises that by speaking about shame and the true feelings associated with shame, expressing emotions, a person builds connections and thereby overcomes and transforms shame.

In an earlier work on shame in families, Fossum and Mason (1989) point out that families need to face shame across generations to overcome and transform shame within the family as a core unit of society. Again, the overall perspective is that shame needs to be uncovered, made visible, and be taken into view to work with it and overcome it, irrespective of whether it is on an individual or family level. Dearing and Tangney (2011), in Shame in the Therapy Hour, provide the reader with many practical and theoretically well-anchored ideas and methods of how to manage shame in therapeutical settings.

Other contributions to transforming shame within different contexts and anchored in different disciplines and theoretical stances have been presented by Vanderheiden and Mayer (2017), as well as in publications by Klinger, Landany, and Kulp (2012), Randles and Tracy (2013), Zhang and Chan (2016), Raposa, Laws, and Ansell (2016), DeYoung (2015), Jacob (2011), and Jacob and Seebauer (2014).

The book at hand expands on previous responses in so far as it takes the cultural contexts, transdisciplinary perspectives, and the very practical applications through reflections, exercises, case studies, and other forms of applications into account, thereby accepting not only the positive psychology movements, but also PP2.0 (Wong, 2011, 2017) as its foundational theoretical approach. Each chapter bases the introduced applications on a sound theoretical footing and refers to a specific cultural, disciplinary, and methodological background. The authors combine their offerings to provide readers with a complex theoretical understanding from different perspectives, which they then demonstrate with practical contextualised, sociocultural adaptive applications. The applications may be directly usable by readers or may require slight adjustments to suit the readers' sociocultural and professional contexts.

Contents and Structure of the Book

The book integrates sociocultural, disciplinary, and transdisciplinary perspectives. All chapters address the topic of how to work with shame, based on a constructive approach to shame and a "growth perspective" which can feed into the self-development and self-actualisation of the reader.

The book opens with a foreword by Paul T. P. Wong, followed by acknowl-edgements and a brief introduction to the editors and contributors. Thereafter, each chapter has a similar structure: first, an abstract is provided, together with five keywords to give an insight into the topic. Then, the introduction refers to shame in the described contexts and the aim of the chapter is expressed. The sections that follow anchor the chapter's content theoretically and contextually. Finally, all chapters provide insights into applied approaches on how to deal with shame in specific contexts by providing an example of an applied method, techniques, and/or applications to deal with shame constructively.

Each of the chapters offers the reader theoretical, methodical, and applied knowledge to create new perspectives, thought patterns, and practical approaches to deal with shame constructively in specific sociocultural contexts.

The book is divided into eight parts and 40 chapters which will be briefly introduced in the following paragraphs, to provide an overview on the discourses and topics covered in this book.

The different parts of the book include selected perspectives on shame, based on, for example, culture, society, organisation, education, health, as well as therapy, counselling and self-development. In the following an introduction to the different parts and chapters will be provided in sequential order.

Part I: Transforming Shame in Cultural Perspectives

The opening of the book deals with shame in the German society (Part 1 and Part 2). The first two chapters present a state-of-the-art approach in German contexts from collective and individual cultural viewpoints. The chapters are written by Claude-Hélène Mayer. The author highlights the development of collective shame in German society in historical and contemporary discourses. The focus on shame in German contexts, Part 2, presents selected research conducted regarding individual shame constructs. It provides a brief overview on topics of shame research with regard to individually experienced shame, referring to science, education, the body, care, clinical conditions, and the military, war, and soldiers.

These two chapters are followed by a chapter from *dharma prakaza zarmA bhAwuk* who describes collectively the process and spiritual journey of "Cultivating lajjA for Self-Realisation: Perspectives from Indian Psychology". The Indian concept of lajjA is explained and developed through a path of self-realisation. The author explains that public confession is the way to live with lajjA and shame, and requires distancing oneself from the physical self, while focusing on a spiritual journey. Lessons learned from this approach are applied in social and organisational contexts.

The insights into an Indian perspective are expanded in a chapter written by Kiyoko Sueda, who explores shame as a health resource in a specific Japanese context, the context of Japanese returnees (kikokushijo) in Japan. These people face various challenges in returning to Japan, and a programme is described which supports these returnees in coping with shame.

Liusheng Wang and Biao Sang then focus on the "The Effect of Regulation on Shame in Adolescence in China" in which they analyse school students' ability to regulate shame and self-blame. The authors present findings of their research and a specific case.

HIV/AIDS are in the focus of the following chapter, in which Busisiwe Nkosi and Paul Rosenblatt discuss shame, stigma, and discrimination in South Africa. The authors refer to the "care gap", arguing that understanding of the sociocultural systems and local contexts is important in transforming shame into a positive experience. They also show the value and use of visual participatory methods as therapeutic tools and for social change and illustrate how these techniques are increasingly used to share intersectional experiences and transform stigma and shame into positive experiences through creative expression.

The author Johana Kunin then provides new insights on shame in a Southern American context and describes how community theatre as a social development activity deals with personal challenges and life experiences. The author describes how many people before participating in community theatre activities feel ashamed and that those participating declare having "lost a sense of shame". The chapter then focuses on how to overcome shame through theatre participation and on how to develop pride.

Coming from the exploration of cultural perspectives, the second part of the book gives insights into shame within the society.

Part II: Transforming Shame in Society

Gail Womersley explores the shame and trauma experiences of refugees entering Europe. She refers to the hidden, yet pervasive role that shame may play in post-traumatic symptomatology. It occurs in the context of torture, sexual violence, and other atrocities experienced in the country of origin of refugees, but also during the asylum-seeking process when culturally informed expectations are not met. The author discusses key implications for clinicians and researchers alike, who work in the context of refugees.

Shame and shaming are highly important aspects of the study of crime, crime sciences, and criminal investigation and restorative justice. Claude-Hélène Mayer takes selected aspects into account and presents state-of-the-art research and practice regarding four questions: (1) How are experiences of shame, crime, and criminal behaviour related? (2) What effect does shaming (sanctions) have in criminal law and regulatory systems? (3) What is reintegrative shaming in the context of crime and criminal justice and how does it impact on crime? (4) How does culture impact on the topics of shame and shaming in the context of criminal law, justice, and criminal (risky) behaviour?

Liv Larsson focuses on shame within the context of conflict management. This chapter demonstrates ways of reclaiming power and choice through transforming shame in mediation. The author presents "The Compass of Needs" tool to transform shame. This tool is based on the principles of non-violent communication, a technique established by Marshall Rosenberg.

Part III: Working with Shame and Gender

According to Sergio A. Silverio, in contemporary society, the body is used as a radical tool with which individuals negotiate their place and status in society. The body has become a form of language in its own right. In Western society in particular, the quest for the "eternal feminine" endures, rendering women passive, sexualised, and objectified, without the opportunity to subvert the shame they are forced to withstand. The aim of this chapter is to advocate the reconstruction of gender in society, allowing for an understanding of fluid gender identity and context-specific gender construction to permit the desexualisation of the body and the removal of body-specific shame.

The following chapter, "Interventions for Shame and Guilt Experienced by Battered Women", is written by Kathryn A. Nel and Sarawathie Govender. They present shame in the context of the battered woman syndrome which is based on a sense of learned helplessness and which reinforces the power and control of her male partner. The authors discuss this syndrome in the context of sub-Saharan Africa, with special regard to lobola (bride price) and shame. The chapter provides new insights on interventions which help women deal with feelings of guilt and shame related to their abuse, and which are based on religious practices and specific therapies such as brain working recursive therapy, to increase self-esteem to change their circumstances.

After having addressed shame in the context of gender, the work with shame in spiritual and religious perspectives follows.

Part IV: Managing Shame in Spiritual and Religious Perspectives

In the following, Christian and Islamic views on the transformation of shame within the context of religious and spiritual approaches are presented to provide the reader with a deepening insight into how shame can be dealt with in the context of spirituality.

Thomas Ryan draws on religious and theological as well as psychological perspectives to build an inclusive approach to spirituality. While understanding prayer as a personal relationship, the author explains the role of emotional transparency with special regard to shame. He views shame's transformative potential in the light of socio-phenomenological theory with its focus on the meaning people attach to events and their impact on a person's life. In the chapter, specific practices, such as biblical texts and strategies in prayer to explore meaning in shame-laden events in two life-contexts, are described. The authors explain that when painful shame is named, accepted, and shared in prayer and interpersonally, it can offer deeper meaning, self-awareness, self-transcendence, and love.

Dini Farhana Baharudin, Melati Sumari, and Suhailiza Md Hamdani report on "Shame Transformation using an Islamic Psycho-Spiritual Approach for Malay Muslims Recovering from Substance Dependence". In their chapter, they describe selected Islamic psychospiritual approaches and practices for transformation and alleviation of shame for Malay Muslims recovering from substance dependence, such as the process of self-audit (muhasabah), repentance, and forgiveness (taw-bah), constructing new narrative of the self, and developing a stronger relationship with Allah (hablum min Allah) and other humans (hablum min annas) as the foundation for healthy recovery.

After the perspectives of shame in the context of society, gender and religion and spirituality are given, and different societal levels have been taken into account, the following Part V of the book illuminates shame within organisational contexts.

Part V: Transforming Shame in Organisational Contexts

Part V opens the perspective on managing shame in organisations with Rudolf Oosthuizen's self-compassionate perspective. The author asks how employees in organisations can cope with shame in organisations, discusses certain maladaptive strategies, and describes how compassionate strategies can improve shameful feelings. In his chapter, he is also touching on mindfulness in organisations.

This chapter is followed by Louise Tonelli's insights on shame from a systems' psychodynamic perspective. The author understands shame as an envious attack resulting from defences against anxiety in groups, organisations, and communities and presents an idea of coaching individuals from an unconscious psychoanalytic stance. The chapter provides the reader with new ideas on how to deal with shame from an unconscious group perspective.

The purpose of the chapter by Dirk Geldenhuys is to explore shame from the neuroscientific perspective within the context of the workplace, leadership, and organisations. The author argues that the neuroscientific perspective can add a unique dimension to the development and implementation of interventions to prevent and address toxic shame. Applied neuroscientific concepts such as the triune brain, neuroplasticity, and epigenetics are discussed. The discussion includes an introduction to the hypothalamic pituitary adrenal (HPA) axis, memory systems, and neuro-psychotherapy as a wellness intervention. Finally, the concept of "brainfit", as an approach for leaders in organisations to deal with shame, is presented.

Clifford Clark and Naomi Takashiro focus in their chapter on the intercultural misunderstandings between Japanese and American managers in their bicultural organisations in Japan and stress that intercultural misunderstandings are often based on feelings of shame related upon perceived inadequacies in adjusting to a new workplace. Intention of their chapter is to present a practical intercultural developmental model that transforms shame through respect, empathy, trust, and social equity to a collective pride in bicultural organisations in Japan.

The third and final chapter on this part is written by Maike Baumann and Anke Handrock. The two authors explain how important it is to build a work culture which goes beyond forgiveness. They explore the influence of shame and anxiety on people when expected to acknowledge their own mistakes or failures in a workplace environment—which often seems to be overlooked—and present crucial aspects of a new approach on how to form an organisational culture where mistakes are not only perceived as forgivable, but are seen as a chance for collective growth and as a possibility to develop excellence.

Part VI: Transforming Shame in Education

The next three chapters in Part VI of this book focus on shame in selected educational contexts.

Michelle May opens Part VI from the perspective of lecturers at a historically "Black" university in South Africa who disown shame through "stay-away actions". The findings of a hermeneutic study illustrate how participation in a stay-away action, and reflexivity about these actions, might move beyond shame dynamics to a new story. The author provides further insights on how shame can be transferred through specific interventions in the described context.

In their chapter, authors Paul A. Wilson and Barbara Lewandowska-Tomaszczyk describe different scenarios of moderating shame cluster emotions in foreign language learners. The focus is in particular on two studies conducted in Poland with different English language scenarios. In the first study, shame was reduced in the learners when they imagined learning scenario evaluations which were more private than public. In the next study, shame was reduced when international email peer cooperation was bound to a more informal cooperation and communication and a more positive linguistic self-evaluation.

Similar assumptions are expressed in the third chapter which focuses on shame in the educational system. Christian Martin Boness describes a macro-didactical concept used in a German school context which aims at integrating students from different cultural backgrounds in school. The Team Ombuds Model (tOm) supports learners in terms of evaluations and social competences which are mediated in learner groups and outputs. The chapter introduces the case of a 16-year-old Chinese immigrant in Germany and demonstrates how shame is transformed in the class context, using tOm.

The following Part VII addresses the question of how shame can be taken into account and transformed in the context of healing and doctor–patient interactions.

Part VII: Transforming Shame in Medical Contexts

The first chapter in Part VII, written by Iris Veit and Kay Spiekermann, focuses on "Dealing with Shame in the Medical Context". The authors highlight that shame is an important emotion in medical contexts which is neither being addressed openly in the training of doctors and medical practitioners, nor is it being addressed in healthcare settings. Shame in the medical interactions and healthcare settings is associated with a restricted personal privacy of patients, questions on the private life, the narration of the medical history, body shame and nakedness, diseases connected to the patient's physical appearance, and/or social stigma. However, medical practitioners also experience shame. The chapter provides insights and ideas on how to reduce and/or transform shame in medical contexts.

The second chapter, written by Ottomar Bahrs and Karl-Heinz Henze, on shame in medical contexts particularly focuses on shame in review dialogues and doctor–patient interaction. The authors highlight that shame is experienced in individuals with chronic conditions through marginalisation and a lack of social support and stigmatisation. The method of review dialogues can support managing shame. A case is described to enhance a deeper understanding of how review dialogues can support coping with and transforming shame.

Part VIII holds the majority of chapters of this book. They deal with the transformation of shame in therapy, counselling, and self-development processes and programmes.

Part VIII: Transforming Shame in Therapy, Counselling and Self-development

Holger Lindemann focuses on shame and pride in the concept of certainty and doubt. The author describes an antogonistic relationship between shame and pride which evaluates certainty and doubt by drawing onto previously experienced (self-) evaluations and judgements. A meta-model is presented that can help in counselling, mediation, consulting, and therapy to manage and transform shame and pride consciously.

Aakriti Malik provides a vivid insight into the widely felt emotion of shame within the context of psychopathology and psychotherapy with clients. Explaining that shame often hides under secondary emotions such as pain, embarrassment, grief, or anger, the author emphasises that the therapist needs skill, patience, and knowledge to uncover and work with shame in therapy. Cases from within the

Indian psychotherapeutical setting are described and discussed, and conclusions on effectively healing shame in psychotherapy are suggested.

Jeff Elison discusses how shame can be treated from an evolutionary perspective, as an adaptive or maladaptive response. Findings on the affective neuroscience of social pain suggest the physical pain system was co-opted for adaptive social functions. Thus, the author argues physical pain is an appropriate analogy for understanding shame, the two sharing many features. He proceeds by explaining that clients understand the functions of physical pain and how it protects us. He suggests how a shame–pain analogy can help clients to understand shame and to then employ transformative actions to prevent further shame from developing.

Another chapter, written by Paul Gilbert, uses an evolutionary analysis to distinguish shame, humiliation, and guilt. The author emphasises that shame is associated with social sanction, stigma, and being diminished in some way, whereas guilt is focused on harm-doing. Shame and guilt have very different evolutionary historical functions which are described in this chapter and which affect the causes of shame and guilt, their psychopathologies, and the effective therapeutic interventions. With regard to practical applications, the author describes an approach to shame through compassion.

The following chapter written by Claude-Hélène Mayer describes "Transforming Shame Experiences in Dreams: Therapeutical Interventions". By working with dreams, therapists can support individuals to transform shame in the context of therapy, aiming at personal growth and self-development. The chapter provides insights into different dream scenarios and how they can be addressed in therapy sessions.

Barbara Buch writes on shame by considering it from a salutogenic and shamanic point of view as an emotional death experience, which, when overcome, can lead to increased strength and empowerment. The author considers intergenerational, unjustified, and toxic shame in the context of female and racial shaming. Different cognitive steps as well as physical processes are suggested to transform toxic shame. Exemplary movement with rhythmic music and body awareness practices with their underlying mechanisms are described, which may be able to rebalance, reassemble, and recreate one's sense of self.

The next chapter by Claude-Hélène Mayer deals with the coaching of an unemployed high achiever using symbol work and active imagination to transform the experiences of shame which are accompanied by traumatic shame experiences. This shame can be overcome through the work with symbols and a dialogue between the unconsciousness and the conscious mind.

"Shame and Forgiveness in Therapy and Coaching" is a topic for Anke Handrock and Maike Baumann. The authors point out that in order to avoid the feeling of shame, behaviours such as aggressive attacks or withdrawal from social relationships are common strategies. In the secure environment of coaching sessions, counselling, or therapy, the client can find ways to disclose feelings of shame and guilt and to forgive. This chapter highlights the general process of a non-religious approach to forgiveness and offers practical exercises referring to schema therapy, positive psychology, and imaginative therapy.

Patricia Sherwood presents "Somatically Based Art Therapy for Transforming Experiences of Shame" through the nonverbal artistic languages of sensing, gesturing, breathing, visualising, and sounding to identify, explore, and transform experiences of shame within individuals and groups. She introduces three artistic exercises which are particularly designed to promote healing from shame experiences and include the shame to self-esteem healing sequence, the cutting negative voices sequence, and the self-parenting sequence. The art therapy exercises have been effectively used in multicultural contexts to explore and transform shame experiences resulting from trauma and abuse within the family, community, and society.

Stephen D. Edwards discusses "HeartMath Techniques for the Transformation of Shame Experiences" which might then develop into a source of resilience and health. The HeartMath system is described as a scientific, evidence-based self-regulation technique which was designed to relieve stress, improve resilience, and promote positive feelings, sense of coherence, health, and performance. The aim of the chapter is to explore a research hypothesis concerning the effectiveness of HeartMath techniques to transform shame feelings. Specific techniques to address negative emotions, manage stress, promote positive feelings, and build resilience are discussed.

"Nothing I Accept about Myself can be Used Against Me to Diminish me— Transforming Shame through Mindfulness" is a chapter by Elisabeth Vanderheiden which recognises mindfulness as a source of well-being which reduces stress symptoms, depression, and shame-based trauma appraisals. The author provides an insight into how mindfulness is able to reduce negative reactions to emotionally charged situations, which can reduce psychological symptoms and emotional reactivity on the one hand, and improve behavioural regulation on the other. This chapter combines these two approaches and offers exercises to transform shame into a positive, constructive, and growth-orientated resource.

The chapter on "Healing Rituals to Transform Shame: An Example of Constellation Work" written by Claude-Hélène Mayer also promotes a mindful and healing-orientated approach to shame through the therapeutic method and rituals of constellation work. The chapter explains the basics of constellation work and provides examples of how shame issues can be explored and addressed on an individual and on a therapeutical group level.

In a second chapter, the authors Kathryn A. Nel and Sarawathic Govender are focusing on shame using the framework and method of appreciative inquiry. They explain how appreciative inquiry can be used to deal with shame and guilt experienced by individuals affected with HIV/AIDS in a sub-Saharan socio-economic context. The four key tenets of appreciative inquiry, namely Discovery (the best of what is), Dream (what might be), Design (what should be), and Destiny (what will be) provide a reflexive approach for use in therapeutic settings.

Len Andrieux contributes a chapter "Facing the Ambivalence of Shame Issues: Exploring the use of Motivational Techniques to Enhance Shame Resilience and

Provoke Behaviour Change". The author examines the use of motivational interviewing techniques in coaching when faced with shame issues, and the ambivalence resulting from the acknowledgement of shame. Her approach is based on a qualitative and hermeneutic research study and emphasises that the ambivalence can be alleviated by use of motivational techniques instead of, or in concert with, other therapeutic approaches.

The following chapter, presented by Rebecca Merkin, updates the literature on shame, guilt, and workplace bullying and introduces different possible cognitive-behavioural approaches that could be used to help remediate the shame underlying bullying in the workplace. She further describes methods to move from shame to guilt by using different cognitive-behavioural approaches, such as promoting pro-social work behaviours, responsibility, and empathy.

Conclusions and Recommendations

This section provides the reader with final conclusions on the topic and gives a prospective for future research and practice on shame. The two editors of this compilation, Claude-Hélène Mayer and Elisabeth Vanderheiden, describe the best practices emphasised in the book and highlight in their postscript the way forward in research on shame as a health research from the different perspectives chosen in this book.

Moving Forward in Transforming Shame

Shame—as a relevant universal emotion with culture-specific expressions and experiences—needs to be addressed and made visible not only at the level of culture, but also on societal, organisational, and individual levels, as shown in the various chapters of this book. Shame needs approaches which go beyond theoretical discourses and which take various perspectives, theories, methodologies and therapeutical approaches and interventions seriously into account. These perspectives are highlighted by the authors of this book who aim at transforming shame from a rather toxic towards a healthier emotion and which can be used transculturally and across disciplines for individual and collective growth.

Acknowledgements

We thank each of our colleagues from all over the world who inspired us by working on exploring the topic of shame as a resource for personal and sociocultural growth. Special thanks go to Prof. Paul T. P. Wong for his focus on meaningfulness across the lifespan and the empowering discourse on PP2.0 which stimulated us to move deeper and forward in our discourse.

Claude-Hélène Mayer
Elisabeth Vanderheiden

References

Andrieux, L. (2012). *Submission for INSEAD Executive Masters Thesis Consulting and Coaching for Change*. (1st ed.).
Bradshaw, J. (2005). *Healing the shame that binds you*. Deerfield Beach: Health Communications, Inc
Brown, B. (2004). *Women & shame: Reaching out, speaking truths & building connection*. Austin, TX: 3C Press.
Brown, B. (2012). *Daring greatly*. New York, NY: Gotham Books.
Casimir, M. J., & Schnegg, M. (2002). Shame across cultures: The evolution, ontogeny and function of a "moral emotion". In H. Keller & Y. H. Poortinga (Eds.), *Between culture and biology: Perspectives on ontogenetic development* (pp. 270–200). New York: Cambridge University Press.
Dearing, R. L., & Tangney, J. P. E. (2011). *Shame in the therapy hour*. Washington, D.C: American Psychological Association.
DeYoung, P. A. (2015). *Understanding and Treating Chronic Shame*. A relational/neurobiological approach. New York: Routledge.
Fossum, M. A., & Mason, M. J. (1989). *Facing shame: Families in recovery*. New York: WW Norton & Company.
Freud, S. (1961/1933). *New introductory lectures on psychoanalysis*. In Strachey, J., (Ed.), The standard edition of the complete psychological works of Sigmund Freud. New York: Norton. vol. 22.
Furukawa, E., Tangney, J., & Higashibara, F. (2012). *Cross-cultural Continuities and Discontinuities in Shame, Guilt, and Pride: A Study of Children Residing in Japan, Korea and the USA. Self And Identity, 11*(1), 90–113. Retrieved from https://doi.org/10.1080/15298868. 2010.512748.
Hernandez, V., & Mendoza, C. (2011). Shame Resilience: A Strategy for Empowering Women in Treatment for Substance Abuse. *Journal of Social Work Practice in the Addictions, 11*(4), 375–393. Retrieved from https://doi.org/10.1080/1533256x.2011.622193.
Hilgers, M. (2013). *Scham*. Göttingen: Vandenhoeck & Ruprecht.
Ivtzan, I., Lomas, T., Hefferon, K., & Worth, P. (2015). Second wave positive psychology: Embracing the dark side of life. London, UK: Routledge.
Jacob, G.A. (2011). Was ist innovativ an der Schematherapie? *Zeitschrift für Psychiatrie, Psychologie und Psychotherapie, 59*, 179–186
Jacob, G.A., & Seebauer, L. (2014). Schematherapie. *Zeitschrift für Klinische Psychologie und Psychotherapie, 43*, 271–278.

Kashdan, T., & Biswas-Diener, R. (2014). The upside of your dark side: Why being your whole self—Not just your "good" self—Drives success and fulfillment. New York, NY: Plume.

Klinger, R. S., Ladany, N., & Kulp, L. E. (2012). It's too late to apologize: Therapist embarressment and shame. *The Counseling Psychologist, 40*(4), 554–574.

Lewis, M. (1992). *Shame*. New York: Free Press.

Lomas, T. (2016). *The positive power of negative emotions: How harnessing your darker feelings can help you see a brighter dawn*. London, England: Piatkus.

Marks, S. (2011). *Scham—die tabuisierte Emotion*. Düsseldorf: Patmos.

Markus, H. M., & Kitayama, S. (1995). *Emotion and culture*. Washington, DC: American Psychological Association.

Mayer, C.-H. (2017). Shame—"A soul feeding emotion": Archetypal work and the transformation of the shadow of shame in a group development process. In Vanderheiden, E. & Mayer, C.-H. (2016). *The Value of Shame—Exploring a Health Resource in Cultural Contexts*. Cham: Springer. pp. 277–302.

Parrott, W. G. (2014). *The positive side of negative emotions*. New York, NY: Guilford.

Röttger-Rössler, B. (2004). *Die kulturelle Modellierung des Gefühls: Ein Beitrag zur Theorie und Methodik ethnologischer Emotionsforschung anhand indonesischer Fallstudien*. Münster: Lit.

Röttger-Rössler, B. (2010). Zur Kulturalität von Emotionen. *Existenzanalyse, 27*(2), 20–27.

Randles, D., & Tracy, J. L. (2013). Nonverbal displays of shame predict relapse and declining health in recovering alcoholics. *Clinical Psychological Science, 1*(2), 149–155.

Raposa, E. B., Laws, H. B., & Ansell, E. B. (2016). Prosocial behavior mitigates the negative effects of stress in everyday life. *Clinical Psychological Science, 4*(4), 691–698.

Ryan (2017). The Positive Function of Shame: Moral and Spiritual Perspectives. In. Vanderheiden, E. & Mayer, C.-H. (2017). *The Value of Shame—Exploring a Health Resource in Cultural Contexts*. Cham: Springer, 87–109.

Scheff, T. (1988). Shame and Conformity: The Deference-Emotion System. *American Sociological Review, 53*(3), 395. https://doi.org/10.2307/2095647.

Scheff, T. (2013). *The S-Word: Shame as a Key to Modern Societies*. Global Summit on Diagnostic Alternatives. http://dxsummit.org/archives/1286. Accessed 1 May 2016.

Starrin, B. (2016). Humiliationstudies.org. Retrieved from http://www.humiliationstudies.org/documents/StarrinShameHumiliationPsychiatricIllHealth.pdf. Accessed 3 April 2018

Tangney, J. & Dearing, R. (2002). *Shame and guilt*. New York: Guilford Press.

Tracy, J. L., & Matsumoto, D. (2008). *The spontaneous expression of pride and shame: Evidence for biologically innate nonverbal displays*. Proceedings of the National Academy of Sciences, *105*(33), 11655–11660. Retrieved from https://doi.org/10.1073/pnas.0802686105.

Vanderheiden, E. & Mayer, C.-H. (2017). *The Value of Shame—Exploring a Health Resource in Cultural Contexts*. Cham: Springer.

Werden, R. (2015). *Schamkultur und Schuldkultur. Revision einer Theorie*. Münster: Aschendorff Verlag.

Wong, P. T. P. (2011). Positive psychology 2.0: Towards a balanced interactive model of the good life. Canadian Psychology, *52*, 69–81.

Wong, P. T. P. (2017). The Positive Psychology of Shame and the Theory of PP2.0. http://www.drpaulwong.com/the-positive-psychology-of-shame-and-the-theory-of-pp20/

Wong, Y. & Tsai, J. L. (2007). Cultural models of shame and guilt. In J. Tracy, R. Robins & J. Tangney (Eds.), *Handbook of Self-Conscious Emotions* (pp. 2010–2023). New York, NW: Guilford Press.

Wurmser, L. (2010). *Die Maske der Scham*. Eschborn/Frankfurt, M.: Klotz.

Zhang, J. W., & Chen, S. (2016). Self-compassion promotes personal involvement from regret experiences via acceptance. *Personality and Social Psychology Bulletin, 42*(2), 244–258.

Part I
Transforming Shame in Cultural Perspectives

Chapter 1
Opening the Black Box Part 1: On Collective Shame in the German Society

Claude-Hélène Mayer

Abstract This chapter is the first of two chapters on shame in German society. It explores collective shame in the German context, thereby, opening the "black box" of shame which is often left closed and stored in the back of collective and individual minds. The chapter explores shame from different German historic and contemporary collective perspectives and provides the reader with an overview of research and state-of-the-art research and practices on collective shame in the context described. It explores how shame is experienced and developed, (re-)constructed, addressed and transformed at these different societal levels. The chapter presents conclusions and recommendations on how to transform collective shame in different German contexts.

Keywords Germany · Historic shame · Politics · Violence · Shame development · Collective · Nation

> Wenn die meisten sich schon
> armseliger Kleider und Möbel schämen,
> wieviel mehr sollten wir uns da erst
> armseliger Ideen und Weltanschauungen schämen.
>
> Albert Einstein[1]

---

[1] Translation by the author: "If most people are already ashamed of their poor clothing and furniture, how much more should we be ashamed of poor ideas and worldviews".

C.-H. Mayer (✉)
Institut für Therapeutische Kommunikation und Sprachgebrauch, Europa Universität Viadrina, Logenstrasse 11, 15230 Frankfurt (Oder), Germany
e-mail: claudemayer@gmx.net

Department of Management, Rhodes University, Drosdy Road, Grahamstown 6139, South Africa

© Springer Nature Switzerland AG 2019
C.-H. Mayer and E. Vanderheiden (eds.), *The Bright Side of Shame*,
https://doi.org/10.1007/978-3-030-13409-9_1

3

1.1   On Opening the Black Box

Shame is a powerful emotion which is often associated with self-condemnation and which impacts strongly on regulating social interaction in which a person or a group has violated a moral or social code (Tangney & Fischer, 1995; Zhang & Chen, 2016; Pettigrove & Parsons, 2008; Rensman, 2004). Shame, is not only the regulating social interaction with regard to an individual and/or social code, but is also a force behind an objectifying self-consciousness (Lotter, 2012).

In the 1980s, Scheff (1988, 400) highlighted the "invisibility of shame in Western cultures", pointing out that shame is viewed as a "master emotion" which is inherent in all communities, and which appears to be invisible in certain societies and cultures. Scheff (1988, 400) refers to these as "low-visibility-shame" societies. In her book on shame, Jacquets (2015) emphasises that shame plays an important influential role in the political arena. She discusses shame and shaming as powerful tools in influencing collectives, and describes seven effective ways to shame others, as well as exploring shaming within virtual realities (Jacquets, 2015).

Germany could be classified as a low-visibility-shame society, according to Scheff (1988, 2013). The topic of shame seems to be strongly taboo in German contexts (Scheff, 2003). In low-visibility shame cultures, shame seems to stay unrecognised, denied or even forgotten (Scheff, 2016).

However, there seems to be a split with regard to shame in German historical and collective contexts: on one hand, people do not seem to wish to talk about shame and collective historical events, while on the other hand, there is a vast amount of literature (Brogle, 2016; Burleigh & Wippermann, 1991; Dresler-Hawke & Lui, 2006; Lu, 2008; Rothe, 2012; Sullivan, 2014a, 2014b) dealing with Germany's past, referring indirectly to past shame, but defining the emotions rather as pain or suffering.

If a shameful event is too difficult to process and is too emotionally laden, it is stored in the unconscious rather than being transformed at conscious levels. This is true for collectively experienced shame, as well as for individual shame (see Mayer, part 2 in this book). When discussing collective shame, it needs to be acknowledged as an emotion that demonstrates flexible and strategic features while negotiating social and relational contexts (Burkitt, 2014). Shame is thereby viewed as an emotion which occurs in response to the judgement of a person, with actions being seen through the eyes of "the other", based on the foundation of the social norms and values of the group (Scheff, 1988).

Collective shame has often been referred to sceptically in the literature which questions how a collective could even have or create a particular emotion (Pettigrove & Parsons, 2012). Smith (2008) observes that collective emotions are usually questioned owing to the difficulty of phenomenological credibility. However, he points out that collective emotions, such as collective shame, often contribute to certain dynamics within and across societies which might lead to conflicts (Smith, 2008). Such shame-based conflict emotions might be addressed through face-saving narrations (Smith, 2008), or by using other strategies such as denial, repression (Lewis, 1971), or the development of collective pride (Sullivan, 2014a, 2014b).

Germany has suffered as a nation from its history and feelings of collective shame and guilt, based on the two world wars (WWI and WWII), the Nazi past, the Holocaust, the split nation and its reunification, as well as from its image of being a domineering and aggressive nation (Sullivan, 2014a, 2014b). WWII and recent German history have been assessed from many different viewpoints around the world and judged in negative ways. This multiple and long-term negative reference might have contributed to strong feelings of shame in German collectives and individuals (Sullivan, 2014a). However, this societal shame is scarcely visible, as is often the case in modern societies (Scheff, 2016). Lotter (2012) argues that shame is a phenomenon that develops out of social practices and cultural forms of life. It is strongly connected to moral and philosophical discourses within a societal setting and opens new access to ethical understanding. In this manner, shame is viewed in terms of its function as a protector within individual and social contexts. Conflicts based on shame experiences are not only protective, but also viewed as important for the moral development (Lotter, 2012) of an individual or collective. Shame is a universal emotion which manifests itself in various ways and practices (Lotter, 2012).

This chapter focuses on the exploration of collective shame in German contexts. In so doing, the "black box" of collective German shame is opened and its transformational aspects in contemporary society are revealed.

The following section provides insight into collective shame in German contexts with regard to historic and contemporary experiences. Applications will then be provided in terms of statements on collective shame in German contemporary contexts, with questions for self-reflection and team discussions. Conclusions are provided and implications for future research and practice are discussed.

1.2 Shame and Shaming Before and During WWI and WWII

Although shame often remains unspoken in contemporary German contexts, shame does play an extraordinary role in German history and in the present (Dresler-Hawke & Lui, 2006). Shame in research in German contexts is often referred to as a collective shame (Brogle, 2016; Dresler-Hawke & Lui, 2006; Rothe, 2012) and has been explored with a strong focus on historical world events, such as WWI (Lu, 2008) and WWII (Burleigh & Wippermann, 1991; Sullivan, 2014a, 2014b) in which Germany played a major role.

Research shows that before WWI, concepts of shame differed strongly according to class and gender in Germany (Frevert, 2014), being transformed during WWI, when shame and honour became emotions of the wartime which impacted strongly on the politics, but also on military actions and gendered concepts. During this time in Germany, shamefulness was considered a virtue for women (Frevert, 2014). Foreign soldiers, the enemies, and the captured, were shamed publicly by being displayed, dishonoured and ashamed in public.

After WWI, the concepts of shame changed again (Frevert, 2014; Lu, 2008). Post-war politics have led to creating reconciliation marked by political and moral transformation based on strong experiences of shame and guilt within the German society (Lu, 2008). Shame and guilt in the post-WWI years covered up a huge part of the national identity, as well as certain societal values and beliefs. These led to strong collective identity transformations and new politics (Lu, 2008), which, under the influence of collective shame, turned out to1 be somewhat defensive, reactionary and violent and were viewed as not necessarily healthy transformation of the collective shame of the previous war (Lu, 2008).

During WWII, a culture of shame was encouraged by Hitler with regard to German warfare: soldiers and superiors who refused to carry out genocide orders were belittled and shamed as being "soft" or "not tough" to carry out the executions of Jews as ordered (Kühne, 2008).

Not only did shame play a role in military actions, but it was also relevant in terms of the implemented shame sanctions which were reinstituted (from WWI) during WWII. Shame sanctions fitted into the Nazi worldview in terms of a "spirit of parade, display and humiliation" (Whitman, 1998, 1085). Nazis used shame sanctions and promoted them as the Nazi punishment of choice, and the pillory and other shame sanctions were (re-)introduced in 1933/1934. However, in the end, Nazi norms did not comply with the shame sanctions and pure humiliation sanctions were rejected by the Nazi regime based on the fear that public shaming would "undermine the ability of the state to control the crowd" (Whitman, 1998, 1085).

Both world wars brought a strong audience effect[2] for Germany, restating and re-emphasising the negative traits within the German society, its culture and its past. This contributed, according to Dresler-Hawke and Lui (2006), to the strong feelings of collective shame which were increased through the long-term negative reference to the German culture, morals and warfare based on the strong focus on Germany's wrongdoings.

1.3 Dealing with and Healing the Shame in Post-war Years

In the post-war German society, research indicates that the younger generation of Germans seemed to dissociate themselves, particularly in the years after the war, from previous generations of active perpetrators and silent acceptors of the Nazi regime (Schlink in Lickel, Schmader, Curtis, Scarnier, & Ames, 2005). One study

---

[2]"A strong audience effect" describes the fact that there was a huge audience to witness Germany's role in the world wars. This audience effect is created by the audience who observes and judges an action, e.g. Germany's actions in the world wars, and thereby affect and re-emphasise the (negative) judgements while feeding them back into German society. The larger, the stronger and more influential the audience (also in the reflection and the perception of "the other"), the more intensive is the effect of the audience on the observed.

by Bar-On (1989) established that 32% of Germans experienced guilt regarding the war in 1951, while in 1967, 62% of Germans experienced feelings of guilt.

This dissociation helped the younger generation to overcome suffering from shame during the years after the war. However, Schlink (in Lickel et al., 2005) emphasises that this dissociation did not necessary help to overcome the shame itself, but rather helped to overcome the suffering (Schlink in Lickel et al., 2005).

Heimannsberg and Schmidt (1993) point out that the shame of victims and perpetrators in WWII has been repressed in silence for several decades, in order to heal the emotional wounds caused during war time. Only after several decades of silence, victims and perpetrators and family members of both groups, could start to open up about the shameful experiences and the silence (Heimannsberg & Schmidt, 1993).

1.4 The German Split and the German and European Reunification

The split that occurred in German society in the years after WWII reinforced the shame about the world wars. Figlio (2011) concludes that the reunification of East and West Germany in particular, allowed the memory of WWII to retreat and enabled Germany to reclaim national identity and self-esteem, while consciously and actively dealing with historic shame, the societal splitting and the broken national identity.

Dresler-Hawke and Lui (2006, 135) contend that contemporary German society deals proactively with healing the shame of historic events, by, for example, playing an active role in the unification movement of Europe. The authors suggest that by focusing on the re-unification of Germany and Europe, German society's approach to dealing with shame can be classified as "reparative model of shame" (Dresler-Hawke & Lui, 2006, 135). The collective shame is thereby transformed through reparative actions at both national and European levels, thereby making restitution for and healing the immoral behaviour of the past.

This political and unifying role which Germany plays on a political level might even counteract the strong audience effect Germany had to carry in the past (Dresler-Hawke & Lui, 2006). Since the end of WWII, it this war is internationally described as the most important event in recent world history, while in this context, Hitler is named as one of the most negatively described people in world history. German citizens, according to Dresler-Hawke and Lui (2006), even in the third generation after WWII, still have to cope constantly with negative images of their country and with historical comparisons which relate to shame, even 70 years after the end of WWII.

1.5   Research on Shame in Contemporary Germany: From 1990s to the Present

Most of the time, contemporary discourses on shame in German contexts refer back to the history of the two created world wars and particularly to the holocaust in WWII (Figlio, 2011; Lu, 2008; Rothe, 2012; Sullivan, 2009, 2014a, 2014b). This shows that in German research and contexts, collective shame plays an important role. This collective shame experience in the post-war generations is transmitted inter-generationally (Rothe, 2012). Rothe (2012) points out that, for example, strong experiences of shame are still transmitted from non-Jewish Germans who, as children, witnessed the deportation of Jews in 1941, to the following generations. Feelings of shame and guilt in these individuals have been transmitted through their children to their grand- and great-grandchildren (Rothe, 2012). Research thereby points out that shame is being dealt with on a collective, but also on a familial level, and is still prevalent within the contemporary society (Dresler-Hawke & Lui, 2006).

According to the authors, this vivid experience of shame in Germany defines German identity, correlating it strongly to a negatively viewed national identity and a problematic collective self-esteem. However, German identity is viewed in a positive light when reparations are made to make up for the past (Dresler-Hawke & Lui, 2006).

Bierbrauer (1992) has studied the experiences of shame and guilt in Germany in generations after the violation of legal, religious and traditional norms, and compares these experiences with other cultures, particularly Kurds and Lebanese. This research suggests that the German reactions to collective historical experiences are guilt-orientated rather than shame-orientated, and that these experiences were still vivid during the 1990s. Another study from the 1990s (Pätzold, 1995), indicates that 50 years after WWII, Germans feel the least historical pride of 23 countries researched.

However, Dresler-Hawke and Lui (2006) find that, for the third generation after the end of WWII, history is no longer a source of guilt, since "to feel a sense of guilt a person must accept responsibility for a moral violation caused by their own action or inaction" (Dresler-Hawke & Lui, 2006, 134), while shame is experienced when being in some way or other "associated or identified with someone who has committed a guilt-involving act" (Goldberg, 1991, 56). Accordingly, shame is still prevalent in this German generation, but guilt is not.

A recent study on shame and guilt with regard to the German past conducted by Rensman (2014), highlights that lower levels of perceived control of self and situations are associated with shame and higher levels of control are associated with guilt (Rensman, 2014). Therefore the feelings of shame regarding the Holocaust are higher in third-generation Germans (65%)—because individuals in the third generation of Germans feel that they can not control the past anymore—compared to the feelings of guilt (41%) which are associated with the ability to control. Lickel, Schmader and Barquissau (2004) agree with these findings, explaining that shame is rather associated with avoidance, escape, distancing and hiding, while guilt is related to reparation and apology (Baumann and Handrock, in this book).

In a survey conducted in 2003 by Langenbacher, 51% of German citizens wished to forget about the past and proceed with a focus on the future, while 41% agreed to a continued debate on the past. This shows a strong split within German society concerning how to go about dealing with guilt and shame and the uncertainty regarding how to heal the past on a long-term basis.

In parallel to these studies, a study by Conrad (2003) indicates that Germany has dealt relatively well with its difficult and challenging past in comparison to other countries. The author (Conrad, 2003) points out that Germans were able to learn more from guilt and shame then people in other countries, such as Japan and Austria. This learning from the history is based on the one hand on an internalised self-criticism which Germans experienced (Conrad, 2003) and on the other hand on the strict monitoring of Germany by other countries. Based on the audience effect described above, and on the influence of the allied international surveillance following the war, it could be assumed that Germany would have been more self-critical and more prepared to learn from its failures than would Austria or Japan. Conrad (2003) suggests that this might be the case owing to Austria in particular claiming its victim status in the context of WWII and therefore not dealing as proactively with the past as Germany.

1.6 The Transformation of Shame 70 Years After WWII

Miller-Idriss and Rothenberg (2012) argue that it is not easy to capture an understanding of German nationhood because of the ambivalence, confusion and contradictory feelings individuals experience in terms of pride and shame regarding the German nation and their national identity 70 years after the end of WWII. The authors highlight that this is still a project in progress and that Germany is still redefining its national identity while individual citizen work on the transformation of their individual identities.

Brogle (2016) points out that German citizens see themselves caught up in between feelings of shame, guilt and pride several decades after the end of WWII. These emotional entanglements lead to heated discourses on national shame and pride within the society. Further, strongly debated topics in German society revolve around guilt, questions regarding the occurrence of a new national consciousness, taboos around national shame and pride, and how to deal with the phenomena of migration, nationality, moral and ethics in the context of shame (Brogle, 2016).

In contrast to Brogle's view, Heinrich (2017), as a political analyst, has recently concluded that Germany seems to have overcome its shame. After having disowned the past in post-war years—even to the point of making it a taboo subject, individuals internationally are now beginning to approach the Third Reich with a kind of distanced fascination, which Heinrich (2017) describes as "Nazination". These contemporary political movements of right-wing extremism need to be contextualised and understood within global contexts and, for example, through the militant organisation of Aryan nations, from which new fascination with fascism is spread (Shaffer, 2017).

The new generation of Germans seems to have overcome the guilt and shame of the previous generations, and is redefining its identity, associating with cosmopolitan, bilingual and tech-savvy values. However, Heinrich (2017) also points out that this societal transformation needs to be monitored in terms of a rebranded socially acceptable Nazism which is promoted by the Alternative für Deutschland (AfD), a new right-wing-orientated political party, which uses core tenets of race and nationalism and which has a voice in parliament in the recent 2017 German elections.

Fear of a new strengthening right-wing movement in the German context has been previously highlighted (Koopmans & Olzak, 2004), and is often based on the new, open expression of politically motivated right-wingers emphasising their pride in the German nation and their idea of exclusiveness of Germany for Germans only (Rau, 2000), often referring back to German history. These new movements are associated with neo-Nazism and with feelings of shame within the society and they are strongly counteracted by anti-right-wing groups and initiatives (Müller-Idriss, 2009).

Koopmans and Olzak (2004) note that the acts of right-wing violence in Germany are commented on in terms of being shameful for the country. Breitenbach (2011) also observes the expression of shame in the German parliament over far-right murder and the Federal President Rau (2000) has pointed out that right-wing extremism is a shame for German patriotism. Clearly, shame is an important topic in German contemporary politics, on the one hand with regard to history, but on the other hand with regard to the current flourishing of right-wing movements in Germany and the nation's way forward in constructing a national identity.

Vollmer (2016) refers to shame not only in relation to Germany, its political structures, backgrounds or political movements, but also in terms of European politics in the context of migration. The author points out that migration and migration politics in Europe contribute to the "shame of Europe", particularly highlighting the role of Germany in border and migration politics based on the irregular migration towards Europe in the years 1973–1999. According to Vollmer (2016), the "shame of Europe" is defined by the conceptual shift of demonising and re-labelling irregular migrants as enemies, logics of urgency, securitisation and normalisation.

1.7 Collective Shame, Migration and Foreignness

During the past years, interest in the study of emotions, and thereby shame, in the context of migration, has grown (Wettergren, 2015) and collective and individual voices on shame in German society have been taken into account. Within the context of migration and the German society, shame is rife on political, as well as individual levels and has been observed and described by individuals from different cultural backgrounds living in Germany, such as immigrants or refugees. According to Wettergren (2015), emotions and shame specifically occur in discourses of "homelands and hostlands", in interactions between migrants and locals, and in the different migration statuses (legal, semi-legal and illegal). In the context of labour migration, migrants have experienced humiliation and shame during the integration process and through the media, racism and the construction of the diaspora and representations of shamed (migrating) nations.

A recent study by Stotz, Elbert, Müller, and Schauer (2015) demonstrates that refugee minors in German contexts experience traumatic stress, shame and guilt as self-conscious emotions (Womersly, in this book). The study shows that shame and guilt correlate with each other and with posttraumatic stress symptom severity. Shame can hinder the processing of the coping with the traumatic event, consequently leading to mental illness such as posttraumatic stress disorder (PTSD) (Muris & Meesters, 2014).

Similar findings have shown that Vietnamese immigrants in Germany experience strong feelings of shame resulting from experiences of alienation which are being reinforced through stereotyping and stigmatisation which they experience in the German society (Bui, 2003). These experiences are usually connected to the refugee status with which they have entered Germany, linked to shameful living conditions, such as the experience of "being forced to life in a ghetto" (Bui, 2003, 74).

Immigrants whose parents or grandparents have moved to Germany and those who have been born in Germany describe the feelings of shame they experience in German contexts owing to their cultural background. From the perspective of immigrants, shame is experienced through the experience of "being different", the perceived "foreignness" or because they speak German with a "foreign accent" (Topcu, Bota, & Pham, 2012, 9).

A publication by Kroth (2010) on narrations of Turkish Muslim male immigrants indicates that these immigrants experience shame within various contexts in Germany. Some examples of these are shame about migrating without money into a rich country, shame about where they come from, shame about getting divorced and shame about being illegal in a foreign country (Kroth, 2010). Another study of Turkish immigrants in Germany concludes that value orientations of Turkish immigrants are highly gendered (Patzke Salgado, 2006). Patzke Salgado (2006) emphasises that for male Turkish immigrants, behaviour relates to the concept of honour, while female Turkish immigrants usually relate their behaviour to shame. Both concepts are associated with the question of how traditional Turkish values and norms are lived and kept while living in the German society. For male Turkish immigrants honour is associated with keeping up traditional Turkish values in the name of the family. Female Turkish immigrants bring shame to the family if they refrain from living according to traditional Turkish values and starting to live according to German societal values and behavioural norms. This potential value change brings shame to the family through the female Turkish family member (Patzke Saldago, 2006) and might even end in an honour killing (Korteweg & Yurdakul, 2009).

A study of Pakistani immigrant women highlights similar findings (Zakar, Zakar, Faist, & Kraemer, 2012), in that the women experience home-based psychological violence from their intimate partners and immigration stressors. These women, however, do not make use of the German formal support and care facilities because of shame-related issues. The study suggests that this might be a consequence of the shame they might bring to the family in case they get divorced (Zakar, Zakar, Faist, & Kraemer, 2012).

A study of the African diaspora in Germany reveals that African immigrants in Germany have to deal with the collective trauma of slavery and colonialism which is strongly connected to shame (Kron, 2009). Also Russian Jews who migrate to Germany experience shame associated with historical events; they are ashamed of admitting their origin, thereby reconnecting to the collective trauma of the past (Becker, 2003).

The views of different studies of shame in cultural contexts show that individuals and members of different groups of immigrants in Germany deal with different topics and issues of shame to varying degrees, always relating to their personal and social backgrounds and the negotiation of values and norms within their social contexts in the past, as well as in the present.

1.8 Transforming Collective Shame Through International Events

Germany is involved in a steady process of transforming its shame on a global level, to such a degree that Sullivan (2014a, 2014b) suggests that other countries witness Germany's collective transformation with regard to shame and pride as an extraordinary positive process. This development of transformation of shame towards pride or other positively experienced emotions can be viewed as a source of healing and reconstruction (Vanderheiden & Mayer, 2017).

Shame and its recent transformation within Germany's cultural contexts has been expressed in the sphere of national sports events with Germany's success in the soccer World Cup of 2006 (Sullivan, 2009, 2014a, 2014b). Sullivan (2014a, 112) affirms that Germany has undergone a long process of transformation of collective shame after WWII, which finally resulted in a transformational experience of a "cosmopolitan national pride through football at the World Cup 2006 and other subsequent international successes".

This transformation of collective shame to pride was supported particularly by the German soccer team playing in an uncharacteristically positive, team-orientated style which was internationally acknowledged (Sullivan, 2009). According to Sullivan (2014a, 116), Germany has used international football to "transform its international image and to rebrand its nation", particularly with its first world victory as a reunified nation. Sullivan (2014b) emphasises that such internationally recognised accomplishments can become indicators of international values and sources of change on a large-scale level of global societies. Germany's transformation has been declared to be an extraordinary example of this transformation.

1.9 Shameless Germany? Political Movements and Shame in the 21st Century

During the past years, societal changes can be observed in Germany based on the increasing numbers of immigrants from different countries such as Syria, Afghanistan, Iran, Iraq and Pakistan. Perceptions of Germany, its political role in Europe and the world, the acceptance of immigrants and foreigners within the country and the image of Germany as a multicultural nation society, seem to be in a concerted process of change (Abadi, 2017).

Underlying this shift in the landscape of the German political party system and the rise of the AfD into parliament, is a major social change in perception, attitude and behaviour. This shift can be recognised in societal discourses on migration, immigration and on certain cultural groups within Germany (Ramm, 2017). There appears to be growing awareness of threat, open statements against immigrants and foreignness, particularly with regard to a rising tide of intolerance towards Muslim immigrants (Erisen & Kentmen-Cin, 2016). Further, discriminative statements including anti-semitism, sexism, cultural and religious intolerance and homophobia are on the rise, are accepted and even rewarded, as in the Echo-Award giving ceremony in April 2018 (Berliner Morgenpost, 2018). However, this shameful event has also led to strong discourses on freedom of speech, artistic expression and shame.

Based on these societal changes, processes of culturalisation of negative examples of behaviour of immigrants and refugees seem to place the question of collective historical shame in Germany and its impact on contemporary behaviour, attitude and perceptions into a new light. The new trend and reactions towards immigration and foreigners in Germany will most certainly test Germany's new definition of shame, shamelessness and guilt.

1.10 Random Statements on Collective Shame in German Therapeutical and Counselling Contexts

Having lived and worked in (West) Germany for many years, I have been able to gradually collect direct statements on collective shame. During the past years, I have also developed a conscious recognition of the circumlocutions on shame (Scheff, 2016) for what they are, namely indirect descriptions of shame by using alternative terms such as pain, suffering, embarrassment, stigma or disrespectful behaviour, as described recently by Scheff (2016).

In the following section, I would like to present selected statements on shame which do not claim to be in any way representative of the entire German society, but which can provide impressions of contemporary ideas on collective shame within the German context. I provide only a few demographic details of the person who has given the statement, for contextualisation.

1. **Woman, 35 years old, German citizen (statement in 2008):**

   I grew up with my grandmother who has survived two world wars. She always talked about the difficult times and how she lost her husband in the war and how she had to rebuild the German society in the post-war years. She talked a lot about the pain and the suffering and often she described her own coping with the war experiences in such a distanced and neutral way that I wondered how this was possible. I could only understand later that this was probably due to the overwhelming emotions and the experience of shame and guilt. So, when I grew up, the war was very close to me, although I was born three decades after it had ended and still today I struggle to say out loud that I am German.

2. **Man, 70 years old, German citizen (statement in 2018):**

   My uncle who was in the resistance in Germany during the second world war was killed by the German Nazis. My father, the brother of this uncle, carried all of the guilt and shame that he had survived during the war without fighting the regime. This led to a complete silence about this uncle and his death in the family. Almost like a family taboo. However, I can still feel the shame which the family carried and the shame how the citizen could let things like that happen within the family and beyond.

3. **Women, 48 years old, German citizen (statement in 2017):**

   Do you know what the worst is? The worst is that: the ideas of the historic ideologies, you still find them in many of the German institutional structures… and during the recent elections in Germany in 2017 we can see that the Neo-Nazis are back. Or have they never been away? It is a shame for the German nation.

4. **Male, 15 years old, German citizen (statement in 2010):**

   I am tired of having to talk about the German history in almost every school year. I have been born over sixty years after WWII and I do not know why I should feel ashamed about the past. I have not been there and there is nothing really that connects me with this past.

5. **Male, 9 years old, German citizen of African descent (statement in 2017):**

   I travelled on the train the other day and the conductor said to me that I was a "black rider"—although I had a ticket. First, I was confused, then I had to laugh, but actually, it was a shame.

6. **Male, 30 years old, German citizen of Turkish descent (statement in 2014):**

   I do not know why most of the Germans are ashamed of themselves and why they hide their pride to be German. I celebrate each and every success of the German football team. And sure, I carry the German flag.

7. **Male, 19 years old, refugee in Germany from Pakistan (statement in 2018):**

   I am ashamed. I am so young and I struggle to find a German girlfriend. I am in this country since two years… but no German girlfriend. It is a shame. See: I am losing my hair, I am growing old and I will only be able to marry when I am white haired. It is such a shame. I am not sure what to do. Looks like I am not saying the right things at the right time to them?

After you have read through these different statements, you can use the statements for reflection on shame with regard to German cultural contexts and/or discuss them within a team. You can use the following questions to lead you through the reflection and/or discussion. It does not matter what your personal background is. You can reflect on the questions from a German or from any other perspective:

1.	How do you experience the different statements on shame? Which one do you judge to be positive, which one do you judge as negative?
2.	With which statement can you agree? With which one do you disagree?
3.	How do you see and how do you experience (if ever) shame in connection to Germany, the German nation, selected aspects within the German society?
4.	How do you think shame can be transferred with regard to each and every statement? Please reflect and if possible, discuss.
5.	What do you think needs to happen in the German society to release shame even more? Or should the German society rather aim at keeping aspects of the collective shame founded in the past?

1.11   Conclusion

This chapter opened the black box of collective shame in Germany and provided a first insight into shame within German cultural contexts. It provides a state-of-the-art view into the development of collectively experienced shame from past to present. It also asks the question how the collective shame develops in contemporary Germany with special regard to collective international (sport) events and the collective (shameless?) responses to migration/immigration. Finally, I provide an application to reflect and discuss individual statements on collective shame in German contexts to further explore options of transformation.

1.12   Implications for Future Research and Practice

Further research is needed to explore the development of collective shame within different generations in Germany. This research should explore the contemporary shame experiences in Germany in terms of nationhood and collective identity, and particularly explore the transformative potential within different subgroups (gender, age-based, professional) to provide a differentiated image of collective shame experiences, developments and transformation in German contexts.

Research on collective and individual shame experiences should explore the connection of shame on both the collective and the individual level, in selected contexts.

In future, the collective shame and shamelessness with regard to collective and societal challenges and how they will be responded to by different sub-collectives and on a national level, might become an important centre of defining the identity of a multicultural Germany.

Only if the taboo on shame is lifted and shame is consciously taken into account with awareness and mindfulness of German historic and contemporary events and group dynamics, then context-specific, sustainable strategies can be developed to transform shame based on transdisciplinary and transcultural approaches across societal and individual German contexts.

The black box of collective shame has been opened and can now be explored further.

Acknowledgements I would kindly like to thank Elisabeth Vanderheiden for awaking the interest on shame in me, for our on-going discussions about shame and culture and for emphasising the importance of exploring and transforming shame within the German society.
With regard to all my chapters in this book, I would kindly like to thank Mrs Ruth Coetzee for her professional and efficient language editing. I would also like to thank Professor Lynette Louw, Department of Management at Rhodes University, Grahamstown, South Africa, for her continuous support of my research activities in my position as a Senior Research Associate in the department.

References

Abadi, D. (2017). *Negotiating group identities in multicultural Germany: The role of mainstream media, discourse relations, and political Alliances*. Lanham: Lexington Books.

Bar-On, D. (1989). *The legacy of silence. Encounters with children of the Third Reich*. Harvard: Harvard University Press.

Becker, F. (2003). Migration and recognition: Russian Jews in Germany. *East European Jewish Affairs, 33*(2), 20–34.

Berliner Morgenpost. (2018). *Kollegha und Campino sorgen für Eklat - Echo für Rapper*. Retrieved from https://www.morgenpost.de/vermischtes/article213985405/Echo-2018-Campino-schiesst-gegen-Kollegah-und-Farid-Bang.html.

Bierbrauer, G. (1992). Reactions to violation of normative standards: A cross-cultural analysis of shame and guilt. *International Journal of Psychology, 27*(2), 181–193.

Breitenbach, D. (2011). *Parliament expresses shame over far-right murder spree in Germany*. Deutsche Welle. November 22.

Brogle, C. (2016). *Deutschland zwischen Schuld, Scham und Stolz. Eine ethische Betrachtung der Gefühle Schuld, Scham und Stolz im Hinblick auf Staatszugehörigkeit*. Norderstedt: GRIN Verlag.

Bui, P. (2003). *Envisioning Vietnamese migrants in Germany: Ethnic stigma, immigrant origin narratives and partial masking*. Münster: LIT.

Burkitt, I. (2014). *Emotions and Social Relations*. London: Sage.

Burleigh, M., & Wippermann, W. (1991). *The racial state. Germany 1933–1945*. Cambridge: Cambridge University Press.

Conrad, S. (2003). Entangled memories: Versions of the past in Germany and Japan, 1945-2001. *Journal of Contemporary History, 38*, 85–99.

Dresler-Hawke, E., & Liu, J. H. (2006). Collective shame and the positioning of German national identity. *Psicología Política, 32*, 131–153.

Erisen, C., & Kentmen-Cin, C. (2016). Tolerance and perceived threat towards Muslim Immigrants in Germany and the Netherlands. *European Union Politics, 18*(1), 73–97.

Figlio, K. (2011). A psychoanalytic reflection on collective memory as a psychosocial enclave: Jews, German national identity, and splitting in the German psyche. *International Social Science Journal, 62*(203–204), 161–177.

Frevert, U. (2014). Wartime emotions: honour, shame and the ecstacy of sacrifice. International Encyclopedia of the First World War. In: U. Daniel, P. Gatrell, O. Janz, H. Jones, J. Keene, A. Kramer, & B. Nasson (Eds.), 1914–1918-online. *International Encyclopedia of the First World War.* Berlin: Freie Universität Berlin.

Goldberg, C. (1991). *Understanding shame.* London: Jason Aronson.

Heimannsberg, B., & Schmidt, C. J. (1993). *The Jossey-Bass social and behavioral science series. The collective silence: German identity and the legacy of shame.* San Francisco, CA, US: Jossey-Bass.

Heinrich, M. (2017). Germany's past: From shame to fascination. *The globalist: Rethinking globalization.* March 18, 2017. Retrieved from International perspectives. Cambridge: Cambridge University Press. https://www.theglobalist.com/germany-past-from-shame-to-fascination-history/.

Jacquet, J. (2015). *Scham. Die politische Kraft eines unterschätzten Gefühls.* Berlin: Fischer.

Koopmans, R., & Olzak, S. (2004). Discursive opportunities and the evolution of right-wing violence in Germany. *American Journal of Sociology, 110*(1), 198–230.

Korteweg, A., & Yurdakul, G. (2009). Islam, gender, and immigrant integration: Boundary drawin in discourses on honour killing in the Netherlands and Germany. *Ethnic and Racial Studies, 32*(2), 218–238.

Kron, S. (2009). Afrikanische Diaspora und Literatur schwarzer Frauen in Deutschland. In Heinrich-Böll-Stiftung (Eds.). *Migrationsliteratur. Eine neue deutsche Literatur?* (pp. 86–93). Online-Dossier. https://heimatkunde.boell.de/sites/default/files/dossier_migrationsliteratur.pdf.

Kroth, I. (2010). *Halbmond-Wahrheiten. Türkische Männer in Deutschland. Innenansichten einer geschlossenen Gesellschaft.* München: Diederichs.

Kühne, T. (2008). Male bonding and shame culture: Hitler's soldiers and the moral basis of genocidal warfare. In: O. Jensen, C.-C. W. Szejnmann, M. L. Davis (Eds.), *Ordinary people as mass murderers* (pp. 55–77). Location: Palgrave Macmillian.

Langenbacher, E. (2003). Changing memory regimes in contemporary Germany? *German Politics and Society, 21*(2), 46–68.

Lewis, B. (1971). Shame and guilt in neurosis. *Psychoanalytic Review, 58*(3), 419.

Lickel, B., Schmader, T., & Barquissau, M. (2004). The evocation of moral emotions in intergroup contexts. In N. R. Branscombe & B. Doosje (Eds.), *Collective guilt: International perspectives.* Cambridge: Cambridge University Press.

Lickel, B., Schmader, T., Curtis, M., Scarnier, M., & Ames, D.R. (2005). Vicarious shame and guilt. *Group Processes & Intergroup Relations, 8*(2),145–157.

Lotter, M.-S. (2012). *Scham, Schuld, Verantwortung. Über die kulturellen Grundlagen der Moral.* Berlin: Suhrkamp.

Lu, C. (2008). Shame, guilt and reconciliation after war. *European Journal of Social Theory, 11*(3), 367–383.

Miller-Idress, C., & Rothenberg, B. (2012). Ambivalence, pride and shame: Conceptuations on German nationhood. *Nations and Nationalism, 18*(1), 132–135.

Muris, P., & Meesters, C. (2014). Small or big in the eyes of the other: On the developmental psychopathology of self-conscious emotions as shame, guilt, and pride. *Clinical Child and Family Psychology Review, 17,* 19–40.

Pätzold, B. (1995). Le cinquantenaire de la victoire sur l'hitlerisme en Allemagne. *Le Monde Diplomatique, 495,* 20.

Patzke Salgado, A. (2006). *Männliche Ehre - weibliche Scham. Analyse immanenter Wertvorstellungen vor dem Hintergrund von Migration.* Berlin: GRIN Verlag.

Pettigrove, G., & Parsons, N. (2008). Shame: a case study of collective emotion. *Social theory and practice, 38*(3), 504–530.

Pettigrove, G., & Parsons, N. (2012). Shame: A case study of collective emotion. *Social Theory and Practice, 38,* 1–27

Ramm, C. (2017). The Muslim-makers: How Germany "Islamizes" Turkish Immigrants. In Mahade-van, J. & Mayer, C.-H. (Eds.). *Muslim minorities, workplace diversity and reflexive HRM* (pp. 47–58). London: Routledge.

Rau, J. (2000). *"Berliner Rede"* von Johannes Rau. Ohne Angst und ohne Träumereien: gemeinsam in Deutschland leben. 12. Mai 2000 im Haus der Kulturen der Welt in Berlin, Germany. Retrieved from http://egora.uni-muenster.de/FmG/fremdenfeindlichkeit/bindata/f_m1201.pdf.

Rensman, L. (2004). Collective guilt, national identity, and political process in contemporary Ger-many. In N.R. Branscombe, N.R., & B. Doosje (Eds.). *Collective guilt.*

Rensman, A. (2014). Let them Speak - Slave Stamouers of South Africa. South African His-tory Online.https://www.sahistory.org.za/archive/let-them-speak-slave-stamouers-south-africa-andre-van-rensburg

Rothe, K. (2012). Anti semitism in Germany today and the intergenerational transmission of guilt and shame. *Psychoanalysis, Culture & Society, 17*(1), 16–34.

Scheff, T. (1988). Shame and conformity. The deference emotion system. *American Sociological Review, 53,* 395–406.

Scheff, T. (2003). Shame in self and society. *Symbolic Interaction, 26*(2), 239–262.

Scheff, T. (2013). *The S-word: Shame as a Key to modern societies. Global summit on diagnostic alternatives.* Retrieved from http://dxsummit.org/archives/1286. Accessed May 1, 2016.

Scheff, T. (2016). The S-word is taboo: shame is invisible in modern societies. *Journal of General Practice, 4*(1), 1–6.

Shaffer, R. (2017). The extreme right and neo-nazism in post-war United States. In: S.C. Cloninger & S.A. Leibo (Eds.). *Understanding angry groups. multidisciplinary perspectives on their moti-vations and effects on society* (pp. 189–208). Santa Barbara, California: Praeger.

Smith, N. (2008). *I was wrong: The meanings of apologies.* Cambridge: Cambridge University Press.

Stotz, S. J., Elbert, T., Müller, V., & Schauer, M. (2015). The relationship between trauma, shame, and guilt: Findings from a community-based study of refugee minors in Germany. *European Journal of Psychotraumatology, 22*(6). Retrieved from https://doi.org/10.3402/ejpt.v6.25863.

Sullivan, G. B. (2009). Germany during the 2006 World Cup: The role of television in creating a national narrative of pride and "party patriotism". In E. Castelló, A. Dhoest, & H. O'Donnell (Eds.), *The nation on screen, discourses of the national in global television* (pp. 235–252). Cambridge: Cambridge Scholars Press.

Sullivan, G. B. (2014a). Collective emotions and the World Cup 2014: The relevance of theories and research on collective pride and shame. *Psicologia e Saber Social, 3*(1), 112–117.

Sullivan, G. B. (Ed.) (2014b). Collective emotions, German national pride and the 2006 World Cup. In G. Sullivan (Ed.). *Understanding collective pride and group identity: New directions in emotion theory, research and practice* (pp. 124–136). London: Routledge.

Tangney, J. P., & Fischer, K. W. (1995). *Self-conscious emotions.* New York: Guilford.

Topcu, Ö., Bota, A., & Pham, K. (2012). *Wir neuen Deutschen.* Berlin: Rowohlt.

Vanderheiden, E., & Mayer, C.-H. (2017). *The Value of shame—Exploring a health resource in cultural contexts.* Cham, Switzerland: Springer.

Vollmer, B. A. (2016). The continuing shame of Europe: Discourses on migration in Germany and the UK. *Migration Studies, 5*(1), 49–64.

Wettergren, A. (2015). Protecting the self again shame and humiliation: unwanted migrant's emo-tional careers. In: J. Kleres J., & Y. Albrecht (Eds.) *Die Ambivalenz der Gefühle.* (pp. 221–245). Springer VS, Wiesbaden.

Whitman, J. Q. (1998). *What is wrong with inflicting shame sanctions?* Faculty scholarship series, paper 655. Retrieved from http://digitalcommons.law.yale.edu/fss_papers/655.

Zakar, R., Zakar, M. Z., Faist, T., & Kraemer, A. (2012). *Intimate partner violence against women and its related immigration stressors in Pakistani immigrant families in Germany.* Springer Plus, 1(5). Retrieved from https://doi.org/10.1186/2193-1801-1-5.

Zhang, J. W., & Chen, S. (2016). Self-compassion promotes personal involvement from regret experiences via acceptance. *Personality and Social Psychology Bulletin, 42*(2), 244–258.

Claude-Hélène Mayer (Dr. habil., PhD, PhD) is a Professor in Industrial and Organisational Psychology at the Department of Industrial Psychology and People Management at the University of Johannesburg, an Adjunct Professor at the Europa Universität Viadrina in Frankfurt (Oder), Germany and a Senior Research Associate in the Department of Management at Rhodes University, Grahamstown, South Africa. She holds a Ph.D. in psychology (University of Pretoria, South Africa), a Ph.D. in management (Rhodes University, South Africa), a Doctorate in political sciences (Georg-August-Universität, Göttingen, Germany), and a Habilitation with a Venia Legendi (Europa Universität Viadrina, Germany) in psychology with focus on work, organizational, and cultural psychology. She has published numerous monographs, edited text books, accredited journal article, and special issues on transcultural mental health, salutogenesis and sense of coherence, shame, transcultural conflict management and mediation, women in leadership in culturally diverse work contexts, constellation work, coaching, and psychobiography.

Chapter 2
Opening the Black Box Part 2: Exploring Individual Shame in German Research

Claude-Hélène Mayer

Abstract This chapter is the second part of two chapters on shame in German contexts. It explores research which focuses on shame in individuals. The question addressed is the following: Which aspects of shame does research highlight with regard to shame in individuals in German contexts? Individually experienced shame in German cultural and contemporary research is explored and reflected on, to provide readers with an insight into shame research in Germany, which is often published in the German language. Practical applications are added with regard to the selected research areas on individual shame. Conclusions are drawn and recommendations for future research and (therapeutical) practice are given.

Keywords Individual shame · German research · Science · Education · Body shame · Care · Clinical conditions · Shame

> Der Tag kennt mehr Scham
> als die Nacht.[1]
> Roman-German idiom from the Middle Ages

2.1 Opening the Black Box of Individual Shame

After having focused on the collective shame in past and present in Germany (Mayer part 1, in this book), this chapter provides an insight into research on individually experienced shame in German contexts.

Research, theoretical and empirical studies have been conducted in German contexts particularly with regard to shame from psychological and therapeutical

---

[1] Translation by the author: "The day knows more shame, than does the night."

C.-H. Mayer (✉)
Institut für Therapeutische Kommunikation und Sprachgebrauch, Europa Universität Viadrina, Logenstrasse 11, 15230 Frankfurt (Oder), Germany
e-mail: claudemayer@gmx.net

Department of Management, Rhodes University, Drosdy Road, Grahamstown 6139, South Africa

© Springer Nature Switzerland AG 2019
C.-H. Mayer and E. Vanderheiden (eds.), *The Bright Side of Shame*,
https://doi.org/10.1007/978-3-030-13409-9_2

perspectives (see Hilgers, 2006; Marks, 2017; Wurmser, 2013), but also from anthropological (Lietzmann, 2007), philosophical, sociological and social science (Simmel, 1986; Landweer, 1999) perspectives. These publications touch on issues such as shame and the body (see Gröning, 2013a), as well as shame and conflict, shame and clinical conditions (Grabhorn & Overbeck, 2005; Rüsch et al., 2007; Scheel, Bender, Tuschen-Caffier, & Jacob, 2013), shame and the healthcare system (Gröning, Feldmann, Bergenthal, Lebeda, & Yardley, 2016; Immenschuh & Marks, 2014) and shame and status (Neckel, 1993).

The insights provided here do not claim to be a complete overview of shame research in German contexts; rather, they offer an indication of the focus and trend of shame studies in this specific cultural context.

This chapter feeds into Scheff's (2016) idea of actively reclaiming shame studies, since shame is one of the less explored and discussed emotions. Studies discussed here are those that have addressed shame directly as shame and not as a circumlocution (Scheff, 2016, 3; see Mayer, Part 1).

This chapter describes selected major foci of German research on shame, specifically shame in science and scientists, in education, in the context of the body, in care, and with regard to clinical conditions. It also includes applications for reflection, a conclusion and a recommendation for future research.

2.2   Shame in Science and Scientists

Friedrich Nietzsche, a German philosopher, cultural critic and poet, pointed out early in his hermeneutics of shame that shame is a form of a practical pre-understanding of the world. According to Nietzsche, as understood by van Tongeren's (2007), a philosopher needs to be "shamelessly fearless" on one hand, and characterised by honour, shame and depth on the other. The same might be said about contemporary scientists.

Nedelmann (2006) explores shame in the context of science. To the author, shame is inherent in the management and handling of science in past and present Germany. He refers to the fact that psychoanalysis and psychoanalytic thought in sciences was forced out of Germany during WWII, and is in the process of rapprochement. This process needs to take German cultural traditions and Jewish thoughts into account, to transform the painful process of dealing with shame when scientists of psychoanalysis lead a discourse. This process of rapprochement is associated with feelings of anger, shame, guilt and sadness (Nedelmann, 2006) and is reflected in the scientific discourse.

2.2.1 Reflection

1.	How is shame experienced and expressed in science and in scientists?
2.	Where is shame shown directly in science?
3.	Where is shame expressed in science as a circumlocution?
4.	How does the topic of shame connect philosophy and science?

2.3 Shame in Education

Shame is not only a topic in science, but also in educational contexts and schools (Haas, 2013; Marks, 2013). Marks (2013) explains that when shame is experienced, the brain retracts into a "survival mode" (Geldenhuys, in this book), therefore educational contexts in particular need to help students to develop tools and mechanisms not to avoid shame, but to deal with shame constructively within their contexts. In order to achieve this, students and teachers need to trust each other and trust the environment in which school and education is experienced, as non-shaming (Marks, 2013; Boness, in this book).

Frenzel, Thrash, Pekrun, and Goetz, (2007) have conducted cross-cultural research on shame in the context of educational achievement and parental achievement expectations, success and failure. In their research, they show that German students experience lower levels of shame and anxiety when it comes to achievement in Mathematics, but they show higher levels of anger in comparison to Chinese students (Frenzel et al. 2007).

Wertenbruch and Röttger-Rössler (2011) state in their research on shame and shaming in German schools that often shame is experienced based on the violation of norms of the peer group of students. According to the authors, shame and shaming are important emotional dimensions in German school routines. Adolescents are primarily affected by feelings of shame because they are in the process of learning how to comply with the social and cultural norms (Wertenbruch & Röttger-Rössler, 2011). The authors further highlight that shame experiences differ based on the socio-cultural background of the individuals in German educational contexts, and on how they define their values and norms in the German school system. Shame becomes an important factor of processes of inclusion and exclusion. Its role also needs to be increasingly recognised in the context of mental health, achievement and coping in multicultural school contexts in Germany (Boness, in this book).

2.4   Shame, the Body and Family Contexts

Studies in Germany have focused on shame and the body and shame in family relations. The Federal Agency for Health Education (BZGA, 2005) has published a foundational study on shame in childhood and on the regulation of shame in families, highlighting the value of shame. According to the study (BZGA, 2005), the perceived value of shame is dependent on the professional status of the father: the higher the father's professional status, the more feelings of shame are valued as impacting positively on the way people live together and as a protective factor for the self and for others. In a study, mothers in German contexts usually judge shame as positive (BZGA, 2005). In addition, it has been pointed out that shame is often associated with sexuality, as well as with nudity in the context of the body (BZGA, 2005, Silverio, in this book).

2.5   Shame in the Context of the Body

Body shame has often been distinguished from research on psychological and mental shame, as well as from social shame (see Hilgers, 2006; Gröning 2014) in German research. In his texts on shame, Simmel (1986), a German sociologist, philosopher and classical shame researcher, highlights that shame is strongly connected to the body, and to the experience of inferiority and nakedness, since the body represents nature, the flesh and the fleeting moments of life.

Köhler (2017) points out that although bodies often touch in post-modern life situations such as in an overcrowded tram, individuals usually do not feel ashamed by this touch because of the framing of definitions of shame within contexts. However, nakedness is still shameful in German contexts, although people are used to see naked bodies (Köhler, 2017). Shame is still connected to eroticism and sexuality, to puberty, body contact, distance and violence (Köhler, 2017).

Ko (2010) has studied the role of body shame in social appearance anxiety, body-checking behaviour and body dissatisfaction, as well as disordered eating behaviour. The author compared German and Korean students, and found that Korean females had higher scores in all of these shame areas than did German females and males. In both cultures, body shame predicted bulimia symptoms, but it did not predict a drive for thinness in either of the female groups. Body shame predicted body dissatisfaction in both cultures.

Another culture-comparative study (Hong, 2011) compared German, Korean and Chinese female students' attitudes towards body shame and intention to change appearance. Findings showed that in the German group of female college students, the body mass index (BMI) was the highest, while scores in public self-consciousness, socio-cultural pressure, ideal appearance attitude, body shame, and appearance change intention were lowest in Germany, highest in Korea. The variables that affected body shame were powerful in the order of appearance internalisation, appearance awareness, socio-cultural pressure, and public self-consciousness in Germany and different from the Chinese and the Korean findings in which socio-cultural appearance was the highest variable that affected appearance change intention. Appearance change intention was powerful in the order of sociocultural pressure in Korea and China in the first place, while the order was appearance internalisation, body shame, and BMI in the German group (Hong, 2011).

Hahn (2016) discusses the impact of the social memory of the body by referring to appearances and perception and memory of shame from a sociological perspective. The author points out that the memory plays a central role in managing social and individual shame: shame can be avoided by keeping it secret and by forgetting. The author interprets social fights regarding the public memory as fights about the question of who can deal with shame and shaming.

2.5.1 Reflection on Body Shame

If you would like to explore your attitude towards body and body shame within your social and cultural context, reflect on the following aspects:

1.	What image of your body do you hold?
2.	How do you feel about this body?
3.	Which parts of your body do you relate to in a positive, which in a negative way?
4.	Where in your body do you feel the most energy flow?
5.	Focusing on your biography, when did you experience shame with regard to your body across your lifespan? Reflect on your childhood, adolescence and adulthood.
6.	Which key situations do you remember with regard to body shame as being the most influential?
7.	Contextualising your body shame, how does your culture, your social and cultural background, your gender, your age, your language abilities, your general abilities/disabilities influence your body shame?
8.	Where are your body's and your body shame boundaries?
9.	How can you help to ensure that your body shame boundaries are being accepted and respected in your contemporary life and in future life situations?

2.6 Shame in the Context of Care

With regard to the German demographical structure and the growing number of Germans above the age of 65 years, shame becomes a specific topic in the context of care of individuals of old age (Gröning, 2014). Hayder-Beichel (2016) points out that patients with urological illnesses—here especially men—experience the treatment of these illnesses and conversations about it as shameful. However, Marks (2011) comments that not only patients in care experience shame, but also their carers (Veit and Bahrs & Henze, in this book). In German contexts they experience shame, because they cannot care for the people in need in the way they want to, owing to time pressure and other work-related restrictions (Marks, 2011).

Several recent German studies refer further to shame in the context of care, care institutions and psychiatric contexts (Gröning et al., 2016). Shame is not only a topic which is generally relevant for Germans in care (Immenschuh & Marks, 2017), but seems also to be particularly relevant with regard to Muslim patients (Von Bose & Terpstra, 2010) and Turkish patients (Ulusoy & Grassel, 2010) in German care and hospitals. According to Ulusoy and Grassel (2010), shame is associated with over-estimation of the self and with language barriers in Turkish migrants, and according to Von Bose and Terpstra (2010), with honour in Muslim migrants.

Generally, shame is strongly linked to nakedness and challenging care situations in gender-specific care, especially with regard to hygiene and shame (Heusinger & Dummert, 2017). However, Gröning (2013b) points out that shame and anxiety are the basic emotions experienced in old age with special regard to "shame of dependence", shame of the changing body, and the shame of being blamed.

2.6.1   Reflection

Please reflect on the question of shame in the context of care, either on your own or in a group, in terms of these questions.

1.	Have you ever experienced shame in the context of care?
2.	If yes, in which role were you experiencing shame—as a carer, a person being cared for, or as a relative or family member?
3.	What kind of shame did you experience?
4.	Thinking of care and shame and culture-specific and/or inter-/transcultural situations, what needs to be considered when working with shame in the context of culture within the German or other societies?
5.	What should be done in care institutions (hospitals, hospices, retirement homes) to transform shame? Are there any programmes, trainings, workshops you can think of which would be helpful?

2.7   Shame and Clinical Conditions in German-Based Research

In German settings, shame is usually researched in individuals with clinical conditions (Grabhorn, Stenner, Standier, & Kaufhold, 2006; Rüsch et al., 2007;

Rummel-Kluge, Pitschel-Walz, Bäuml, & Kissling, 2006), since shame is a meaningful self-reflexive emotion in the context of the exploration of mental disorders (Kämmerer, 2010). Only a few such selected studies are presented in this chapter. Hilgers (2006) provides an extensive overview of shame in terms of singular psychological problems such as social phobia, schizophrenia, suicidal syndromes, depression, borderline personality disorders, eating disorders, hysteria, post-traumatic stress disorder (PTSD) or psychophobia. Hilgers (2006) also offers insight into conflicts based on shame in somatic illnesses, and with regard to managing shame conflicts in therapy, and in counter-transfer situations between therapist and client/patient in individual therapy settings. The author also gives advice on how to deal with shame in group-psychotherapy.

Research focusing on a sample of German native speakers shows that shame-proneness and self-report of shame is higher in women with borderline personality disorder than in women with social phobia and healthy women (Rüsch et al., 2007). For the women with borderline personality disorders, shame is strongly associated with the self (Rüsch et al., 2007) and with existential shame. In their article on the development of a German questionnaire on shame, Scheel et al. (2013) highlight that shame is strongly associated with borderline personality disorder and with the adjustment to social norms and self-regulation processes. Scheel et al. (2013) contend that the experience of physical and cognitive shame can be viewed as functional, while existential shame is viewed as maladaptive.

Apart from the finding that shame is a meaningful construct to understand eating disorders (Albohn-Kühne & Rief, 2011; Grabhorn, Stenner, Standier, & Kaufhold, 2006), a recent study by Borgart, Popescu, and Meermann (2016) suggests that bulimia nervosa is associated with depression and shame in German contexts and relates to self-perception and body image. Individuals with anorexia and bulimia nervosa are found to have higher scores in global shame than do individuals with anxiety disorders and depressions (Grabhorn et al., 2006). Feelings such as shame, sadness, and anxiety need to be experienced by awareness of one's self, feeling through body awareness (Gugutzer, 2015).

Other studies in Germany show that shame has been identified as the key emotional symptom in the link between social anxiety and social phobia (Bandelow & Michaelis, 2015). Shame makes an important difference in explaining social anxieties; these authors highlight that therapeutic strategies need to target the transformation of shame and social anxiety.

Another German study (Rummel-Kluge et al., 2006) compares psychoeducation in schizophrenia in Germany, with the same in Austria and Switzerland, indicating that guilt and shame are topics discussed during psychoeducation in the three countries. The study concludes that the most discussed topic is stigmatisation (80%), followed by isolation (83%) and guilt and shame (70%). No differences could be found between the findings from the three countries. Shame is therefore a particularly important topic in German-speaking populations of patients suffering from schizophrenia, a topic which needs to be dealt with proactively.

2.8   Shame in the Context of Military, War and Soldiers

Finally, it is noteworthy that very recent research (Alliger-Horn, Zimmermann, Herr, Danke-Hopfe, & Willmud, 2017; Zimmermann, 2015) also focuses on shame and PTSD in German soldiers who suffer from shame and guilt as a result of war experiences. These recent studies explain how to minimise shame effectively during therapeutical interventions. Another study in the German military context (Siegel et al., 2017), however, finds that veterans often do not seek psychotherapeutic advice owing to experiences and fear of discrimination, stigmatisation and shame. The authors suggest that these barriers to seeking advice and therapy are an international phenomenon, while the existence of complex and intimidating structures to seek psycho-medical support seem to be specific to Germany (Siegel et al., 2017). Working with shame, particularly in individuals with PTSD, can become a key to managing PTSD in therapy and therefore should be addressed (Schoenleber et al., 2015).

2.9   Working with Shame in the Context of Clinical Conditions

Based on the research on shame in German clinical conditions as described above, the following factors can be taken into account when working with shame in the context of counselling and/or therapy:

1. The basis on which to transforming shame is the creation of a warm and safe place in counselling and therapy to explore individual and collective shame on a deeper level. There needs to be general openness to self-reflection and to work with shame on different levels, such as with the feeling of shame (body) and the memory of shame (psychology) (Gugutzer, 2015; Hahn, 2016).
2. Accept shame as a part of the shadow and take this general acceptance as a foundation to accept that shame can be transformed to become functional, and work with shame and transform it for personal growth (Mayer, 2017).
3. As in every other therapeutical context, the relationship of the therapist and the client needs to one of trust; the therapist needs to remain highly conscious and aware of how to explore shame while dealing with other clinical conditions. It can be helpful to the therapist to remember that the experience of shame in a therapeutical context is normal (Klinger, Ladany, & Kulp, 2012). Mayer & Oosthuizen (2018, in press) point out that therapists and therapist trainees should focus on developing their own mental health and self-care and thereby encourage and promote mental health in their clients.
4. Shame can be explored in individual and group therapy sessions depending on the clinical conditions and the aims of the therapy (Mayer, 2017; Mayer healing rituals, in this book). While working with shame, verbal and non-verbal expressions of shame should be taken into account and made conscious to develop an

improved understanding of the impact of shame (Randles & Tracy, 2013). Non-verbal keys to shame can particularly be observed in intervention techniques like constellation work (Mayer healing rituals, in this book), or sculpture work (Virginia Satir).

5. Therapeutical interventions such as dream work, self-compassion, mindfulness and other self-accepting attitudes and their development within the client and therapist can become a key to exploring and transforming shame (Zhang & Chan, 2016; see Vanderheiden, Gilbert, Mayer 2018 dream work, in this book).

6. The development of pro-social behaviour in clients can reduce stress and support a constructive management and transformation of shame (see Raposa, Laws, & Ansell, 2016).

7. Meditation exercises, as well as creative expression such as dance, can help to deal with self-criticism and shame (see Buch, Edwards, Vanderheiden, in this book).

8. Make use of specific therapeutical interventions or therapies which have been viewed as innovative methods to transform shame in the context of specific mental disorder, such as schematherapy (Jacob, 2011) which integrates cognitive, emotional and behavioural methods from various schools of therapy. In the German context, schematherapy has only gained increasing interest in the beginning of the new century and is still in its exploration and development (Jacob & Seebauer, 2014).

9. These aspects can be respected as foundational when working with shame in the context of dealing with clients with clinical conditions, but also in other counselling contexts. For further explorations of how to deal with shame within therapy contexts see, for example, Dearing and Tangney (2011) or DeYoung (2015), Jacob (2011) and Jacob and Seebauer (2014).

2.10   Conclusion

This chapter provided an insight into shame within German research and cultural contexts particularly with regard to experiences of individual shame from the perspective of German researchers and in German-based research. The chapter does not stake out the claim of an entire overview of the literature on individually experienced shame in German contexts, but provides the reader with an insight in shame research in Germany. Further, the chapter presents reflections and practical applications of working with shame based on the research reviewed.

2.11   Implications for Future Research and Practice

Future research on individually experienced shame in German contexts should focus on the interrelationship of shame, psychological and body shame and study shame not only with regard to clinical samples, but also with regard to non-clinical samples. Areas which seem to be underrepresented with regard to studies on shame in German contexts are areas such as: shame in the workplace, shame in education, shame with regard to science. Further, shame should be researched with regard to specifically defined sub-contexts in the German society and, for example, bicultural individuals as well as individuals acting in specific professional contexts, following our earlier call for increasing intercultural, culture-specific and transcultural studies on shame (Vanderheiden & Mayer, 2017). Gender and culture should be addressed more intensively in terms of the question if gender and culture make a difference when opening the black box of individually experienced shame in different German contexts.

Acknowledgements I warm-heartedly thank my friend and colleague Elisabeth Vanderheiden for her inputs and discussions regarding this chapter.

References

Albohn-Kühne, C., & Rief, W. (2011). Scham, Schuld und soziale Angst bei Adipositas mit "Binge-Eating"-Störung. *Psychotherapie, Psychosomatik, Medizinische Psychotherapie, 61*(09/10), 412–417.

Alliger-Horn, C., Zimmermann, P., Herr, K., Danke-Hopfe, H., & Willmud, G. (2017). Adaptierte, stationäre Alptraumtherapie mit Imagery Rehearsal Therapy bei chronisch kriegstraumatisierten deutschen Soldaten mit PTBS. *Zeitschrift für Psychiatrie, Psychologie und Psychotherapie, 65,* 251–260.

Bandelow, B., & Michaelis, S. (2015). Epidemiology of anxiety disorders in the 21st century. *Dialogues in Clinical Neuroscience, 17*(3), 327–335.

Borgart, E. J., Popescu, C., & Meermann, R. (2016). Bulimia nervosa. Essen und Brechen aus Frust und Scham. MMW - Fortschritte der Medizin (2016) 158: 43. Retrieved from https://doi.org/10.1007/s15006-016-7753-8.

BZGA. (2005). *Kindliche Körperscham und Familiale Schamregeln.* Köln: BZGA.

Dearing, R. L., & Tangney, J. P. (2011). *Shame in the therapy hour.* Washington, D.C: American Psychology Association.

DeYoung, P. A. (2015). *Understanding and Treating Chronic Shame. A relational/neurobio-logical approach.* New York: Routledge.

Frenzel, A. C., Thrash, T. M., Pekrun, R., & Goetz, T. (2007). Achievement emotions in Germany and China. A cross-cultural validation of the Academic Emotions Questionnaire—Mathematics. *Journal of Cross-Cultural Psychology, 38*(3), 302–309.

Grabhorn, R., & Overbeck, G. (2005). Scham und soziale Angst bei Anorexia und Bulimia nervosa. *Zeitschrift für Psychosomatische Medizin und Psychotherapie*: Band 51, Ausgabe 2, S. pp. 179–193. Retrieved from https://doi.org/10.13109/zptm.2005.51.2.179.

Grabhorn, R., Stenner, H., Stangier, U. & Kaufhold, J. (2006). Social anxiety in anorexia and bulimia nervosa: The mediating role of shame. *Clinical Psychology and Psychotherapy, 13*(1). https://onlinelibrary.wiley.com/doi/abs/10.1002/cpp.463.

Gröning, K. (2013a). Der verlorene Körper. Theorien von Körperbild, Körperselbst und Scham. In: D. Nittel, A. Seltrecht (Eds.) Krankheit: *Lernen im Ausnahmezustand? Brustkrebs und Herzinfarkt aus interdisziplinärer Perspektive.* Berlin: Springer.

Gröninger, K. (2013b). Alter und Scham. *Soziale Passage, 5*(1), 51–58.

Gröning, K. (2014). *Entweihung und Scham: Grenzsituationen bei der Pflege alter Menschen.* 6, überarb. Aufl. Frankfurt a. M.: Mabuse-Verlag.

Gröning, K., Feldmann, M., Bergenthal, S., Lebeda, D., & Yardley, Y. (2016). *Somatische Kultur und psychiatrische Pflege.* Universität Bielefeld. Retrieved from https://www. uni-bielefeld.de/erziehungswissenschaft/ag7/familiale_pflege/materialien/studienbriefe/StB_ somatik-psychiatrische-pflegekultur.pdf.

Gugutzer, R. (2015). *Soziologie des Körpers.* 5. vollstndig überarbeitete Auflage. Bielefeld: transcript.

Haas, D. (2013). *Das Phänomen Scham: Impulse für einen lebensförderlichen Umgang mit Scham im Kontext von Schule und Unterricht.* Stuttgart: Kohlhammer Verlag.

Hahn A. (2016) Scham, Körper, Geheimnis und Gedächtnis. In: Heinlein M., Dimbath O., Schindler L., & Wehling P. (Eds.), *Der Körper als soziales Gedächtnis. Soziales Gedächtnis, Erinnern und Vergessen – Memory Studies.* Springer VS, Wiesbaden.

Hayder-Beichel, D. (2016). Privat. Intim. Peinlich? *Heilberufe, 68*(4), 14–16.

Heusinger, J., & Dummert, S. (2017). Scham und Nacktheit bei der Körperpflege im Heim. *Heilberufe, 69*(4), 16–18.

Hilgers, M. (2006). *Scham.: Gesichter eines Affekts* (4th ed.). Göttingen: Vandenhoeck & Ruprecht.

Hong, K.-H. (2011). A study on the variables influencing female college students' body shame and appearance change intention: Comparison of Korea, China and Germany. *Fashion and Textile Research Journal, 13*(4), 523–530.

Immenschuh, U., & Marks, S. (2014). *Würde und Scham - ein Thema für die Pflege.* Frankfurt: Mabuse Verlag.

Jacob, G. A. (2011). Was ist innovativ an der Schematherapie? *Zeitschrift für Psychiatrie, Psychologie und Psychotherapie, 59,* 179–186.

Jacob, G. A., & Seebauer, L. (2014). Schematherapie. *Zeitschrift für Klinische Psychologie und Psychotherapie, 43,* 271–278.

Kämmerer, A. (2010). Zur Intensität des erlebens von Schamgefühlen bei psychischen Störungen. *Psychotherapie, Psychosomatik, Medizinische Psychologie, 60*(7), 262–270.

Klinger, R. S., Ladany, N., & Kulp, L. E. (2012). It's too late to apologize: Therapist embarrassment and shame. *The Counseling Psychologist, 40*(4), 554–574.

Ko, N. (2010). *The role of body shame, social appearance anxiety, and body checking behaviour on body dissatisfaction and disordered eating behaviours: A cross-cultural study in Germany and Korea.* Dissertation, Freiburg, Germany. Retrieved from https://d-nb.info/1009955454/34.

Köhler, A. (2017). *Scham. Vom Paradies zum Dschungelcamp.* zu Klampen.

Landweer, H. (1999). *Scham und Macht. Phänomenologische Untersuchungen zur Sozialität eines Gefühls.* Tübingen: Mohr Siebeck.

Lietzmann, A. (2007). *Theorie der Scham. Eine anthropologische Perspektive auf ein menschliches Charakteristikum.* Hamburg: Verlag Dr. Kovac.

Marks, S. (2011). *Menschenwürde und Scham. Vortrag, Herbsttagung.* Zürich, November 5, 2018.

Marks, S. (2013). Scham im Kontext von Schule. *Soziale Passagen, 5*(1), 37–49.

Marks, S. (2017). *Scham - die tabuisierte Emotion* (7th ed.). Ostfildern: Patmos Verlag.

Mayer, C.-H. (2017). Shame—"A soul feeding emotion": Archetypal work and the transformation of the shadow of shame in a group development process. In: E. Vanderheidenn & C.-H. Mayer (Eds.), *The value of shame—Exploring a health resource in cultural contexts* (pp. 277–302). Cham, Switzerland: Springer.

Mayer, C.-H., & Oousthuizen, R. (2018, in preparation). *"What contributes to family therapist trainees health and well-being?" A preliminary, longitudinal investigation.* ORT & Verlag.

Nedelmann, C. (2006). Psychoanalytische Identität in Deutschland. *Tradition und Wiederannäherung. Forum der Psychoanalyse, 22*(2), 182–189.

Neckel, S. (1993). Achtungsverlust und Scham. Die soziale Gestalt eines existentiellen Gefühls. In: Hinrich Fink-Eitel & Georg Lohmann (Hg.): *Zur Philosophie der Gefühle.* (pp. 244–265) Frankfurt am Main: Suhrkamp.

Randles, D., & Tracy, J. L. (2013). Nonverbal displays of shame predict relapse and declining health in recovering alcoholics. *Clinical Psychological Science, 1*(2), 149–155.

Raposa, E. B., Laws, H. B., & Ansell, E. B. (2016). Prosocial behavior mitigates the negative effects of stress in everyday life. *Clinical Psychological Science, 4*(4), 691–698.

Rüsch, N., Lieb, K., Göttler, I., et al. (2007). Shame and implicit self-concept in women with borderline personality disorder. *The American Journal of Psychiatry, 164*(3), 500–508.

Rummel-Kluge, C., Pitschel-Walz, G., Bäuml, J., & Kissling, W. (2006). Psychoeducation in Schizophrenia—Results of a survey of all psychiatric institutions in Germany, Austria, and Switzerland. *Schizophrenia Bulletin, 32*(4), 765–775.

Scheel, C. N., Bender, C., Tuschen-Caffier, B., & Jacob, G. A. (2013). SHAME—Entwicklung eines Fragebogens zur Erfassung positiver und negativer Aspekte von Scham. *Zeitschrift für Klinische Psychologie und Psychotherapie, 42*(4), 280–290.

Scheff, T. (2016). The S-word is taboo: shame is invisible in modern societies. *Journal of General Practice, 4*(1), 1–6.

Schoenleber, M., Sippel, L. M., Jakupcak, M., & Tull, M. T. (2015). Role of trait shame in the association between posttraumatic stress and aggression among men with a history of interpersonal trauma. *Psychological Trauma: Theory, Research, Practice, and Policy, 7*(1), 43–49.

Siegel, S., Rau, H., Dors, S., Brants, L., Börner, M., Mahnke, M., et al. (2017). Barrieren der Inanspruchnahme von Psychotherapie ehemaliger Soldatinnen und Soldaten der Bundeswehr (Veteranen). Eine Expertenbefragung. *Zeitschrift für Evidenz, Fortbildung und Qualität im Gesundheitswesen, 125,* 30–37.

Simmel, G.(1901/1986): *Psychologie der Scham.* In: Schriften zur Soziologie, hg. v. J. Dahme, O. Rammstedt (pp. 151–158). Frankfurt a. M.: Suhrkamp.

Ulusoy, N., & Gräßel, E. (2010). Türkische Migranten in Deutschland. *Zeitschrift für Gerontologie und Geriatrie, 43*(5), 330–338.

Vanderheiden, E., & Mayer, C.-H. (2017). *The value of shame—Exploring a health resource in cultural contexts.* Cham: Springer.

Van Tongeren, P. (2007). Nietzsches Hermeneutik der Scham. In C. J. von Emden, H. Heit, V. Lemm, & C. Zittel (Eds.), *Nietzsches Studien 36* (pp. 131–154). Boston: DeGruyter.

Von Bose, A., & Terpstra, J. (2010). *Muslimische Patienten pflegen. Praxisbuch für Betreuung und Kommunikation.* Cham: Springer.

Wertenbruch, M., & Röttger-Rössler, B. (2011). Emotionsethnologische Untersuchung zu Scham und Beschämung in der Schule. *Zeitschrift für Erziehungswissenschaft, 14*(2), 241–257.

Wurmser, L. (2013). *Die Maske der Scham: Die Psychoanalyse von Schamaffekten und Schamkonflikten* (2nd ed.). Berlin: Springer.

Zhang, J. W., & Chen, S. (2016). Self-compassion promotes personal involvement from regret experiences via acceptance. *Personality and Social Psychology Bulletin, 42*(2), 244–258.

Zimmermann, P. (2015). Einsatz, Werte und psychische Gesundheit bei Bundeswehrsoldaten. In: M. Gillner, & V. Stümke (Eds.), *Kollateralopfer. Die Tötung von Unschuldigen als rechtliches und moralisches Problem* (pp. 173 – 194). Münster: Aschendorff Verlag.

Claude-Hélène Mayer (Dr. habil., PhD, PhD) is a Professor in Industrial and Organisational Psychology at the Department of Industrial Psychology and People Management at the University of Johannesburg, an Adjunct Professor at the Europa Universität Viadrina in Frankfurt (Oder), Germany and a Senior Research Associate in the Department of Management at Rhodes University, Grahamstown, South Africa. She holds a Ph.D. in psychology (University of Pretoria, South Africa), a Ph.D. in management (Rhodes University, South Africa), a Doctorate in political sciences (Georg-August-Universität, Göttingen, Germany), and a Habilitation with a Venia Legendi

(Europa Universität Viadrina, Germany) in psychology with focus on work, organizational, and cultural psychology. She has published numerous monographs, edited text books, accredited journal article, and special issues on transcultural mental health, salutogenesis and sense of coherence, shame, transcultural conflict management and mediation, women in leadership in culturally diverse work contexts, constellation work, coaching, and psychobiography.

Chapter 3
lajjA: Learning, Unlearning and Relearning

Dharm P. S. Bhawuk

Abstract *lajjA* is a personal virtue to be cultivated, not a social sanction to be avoided, to lead a noble life. It guides us in life by (1) prescribing what we ought to do and (2) proscribing what we ought not do. It is cultivated through cultural socialization process from early childhood, but as young adults we make choices that leads to further learning, unlearning, and relearning *lajjA* in multiple social contexts. In this paper, I employ autoethnography to show how I learned, unlearned, and relearned *lajjA* hoping to throw some light on the developmental trajectory of this construct.

Keywords lajjA · Shame · Autoethnography · Religious scriptures and practice · India · Nepal

Harvard-Kyoto protocol for transliteration for *devanagarI* is used for all *saMskRtaM* and *hindI* words and names, and the first letters of names are not capitalized. All non-English words are italicized.

अ a आ A इ i ई I उ u ऊ U ए e ऐ ai ओ o औ au ऋ R ॠ RR ल IR ऌ

IRR अं M अः H क ka ख kha ग ga घ kha ङ Ga च ca छ cha ज ja झ jha ञ

Ja ट Ta ठ Tha ड Da ढ Dha ण Na त ta थ tha द da ध dha न na प pa फ

pha ब ba भ bha म ma य ya र ra ल la व va श za ष Sa स sa ह ha

क्ष kSa त्र tra ज्ञ jJa श्र zra

D. P. S. Bhawuk (✉)
2404 Maile Way, Honolulu, HI 96822, USA
e-mail: bhawuk@hawaii.edu

© Springer Nature Switzerland AG 2019
C.-H. Mayer and E. Vanderheiden (eds.), *The Bright Side of Shame*,
https://doi.org/10.1007/978-3-030-13409-9_3

3.1 *lajjA*: Learning, Unlearning, and Relearning

Menon and Shweder (1994, 2003), concluded that *lajjA* is associated with being shy, having modesty, and showing deference to elders. Having *lajjA* is akin to being a civilized person who knows his or her place in the society and acts properly as demanded by one's duties and responsibilities. Thus, *lajjA* prevents people from any transgression. Employing films, advertisements, conversations, and written narratives, Sinha and Chauhan (2013) identified the behavioral representations of the construct of *lajjA*, and showed how it is used by women in defining their identity in India. For example, one of the participants stated that *lajjA* provides a woman beauty and gracefulness without robbing her of determination or ambition.[1] They noted that *lajjA* not only seems to be the core of womanhood in India, but also can be used as a manipulative tool against women in certain situations.

I examined dictionary meanings, synonyms, and antonyms of *lajjA* in *saMskRtaM* and *hindI*, and analyzed the usage of the word in two popular scriptural texts, namely, the *bhagavadgItA* and *drugA saptazatI* (Bhawuk, 2017). In that paper, I further examined uses of *lajjA* in the literature in *kAmAyanI*, a modern *hindi mahAkAvya* or epic as well as in daily communications and proverbs. This multi-method approach resulted in a thick-description of the construct, showing that *lajjA* is one of the 26 virtues enumerated in the *bhagavadgItA* that guides human behavior, and has both internal and external aspects, or guilt and shame elements. Such a structure is at odds with the Western literature that views guilt and shame as distinct and independent constructs (Creighton, 1990; Lewis, 1971; Tracy & Robins, 2006). There is evidence that, *lajjA* is an important virtue that guides human behavior in Asia (for example, Fung, 1999; Lebra, 1983); in general and India in particular (Bhawuk, 2017; Menon & Shweder, 1994, 2003; Sinha & Chauhan, 2013). However, it is not clear how *lajjA* is learned or unlearned. This paper fills that lacuna.

In this paper, I trace how *lajjA* is learned through the socialization process from childhood so that we can develop a sense of right and wrong. I also document how *lajjA* is unlearned or relearned. I reflect on my personal experience and present critical incidents that help understand the social and cultural processes of acquisition of *lajjA*. I hope the paper contributes not only to the indigenous literature but also to the nuanced understanding of global psychology of shame and guilt.

3.2 Methodology

Through reflexive investigation, autoethnography (Anderson, 2006; Bhawuk, 2009; Ellis, 1997, 2004; Ellis & Bochner, 2000) allows us to use the lived experience of an individual to examine cultural phenomena by presenting insightful evidence

---

[1] "*lajjA* makes me feel like a woman. Having *lajjA* does not make me any less determined, any less ambitious or any less strong as a human being. It just makes me graceful in my mannerisms and I appreciate the beauty in that (Sinha & Chauhan, 2013, p. 134)".

connecting the experience of the individual to the cultural level construct. It can be a necessary first step in understanding the process of how an indigenous phenomenon operates or how a cultural skill is acquired over time. Therefore, I reflected on my own life experiences to map the process of learning, unlearning, and relearning *lajjA*. I provide some examples from my school days but focus mainly on my experience during college years. Further, I corroborated the results of autoethnography using comments from colleagues, and synthesized their ideas to enrich the findings with multiple perspectives. This autoethnographic approach complements my previous work (Bhawuk, 2017), and further enriches the understanding of the construct of *lajjA*.

I focused on college years for three reasons. First, often going to college entails living away from the sheltered environment of home and family for the first time except for those who go to boarding school from childhood. In college we are forced to make decisions building on the values learned at home and in school. Second, we are legally considered responsible adults who can make their own decisions and face the related consequences. Finally, these four or five years are considered formative and shape how we act in later life. A fuller description of my childhood experience and how it shaped my college years, and how the college years shaped my later adult years will be discussed in another paper presenting a multiphase longitudinal perspective on the learning, unlearning, and relearning of *lajjA*.

3.3 Learning *lajjA*

I learned from the experience of my four elder siblings that in our family academic excellence was rewarded, so I studied hard. My father was a historian, but an intuitive Skinnerian. He rewarded me nickels and dimes for memorizing texts, and told me that it will help me assimilate the language of the text as my own. It helped me form good study habits. Outside of studies, behaving appropriately, which included speech and action, was an important lesson that I learned from my parents, uncles, aunts, siblings, teachers, and village elders. I was scolded if my speech or behavior was not proper, and avoided punishment by learning from the mistakes of my siblings.

lajjA was used in multiple ways in my socialization process. My parents used the idiom, "*zarma nahiM AtI hai?*" in *hindI* or "*lAja lagdaina?*" in *nepAlI* (since we are multi-linguals we used whatever came to us naturally) as a question (Aren't you ashamed?), which implies that I should be ashamed of what I did. If a child takes more than his share of food on many occasions, then the parents may use this expression to chide him or her. I had a weakness for sweets and sneaked sweets on many occasions. I received my fair share of shaming for it. Another expression *zarma se pAnI-pAnI ho gayA/gayI* is used when one is thoroughly embarrassed for not doing something or doing something that should not have been done. The target person is so embarrassed that he or she would like to hide from everybody.

I was also aware of the expression, *cullu bhar pAnI me dUba maro* (drown yourself in the water in your cupped hand, meaning the person should be ashamed of himself or herself). This is what an elder tells a youngster who is constantly failing to do something, often a weak student hears this in relation to studies, and a problem child hears this in relation to social embarrassment that he or she constantly causes. I was aware of it and avoided such situations.

The earliest incidents in which I experienced *lajjA* pertained to incontinence (bed-wetting and diarrhea related soiling of my pants because of eating too many mangoes). I can still recall felling really small and wanting to vanish from the eyes of others. Fortunately, these problems happened only a few times, and I naturally grew out of them before I was seven years old.

I remember feeling extreme *lajjA* when my father caught my lie when I was about 14 years old. Two teams of boys played a football match. Our team lost, but the goal was disputed, and the match could be called a tie game. So we refused to pay the bet money to the other team. Things got rough, and I ran away since the money was with me. When somebody from the other team complained to my father, he asked me if I had run away with the bet money. I told him that I did not have the money, not to let down my team. The following day my lie was exposed, and he showed strong displeasure that I had lied to him. I felt like drowning myself in the water in my cupped hand (or *cullu bhar pAnI me dUba maranA*), the proverbial case of feeling extreme *lajjA*. I gave the money to the captain of the other team. I don't think I lied ever after that.

Another time at an embassy social event at a public auditorium some of us sitting behind a family were not proper with our language. The couple in the front asked us to behave properly. Shortly after the intermission, the couple left. After the show was over I learned that my friend's older brothers had whispered something to scare them and that is why they left before the program was over. The next day in the evening when my father came home from work he told me that one of his colleagues who knew me had complained to him about how I had misbehaved at the event. He said he was embarrassed, and I felt the proverbial *lajjA - zarma se pAnI-pAnI ho gayA*. I was about 16 years old then.

I picked up a few swear words in Nepali and Hindi, and used them among my peers in school. But I avoided using swear words in the presence of the elders. I was raised non-vegetarian and we ate mutton and chicken at home, but no pork or beef. I did sneak a sip of whisky at home during a party when I was sixteen. I also smoked a few times in the company of older cousins but did not pick it up as a habit. I did get into some fights at school, but they were not serious enough to be reported to my parents. While living at home, I was always careful and avoided trouble so that no report of bad behavior reached home. I had a sense of appropriate and inappropriate behaviors, and was able to act properly to avoid causing *lajjA* to my family or myself.

The incidents I presented show that *lajjA* is caused when one does something inappropriate—bed-wetting, not managing diarrhea well, lying, and using inappropriate language. Incontinence is physical and messy, but usually one may receive some sympathy from others as one is helpless. However, lying and using inappropriate language are avoidable, and we are likely to receive disapprobation from other people. Therefore, *lajjA* is always associated with *akaraNIya* or ought not to do actions, but some of these actions are rather involuntary whereas others are choice behaviors (see choice theory by Glasser, 1998). One experiences *lajjA* in either case, but in case of choice behaviors one is responsible and likely to feel extreme *lajjA*.

3.4   Unlearning *lajjA*

I went to the Indian Institute of Technology, Kharagpur ((IITKh), in August 1974 to study mechanical engineering. It was a five-year program. This was the first time I was living by myself in a dormitory. I got to visit home (i.e., Kathmandu) during the winter break only as I used the summer break for doing internship. My first shocking experience was with hazing (or ragging as it is known in India), which lasted for about a month. The senior students who ragged us became our friends at the end of the month, which was quite exciting.

I noticed that the norm for students was to use abusive language, and the four letter word (f***) was generously used to create a variety of phrases such as f*** it, f*** that, f*** him, f*** off, f*** knows, I got f***ed (did not do well on examination or test), and so forth. It was as if the only way to emphasize anything was to use the f-word. For example, it was not enough to say "What is wrong with you!" and it had to be "What the f*** is wrong with you!" What used to be boring became "f***ing boring"; what was exciting became "f***ing exciting"; and so forth. Thus, foul language became casual conversational habit (Jay, 2009). If a fellow female student said,"I got f***ed," meaning she did not do well on the test, she was considered emancipated. The f-word became a part of my language. One could make a dictionary of unprintable words and phrases that I had acquired during my stay at IIT-Kh. Using swearwords in our language is acquired implicitly in childhood by watching adults, and speech pollution marks the opening ground for shedding some *lajjA*. The institute had not only imparted a world-class engineering education but also provided the social context for opening the flood gate for foul language, and other socially undesirable behaviors causing the loss of *lajjA*.

There was a wide range of individual differences in shedding *lajjA*. For example, some of my peers remained cautious in their choice of words and expressions. On the other hand some students used to call even their best friend a son-of-a-b****. Interestingly, the measure of closeness between two friends was the extent to which they could hurl insults at each other! Thus, a person like me who was intolerant of those using an abusive term for his or her own mother or someone's mother became tolerant of such abusive words. I lost a lot of *lajjA* in those five years (1974–79) at IIT-Kh. I take full responsibility for my own transformation. Until I started working on *lajjA* and took up writing this paper, I never realized that I had actually lost a lot of *lajjA* becoming coarse, harsh, and insensitive in many ways.

I shared the draft of this paper with some colleagues and students. Two students from IIT-K (Kanpur) noted that while they had acquired the use of foul language after coming to IIT-K, their friends back home had not changed. Thus, there is some support that academic institutions provide an environment for students to cultivate the use of foul language and they lose *lajjA* in the process. A female colleague who went to another engineering college reported that in her college women called each other stupid or *cudail* (or witch) and that was the extent to which they used inappropriate language. Thus, there is a range of variation among students, and there are also some gender differences.

I also picked up some inappropriate behaviors like smoking and drinking alcohol at IIT-Kh. Many of my friends tried some other inappropriate behaviors and clearly each person chose what he or she wanted to do. I would like to note two caveats. First, it seems that it is conformity and peer pressure that leads people to pick-up vices. However, there is much more interaction between person and environment, and personal choice plays an equally important role. Second, we all picked up many positive skills in each other's company and developed life-long friendships. So, loss of *lajjA*, though a serious drawback, there were other qualities that we developed, which counter balanced the loss. For example, I had full support of my friends when I led an ascetic life in the final year at IIT-Kh, which included, among other practices, having one salt-less meal a day at lunch time, wearing clogs, not taking a haircut, not looking into a mirror, and leading the life of a recluse right in the dormitory!

3.5 Relearning *lajjA*

In aSTAGgaYoga or the eight-fold path of yoga,[2] the practitioner is first required to exercise five controls (or *yamas*), namely, *ahiMsA* (non-violence), *satya* (truth), *asteya* (non-stealing), *aparigraha* (non-accummulation), and *bramhacarya* (pursuing *bramha;* practice of celibacy for single people and fidelity for married people). Next, one has to practise five *niyamas* or additional restraints including *zauca* (purification), *santoSa* (contentment), *tapaH* (austerities), *svadhyAya* (self study), and *IzvarpraNidhAna* (contemplation on *bramha* or the formless God). These ten practices are to be practiced at three levels, at the level of *karma* (or action), *vacana* (or speech), and *vicAra* (or thought). The three levels are not independent, and purification at one level could lead to positive change in the other two. Similarly, dilution at one level could lead to pollution at the other two levels.

The ten practices covered by *yama* and *niyama* are used by all spiritual aspirants irrespective what path they follow, including Buddhism, Jainism, and Sikhism.

lajjA is the virtue that guides behavior. It helps us avoid doing inappropriate behavior and also prevents us from shying away from what is our duty even if the situation is burdensome. Therefore, *lajjA* is the gentle virtue that is needed in cultivating any virtue (see Bhawuk, 2017) including the *yamas* and *niyamas* discussed above. Therefore, to relearn *lajjA*, we will need to cultivate virtues, and the *yamas*

---

[2]*asTAGgayoga* or the eight-fold path of yoga includes the following eight practices: *yama* (or controls), *niyama* (or restraints), *Asana* (or control of posture with effort), *prANAyAma* (or control of breath with effort), *pratyAhAra* (control of senses with effort), *dhAraNA* (holding of *manas* with effort), *dhyAna* (holding of *buddhi* with effort), and *samAdhi* (*buddhi* is in equanimity without effort).

and *niyamas* being the foundation of all *sAdhanAs* (or spiritual practices), cultivating them will slowly regenerate the lost *lajjA*.

Failure is the first step in learning of any skill. No project can be completed without facing unexpected and undesirable outcomes. A spiritual journey is analogous to walking on the razor's edge,[3] and so lapses are natural and many. There are stories in Indian scriptures about how many noble aspirants experienced failure in their spiritual journey, but they kept trying without letting the failures hold them back.

A wise saint ("Cloudburst," 2008) advised spiritual practitioners to confess their mistakes publicly, without hesitation because hiding the act binds one to it but not hiding it frees one of the karmic bondage. Public confession not only helps to develop the ability to take responsibility for one's failure (an internal process), but also forces one to face others in making amends (an external process). In group therapy, it is possible to pursue growth through shame and humiliation (Rutan, 2000). It is also plausible that a self-reflective person can grow by dealing with humiliation in his or her own unique way as I did (Bhawuk, 2009). It is not surprising, therefore, that Tony Robbins (Robbins, 2016; see the Netflix documentary that is publicly available on YouTube) uses public shame to treat distressed people. Once people accept their weaknesses, wrong doings, or how others exploited them, they possibly free themselves from the burden of covering it. Thus, *lajjA* can be relearned by (i) cultivating the ten practices of *yama* and *niyama*, and (ii) publicly acknowledging one's short comings and working on them. I have adopted both the strategies and find them to bear fruits.

I started my journey by announcing to my family that I had become a *vaiznava* sometime in 1998. The *vaiznavas* are devotees of Lord *viSNu*, the protector god of the trinity of creator (*bramhA*), protector (*viSNu*), and destroyer (*ziva*), who are not supposed to get angry with anybody. Controlling one's anger is a form of the practice of *ahiMsA*. I started with speech purification and making effort not to get angry with anybody. My family became the mirror to show my failures and encouraged and supported me in my journey. I used the f-word to show my extreme displeasure with my sons, what they called the f-bomb, when things got really bad. When I did that they knew the matter was really serious, and they needed to change their behavior. With practice, I was able to let go of my anger and stop using the f-word, and still could negotiate with them that they needed to change their behavior. For the past few years, I have been working on annoyance, which is the subtlest form of anger and violence.

---

[3] *uttiSTha   jAgrata   prApya   varAnnibodhata,   kSurasya   dhArA   nizitA duratyayA   durgaM   pathastatkavayo   vadanti   (kathopaniSada: 1.3.14)—*
उत्तिष्ठ जाग्रत प्राप्य वरान्निबोधत | क्षुरस्य धारानिशिता दुरत्यया दुर्ग पथस्तत्कवयो वदन्ति॥
Finding a teacher, rise, wake up, and realize. The wise say that the path is like a razor's edge, difficult to walk on.

3.6 Discussion

lajjA is a social psychological construct, and so it is plausible that we learn it through the socialization process (see Fung, 1999, for how shame is used to socialize children in China so that they can develop a sense of right or wrong) (Wang and Sang, in this book). This fits well with my own personal experience. When we examine my college experience, we could be satisfied with the socialization argument and even add the conformity argument (Asch, 1955, 1956). However, I contend that I learned as well as unlearned *lajjA* not only through the socialization process but I also exercised a personal choice, or what Asch (1955, 1956) called independence. There is interaction between socialization, conformity, and personal choice in our learning, unlearning, and relearning of *lajjA*. I would like to present some other examples.

Smoking was a taboo when I was growing up. My father never smoked, nor did my elder bother. The latter did not drink either. Nevertheless, I did smoke sometimes in my early adulthood. Given those role models, I should not have smoked. That I did smoke suggests that conformity to the majority alone is not sufficient for acquisition or loss of *lajjA*. Personal choice is also necessary and no less important in acquisition and extinction of *lajjA*. Researchers have given more importance to conformity and neglected the importance Asch ascribed to independence in the face of pressure from the group (see also Friend, Rafferty, & Bramel, 1990).

Greasing palms of civil servants is a normative behavior in collectivistic cultures (Hellman, 2017). During my professional career in Nepal (1979–91), a collectivistic culture (Bhawuk & Udas, 1996), I did not accept any kickback. When deciding about what branch of engineering to pursue, I was advised by many to study civil engineering. However, I took a stand and chose mechanical instead of civil engineering (CE), because CE was well-known for generating kickbacks. Since I could do it at the age of 17, personal choice or independence does play a role in learning or unlearning *lajjA*.

When I was 25 years old, a friend and I joined my father and uncles in drinking at a family gathering. My elder brother told me after the event that the embarrassment our elders experienced was palpable. However, I was unaffected as if I had not only unlearned *lajjA* but also took pride in being *lajjA-hIna* (one devoid of *lajjA* or *bezaram*). A female colleague noted that Indian women sometimes hide their drinking habit from their in-laws but not their parents, highlighting gender diffcrences in drinking behvaior. Athough *lajjA* is a general guideline against doing what is inappropriate and not doing what is appropriate as scriptures define (see Bhawuk, 2017), one can engage oneself in some inappropriate behaviors but not others or choose some appropriate behaviors over others. Thus, *lajjA* is learned and unlearned by one's personal choice under certain behavioral settings, given that the social environment is conducive to such changes. As noted above, without the supportive environment provided by the academic institution of IIT-Kh, I could not have imbibed the abusive language, or picked up smoking or drinking alcohol.

A female colleague pointed out that while going to college in the 1980s, she felt that she was expected to show *lajjA* as a woman following the dictum, *lajjA narI kA zRGgAra hai* or *lajjA* makes a woman look good (or it is the makeup she should always wear). She noted that as her daughter has grown to be an adult, her daughter has empowered her to be more of herself, and so she is able to shed *lajjA* in many domains. However, she observed that her daughter does not use foul language or raise her voice, and conjectured that perhaps *lajjA* runs deep in the Indian female blood. Her observations provide much insight from Indian women's perspective.

I may also have an idiosyncratic reason for acting the way I did. I considered feeling guilt for any transgression unhealthy. As a consequence, I consciously cultivated the skill of suppressing guilt (Wenzlaff & Wegner, 2000) right from my adolescent years. This skill might have been an outcome of a story narrated to me by my father about Motilal Nehru (ML), the father of Jawaharlal Nehru (JL), the first prime minister of India. ML was a successful and affluent barrister who could afford a wealthy western lifestyle during 1900–1930, before he gave up much of his wealth and legal practice to join the freedom movement of India, accepting the leadership of Gandhiji. He sent JL to England to study, and his two daughters also received Western education in India and had European governesses. He entertained guests at his large home, was known to be non-vegetarian, and consumed alcohol socially (Nanda, 1962). When he joined politics, his love of drinking and entertaining others was not viewed positively by Gandhiji, who suggested that if he could not stop drinking, he should at least not drink in public. ML felt strongly about hiding it from the public eyes, and thought it would be twice wrong to do so. The moral of this story[4] for me was that one should neither hide a seeming wrongdoing nor feel guilty about it. My father acted in the same spirit in his own social interactions. In hindsight, this moral lesson might have laid the foundation of my unlearning of *lajjA*.

In Indian philosophy, spiritual aspirants (or *sAdhakas*) monitor themselves at the levels of *vicAra* (i.e., thoughts, the *manas*[5] referred to as *manasA*), *vacana* (words or vAcA), and *karma* or actions (*karma* done by the *kAyA* or actions done by the body). As in the Western psychology, *karma* is an overt response but *vicAra* is a covert response. *vacana* falls in between and supposedly translates *vicAra* into *karma*.

---

[4]I have not been able to find a written evidence of this episode, though more than one person has reported hearing about it. In my studies of the biographies of ML, JL, and Gandhiji (Nanda, 1962; Gandhi, 1957/1993; Nehru, 1942) it is clear that ML was a very strong person who could publicly disagree with Gandhiji on issues and defend his position. I do not mean to slight either ML or Gandhiji. My father never slighted other people, and admired ML, JL, and Gandhiji. So, I believe the incident is likely to be true. The story is an important part of my development process even if it were made up.

[5]*manas* in *sanskrit* or *mana* in *hindi* is the center for cognition, affect, and behavior (Bhawuk, 2011), and, therefore, it is difficult to translate it in English. Mind is a widely used translation, which only captures the cognitive function of *manas*, but not the affective and behavioral functions. Therefore, I use *manas* in my writing, and use "*manas* or mind" from time to time to remind the readers of the translation issue. See b*hAwuk*, 2011, Chap. 4, for a definition and discussion of *manas*, *buddhi*, *ahaGkAra*, and *antaHkaraNa*. The closest translation of *ahaGkAra* would be ego, which comes at the cost of much loss of meaning. People often use mind for *manas*, which is simply wrong, since *manas* is the locus of cognition, affect and behavior, whereas mind is only cognitive. And *buddhi* is closest to the super-ego in Freudian parlance, but without ego, which makes the similarity rather superficial. And *antaHkaraNa* is the composite internal organ or agent combining *manas*, *buddhi*, and *ahaGkAra*.

lajjA guides people at all the three levels. Awareness of one's motives and intentions is purely internal; crafting one's words and deeds are seen by observers and are external. Smoking, drinking, disrespecting elders, and neglecting one's duties to the needy are examples of socially undesirable behaviors. When one displays such acts, he or she is effectively snubbing *lajjA* as if *buddhi* (see Footnote 2) is unable to guide *manas*.

The use of foul language is *akaraNiya* (or something we ought not to do) and evokes *lajjA*. Similarly, one's failure to deliver on the promise would evoke *lajjA*. I have experienced *lajjA* on the occasion of not delivering a paper on time or not attending a committee meeting. Similarly, a parent would experience *lajjA* when he or she is unable to provide what is promised to his or her child. All these scenarios entail behavior but the cause of *lajjA* is not behavior per se but the target's inability to fulfill one's promise. In the *rAmacaritamAnasa*, *tulsidAsa* creates an exemplar in king *dasaratha* who gives up his life but honors the word he had given to his queen—*raghukul rIta sadA calI Ayi, prANA jAye par vacana na jAye (the great tradition of the descendants of king raghu is that, they would rather die than go back on their word).*

Socially unacceptable behaviors like smoking, drinking, going to a prostitute, and adultery ought to cause *lajjA*. In the Indian worldview, there are six enemies of spiritual practice - *kAma* (desire), *krodha* (anger), *lobha* (greed), *moha* (attachment), *ahaGkAra* (ego), and *mAtsarya* (jealousy) (see Bhawuk, 2011, Chap. 7; Fig. 7.1). Those who cannot detach themselves from these evils would experience *lajjA* themselves and would also cause *lajjA* to their families.

lajjA can operate at the level of *manas also*. Whenever a person does a wrong, he might feel angry, guilty, envious, or jealous merely because of the awareness of that misdeed. A reflective person can recognize the loci of such feelings and work on them to deal with those thoughts and feelings. Thought suppression and diverting attention (Wenzlaff & Wegner, 2000) are likely to be ways of coping with ideas that transpire *lajjA* in both short- and long-term. One's *buddhi* is the citadel of *lajjA*. *buddhi* uses *lajjA* to guide behaviors, such as choosing right over wrong or healthy over unhealthy. As *lajjA* is a *sancarI bhAva* or a fleeting emotion (Bhawuk, 2017), it stops appearing in our *manas* when it is ignored or flouted a few times by indulging in behaviors that are improper. Therefore, if our speech and acts are polluted, our thoughts will be polluted. And if our speech and acts are polluted in a wide range of domains, our thoughts are likely to be equally polluted. Purifying the thoughts would require the purification of actions and speech. Hence, the emphasis on the three levels, thought, speech, and action, for spiritual aspirants. Relearning *lajjA* would require a public commitment to a set of proper behaviors, which constitute performing actions that are proper, and not performing actions that are improper.

There is a need to differentiate between *lajjA* and *viveka* (or discretion). They are similar in that they guide us to make right or ethical decisions in doing what we ought to do (*karaNIya*) and not doing what we ought not to do (*akaraNIya*). Ideally, when *viveka* guides us properly, we do not experience *lajjA*. However, our *viveka* may be clouded by desires for certain outcomes or for favoring people we love. These are the situations where we are likely to experience *lajjA* both while making the decision and later when we face the outcome. But if we consider such situations as having absence of *viveka* (or we are being *vivekahIna*), then we could say that absence of *viveka (or vivekahInatA)* leads to *lajjA*.

We often use *viveka* in making decisions about how to approach a problem, since a problem can be solved in many ways. We use *viveka* in deciding if we should cross a river or not based on our estimate of how good a swimmer we are and how strong the current is. We use *viveka* in choosing what to say to people to make friends. We use *viveka* in guiding our students. There are many situations like these where *viveka* is the instrument of *buddhi*, and *lajjA* is not salient, primarily because we are choosing from a pool of right decisions (i.e., none of the decisions would cause *lajjA*) of which one may be better. Sometimes choosing one decision may lead to poorer outcome, and the outcome may be a cause of *lajjA*. But in the selection of the decision itself *lajjA* need not be salient.

For example, using *viveka*, I would be able to guide myself on a test—(i) I should not be stuck on a problem that I am not able to solve; (ii) I should move on to another problem, and return to it if I have time at the end; (iii) I may not be able to solve all the problems on the test, if I spent too much time on a problem I am not able to solve; (iv) I am likely to get a poor grade because of this. If I did not have *viveka*, I would get a poor grade choosing the less efficient process. Thus, *lajjA* may be associated with the outcome, whereas *viveka* is associated with the process only.

When we want something that *viveka* does not recommend, because it is not right for the other person to do it, because it is burdening the other person, and so forth, we are becoming selfish and we may experience *lajjA* in the situation. We find parents begging for forgiveness for their children's wrong doing so that the kids do not face stiff penalties. Parents rationalize their behavior because it is to protect their children. Parents may punish the children later, in the privacy of their home, for causing them extreme *lajjA*. We may find subordinates asking for favors from their superiors even when they know they do not deserve them. Superiors may concede to the groveling subordinates, causing *lajjA* to both of them, for the one for obliging and for the other for asking.

I noted that *lajjA* is an instrument of *buddhi,* and it is associated with *buddhi* in mediating thought and action (Bhawuk, 2017). It is a fleeting emotion (or a *saJcarI bhAva*). Metaphorically, *lajjA* is the wife of *dharma*, and so it is always present where *dharma* is present (see Bhawuk, 2017 for a discussion). Both *viveka* and *lajjA* are instruments of *buddhi*, but whereas *lajjA* is asscoiated with emotion, *viveka* does not seem to be associated with emotion and is rather associated with *tejas* (fiery energy, vital power, or efficacy)—*viveka* is associated with discriminating the spiritual from the material, and, therefore, it does not get confounded with desires and passions.

Therefore, there will be difference in the *viveka* of a worldly and that of an enlightened person, and using their *viveka* two people could come to two different decisions in the same situation. We found this in the battlefield of *mahAbhArata* when *arjuna* used his *viveka* and decided not to fight the battle because wars destroy the families and societies. His anti-war arguments presented in the first canto of the *bhagavadgItA* are quite convincing. Using his *viveka*, on the other hand, *kRSNa*, presented multiple arguments that countered *arjuna*'s, and convinced him to fight the battle. *viveka* often is related to quality rather than appropriateness of decisions.

3.7   *ahiMsA* in Speech: A Practice

Citing his personal experience, *gAandhiji* concluded his autobiography (Gandhi, 1957) by stating that there was no other God than truth, and the only way to God was through the practice of *ahiMsA* or nonviolence. The test of such a practice lies in one's daily behavior of loving the smallest living entity as oneself. Identifying with all living beings[6] calls for self-purification in all walks of life by becoming "absolutely passion-free in thought, speech and action; to rise above the opposing currents of love and hatred, attachment and repulsion.[7]" He further extolled the practice of *ahiMsA* by stating that it was "the farthest limit of humility," and it could only be achieved when one puts oneself last. His stated goal for writing the autobiography was to describe truth so that common people's faith in truth and *ahiMsA* would be restored, and he recommended only one practice for the realization of truth, that of *ahiMsA*. He even entreated the readers to pray for him[8] so that he could master *ahiMsA;* such was his faith in the practice of *ahiMsA*.

Following Gandhiji, I too would like to recommend only one practice for the cultivation of *lajjA*, *ahiMsA* in speech. I think purification of speech will lead to the purification of actions and finally the cleansing of thoughts. Of course, if one is a violent person, then therapy would be needed to curb the violent behaviors first. But often in interpersonal interactions it is violence of speech that leads to physical violence. If violence in speech can be controlled, violence of action can be avoided. Focusing on purifying thoughts would be relevant for a person who has mastered nonviolence in action and speech. Further, the practice of affirmation, using positive words, could be a positive psychological practice that could help cultivate purification

---

[6]Gandhiji is instinctively quoting *bhagavadgItA* verse 6.29 that captures the idea of *samadarzana* or harmonious perspective where one sees the self in others and others in the self. Verse 6.29: *sarvabhUtasthamAtmAnaM sarvabhUtAni cAtmani, IkSate yogayuktAtmA sarvatra samadarzanaH*. One who sees the self in all beings and all beings in oneself, such a person, who is absorbed in yoga, has a harmonious global perspective.

[7]Gandhiji is instinctively quoting *bhagavadgItA* verses 2.56 and 2.57 that describe the person whose *buddhi* is in equanimity or one who is free of all passions, a *sthitaprajJa*. 2.56: *duHkheSvanudvignamanAH sukheSu vigatsprihaH, vItarAgabhayakrodhaH sthitdhIrmunirucyate*. When facing sorrow one's *manas* is not agitated, and when facing pleasure one does not desire more; one who has transcended attachment, fear, and anger is said to be in equanimity by the seers. 2.57: *yaH sarvatrAnabhisnehastattatprApya zubhAzubham, nAbhinandati na dveSTi tasya prajJA pratiSThitA*. One who is without attachment or fondness in all situations, and neither celebrates the appearance of what is pleasurable nor mourns the appearance of what is detestable; such a person's *buddhi* is in equanimity.

[8]"In bidding farewell to the reader, for the time being at any rate, I ask him to join with me in prayer to the God of Truth that He may grant me the boon of *ahiMsA* in mind, word and deed." (Gandhi, 1957).

of speech. Cultivating *ahiMsA* in speech and the practice of affirmation have both been rewarding for me on my spiritual journey, and in the cultivation of *lajjA* and other virtues. I have not used the f-word, even for dramatization, in more than a decade. However, I still think one should be able to use it without feeling guilty, and then not use it as self-discipline.

3.8 Coda

I presented an account of my subjective experiences in learning, unlearning, and relearning of *lajjA*, using autoethnography as the method. I also corroborated the findings with the experience of others, and synthesized the comments of colleagues to enrich the narrative. Reflecting on how *lajjA* was learned, unlearned, and relearned helped me demonstrate the role of socialization, conformity, and personal choice in the cultivation of *lajjA*. Institutions provide the socio-psychological space that is necessary for learning or unlearning *lajjA*, which has important implications for creating positive workplace environment. Relearning *lajjA* requires personal commitment and the support of one's social group, and cultivating the ten practices of *yama* and *niyama* and practicing affirmation can facilitate the process.

The value of cultivated *lajjA* is highlighted in other cultures too. Fung (1999, p. 180) presented the pedigree (and Familial Instructions) of the Zhou Clan

> What distinguishes the human being from the animal is shame. When a person does not know shame, his/her conscience would vanish. For such a person parents would have no way to discipline; teachers and friends would have no way to advise. Without the will to strive upward, how could one improve? To be an official without shame is treacherous; how could he be loyal? To be a son without shame is disobedient; how could he be filial? To be a neighbor without shame is wicked; how could he be kind? … As one knows shame, the sense of right and wrong would be realized, and his dying conscience would have a chance to revive.

The Chinese wisdom is consistent with how Prophet Mohammad emphasized the role of *hayA* or *lajjA* in shaping human behavior—If you don't feel *hayA* do whatever you like (see Bhawuk, 2017).

After leaving IIT-Kh, I had stopped using *lajjA* as a guide and used conscience instead. I visualized conscience as a multifaceted diamond that pricks us when we do something inappropriate. When we insist on continuing with such inappropriate behaviors, we grind away that facet of the diamond. Ultimately, a person may end up having a spherical shaped conscience that does not prick at all, whatever the person does. I have met some people in my life who could rationalize everything they did, and have no *lajjA*. Conscience worked for me for many years as an organizing framework, but now I am cultivating *lajjA* all over again since it is a richer construct consisting of both internal and external elements. *lajjA* is a virtue that nurtures a tender heart. Since conscience lies in a tender heart, *lajjA* can be an instrument to cultivate and nurture conscience. I hope that future indigenous researchers will develop other culture-specific constructs similar to *lajjA* that can enrich the literature on behavior, culture, and management, and help create a more conscientious global village.

Acknowledgements I would like to thank Professors Jai B. P. Sinha, Ramadhar Singh, Braj Bhushan, Smriti Anand, Richa Awasthy, Chandra P. Sharma, Dr. Om P. Sharma, Anand C. Narayanan, Vikram Patel, Ajay Chugh, Rekhanshi Varma, and Robin Singh for their insightful comments that helped improve the paper. An earlier draft of the paper was presented at the International Congress of International Association for Cross-Cultural Psychology, Guelph, Canada, July 1 to July 5, 2018.

References

Anderson, L. (2006). Analytic autoethnography. *Journal of Contemporary Ethnography, 35*(4), 373–395.

Asch, S. E. (1955). Opinions and social pressure. *Scientific American, 193*(5), 33–35.

Asch, S. E. (1956). Studies of independence and conformity: I. A minority of one against a unanimous majority. *Psychological monographs: General and applied, 70*(9, Whole No. 416), 1.

Bhawuk, D. P. S. (2009). Humiliation and human rights in diverse societies: Forgiveness & some other solutions from cross-cultural research. *Psychological Studies, 54*(2), 1–10.

Bhawuk, D. P. S. (2011). *Spirituality and Indian psychology: Lessons from the Bhagavad-Gita.* New York: Springer.

Bhawuk, D. P. S. (2017). *lajjA* in indian psychology: Spiritual, social, and literary perspectives. In Elisabeth Vanderheiden & Claude-Hélène Mayer (Eds.), *The value of shame—Exploring a health resource across cultures* (pp. 109–134). New York: Springer.

Bhawuk, D. P. S., & Udas, A. (1996). Entrepreneurship and collectivism: A study of Nepalese entrepreneurs. In J. Pandey, D. Sinha, & D. P. S. Bhawuk (Eds.), *Asian contributions to cross-cultural psychology* (pp. 307–317). New Delhi: Sage.

"Cloudburst" (2008). *Cloudburst of a thousand suns.* The vaani of Sri Sri Sitaramdas Omkarnath. Originally compiled by Tridandi Swami Madhava Ramanuja Jeur. Rendered in English by Raj Supe Kinkar Vishwashreyananda. Delhi: Jay Guru Sampradaya.

Creighton, M. R. (1990). Revisiting shame and guilt cultures: A Forty-Year Pilgrimage. *Ethos, 18*(3), 279–307.

Ellis, C. (1997). Evocative autoethnography: Writing emotionally about our lives. In W. G. Tierney & Y. S. Lincoln (Eds.), *Representation and the text: Reframing the narrative voice* (pp. 116–139). Albany: State University of New York Press.

Ellis, C. (2004). *The ethnographic I: A methodological novel about teaching and doing autoethnography.* Walnut Creek, CA: AltaMira.

Ellis, C., & Bochner, A. P. (2000). Autoethnography, personal narrative, reflexivity: Researcher as subject. In N. K. Denzin & Y. S. Lincoln (Eds.), *Handbook of qualitative research* (2nd ed., pp. 733–768). Thousand Oaks, CA: Sage.

Fung, H. (1999). Becoming a moral child: The socialization of shame among young Chinese Children. *Ethos, 27*(2), 180–209.

Friend, R., Rafferty, Y., & Bramel, D. (1990). A puzzling misinterpretation of the Asch 'conformity' study. *European Journal of Social Psychology, 20*(1), 29–44.

Gandhi, M. (1957/1993). *Autobiography: The story of my experiments with truth.* Boston, MA: Beacon Press.

Glasser, W. (1998). *Choice theory: A new psychology of personal freedom.* New York, NY: Harper Collins.

Hellmann, O. (2017). The historical origins of corruption in the developing world: a comparative analysis of East Asia. *Crime Law and Social Change, 68*(1–2), 145–165. https://doi.org/10.1007/s10611-016-9679-6.

Jay, T. (2009). The utility and ubiquity of taboo words. *Perspectives on Psychological Science, 4*(2), 153–161.

Lebra, T. S. (1983). Shame and Guilt: A Psychocultural View of the Japanese Self. *Ethos, 11*(3), 192–209.

Lewis, H. B. (1971). Shame and guilt in neurosis. *Psychoanalytic Review, 58*(3), 419.

Menon, U., & Shweder, R. (1994). Kali's Tongue: Cultural Psychology and the Power of "Shame" in Orissa, India. In S. Kitayama & H. Markus (Eds.), *Emotion and culture: Empirical studies of mutual influence*. Washington, D.C.: American Psychological Association.

Menon, U., & Shweder, R. (2003). Dominating Kali: Hindu family values and tantric power. In R. McDermott & J. Kripal (Eds.), *Encountering Kali: In the margins, at the center, in the west*. Los Angeles, CA: University of California Press.

Nanda, B. R. (1962). *The Nehrus: Motilal and Jawahrlal*. New Delhi, India: Oxford University Press.

Nehru, J. (1942). *Toward freedom: The autobiography of Jawaharlal Nehru*. New York, JY: The John Day Co.

Robbins, A. (2016). *I am not your guru*. https://www.youtube.com/watch?v=VQCg411Sn2g.

Rutan, J. S. (2000). Growth through shame and humiliation. *International Journal of Group Psychotherapy, 50*(4), 511–516.

Sinha, M., & Chauhan, V. (2013). Deconstructing *LajjA* as a marker of Indian Womanhood. *Psychology and Developing Societies, 25*(1), 133–163.

Tracy, J. L., & Robins, R. W. (2006). Appraisal antecedents of shame and guilt: Support for a theoretical model. *Personality and Social Psychology Bulletin, 32*(10), 1339–1351.

Wenzlaff, R. M., & Wegner, D. M. (2000). Thought suppression. *Annual Review of Psychology, 51*(1), 59–91.

Dharm P. S. Bhawuk (Ph.D.), is a professor of Management and Culture and Community Psychology at the University of Hawaii at Manoa. He brings with him the experience of living and growing in a developing economy, Nepal. He started his intercultural journey with a month at international children's camp in Artek, USSR, in 1972. His interdisciplinary training includes a Bachelor of Technology (B.Tech., Honors) from the Indian Institute of Technology, Kharagpur, in mechanical engineering, a Master of Business Administration (MBA) from the University of Hawaii at Manoa with a Fellowship from the East-West Center, where he did research with Prof. Richard W. Brislin in the area of intercultural training, and a Ph.D. in industrial relations with specialization in human resource management and cross-cultural psychology under the guidance of Prof. Harry C. Triandis at the University of Illinois at Urbana-Champaign.

Chapter 4
Shame as a Health Resource for the Repatriation Training of Japanese Returnees (*kikokushijo*) in Japan

Kiyoko Sueda

Abstract The purpose of this chapter is to apply the concept of shame as a health resource (Vanderheiden and Mayer in The value of shame: exploring a health resource in cultural contexts. Springer, Cham, 2017) to the field of intercultural training and to propose a repatriation-training programme for Japanese returnees (*kikokushijo*) who have spent considerable time overseas due to their parents' jobs. Given that most returnees are fluent in English, they have often been perceived as privileged and as a valuable resource for globalisation in Japan. However, at the same time, returnees feel disadvantaged because of the difficulties they face in readjusting to the school environment in Japan. Although returnees have been in different situations and have had different experiences, they are not perceived based on 'who they are' but 'who they should be like'. Therefore, returnees often go through face-threatening incidents, with their shame tending to remain unacknowledged or bypassed for a long time. The importance of repatriation training has been recognised for several decades; however, little substantial repatriation training has been provided for Japanese returnees. The proposed programme focuses on affective training sessions where returnees reflect on the face-threatening or negative experiences they have encountered upon returning to Japan. The programme should benefit participants by helping them to: (1) acknowledge their shame by fully attending to their own judgements about their face-threatening experiences, emotions and physical sensations, (2) think about ways to cultivate stillness and remove shame and (3) devise ways to make the school environment friendlier.

Keywords Japanese returnees · Repatriation training · Face · Shame · Pride

I would like to express my appreciation to Professor Eriko Katsumata for assisting me with needs assessment and to Ms Katsuko Sugiyama, Personal Leadership Senior Facilitator, Dr. Adair Linn Nagata, Professor Jin Abe, and those in the Personal Leadership Facilitators' Community of Practice for their valuable suggestions and insights.

K. Sueda (✉)
Department of International Communication, School of International Politics, Economics, and Communication, Aoyama Gakuin University, 4-4-25, Shibuya, Tokyo 150-8366, Japan
e-mail: sueda@sipeb.aoyama.ac.jp

4.1 Introduction

Face is defined as 'an image of self delineated in terms of approved social attributes' (Goffman, 1967, 5). Based on Goffman's premises (1959, 1967), people save one's own and the other's face in daily interactions in maintaining amicable relationships with one another. Therefore, when one loses face, one tries to restore one's own face, and the other party present in the situation attempts to help the first party re-establish the lost face. A failing to save one's own and the other party's face could be detrimental to the relationship at all levels. This 'interaction ritual' hints at the presence of shame, but Goffman does not highlight the affective aspects of face.

Scheff (1997) has discussed the importance of shame and addresses shame as 'the master of emotion' (12). In agreement with Scheff, I conceive shame as containing a larger range of meaning than the Japanese terms *haji* (shame), *hazukashii*[1] (embarrassed) or *kuyashii* (chagrin), and treat shame as an emotion involving reactions to rejection, denial, feelings of failure, insufficiency or inadequacy. By contrast, pride refers to our sense of comfort and contentment with oneself and others (Scheff, 1977). Pride does not concern arrogance or boastfulness.

In relationships at all levels, whether interpersonal, intergroup, intercultural or international, shame and pride play crucial roles. Pride engenders a secure bond and shame provokes a threatened bond (Nathanson, 1992; Scheff, 1994). Excessive shame causes isolation or alienation while insufficient shame causes engulfment (Scheff, 1994). In other words, when we are too ashamed of ourselves or made to feel ashamed by society, we become isolated or even alienated. Conversely, when we have a sense of pride as a member of society, we feel integrated in the society.

Living in a totally new environment is a challenge for anyone. Likewise, returning to one's own country involves psychological stress. In an earlier study (Sueda 2014), I evaluated how Japanese returnees' exclusion from a given group or society, judgement based on stereotypes, or improper evaluation of their abilities threatened their face and caused emotional responses such as feelings of failure or insufficiency. This finding suggests that examining the affective aspects of face, shame and pride, is crucial. However, systematic repatriation training is generally scarce in Japan, and repatriation training for Japanese returnees (*kikokushijo*)[2] continues to be limited. Some returnees' shame tends to remain unacknowledged or bypassed for a long time.

---

[1] The English term 'embarrass' was found to be semantically closer to the Japanese term '*hazukashii*' than the English term shame (Rusch, 2004). As expressing self is not as emphasized in Japan as in Western societies, Japanese people are likely to become highly conscious of how others perceive them. Therefore, giving a presentation in front of a large audience can potentially generate a feeling of *hazukashii* or embarrassment. Japanese people tend to experience *hazukashii* in their daily lives due to anxiety or having to be the centre of attention.

[2] Japanese returnees or *kikokushijo* are defined as 'all Japanese children under the age of 20 who, because of one or both of their parents' jobs, have at some time in their lives spent at least 3 months overseas and have returned to continue their education in the mainstream education system' (Goodman, 1990, 15).

Below is a comment made by a student at my university. Even though 15 years have passed since she returned to Japan, she still struggles to find a way to assert herself and be authentic:

> Although I can behave so as not to 'stand out' from my peers in Japan, it does not necessarily mean that I am comfortable with the way I am. However, when I went to the USA, where I used to live for 3 years, I realise how Japanese I am for being sensitive and reading the air too much. So far, I have not found any place where I feel comfortable about being myself. Thus, I may not be able to say that I have resolved my difficulties with adjusting to Japan.

This chapter highlights a paradigmatic shift made by Vanderheiden and Mayer (2017) from 'shame as a negative emotion' to 'shame as a health resource' and applies this new understanding to a repatriation-training programme for Japanese returnees (*kikokushijo*) who have spent a considerable amount of time overseas because of their parents' jobs. By being provided a safe environment in which to share shameful experiences in their host country and work with their shame about returning to their home country, returnees can discharge emotional stress, pain and shame, build sound interpersonal relationships with those around them and make their school environment more comfortable.

4.2 Theoretical Framework

4.2.1 Face-Threatening Incidents and the Reintegration of Shame

Taking up Goffman's concept of face, Brown and Levinson (1978) make a distinction between positive face and negative face. The former refers to a fundamental claim over a socially accepted self-image. The latter refers to a basic claim to territories, resources and rights to non-distraction. Lim and Bowers (1991) re-categorise Brown and Levinson's positive face into two concepts: fellowship face and competence face. Fellowship face relates to one's needs to be included and competence face concerns one's needs to have one's abilities appreciated. Lim and Bowers preserve Brown and Levinson's (1978) notion of negative face and rename it autonomy face.

In my previous work, I have illustrated face-threatening incidents experienced by Japanese returnee students and former returnees (Sueda, 2014). Most of the returnees felt lonely due to not being a part of their new school environments. Not knowing the rules and rituals of Japanese schools threatened their fellowship face. Japanese was not the dominant language of those who attended a local or an international school in their host country and not being able to express themselves in classes could threaten their competence face. Moreover, although their length of stay, their host countries and the types of schools attended varies, the general Japanese public tends to hold negative stereotypes about *kikokushijo* as knowing little about Japanese culture or having poor Japanese language skills and having difficulty building interpersonal

relationships in Japan. These negative stereotypes could threaten returnees' autonomy face, as they would rather be identified as an individual or a member of another
group instead of being treated as 'who they should be like'.

Scheff (1990, 1994, 1997) highlights three kinds of shame: acknowledged, unacknowledged and bypassed.[3] Shame is acknowledged when both parties share the
first party's shame. Shame is unacknowledged when it is experienced as emotional
distress but not named as shame. Shame is bypassed when it is actively avoided and
unacknowledged by the other through its expression as some other emotion, such as
anger. I view bypassed shame as a complex response in that the outbreak and esca-
lation of conflict may be attributed to accumulated bypassed shame (Lewis, 1971;
Lynd, 1961; Retzinger, 1991; Scheff, 1994, 1997). Scheff regards shame as commonly hidden and denied in modern society; both unacknowledged and bypassed
shame are unhealthy yet common in human interaction. Yet, shame can also be a
health resource (Vanderheiden & Mayer, 2017) once it is acknowledged and reintegrated in interaction.

When shame and pride are well balanced, we are normally unaware of the existence of face. However, when face-threatening incidents take place, the balance
between shame and pride is lost and we must wipe off shame and restore pride to
return to a balanced state (Sueda, 2014). This mechanism echoes Braithwaite's (1989)
theory of reintegrative shaming in crime control. He claims that crime is best controlled when community members actively shame offenders and that, once shame is
acknowledged by offenders, community members also actively help offenders rein-
tegrate into the community (Mayer's chapter on crime and shame, in this book). In
Braithwaite's argument, Japan's relative low crime rate among developed countries
is explained by the country's success in institutionalising both shame and reintegration. This argument applies when sojourners from any society are rejected or denied
by their home environments, leading them to feeling a sense of shame. How well
their shame is wiped off and pride restored can be a key to mental health and sound
interpersonal relationships.

4.2.2   Current Repatriation Training

The repatriation process has been considered a crucial part of intercultural training
since the early 1980s (Adler, 1981; Sussman, 1986). However, with the exception
of a limited number of studies suggesting a module for repatriation training (e.g.
Martin & Harrell, 2004), research on repatriation training for expatriates and student
expatriates remains scarce (Szkudlarek, 2010).

The majority of the existing training programme, as exhibited in Martin and
Harrell (2004), consists of cognitive and behavioural training. However, there is

---

[3]I would like to express my sincere appreciation to Professor Emeritus David Smith at Lancaster
University for assisting my understanding of shame through personal communications (18 August
2017).

also a potential need for affective training as suggested (Gorp et al., 2017; Ra & Trusty, 2015). Ra and Trusty (2015) claim that emotion-oriented coping strategies help Asian international students in the USA cope with acculturative stress. Furthermore, it is suggested that emotional support from friends or relatives in the home country facilitates repatriates' psychological as well as sociocultural adjustment to the home environment (Gorp et al., 2017; Yoshida et al., 2009).

4.2.3 Repatriation Training for Japanese Returnees

Some private high schools offer remedial Japanese language lessons and peer support discussion tables in which returnees can participate once or twice every year. Some private universities offer remedial Japanese language and culture courses prior to returnees' entry into Japanese universities (Yoshida, Hayashi, & Uno, 1999). However, as Yoshida et al. (1999) have noted, systematic repatriation training for Japanese returnees remains scarce at formal educational institutions. They have thus proposed a training programme for returnees. Their programme is significant for two reasons. First, it aims to nurture an awareness of self and others and help returnees understand the differences in shared values, norms and communication styles between their host culture and Japan. Second, Yoshida et al.'s programme incorporates intercultural sensitisers that are highly relevant to returnees' experiences.

This repatriation-training programme, however, still has room for an affective aspect of training because it has been found that success in removing shame and restoring pride influences Japanese returnees' psychological and sociocultural adjustment to their environment and their sense of self (Sueda, 2014). In therapeutic practice with shame, it is crucial to assist clients in acknowledging shame, expressing shame and separating the self from shame by attending to the client's verbal and non-verbal cues (Sinha, 2017; Sueda 2005). Following the process suggested by Sinha (2017), the programme should meet the following criteria: first, participants' non-verbal and verbal messages are to be carefully observed and utilised by both participants and facilitators. As discussed above, shame is difficult to recognise or express and training requires us to make maximum use of non-verbal messages. Second, existing training approaches tend to put Japanese returnees into a mould. After understanding the differences in communication styles between Japan and their host countries conceptually, returnees tend to be expected to accommodate the 'Japanese way'. Forcing returnees to fit a certain way of acting, which they do not relate to, brings on extra psychological stress and shame. A training programme that involves verbal and non-verbal cues and more creative solutions is thus necessary.

4.3 Contextual Description of Working with Japanese Returnees (*kikokushijo*)[4]

4.3.1 Japanese Returnees

According to statistics provided by the Ministry of Foreign Affairs of Japan (6 July 2016), as of April 2015, the total number of children of compulsory education age who have lived abroad was 79,251, of whom 58,227 were in elementary school and 21,021 in junior high school. In terms of destination, Asia (31,383 = 39.6%) has hosted the largest population of Japanese children, followed by North America (25,030 = 31.6%), Europe (16,682 = 21.1%), Oceania (2,552 = 3.2%), Central & Southern America (1,847 = 2.3%), the Middle East (1,068 = 1.3%) and Africa (689 = 0.8%).

The number of returnee students reached its peak of 13,777 in 1992 and decreased by 2011, down to 9,990 in total. In the past ten years, however, the number fluctuated at around 10,000. As of 2015, the total number of returnees was 12,527, including those who in elementary school, junior high school and high school, including six-year secondary schools (e-stat, 2017).

As I have claimed in earlier work (Sueda, 2014), returnees may face difficulties in readjusting themselves to Japan for two main reasons. First, the English or the Japanese language either actually or symbolically demarcates a boundary between returnees and non-returnees. For those who were born overseas and/or mainly educated in English at a local or an international school in their host country, English[5] tends to be their dominant language and they are comfortable with the communication styles of their host countries. Thus, it may be difficult for these students to keep pace in classes taught in Japanese. Although some returnees went to a Japanese school in their host countries and have no problem with classes conducted in Japanese, they are still expected to speak fluent English and poor Japanese.

Second, as Goodman (1990) has noted, *kikokushijo* (returnees) reproduce their parents' relatively high social status and at the same time, acquire some added value: *kokusaisei* (internationality). In other words, returnees are expected to become as 'elite' as their domestically nurtured parents and eventually go beyond them. Thus, those returnees who retain 'Japaneseness', while being fluent in a foreign language (mostly English) tend to be esteemed by their peers and teachers. By contrast, those who have the communication styles of their host country and have lost 'Japaneseness' may not be well regarded by their peers and teachers.

---

[4]Some of the participants in my needs analysis are over 20 years old, but they all shared their experience of returning to Japanese elementary, junior and senior high schools. I thus use the term Japanese returnees or returnees even if participants are over 20.

[5]For some of those who stayed in European countries, other languages than English such as French, German and Spanish could be a possible communication tool. Those who stayed in Asian countries tended not to go to local schools but either Japanese or international schools. Thus, learning a language from locals is very limited in Asian countries.

4.3.2 Difficulties Faced by Japanese Returnees: Open-Ended Questionnaire for Needs Analysis

4.3.2.1 Purpose

To identify the most recent situation surrounding Japanese returnees and assess training needs, an open-ended questionnaire was administered. In addition to demographic data, participants were asked the following questions:

1. Upon returning to Japan, what was emotionally difficult or painful[6] for you (or them[7])at school?
2. What or who helped you (or them) cope with difficulties or emotional pain?

Participants were also encouraged to share any suggestions concerning supporting returnees.

4.3.2.2 Participants

Between the middle of September and the first week of October 2017, 47 university students ($M = 9, F = 38$) at a private university in Tokyo completed the questionnaire for needs assessment. The participants included returnees, those who had studied overseas for nearly one year in a university exchange program[8] and their former or current classmates who had experienced the returnees' difficulties by proxy. The areas in which returnees lived include Asia, Europe, North America and Oceania as shown in Sect. 4.3.1. The period of a single stay ranged from one to 10 years. Several participants stayed overseas more than once, with an average first period of 4.33 years and an average second stay of 2.3 years.

4.3.2.3 Nature of Difficulties

The answers to the first question (Upon returning to Japan, what was emotionally difficult for you at school?) shown in Sect. 4.3.2.1 were analysed using thematic analysis (Gibson & Brown, 2011; Lapadat, 2012; Postăvaru, & Marczak, 2016) with six themes drawn out: (1) Difficulty of dealing with an unfamiliar school environment; (2) Difficulty of adapting to Japanese communication styles; (3) Not sharing much with the surrounding people; (4) Loneliness; (5) Negative consequences of being good at English and (6) Difficulty of Japanese language. Among these six themes, this analysis will focus on the first three because these themes echo the major factors

---

[6]I intentionally try not to use the terms such as 'shame' 'face' as some respondents might not relate to these terms.

[7]'Them' is used for returnees' current or former classmates.

[8]Those who participated in the exchange program were not excluded because some had stayed abroad due to their parents' jobs.

that cause friction between returnees and non-returnees discussed in the literature (e.g. Minoura, 1984; Nakanishi, 1992; Sueda, 2014; Yoshida et al. 1999). Specific examples of the first three themes are given below.

① **Difficulty of dealing with an unfamiliar school environment**

Participant #A, a female student who lived in the UK for 2 years, then went to the USA for 3 years and spent a year in the USA as an exchange student said,

> I wanted to raise my hand and volunteer to speak up in class when I understand the answers, but in a Japanese classroom, if you do so too often, you would be perceived as being 'obtrusive'. In order to avoid being different from the rest of the class, I could not speak up. In Japan, people read the air (*kuh ki o yomu*) and sense how the other party feels before being told so. So, I struggled to understand what was wrong with me and why people did not like me. At the same time, it was truly a pain to think about the 'right' behaviour by reflecting how the other would feel or what caused others to hate me.

② **Difficulty of adapting to Japanese communication styles**

Participant #A also shared her experience of participating in extracurricular activities at school and feeling awkward about the hierarchical relationships existing even among students, *sempai* (elder students) and *kohhai* (younger students). She felt she had to answer with a response that met her seniors' expectations instead of with what she really wanted to say. In both situations, it appears that a part of her felt a sense of shame in following suit and not being authentic:

> At school or extracurricular activities, we often get asked by senior students, 'What do you want?' or 'What do you think?' I know that what I have to do is not to state my opinion honestly but to come up with the 'answer' that the senior students expect me to answer. Also, behaving in my own way might ruin the group's harmony and trying to fit into what everyone else does was really a pain for me.

Participant #B, a male student who spent six years of elementary school in the USA, mentioned his difficulty with dealing with *nori* (maintaining the same wave length as friends). Being forced to 'be on the same wave length' threatens his autonomy face:

> Entering a junior high school in Japan, there were more and more occasions where *nori* 'being on the same wave length', which was seen on TV, was required. That was a pain. To begin with, I hardly watched TV and hated it as an unproductive way of spending time. Dealing with interactions that were as if copied from a variety show on TV, which reflects the Japanese social hierarchy, was very uncomfortable. This annoys me even now.

③ **Not sharing much with the surrounding people**

Participant #C, who lived in Germany for four years from Grade 1 in elementary school and studied on an exchange programme in the USA for two semesters, commented:

> As I have changed a lot mentally, I was afraid that I could not share my feelings even with my family or close friends. I was often afraid that no one would want to listen to my stories about my overseas experience and unless I got asked, I kept silent about my experiences overseas.

4.3.2.4   Solutions

In the answer to the second question (What or who helped you cope with difficulties or emotional pain?) shown in Sect. 4.3.2.1, the majority of the participants indicated that they did not do anything, or that they let time resolve the difficulty. There are several comments that deserve attention as expressing a way to address difficulties or transform negative feelings into positive feelings. Participant #A was relieved from her emotional pain when her parents showed her the many options available to her, other than being confined to Japan:

> During a long holiday, my parents brought me on a trip overseas and when they sent letters to our family friends overseas, they included my messages. That made me think that I do not have to belong in Japan. Even when I have difficulties in Japan, I could imagine that there exist various cultural values in the world, and I am happy to think that I can go anywhere if I wish.

Participant #C mentioned the importance of parents, friends with or without overseas experience and teachers with significant experience helping returnees:

> When I returned from Germany, my family members helped me get adjusted to Japan, and after returning from the USA, either former exchange students or professors helped me to cope with the difficulties of readjustment. Gradually, whenever I wanted to talk about my overseas experience, I talked about it with people.

Participant #D, a female participant who spent 3 years in the UK from the 4th–6th grades, pointed out the importance of releasing the stress of going to a Japanese school upon returning back to Japan:

> My mother listened to me very attentively. But as my mother herself is not a returnee, I could not share my pain with her. Instead, I could do so with my friends who had overseas experience.

She continues:

> Once a week, I went to a foreign language retention programme where returnees try to retain their foreign language (English) ability. Even if I had difficulties at my Japanese school, meeting and interacting with other returnees once a week rebooted my mind. Listening to English songs also helped me feel better.

4.3.2.5   Implications for a Repatriation-Training Programme

Thus, a repatriation-training programme where participants can wipe off shame and shift a negative experience into a positive experience is necessary because relieving emotional pain due to repatriation enables returnees to reflect on and appreciate the cultural differences between their host country and home. Participant #C, a returnee who also studied abroad on an exchange program, shared her insight as follows:

> There are few chances for returnees to share overseas experiences with others. At university, I learned about re-entry shock, and I knew what was expected of me. But that does not mean that I can resolve this difficulty by myself. I think it is also essential to have a vision for

utilising my experience in the future. By understanding how I have changed or grown, how
my values have changed, I could be more mindful about the people around me.

It should also be noted that forcing returnees to follow a 'safe Japanese way'
fosters a sense of shame. The shame felt by returnees could be shared in a classroom
so that both returnees and non-returnee classmates sensitise themselves to cultural
differences.

4.4 Proposed Repatriation-Training Programme for Japanese Returnees

4.4.1 Characteristics of Programme

To assist Japanese returnees experiencing a difficult or painful readjustment process,
the two principles and six practices of Personal Leadership[9] (PL) (Schaetti, Ramsey,
& Watanabe, 2008) are applied for two reasons. First, being mindful, one of the PL
principles, requires utilising various communication resources, such as physical sensation and non-verbal messages. Although some of the existing training programmes
incorporate non-verbal communication, the PL programme actively uses the body
and physical sensations to identify participants' emotional state. Second, being creative, the other PL principle, enables participants to go beyond a limited set of options
and to craft their own way of behaving in accordance with their own vision. Thus,
there is not always 'a right choice' but room for 'your own creative answer'.

Abe's (2013) handouts and information anchored my planning of the training
proposal described below. Abe conducted a two-day workshop in Kawasaki City for
Japanese 5th–10th graders, which aimed to enable students to better relate to those
who are 'different'. In the workshop, six[10] PL practices (1. attending to judgement,
2. attending to emotion, 3. attending to physical sensation, 4. cultivating stillness, 5.
engaging ambiguity, 6. aligning with vision) were applied, but for 5th–10th graders,
they were not presented in the standard PL vocabularies nor they were named as PL.
Instead, workshop participants were asked to read the PL practices and definitions and
apply them to their current social or personal situations after reading an age relevant
story (Abe, pc on 24 August 2017). Although the programme was not targeted to
returnees, it is encouraging to find that PL works for Japanese youth dealing with
diversity.

---

[9]Leadership in this context means 'understanding and managing our own internal experience'
(Schaetti, Ramsey & Watanabe, 2008, p. 4). Personal Leadership will hereafter be abbreviated as
PL.

[10]The practices appear here in the order they are written in in the book (Schaetti, Ramsey, &
Watanabe, 2008), but these numbers are arbitrarily applied. In PL practice, these principles might
not necessarily appear in this order.

4.4.2 Programme Design

4.4.2.1 Participants

Potential participants in the repatriation-training programme would be approximately 30 returnees between the 5th and the 10th grades.[11] The number of participants should be flexible and mentoring should be made available for those who prefer a private session to a discussion with peers.

4.4.2.2 Overview

The programme consists of two parts. In the first part, a hypothetical case as shown in Fig. 4.1 is given to participants. To actively discuss the case study, the participants are divided into several groups. I created a hypothetical case based on the experiences shared above in Sect. 4.3.2.3 and on one of the critical incidents in Yoshida et al. (1999, p. 513), 'volunteering in class'. This case is highly relevant to the participants' own experiences. The purpose of discussing the case before sharing their own experiences is to assist the participants in building rapport and creating a safe atmosphere to share their feelings and state their thoughts. In this part of the programme, participants are expected to become mindful about their own physical sensations, feelings and ways to calm themselves and ease their emotional pain.

In the second part of the programme, participants are encouraged to share their own experiences with one another, attend to their own judgement of the situation and their emotional pain and come up with a way to resolve their difficulties along with their vision.

4.4.2.3 Part One: A Case Study

The case shown in Fig. 4.1 is provided to participants.

After the participants read the case, they will be asked questions below.

Q1: What is happening?

Q1 helps the participants perceive the situation from multiple perspectives.

(Sample answer) Yumiko was very concerned with maintaining a good relationship with Yuka and becoming a competent student in class. She wanted to be independent and did not want others to control her behaviour. Yuka was concerned about how Yumiko would be accepted as a member in class.

Q2: What did her physical reactions tell Yumiko when she was stopped from volunteering in class?

---

[11] In the Japanese school system, the ages of the participants range from 10 to 15 years old.

Yumiko: Volunteering in class

I spent 10 years in the USA and came back to attend the Japanese public junior-high
school, which Yuka, my best friend from elementary school, attends. I was excited
to be in the same class as Yuka. Since the day I came back to school, we spent a lot
of time catching up together.

These days, however, I am confused about her reactions to what I do in class, and
I am afraid that we are not good friends anymore.I want to raise my hand and volunteer
to speak up in class when I know the answer, but every time I try to volunteer, Yuka
stops me. In our last class, I felt my face turning red and heart beating fast, but
I courageously volunteered. Everyone in class looked at me. I am sure that volunteering
in class is good. Isn't it good here too?

During the lunch break, instead of staying in the classroom and chatting with my
classmates, I walked around the school playground and got some fresh air. I felt myself
calming down. Did I do something wrong? Why did Yuka stop me from volunteering? Is
she jealous of me? Should I leave the unknown as it is? Well, I would not know unless
I ask her. Yes, I always clarify things by asking the person involved directly. Does
she mind me asking questions? Does that bother her? I am courageous enough to ask her.
On the way home, I talked to Yuka and asked her about what was going on. I discovered
that she 'saved' me from being obtrusive by volunteering too much. I am glad that
Yuka did that for me. Also, I am glad that she saw the value of volunteering in class,
but she told me that people might feel bad about me taking the floor all the time.
So, I should volunteer in class but be mindful about my classmates.

Fig. 4.1 A sample case

Q2 sensitises the participants to physical reactions.

(Sample answer) Yumiko felt that her face turned red and heart started beating
quickly. These physical reactions told her that she was confused, frustrated and
embarrassed.

Q3: How did Yumiko feel when she was stopped from volunteering in class?

Q3 sensitises the participants to feelings.

(Sample answer) Yumiko may have felt embarrassed about becoming the centre of
attention when Yuka stopped her from volunteering in class. She was also confused
by Yuka's behaviour and might have been sad and thinking that no one understood
her. Yumiko might have felt lonely as she felt out of place not reading unstated rules
in class.

Q4: How could Yumiko calm herself?

Q4 leads the participants to find a way to cultivate stillness for resolving difficulties.
(Sample answer) Yumiko walked around the school playground and got some fresh air to clear her mind.

Q5: What is important for Yumiko? Or, what is Yumiko's vision?

Q6: What did Yumiko do based on her vision?

Q5 and Q6 lead the participants to realise the importance of crafting vision and behaving in accordance with their vision.
(Sample answer) Yumiko's vision is to clarify things by asking questions directly to the person involved. Thus, instead of leaving the unknown as it is, Yumiko asked Yuka directly and understood the reason behind Yuka's behaviour, and Yuka also learned that Yumiko tried to volunteer in class as actively as she did in the USA. Instead of fitting into a 'Japanese custom of not sticking out', she can be creative: she volunteers in class and makes sure not to take the floor all the time. Eventually her classmates may realise the value of volunteering in class.

Q7: What would you do if you were Yumiko?

Q7 helps the participants to put themselves in Yumiko's situation, and helps with the transition to the second part of the programme.

4.4.2.4 Part Two: Sharing Their Experiences

After discussing Yumiko's case and having established a peer support environment, participants are asked to recall their own experiences of difficulties at school upon returning to Japan. The participants are then divided into pairs and ask one another questions in Fig. 4.2.
After this pair work, the participants are brought back into a group and discuss how they felt about the training programme and what they learned.

Q1: What was happening?

Q2: What was your physical reaction to the situation?

Q3: How did you feel about the situation?

Q4: How did you calm yourself? or What could you have done to calm yourself?

Q5: What is important for you?

Q6: How do you change your behaviour to suit your vision?

Fig. 4.2 Questions for pair work

Sharing difficult situations and feelings toward the situations with other participants should help the participants reduce their shame and restore pride. They could also be creative in thinking about how to behave instead of fitting into 'the Japanese way of behaving'.

In the session, participants need to be encouraged to attend to their physical sensations and emotions. As Japanese people are likely to restrain their emotions (Strumska-Cylwik, 2013), this process should be carefully administered. This programme could be conducted as an independent session or together with cognitive or behavioural training. It could also be performed as a daily practice.

4.5   Conclusion

This chapter applies the concept of shame as a health resource (Vanderheiden & Mayer, 2017) to a repatriation-training programme for Japanese returnees (*kikokushijo*) who have spent considerable time overseas because of their parents' jobs. The goal of the proposed programme is to assist returnees with addressing their shame, restoring pride and making their environment friendlier. The chapter could offer a new option for repatriation training, which allows returnees to be creative in approaching their life and environment.

Although further practice and research is necessary, dealing with shame in intercultural training can be applied at least in three ways. First, it can be applied to diversity training in Japanese educational institutions. For example, including non-returnees as participants, the proposed programme in this chapter could be stretched to diversity training and assisting students to better relate with those who are 'different'. Second, this approach can be applied to the business context in Japan. Although Japanese business organisations pay less attention to repatriation training than pre-departure training, removing shame and restoring pride upon returning is crucial to making the maximum use of repatriates' experiences and improving their performance. Last but not least, this approach could be applied to any expatriation or repatriation training in any country, as having lost any familiar situation and integrating old and new value systems and ways of thinking is challenging for anyone.

References

Abe, J. (2013). *Handout distributed at the first session of Children's right symposium, "Kotonaru-mono to umaku kakawaru meijin: 6 tsu no shuhkan* [Expert dealing with differences: 6 practices]" on 7 December 2013 in Kawasaki city.

Adler, N. (1981). Re-entry: Managing cross-cultural transitions. *Group & Organization Studies, 6,* 341–356.

Braithwaite, J. (1989). *Crime, shame and reintegration.* Cambridge: Cambridge University Press.

Brown, P., & Levinson, S. (1978). Universals in language usage: Politeness phenomena. In E. N. Goody (Ed.), *Questions and politeness: Strategies in social interaction* (pp. 56–289). New York: Cambridge University Press.

e-stat. (2017). *Kikoku jidoh seitosuh [The number of returnees at elementary school, junior-high school and high school]*. Retrieved from http://www.e-stat.go.jp/SG1/estat/List.do?bid=000001015843 Accessed 16 December 2017.

Gibson, W.J., & Brown, A. (2011). *Identifying themes, codes and hypotheses. Working with Qualitative Data* (pp. 127–144). London: Sage. Retrieved from http://dx.doi.org/10.4135/9780857029041.

Goffman, E. (1959). *The presentation of self in everyday life*. Garden City, NY: Doubleday.

Goffman, E. (1967). *Interaction ritual: Essays on face-to-face behavior*. Chicago: Aldine.

Goodman, R. (1990). *Japan's 'international youth': The emergence of a new class of schoolchildren*. Oxford: Oxford University Press.

Gorp, L. V., Boroşb, S., Brackea, P., & Stevens, P. A. J. (2017). Emotional support on re-entry into the home country: Does it matter for repatriates' adjustment who the providers are? *International Journal of Intercultural Relations, 58,* 54–68.

Lapadat, J. C. (2012). Thematic analysis. In A. J. Milles, G. Durepos, & E. Wiebe (Eds.,) *Encyclopedia of case study research*, (pp. 926–927). Thousand Oaks, CA: Sage. doi:http://dx.doi.org/10.4135/9781412957397.n342.

Lewis, H. B. (1971). *Shame and guilt in neurosis*. New York: International Universities Press.

Lim, T., & Bowers, J. W. (1991). Facework: Solidarity, approbation, and tact. *Human Communication Research, 17,* 415–450.

Lynd, H. M. (1961). *On shame and the search for identity*. New York: Science Editions.

Martin, J. N., & Harrell, T. (2004). Intercultural reentry of students and professionals: Theory and practice. In D. Landis, J. M. Bennett, & M. J. Bennett (Eds.), *Handbook of intercultural training* (pp. 309–336). Thousand Oaks, CA: Sage.

Ministry of Foreign Affairs of Japan. (6 July 2016). *Jairyuh hohjin gakuseiki shijosuh [Number of Japanese children of compulsory education age]*. Retrieved from http://www.mofa.go.jp/mofaj/files/000171467.pdf Accessed December 16, 2017.

Minoura, Y. (1984). *Kodomo no ibunka taiken: Jinkaku keisei katei no shinrijinruigaku kenkyuh [Children's intercultural experience: Psychological anthropological study on their personality development]*. Tokyo: Shisakusha.

Nakanishi, A. (1992). Kodomo no ibunkasesshoku to kyohiku no shomondai [Children's intercultural encounter and educational problems]. *Ibunkakan kyohiku [Intercultural Education], 6,* 4–10.

Nathanson, D. L. (1992). *Shame and pride: Affect, sex, and the birth of the self*. New York: W. W. Norton & Company.

Postăvaru, G., & Marczak, M. (2016). *A thematic analysis of interviews with women with breast cancer. Sage research methods cases*. London: Sage. Retrieved from http://dx.doi.org/10.4135/9781473992733.

Ra, Y., & Trusty, J. (2015). Coping strategies for managing acculturative stress among Asian international students. *International Journal for the Advancement of Counselling, 37,* 319–329.

Retzinger, S. M. (1991). *Violent emotions: Shame and rage in marital quarrels*. Newbury Park, CA: Sage.

Rusch, C. D. (2004). Cross-cultural variability of the semantic domain of emotion terms: An examination of English shame and embarrass with Japanese hazukashii. *Cross-Cultural Research, 38,* 236–248.

Schaetti, B. F., Ramsey, S. J., & Watanabe, G. C. (2008). *Personal leadership: A methodology of two principles and six practices*. Seattle, WA: FlyingKite.

Scheff, T. J. (1977). The distancing of emotion in ritual. *Current Anthropology, 18,* 483–490.

Scheff, T. J. (1990). *Microsociology: Discourse, emotion, and social structure*. Chicago: The University of Chicago Press.

Scheff, T. J. (1994). *Bloody revenge: Emotions, nationalism, and war*. Boulder, CO: Westview Press.

Scheff, T. J. (1997). *Emotions, the social bond, and human reality: Part/whole analysis*. Cambridge: Cambridge University Press.

Sinha, M. (2017). Shame and psychotherapy: Theory, method and practice. In E. Vanderheiden & C. Mayer (Eds.), *The value of shame: Exploring a health resource in cultural context* (pp. 251–274). Cham: Springer.

Strumska-Cylwik, L. (2013). Communication and emotions-emotional expressiveness or emotional restraint? *International Journal of Arts and Sciences, 6*, 331–350.

Sueda, K. (2005). Helping juvenile offenders reconstruct their identities: Analysis of a case study in Japan. *Human Communication, 8*(1), 1–23.

Sueda, K. (2014). *Negotiating multiple identities: Shame and pride among Japanese returnees*. Singapore: Springer.

Sussman, N. M. (1986). Re-entry research & training: Methods and implications. *International Journal of Intercultural Relations, 10*, 235–254.

Szkudlarek, B. (2010). Reentry—A review of the literature. *International Journal of Intercultural Relations, 34*, 1–21.

Vanderheiden, E., & Mayer, C. (2017). *The value of shame: Exploring a health resource in cultural contexts*. Cham: Springer.

Yoshida, T., Hayashi, Y., & Uno, M. (1999). Identity issues and reentry training. *International Journal of Intercultural Relations, 23*, 493–525.

Yoshida, T., Matsumoto, D., Akashi, S., Akiyama, T., Furuiye, A., Ishii, C., et al. (2009). Contrasting experiences in Japanese returnee adjustment: Those who adjust easily and those who do not. *International Journal of Intercultural Relations, 33*, 265–276.

Kiyoko Sueda (Ph.D.) is Professor at School of International Politics, Economics and Communication, Aoyama Gakuin University and teaches interpersonal and intercultural communication. She served SIETAR Japan as Vice President from 1998–2001 and 2002–2004. Her co-authored book, "*Komyunikeishon gaku: Sono tenboh to shiten* (Communication studies: Perspectives and prospects)" is one of the best sellers among textbooks on communication studies in Japan. Her co-edited book, "*Komyunikeishon kenkyu hoh* (Research methods in communication studies)" was nominated by the Communication Association of Japan as the most outstanding book published in 2011. Her most recent book, "Negotiating multiple identities: Shame and pride among Japanese returnees" was published in 2014 (Springer). Her research interests include face (social), identities, shame and pride in interpersonal and intercultural communication.

Chapter 5
The Effect of Regulation on Shame in Adolescence in China

Liusheng Wang and Biao Sang

Abstract Shame is a kind of self-conscious emotions which creates feelings of powerless, inferior, and depressed affections, particularly when a person transgresses the social norms. It is necessary to self-regulate shame using specific strategies for adolescents in the social life. The aim of the study was to examine the effects of shame regulation, and apply it to counseling. Seventy-two students in Grade 7, average age of 13.92, were required to regulate their shame emotion using either re-planning or self-blaming strategy. The results showed that re-planning or self-blaming strategy could enhance adolescents' intensity of shame, and the effect sizes of regulation were up to medium level which evidenced that individuals could self-regulate their intensity of shame by using counseling strategies.

Keywords Shame · Emotion regulation · Re-planning strategy · Self-blaming strategy · Adolescent

5.1 Introduction

Shame regulation is to enhance, attenuate or maintain the intensity of shame by using some strategies (Wang, 2017). One longitudinal analysis reveals that shame-focused coping is the mediator of the relationship between shame-proneness and depression in high school students (Ding, Gao, Zhang, & Qian, 2012). Higher use of emo-

L. Wang (✉)
Department of Psychology, Nantong University, 9 Seyuan Road, Nantong, Jiangsu, People's Republic of China
e-mail: willow76@ntu.edu.cn

B. Sang
School of Psychology and Cognitive Science, East China Normal University,
3663 N. Zhongshan Road, Shanghai, People's Republic of China
e-mail: bsang@psy.ecnu.edu.cn

© Springer Nature Switzerland AG 2019
C.-H. Mayer and E. Vanderheiden (eds.), *The Bright Side of Shame*,
https://doi.org/10.1007/978-3-030-13409-9_5

tion regulation strategies are positively associated with shame-proneness (Schmahl, Szentágotai-Tătar, & Miu, 2016), which indicates the power of regulation strategies to regulate shame.

Direct evidence of shame regulation is provided by Gao and her colleagues (Gao, Zhao, Wang, Dai, & Qian, 2012). The shame regulation strategies for college students could be broadly divided into two categories and four sub-categories, including reparative strategies, like self-modification strategy and positive reappraisal, and defensive strategies, like deny-attack and avoidance-retreat strategy (Gao et al., 2012). Compared with the general negative emotions, college students seldom use acceptance, putting-into-perspective, rumination, positive reappraisal and refocus-on-planning strategies to regulate shame emotion (Gao, Qian, & Wang, 2011; Garnefski, Kraaij, & Spinhoven, 2001).

Based on the experiment of between-subject design, re-planning strategy and putting-into-perspective strategy could effectively regulate shame experience for college students, in which re-planning strategy promotes participants to show constructive and make-up behavioral tendencies, and putting-into-perspective strategy could better reduce the intensity of negative emotion; however, self-blaming strategy and blaming others strategy are less effective (Gao, 2016).

The most researches on shame regulation mainly focus on adults. Unlike adults, adolescents are at the second stage of physical and psychological acceleration in their lives, and experience biological transition, cognitive transition and social transition. During the adolescence, the interactions among self, the outside world and others increase obviously. The changes of the outside world and self-development could be reflected in the self-shame regulation. Moreover, shame is a self-conscious emotion. Between-subject design may mask the psychological processing characteristics of some individuals (Lanteigne, Flynn, Eastabrook, & Hollenstein, 2014).

This chapter deals with shame regulation in the context of Chinese culture, presenting the effect of experiment-based shame regulation using the specific strategies. Readers are provided with an example of counseling case using the regulation strategies to explore the value of shame transformations in Application.

5.1.1   Regulation Strategies and Shame Regulation

Re-planning strategy and self-blaming strategy are commonly used to regulate shame emotion by adolescents (Wang, 2017). According to Gross' Emotional Regulation Process Model (2015), re-planning strategy is taken as antecedent-focused regulation of emotion, and self-blaming strategy is one of response-focused regulation of emotion. Re-planning strategy refers to the strategy by which one would find out a new way to copy with shame situation, while self-blaming strategy is the regulation strategy by which one would blame himself/herself for the shame incident (Gao et al., 2011). These two strategies could affect the shame emotion of college students (Gao, 2016). Self-blaming is also a kind of external manifestations of aggression in the Compass of Shame (Nathanson, 1992), in which shame regulation styles include Attack self, Attack other, Withdrawal, and Avoidance styles (reference to the chapter of Elison in this book). In addition, Chinese adolescents are increasingly encouraged to develop their career planning skills at schools. In DaXue, one of the classic works written in Warring States Period (453BC-221BC), which describes the theory, principles and methods of moral cultivation by a number of Confucian and Neo-Confucian scholars. Chinese has always advocated the spirit of *"cultivating self, family-discipline, governing the country and maintaining the world peace"* (In Chinese, 修身, 齐家, 治国, 平天下). Individuals pay more attention to self-cultivation and their own responsibilities for their behaviors. Even in non-Asian culture, higher use of self-blaming strategy is positively associated with shame-proneness for adolescents aged 13 to 17 years (Schmahl et al., 2016). Therefore, the current study takes the re-planning strategy and self-blaming strategy as the regulation strategies to investigate the effect of regulation strategy on adolescents' shame emotion.

5.2 Method

The study is a within-subject design in which all the participants used three regulation strategies respectively, including re-planning, self-blaming and non-regulation.

5.2.1 Participants

Seventy-two students in Grade 7 of a public junior high school in Jiangsu, Yangtze River Delta region of China, participated in the experiment using a convenient sampling method. The data of 61 participants was analyzed, aged M = 13.92, SD = 0.61, 28 boys. All participants reported no mental disorder history.

5.2.2 Materials

5.2.2.1 Regulation Strategy

In current study, these strategies are expressed as specific and clear instructions, such as, "You will read some words on the screen representing one of regulation strategy. Please use this strategy to regulate your own shame emotion".

Three strategies are as following, (1) Self-blaming is expressed as "I blame myself". For example, "I should be blamed"; "I should take responsibility for what had happened"; "in this case, I was wrong"; "I was the main reason for this fault". (2) Re-planning is expressed as "I managed to do it better". For example, "I think how to do it better"; "I think how best to deal with these situations"; "I think how to change this situation"; "I want a better plan to do it". (3) Non-regulation means the participants do nothing, just looking at the screen of the computer. Before the experiment, participants were informed about the process and well known about these strategies. The participants were required to use one of the above three strategies to regulate these emotion and after that, the participants self-rated shame intensity.

5.2.2.2 Shame Situation Story

(1) The assessment of shame story. Based on the interview and open survey, three homogencous virtual stories have been built involving behavior, body and family topics in everyday life situation (Wang, 2017). Here is an example for body odor situation:

> My body has a faint smell of body odor. When summer comes, the unpleasant smell spreads after I have done even a little exercise. At the moment, people who know me will secretly cover their noses with a frown, and people who do not know me will directly blurt out, "Who's so smelly?" By seeing this disgusting expression and hearing the impolite tones, I feel embarrassed with the unpleasant smell of mybody.

Thirty-eight graduates, 28 females, aged M = 20.50, SD = 1.41, were required to assess the homogeneous materials on Likert 7-point scale. A higher score meant the more similar. The results showed the score of the similarity among the three sets of materials was above point 5. The results of single-sample t-test with 4 (midpoint on Likert 7-point scale) revealed the significant different from point 4. The situations of story were used to rate the shame intensity or guilt intensity experienced by the story protagonist. The higher the score, the stronger the emotional intensity was. Paired-sample t-test showed that the shame scores for all story situations were significantly higher than the guilt scores, ps < 0.001. (2) Transformations of shame story. All the texts of the situations were read by a radio broadcaster, and recorded in MP3 format. The audio file duration, M = 40.56 seconds, SD = 5.93 seconds. Also, one graduate in Department of Art drew pencil sketches based on the core content of the story. These sketches were converted to electronic version with JPG format in 640 × 470 pixels.

5.2.2.3 Pictures and Music for Relaxation

Six neutral images were selected from the International Affective Picture System (IAPS) for relaxation during the experiment. Valence of the image, M = 4.97, SD = 0.12; arousal score, M = 2.52, SD = 0.42. Eight college students were required to rate soothing degree of light music on 7-point scale, and the piece from "Dancing with the Neon Light" was 1.38, indicating the fragments of music is soothing.

5.2.3 Procedure

The situation-induced method is to induce the shame of the participants (Gao et al., 2012; Roth, Kaffenberger, Herwig, & Bruhl, 2014; Sznycer, Tooby, Cosmides, Porat, Shalvi, & Halperin, 2016), and it is also a paradigm of negative emotion regulation (Deng, Sang, & Ruan, 2013; Gyurak, Goodkind, Kramer, Miller, & Levenson, 2012). Audio-induced method has good effect on inducement (Yao, Wang, & Li, 2019).

All the situations of the story were presented in three blocks by E-prime soft program. The order of blocks was randomized, and the order of situations in blocks was also balanced. Each block only used one kind of regulation strategy. Intervals among blocks were 120 s of relaxing music for participants to listening to. The rest time between blocks was 3 minutes.

Trial procedure was as followed (Deng et al., 2013; Gao et al., 2012), (1) Fixation. The center of the screen showed the "up arrow", "down arrow", or "short horizontal symbol", suggesting that participants would regulate their shame emotion with corresponding re-planning, self-blaming, or non-regulation strategy. Duration lasted 2 seconds. (2) Inducement. The screen presented a sketch of the picture, while the participants wore headsets to listen to the voice corresponding to the pictures of story. The participants were instructed to fully imagine themselves as the protagonists in the story situation so as to fully experience shame emotions. After the audio ended, the picture disappeared. The average duration was about 41 seconds. (3) Regulation. One symbol was presented on the screen. There was only one type of regulation strategy in one block. Regulation strategies included re-planning strategy, self-blaming strategy and non-regulation strategy. The screen displayed the instructions as followed: "↓"stood for "I managed to do it better"; "↑" stood for "I blame it on myself"; and "-" stood for "non-regulation". Participants regulated themselves in accordance with the instructions before the experiment. Duration was 5 seconds. (4) Assessment. Participants self-rated their shame intensity on 4-point scale by pressing the number keys of the computer. (5) Relaxation. The screen showed a neutral emotion picture, while listening to light music to relax by headsets.

5.3 Results

The reaction time of the participants was recorded in the evaluation phase. The data was retained according to the following criteria: reaction time was more than 300 ms and less than 10000 ms, and the data of three regulation strategies was not missing. 85% of data was kept to analyze.

Repeated-measures ANOVA showed a significant main effect of the regulation strategies, $F(2228) = 4.762$, $p < 0.01$, indicating the regulation strategies could affect the intensity of shame experienced. By multiple comparisons, the shame intensities after re-planning strategy($M = 2.79$, $SD = 1.05$) and self-blaming strategy ($M = 2.78$, $SD = 1.12$) were significantly stronger than that of non-regulation condition

(M = 2.47, SD = 1.12), ps < 0.05. The main effect of gender was not significant, F (1114) = 0.231, p > 0.05. The interaction between regulation strategy and gender was not significant, F (2228) = 0.003, p > 0.05.Taking non-regulation condition as the baseline, the Cohen's d as an indicator of effect size, regulation effect was calculated for re-planning strategy and self-blaming strategy. The results showed Cohen's d was 0.29 for re-planning strategy, and 0.28 for self-blaming strategy, which were up to the medium level.

5.4 Discussion

Overall, re-planning strategy and self-blaming strategy could enhance the adolescents' shame intensity. This is not entirely consistent with the results of the Gao's between-subject design study, in which re-planning strategy could effectively affect the shame of college students, while self-blaming strategy did not affect the shame experience (Gao, 2016), and in the line with the study by Schmahl and his colleagues (2016). This revolves the specific operational focus of the self-blaming strategy. In current study, the self-blaming strategy focuses on emotional remorse, which is different from Gao's study focusing on rationality.

Re-planning strategy is in the antecedent-focused phase, while self-blaming strategy is in the response-focused phase in Gross' Emotion Regulation Process Model (2015). Although the two strategies focuses on different stages of shame emotions, they could both affect the experience of shame emotions, and exert a similar regulation effect. Self-blaming is one of the external manifestations of aggression in Compass of Shame Model (Nathanson, 1992). In a shameful situation, adolescents experience self-loathing, contempt, helplessness and alienation, assuming the role of loser and experiencing more shame. Re-planning strategy attempts to reinstate the shame and then make a person choose a better way to avoid the current state. However, the remedial measures after the incident are only hypotheses. Instead, they induce self-incapacity and helplessness, leading to more shame. The self-blaming strategy targets the affective response in shameful situation, which is a direct intervention, leading to individual's change of feeling.

5.5 Application

In counseling with adolescents, some clients ignore the responsibility for their behaviors, lacking the feeling of shame. The counselor can use the guidance to help the clients reflect on their actions, making the client self-blame to enhance the intensity of his/her shame intensity. Here, Xiao Ming's (M) case about ability of shame transformation would be illustrated. M never completed his school assignments on time, and did not concern about the teachers' criticism. He has low academic achievements, but he never felt ashamed of it. Accompanied by her mother, M came to the school's counseling center for help.

From the ancient idiom of "Three Migrations of Mencius' Mother"(孟母三迁, Mencius's mother moved houses three times to provide his son, Mencius, a good education envirnment) to the current phenomenon of "school district housing" (学区房, only the children whose parents bought houses in school district can go to the famous school to accept better education), Chinese parents have always valued their children's academic achievements, which is not only the child's own matter, but also the parents' face (面子) or respects and the honor of the extended family. What's more, in Chinese culture, good academic achievements may even glorify his ancestors (**光宗耀祖**). Based on the basic profile of M, the counselor speculated that M was smarter and his intelligence was normal. M's poor academic performance was due to poor learning attitude and lacked of shame. As a result, the counselor decided to allow M to recognize the significance of his academic performance and the impact of his poor school performance on himself, parents, and his family from the aspects of cognition, emotion, and behavior. By guiding him to apply self-blaming strategy, it ultimately increased M's feeling of shame. And then he transformed the shame, and thereby converted his learning attitudes. In addition, the self-blaming strategy emphasized individual self-regulation and self-motivation, which was a way of self-meditation. This strategy fit well with the concept of traditional Chinese Confucians, which is "cultivating self"(修身). The aim of cultivation is to focus the individual's inner growth.

The following process can show how self-blaming strategy functions:

- What are the reasons for your poor academic achievements? Who should be responsible for it, you, your teachers, or your parents?
- How do you behave in class and in complete your school assignments?
- How do you evaluate your own learning attitude (e.g. I don't have active learning attitude and I am sloppy in handling assignments).
- How are you ranked in each exam?
- When you know that you are ranked behind in the class. How do you feel?
- How do your parents think about your poor performance? Do you think your parents will feel embarrassed about that? Under what circumstances, your parents will be particularly embarrassed?

(M recalls that each time when the parent meeting is held, the teacher talks about his low performance with his parents. Both he and his parents will feel shamed. In China, when the family and friends gather together, the children's academic performance is always the focus topic they will talk about. At that time, if the child has good academic achievements, he and his parents will both feel glorified. However, due to M's poor grades, his parents are in embarrassment in front of relatives and friends).

- Now imagine that when teachers say that your performance is the worst. Please close your eyes and do simple meditation, "My performance is very poor. I should be blamed, for I should take responsibilities for my poor performance. I cannot blame the teacher, because it's my own fault".

- At the moment, continue to imagine that this is a traditional Chinese Festival in which all the family relatives gather for dinner. The elders spontaneously chat about my performance. Because my grades are the worst among all brothers and sisters, my parents feel very embarrassed. I am so ashamed that I want to find in a hole and hide in it. Please close your eyes and do simple meditation, "My performance is very poor that I should be blamed, for I should take responsibilities for my poor performance. I cannot blame my parents, because it's my fault. Because of my faulty, I make myself, as well as my parents, embarrassed".

- Please open your eyes and stop meditation. Talk about how will you treat your own learning in the future.

The above process is gradually guided, focusing on the three aspects of M's cognitive, emotional and behavioral aspects. It cognitively (step 1–3) changes the original mode of attribution. He attributes the reasons for his poor academic performance to the neglect of the importance of his academic performance and his own passive learning attitude. From the emotional aspect (step 4–6), he experiences that both his parents and himself felt embarrassed because of his poor academic performance. In the behavioral aspect (step 7–9), individual meditation and self-blaming generate or enhance a sense of shame, and thus transform shame.

Acknowledgements This research was supported by The Key Project of Philosophy and Social Science Research in Colleges and Universities in Jiangsu Province Grant 2017ZDIXM134.

References

Deng, X., Sang, B., & Luan, Z. (2013). Up- and down-regulation of daily emotion: An experience sampling study of Chinese adolescents' regulatory tendency and effects. *Psychological Reports, 113*(2), 552–565.

Ding, X., Gao, J., Zhang, Z., & Qian, M. (2012). Mediation role of shame-focused coping between shame and depression in high school students. *Chinese Mental Health Journal, 26*(6), 450–454.

Gao, J. (2016). *The regulation of shame emotion*. Beijing: Intellectual Property Publishing House.

Gao, J., Qian, M., & Wang, W. (2011). Cognitive emotion regulation of shame and negative emotion. *Chinese Journal of Clinical Psychology, 19*(6), 807–809.

Gao, J., Zhao, Q., Wang, M., Dai, Y., & Qian, M. (2012). Selection of cognitive emotion regulation strategy on shame: Impact of self appraisals. *Chinese Journal of Clinical Psychology, 20*(4), 469–473.

Garnefski, N., Kraaij, V., & Spinhoven, P. (2001). Negative life events, cognitive emotion regulation and emotional problems. *Personality and Individual Differences, 30*(8), 1311–1327.

Gross, J. J. (2015). Emotion regulation: Current status and future prospects. *Psychological Inquiry, 26*(1), 1–26.

Gyurak, A., Goodkind, M. S., Kramer, J. H., Miller, B. L., & Levenson, R. W. (2012). Executive functions and the down-regulation and up-regulation of emotion. *Cognition and Emotion, 26*(1), 103–118.

Lanteigne, D. M., Flynn, J. J., Eastabrook, J. M., & Hollenstein, T. (2014). Discordant patterns among emotional experience, arousal, and expression in adolescence: Relations with emotion regulation and internalizing problems. *Canadian Journal of Behavioural Science/Revue canadienne des sciences du comportement, 46*(1), 29.

Nathanson, D. L. (1992). *Shame and pride: Affect, sex, and the birth of the self*. New York: W W Norton.

Roth, L., Kaffenberger, T., Herwig, U., & Bruhl, A. B. (2014). Brain activation associated with pride and shame. *Neuropsychobiology, 69*(2), 95–106.

Schmahl, C., Szentágotai-Tătar, A., & Miu, A. C. (2016). Individual Differences in Emotion Regulation, Childhood Trauma and Proneness to Shame and Guilt in Adolescence. *PLoS ONE, 11*(11), e0167299.

Sznycer, D., Tooby, J., Cosmides, L., Porat, R., Shalvi, S., & Halperin, E. (2016). Shame closely tracks the threat of devaluation by others, even across cultures. In *Proceedings of the National Academy of Sciences* (pp. 201514699).

Wang, L. (2017). *The regulation of shame emotion in adolescence*. East China Normal University.

Yao, W., Wang, L., & Li, H. (2019). The effect of college students' shame on prosocial behavior. *Psychology: Techniques and Applications, 7*(1),34-38.

Liusheng Wang (Dr.) is an associate professor at Department of Psychology in Nantong University, Jiangsu, China. He holds Master degree in Educational Science, a Doctorate in Psychology. He has published books and journal articles in the context of emotion, shame, embodied cognition, development of adolescents.

Biao Sang (Dr.) is a professor at School of Psychology and Cognitive Science in East China Normal University, Shanghai, China, and an executive committee of International Society for the Study of Behavioral Development (ISSBD), an executive committee of Chinese Psychological Society, an executive deputy editor-in-chief of Journal of Psychological Science. He holds a Master degree and a Doctorate degree in Psychology. He has published several monographs, accredited journal articles and special issues on personality and social development, emotion, and applied social psychology.

Chapter 6
From 'Death Sentence to Hope', HIV and AIDS in South Africa: Transforming Shame in Context

Busisiwe Nkosi and Paul C. Rosenblatt

Abstract HIV/AIDS is one of the most stigmatized illnesses in history. People living with HIV and AIDS have been experiencing shame, stigma and discrimination and this fuelled the epidemic especially in sub-Saharan Africa including South Africa. For a long period, HIV and AIDS seemed like a death sentence. The association of HIV/AIDS with personal moral failures intensified the stigma and shame associated with HIV and undermines the rights of individuals to effective health care. And, deservingness to receive health services based on social and moral grounds discourages and marginalises individuals infected and affected by the HIV epidemic. Support groups for people living with HIV and AIDS offer arenas for addressing psychosocial issues, enabling them to resist and overcome negative stereotypes, shame, guilt and stigma. The significance and complexity of the work done by the support groups highlights the perceived lack of effective response by government to the HIV and AIDS care needs confronting communities which has left a 'care gap' that support groups fill. The transformative potential of HIV/AIDS is encountered in a much more localised and personalised space in support groups and those groups have evolved into major social and political movements in South Africa. First, this chapter contextualizes HIV stigma as a socio-political process. It demonstrates that HIV stigma and shame expressed and experienced by people infected by the HIV epidemic varies and that gender influences the way men and women deal with HIV/AIDS shame, and how this colours their participation in support groups. This chapter argues that more HIV healthcare resources should be channelled to non-biomedical and interactive dimensions of stigma and discrimination with psycho-social support interventions provided by the support group which is often in the periphery of health care systems. We also argue that the local contexts and understanding of the socio-cultural systems is important in transforming shame into a positive experience. We show this by

B. Nkosi
Africa Centre Building, Africa Health Research Institute, via R618 to Hlabisa Somkhele, 198, Mtubatuba 3935, South Africa
e-mail: BNkosi@ahri.org

P. C. Rosenblatt (✉)
Department of Family Social Science, University of Minnesota, 290 McNeal Hall, 1985 Buford Avenue, St. Paul, Minneapolis, MN 55108-6140, USA
e-mail: prosenbl@umn.edu

© Springer Nature Switzerland AG 2019
C.-H. Mayer and E. Vanderheiden (eds.), *The Bright Side of Shame*,
https://doi.org/10.1007/978-3-030-13409-9_6

demonstrating how support groups initiated by local members often in the periphery of health systems without access to specialised therapists transformed the adversities resulting from HIV into major social change and public discourse, while influencing their own lives and that of many in positive ways. We also show the value and use of visual participatory methods as therapeutic tools and for social change and illustrate how these techniques are increasingly used to share intersectional experiences and transform stigma and shame into positive experiences through creative expression.

Keywords HIV/AIDS shame · Support groups · South Africa · Visual participatory methods

6.1 Shame and HIV and AIDS

HIV and AIDS is one of the most stigmatised illnesses in history (see Nel's and Govender's chapter on Appreciative Inquiry in this book) globally, and particularly in sub-Saharan Africa (Mfecane, 2012; Pettit, 2008). The misperceptions and myths about the origins of the HIV epidemic compounded by the misunderstanding about how HIV is contracted can be sees as the cause and effect of shame and stigma associated with HIV. The labelling and ascribing HIV and AIDS as a 'gay disease', immoral failure and personal irresponsibility have fuelled the spread of the HIV/AIDS epidemic. The socially-constructed views of HIV and AIDS are assimilated and internalised by HIV infected persons, leading them to avoid seeking treatment or care; to engage in risky behaviours such as unsafe sex practices; and to experience feelings of emotional distress, isolation, and self-loathing (Dolezal & Lyons, 2017). While privacy can be both appropriate and desirable, the stigma associated with HIV makes individuals feel shameful and has driven them into secrecy, therefore posing serious impediments to addressing HIV and AIDS among people living with HIV and AIDS (PLWHA).

Although, shame and stigma associated with HIV and AIDS is widely spread across different groups, it is concentrated among women, often with low socio-economic status (Bennett et al., 2016; Dageid, 2014; Walker, Ailber, & Nkosi, 2008). The lack of anti-retroviral therapies in the public health system during the 1990s in South Africa and other sub-Saharan countries reinforced the false notion that HIV and AIDS is 'a death sentence'. Then again, despite the high prevalence of HIV and AIDS in the region and the co-morbidity with mental distress and psychosocial disadvantages, mental and psychosocial health services in sub-Saharan Africa generally have low priority in the public health system (Dageid, 2014). Similarly, individuals providing care for people who are infected and dying of HIV and AIDS have done so in the periphery of the public health system often facing shame themselves (Casale, Wild, Cluver, & Kuo, 2014). Interventions dealing with HIV and AIDS have been explicit about addressing the stigma, while shame has remained in the background in public health discourse. Yet, the influence of shame on health behaviours—failure to disclose one's ill health, poor health behaviours including failure to seek health care, and adherence to treatment remains pervasive and pernicious.

The rapidly increasing care needs generated by the HIV/AIDS epidemic and the accelerating human resource crises in many African countries have shifted the burden of care to families (Friedman, 2005). Consequently, families and community informal networks, have for the most part shouldered the burden of care for HIV infected and other illnesses in the communities outside of the formal health care system. Psychosocial support and health care for PLWHA remains inadequate especially in scarce resource settings (Dageid, 2014; Patel et al., 2012) and support groups have been one of the most formidable sources of care providing a bridge between PLWHA, and the formal health care system.

6.1.1   Support Groups

In South Africa, support groups emerged as a result of the need for wider human resources for dealing with health crisis and that gave rise to the community-based services care workforce. Support groups are highly variable, and depending on the level of sophistication, some are registered as a legal entity and linked to a government department such as Department of Social Development and Department of Health to leverage resources and specialised support, while others exist as informal loosely structured networks. Support groups include individuals who are affected by the HIV epidemic themselves or have a family member/s affected by HIV and can be a small civic group or religious organisation offering arenas where psychosocial issues are addressed. Regardless of type of structure, support groups operate organically in response to poor or absence of HIV services in their communities. Their lack of status for active support group participation as formally employed or as professionals means that they have to work hard to gain recognition, and they are constantly in a position of having to negotiate their status. It was not until the late 1990s and early 2000s that there was mobilisation in South Africa for strong social movements and funding for HIV and AIDS community based programmes, as well as greater levels of cooperation between the state and civil society to deal with the HIV epidemic (Ginneken, Lewin, & Berridge, 2010). While progress has been made, support groups continue to work in the margins and periphery of the health care system without adequate resources as they support families and communities to deal with HIV and associated stigma and shame. Indeed, the transformative potential of HIV is encountered not in the context of the medical system but in the context of a much more localised and personalised space.

PLWHA and their families face a range of psychosocial challenges and adverse life situations. Support groups for PLWHA offer an opportunity for ongoing psychosocial support that is insufficiently covered in the public health settings especially during voluntary counselling and testing (VCT) often linked to public health facilities. The role of VCT as a therapeutic support intervention is limited in terms of operational hours, distances to the health facilities, and costs associated with transport. Also, many PLWHA tend to avoid going to the health facilities for fear of being seen in the health facilities, a situation compounded by negative health provider's attitudes in dealing with PLWHA (Hargreaves et al., 2016; Casale et al., 2014; Duby, Nkosi, Scheibe, Brown, & Bekker, 2018). Community-based support groups have the potential to reach more people faster because they are organic, readily accessible and available, and they are driven by the individuals without any red tape. The past few years have seen efforts made to provide VCT services within the community settings to bring HIV services closer to the communities and reduce HIV stigma and shame. That said, a continued need exists to strengthen HIV services at a tertiary level, particularly for severe cases of physical and mental distress, and treatment in community and primary health care settings.

The literature indicates that belonging to a support group is often associated with better health outcomes among different populations including adults infected with HIV and AIDS (Dageid, 2014; Walker et al., 2008), caregivers of children infected with the illness (Casale et al., 2014), and that support groups provide a protective factor for families with mentally ill patients. PLWHA showed significant improvement in mental health and psychosocial wellbeing, ART adherence and HIV sero-status disclosure resulting from group attendance (Casale et al., 2014). Therefore, support groups may leverage clinical outcomes and rejuvenate the well-being of HIV-infected individuals with depressive symptoms.

A study exploring reasons why individuals join support groups in a rural province of South Africa reported that individuals who joined a support group hoped to gain information and learn to cope, and that women were more likely to join to get support and deal with stress, while men joined to stay active and educate others (Dageid, 2014). PLWHA in support groups indicated experiencing high mental, physical and social distress which they hoped to have help with. Support groups therefore could be important links in the chain of comprehensive HIV health service delivery, given that they manage to recruit and meet the needs of PLWHA. Others formed and/joined support groups for altruistic reasons, to instil hope, and change family and friends' attitude towards the illness, and reduce shame and anxieties among their peers. The reasons for not having joined a support groups were lack of knowledge and understanding about the support group and time constraints (Dageid, 2014). These challenges point to a need for other levels of support such as increasing awareness in hard to reach areas.

6.1.2   Shame and Gender

Shame is a social process rooted in social power relations, and manifests differently across cultural groups and it is influenced by one's background, family experiences, and the immediate context (Dageid, 2014) (see also Silverio's chapter in this book). In various cultural contexts, shame affects men and women differently. Studies report a marked gender imbalance in how much people talk about shame (Dageid, 2014; Mburu et al., 2014; Mfecane, 2012). This imbalance may be attributed to the interplay of several social and cultural factors including gender inequality and the inability of women to negotiate safe sex with their partners and men's unwillingness to use condoms. Women who demand condom use often endure the shame of being perceived as promiscuous and cannot be trusted. In the Zulu culture for example, men with multiple concurrent partners namely 'isoka' tend to be accepted and have a good social standing in their communities, while women are never afforded such a standing in the community. Consequently, men and women respond differently to support groups and uptake of HIV prevention and treatment programmes with men joining support groups to the extent that participation is consistent with the notions of masculinity, joining support groups when there are opportunities for economic opportunities to preserve their image as providers (Mburu et al., 2014; Dageid, Govender, & Gordon, 2012).

Women are generally over-represented in the support groups, and often join support groups for psychosocial support and are more likely to utilise HIV programmes compared to men (Mburu et al., 2014). Reasons for women not joining the support groups include transport costs, having to ask permission from spouse, taking care of ill family members, and lack of knowledge about existing support groups (Dageid, 2014). The traditional notions of masculine identity that portray men as strong, healthy and productive, often keep men from admitting that they are sick, vulnerable, and in need of health services, and make them feel ashamed of utilising health services, especially services where they are with the women. Despite the high prevalence of the epidemic in today's South Africa, the traditional hegemony of masculine ideals still dictates that a man should earn an income to provide for his family. Men are also expected to be actively seeking solutions to problems, including health problems. One mechanism by which HIV stigma was perceived to interact with masculinity to prevent men from accessing services was linked to a sense of shame, secrecy, powerlessness and a loss of respect, qualities that were all contrary to masculine notions of respect. Men living with HIV and AIDS tend to be interested in activities that reinforce their masculinity and social respect including leadership roles, financial incentives or income generating activities rather than solve their problems through talking (Dageid et al., 2012; Mburu et al., 2014; Mfecane, 2012). Indeed, studies in South Africa and Uganda point out that men tended to be motivated by the chance of empowerment through work and community outreach to maintain their identity more than women were (Dageid, 2014; Mburu et al., 2014). Therefore, it is common for men to wait until they were in advanced stages of HIV disease to seek medical assistance to avoid being labelled as weak, and shameful.

6.2 Support Groups: Transforming Shame in Context

By their very nature, support groups create an enabling environment for the PLWHA to address myths, attitudes, shame and stigma associated with HIV and AIDS, a service that is valued by PLWHA, who otherwise feel stuck, defeated and abandoned. Support groups members speak the same languages, are from the same culture, have had to deal with more or less the same kind of shame and stigma therefore they understand cultural nuances, and this enables them to connect with the members in dealing with shame, and related loss. Other than being infected with HIV, some if not most of the support group members had previously lost someone to HIV/AIDS related illnesses, and they find volunteering as a way of relieving their hurt and turning it into a positive energy. Members range between 12 and 20 individuals and meet regularly, often once a week. Regardless of form or level of sophistication, support groups are inclusive and do not have requirements such as literacy. Members decide the aims and activities of the group, and it is important to make sure that no one dominates the group and that no one is left out. Support groups operate in a fluid terrain involving wide interpretations of the need for care of PLWHA. Therefore, their activities are varied and take a more open-ended approach to individuals, households and community needs. These various forms of lay work merge into a plural and complex local environment of healing and can be understood within four focus areas:

- Therapeutic functions and emotional support: Debriefing sessions are central to support groups. Members share their own experiences and testimonials to motivate, comfort and encourage the members to avoid the victim role. Members draw on a higher power, mainly through prayer, and singing to make sense of their conditions and reduce negative feelings and debunk myths such as perceptions of HIV and AIDS as punishment for their wrongdoing or acts of witchcraft. Members make friends in groups, allowing members to call for help and support when the group is not running. Thus, people who are excluded by their community can recreate 'family' and community networks and a sense of belonging through support groups. For most individuals support groups provide a safe space where they do not feel judged and they can disclose their HIV status to the support group members before disclosing to the family (Casale et al., 2013, 2014; Dageid, 2014). For many individuals who belong to a support group, the therapeutic experience gained helps them confront the prejudice, and shame that they experience, and they use the experience to empower other members of the community (Walker et al., 2008).
- Instrumental support: Support group members provide different forms of practical assistance services including routine and structure. They encourage ways to restore dignity and pride among themselves and encourage economic self-reliance activities. Balancing their roles as advocates for PLWHA, members act as intermediaries among health and social services and the communities, promoting rights-based approaches to access and inter-sectoral action. This is critical for families and communities living in environments where formal health services are inaccessible. Where people are poor or are located on the periphery, members act for themselves speaking from the vantage point of the community, enhancing coping skills, supporting medication adherence and improved retention in HIV care, mobilising them to deal with a range of challenges such as gender based violence, and developing income generating schemes (Swaminatha, Ashburn, Kes & Duvvury, 2008). In some instances, registered and formalised structures become a resource for people to 'drop in', to receive information, publications, telephone

counselling, uptake of HIV interventions and referrals to professionals. Examples of successful support groups programmes are demonstrated in the wake of community mobilization efforts, either as part of large-scale political transformation, or through local mobilization, often facilitated by nongovernmental, community-based or faith-based organizations (Dageid, Sliep, & Akintola, 2011) Voluntary counselling and HIV testing and the ongoing counselling provided at clinic and hospital level must be accompanied by broader psychosocial support interventions to meet the needs of PLWHA. Also, HIV positive individuals are likely to have among others emotional, physical, practical and legal issues to deal with, and may thus not be able to register all information or make use of the psychosocial counselling given at a time-constrained counselling session (Dageid, 2014). Support groups thus strategically fill this critical role.

- Informational support: Support groups provide advice on a range of topics including treatment literacy, translating biomedical concepts into the local idioms and overcoming the stereotypes and over generalisations about PLWHA. They use their stories and experiences to equip members and the broader community in how to deal with and overcome the stigma and shame and forms of adversity resulting from HIV and AIDS. They raise awareness and educate communities in various forums including political rallies, schools, and community meetings. They become role models, activists and advocates for PLWHA and communities. As more people use and access and talk about HIV, it gains wider acceptance and there is reduced stigma and shame associated with HIV.

- Appraisal support: Support groups foster a positive identity, sense of hope, belonging, and self-worth to help the members break through cycles of negative coping. Thus, members encourage open communication and make it as safe and comfortable as possible for people to speak about difficult issues. A study conducted on the role of support groups pointed out that some women in support groups identified positive psychological and physical changes as well as behaviour changes in relationships with men, which they attributed to appraisal support from group attendance (Dageid, 2014).

Despite existing on the periphery of the formal health systems, often without the wherewithal to lobby and advocate their cause, support groups by and large remain resilient. Integrating support groups in the established chain of health care services could be a cost-efficient, relatively fast and far-reaching way of addressing psychosocial distress among PLWHAs in sub-Saharan Africa. Indeed, support groups have demonstrated that HIV is not a death sentence.

6.2.1   Visual Participatory Methods

Visual participatory methods (VPM) are increasingly used as a change agents and therapeutic tools in health research and clinical psychology (Gastaldo, Magalhães, Carrasco, & Davy, 2012), and as empowerment tools for stigmatised and marginalised groups. VPM include a range of artistic strategies including photovoice, digital sto-rytelling, theatre, drama, and drawing techniques such as body-maps hand-mapping techniques (Betancourt, 2016; Gastaldo et al., 2012; Jager, Fogarty, Tewson, Lenette, & Boydell, 2017; Lapum et al., 2015). VPM have been used to explore intersection-ality of identities, power dynamics, class, sexuality, and has been used with diverse populations including children, orphaned children, youth, and men who have sex with men (MSM), to explore a range of topics such as STIs, HIV prevention, teenage pregnancies and related topics that have potential to marginalise and or stigmatise certain groups and individuals. One of the strengths of VPM is the ability to engage participants to play an active role in making decisions about how to represent their experiences in a highly personalized manner, and to communicate their stories cre-atively through a deeper, more reflexive process.

In HIV prevention, VPM have been used to explore and identify interconnec-tions with wider issues around stigma and discrimination, shame, care and support, livelihoods and family. In health research, VPM add depth to traditional qualitative methods through creative expression. Strategies such as body-maps and hand-maps illustrate emotions, what the participants can and cannot do regarding adversaries, as well as illustrate life events and health trajectories. By relying less on the language, they are suitable in settings where participants have low literacy skills. The resulting images often illustrate the way the participants give meaning and interpret their life experiences. Participants develop their scripts, and storylines and what they con-sider as the priority. The analysis process awakens and deepens the level of creative engagement, allowing participants to see themselves in a positive light. The final production can either be used as an educational, or advocacy tool, or participant's property in which they decide its use. For many participants, the act of being seen in the final production (whether for education, or exhibit) is regarded by many partic-ipants as a transforming process, providing pleasure in a new perception of self, as well as the seizing of opportunities.

Like all forms of research, VPM must be planned carefully and follow ethical guidelines including privacy, confidentiality. VPM strategies can be done without identifying participants' faces, or related identifiable features. Support services such as counselling and therapy should ideally be available especially when involving sensitive issues with vulnerable individuals sharing intersectional experiences such as children and women who experience violence in addition to dealing with HIV/AIDS.

6.3 Conclusion

Our chapter builds on the literature demonstrating how social constructs of shame, and stigma interact with culturally based gender issues, such as respectability, risk-taking, independence and emotional control, to help to illuminate how and why a stigmatising and shaming health care system which narrowly defines HIV/AIDS treatment as solely biomedical disadvantages women and men's health. Support groups and participatory strategies provide therapeutic space for individuals experiencing shame due to HIV or socio-economic conditions. These strategies are organic, and key focus areas are developed by the individuals as a means of empowerment.

6.3.1   Implications for Positive Therapy

6.3.1.1   Support Groups

For many individuals involved in HIV support groups, HIV positive status could be a life-changing experience, prompting them to review their personal priorities and try to take stronger control over the direction of their lives and abandon abusive relationships. The transformative potential of HIV was encountered not in the context of a major social movement but in a much more localised and personalised space, and this model seemed effective and can be replicated in other areas where individuals confront shame. Interventions that strengthen social support networks, such as their families, close friends and peers, should be bolstered to help men and women cope with the shame associated with HIV. Given the high prevalence of HIV/AIDS and the related mental, physical and social distress, more HIV healthcare resources should be channelled to psycho-social support interventions in South Africa. People are very vulnerable unless they are firmly embedded and supported by communities and health systems. These local contexts become characterized by the value systems and ideologies of care, all of which powerfully shape the ability of support groups to respond to health and other needs 'on the ground'.

6.3.1.2   Visual Participatory Methods

The application of visual methods in community settings enables individuals to make constructive connections with issues and behaviours deemed shameful and equips them to transform the negative life experiences into hope and positive resource through arts and creative expressions. Whether in research or community setting, there is a need for strategies that are able to help people think about their own lives and identities, and what influences them and what tools they use in that thinking, because those things are the building blocks of social change and can be instrumental in transforming shame into a positive resource.

References

Bennett, D. S., Traub, K., Mace, L., Juarascio, A., Virginia, C., & Hall, S. (2016). *Shame among people living with HIV : A literature review, 28*(1), 87–91. Retrieved from https://doi.org/10.1080/09540121.2015.1066749.

Betancourt, G. (2016). Hand mapping a qualitative method to inquire about La Passion: Sexual desires, pleasures and passions of Latino Gay men in North America. Presentation, Sexuality and Social Work Conference 2016, August 18, 2016.

Casale, M., Wild, L., Cluver, L., & Kuo, C. (2014). The relationship between social support and anxiety among caregivers of children in HIV-endemic South Africa. *Psychology, Health and Medicine, 19*(4), 490–503. Retrieved from https://doi.org/10.1080/13548506.2013.832780.

Casale, M., Wild, L., & Kuo, C. (2013). "They give us hope": HIV-positive caregivers' perspectives on the role of social support for health. *AIDS Care, 25*(10), 1203–1209. Retrieved from https://doi.org/10.1080/09540121.2013.763893.

De Jager, A., Fogarty, A., Tewson, A., Lenette, C., & Boydell, K. M. (2017). Digital storytelling in research: A systematic review. *The Qualitative Report, 22*(10), 2548–2582. Retrieved from http://nsuworks.nova.edu/tqr/vol22/iss10/3/.

Dageid, W., Sliep, Y, Akintola, O., & Duckert, F. (2011). *Response-ability in the era of AIDS*: Building social capital in community care and support. Matieland, South Africa: AFRICAN SUN MeDIA Press.

Dageid, W. (2014). Support groups for HIV-positive people in South Africa: Who joins, who does not, and why? *African Journal of AIDS Research, 13*(1), 1–11. Retrieved from https://doi.org/10.2989/16085906.2014.886601.

Dageid, W., Govender, K., & Gordon, S. F. (2012). Masculinity and HIV disclosure among heterosexual South African men: Implications for HIV/AIDS intervention. *Culture, Health and Sexuality, 14*(8), 925–940. Retrieved from https://doi.org/10.1080/13691058.2012.710337.

Dolezal, L., & Lyons, B. (2017). Health-related shame : An affective determinant of health? (pp. 1–7). Retrieved from https://doi.org/10.1136/medhum-2017-011186.

Duby, Z., Nkosi, B., Scheibe, A., Brown B, Bekker, L.-G. (2018). *"Scared of going to the clinic"*: Contextualising healthcare access for men who have sex with men, female sex workers and people who use drugs in two South African cities (pp. 1–8).

Friedman, I. (2005, January). CHWs and community care givers: Towards a unified model of practice. *South African Health Review, 2005*(1), 176–188.

Gastaldo, D., Magalhães, L., Carrasco, C., & Davy, C. (2012). *Body-Map*. Retrieved from http://livelihoods.org.za/projects/usaid-i.

Ginneken, N. Van, Lewin, S., & Berridge, V. (2010). Social Science & Medicine. The emergence of community health worker programmes in the late apartheid era in South Africa : An historical analysis. *Social Science & Medicine, 71*(6), 1110–1118. Retrieved from https://doi.org/10.1016/j.socscimed.2010.06.009.

Hargreaves, J., Stangl, A., Bond, V., Hoddinott, G., Krishnaratne, S., & Mathema, H. et al. (2016). HIV-related stigma and universal testing and treatment for HIV prevention and care: Design of an implementation science evaluation nested in the HPTN 071 (PopART) cluster-randomized trial in Zambia and South Africa. *Health Policy and Planning, 31*(10), 1342–1354. Retrieved from https://doi.org/10.1093/heapol/czw071.

Lapum, J., Liu, L., Hume, S., Wang, S., Nguyen, M., & Harding, B. et al. (2015). Pictorial narrative mapping as a qualitative analytic technique. *International Journal of Qualitative Methods, 14*(5), 160940691562140. Retrieved from https://doi.org/10.1177/1609406915621408.

Mburu, G., Ram, M., Siu, G., Bitira, D., Skovdal, M., & Holland, P. (2014). Intersectionality of HIV stigma and masculinity in eastern Uganda: implications for involving men in HIV programmes. *BMC Public Health, 14*, 1061. Retrieved from https://doi.org/10.1186/1471-2458-14-1061.

Mfecane, S. (2012). Narratives of HIV disclosure and masculinity in a South African village. *Culture, Health and Sexuality, 14*(sup 1). Retrieved from https://doi.org/10.1080/13691058.2011.647081.

Patel, A., Varilly, P., Jamadagni, S., Hagan, M., Chandler, D., & Garde, S. (2012). Sitting at the edge: How biomolecules use hydrophobicity to tune their interactions and function. *The Journal Of Physical Chemistry B, 116*(8), 2498–2503. https://doi.org/10.1021/jp2107523.

Pettit, M. L. (2008). Disease and stigma: A review of literature. *The Health Educator, 40*(2), 70–76.

Swaminatha, H., Ashburn, K., Kes, A., & Duvvury, N. (2008). *Women's property rights HIV and AIDS & domestic violence. Research findings from two rural districts in South Africa and Uganda.* Cape Town: HSRC Press.

Walker, C., Ailber, M., & Nkosi, B. (2008). Research findings from Amajuba, South Africa. In S. Swaminathan, K. Ashburn, A. Kes, N. Duvvury, C. Walker, M. Aliber, B. Nkosi, M. A. Rugadya & K. Herbert (Eds.), *Women's property rights, HIV and AIDS, and domestic violence* (pp. 15–84). Cape Town, South Africa: HSRC Press.

Busisiwe Nkosi (Ph.D.) is a Senior Social Scientist at the Africa Health Research Institute, KwaZulu Natal Province, South Africa. Her interest includes action research focusing on a range of topics including vulnerability, research ethics, HIV prevention, domestic and gender-based violence and community-based services.

Paul C. Rosenblatt (Ph.D.) is Professor Emeritus of Family Social Science at the University of Minnesota. He has a Ph.D. in Psychology from Northwestern University and has authored or co-authored 14 books, 84 refereed journal articles, and 120 other academic publications. As an interdisciplinary scholar he has taught not only in the family field but also in psychology, anthropology, and sociology. Much of his work focuses on individuals, couples, and families dealing with difficulties, and his research often involves qualitative methods and sensitivity to cultural issues.

Chapter 7
"The Group Is that Who Protects You in the Face of Shame": Self-change and Community Theater Participation in an Argentine Agro-City

Johana Kunin

Abstract Community theatre is a social development activity where amateur actors form a diverse group to create and act out stories that result from improvisations related to their personal difficulties and life experiences. Community theatre is a source of reflection, self-knowledge and self-development. But, in the conservative agricultural town in Argentina studied in this chapter, very few people dare to participate in community theatre. Most of the population feels "embarrassment" and "shame" when participating, given that the metropolitan habits of performing leisure activities outside home or work are not common practice. Nor is it common to manifest public protest or dissent. Those who do venture to take part in community theatre express that they have lost their sense of "shame". A new subjectivity is developed by the individual who manages to "cleanse" his problems, to be the "owner" of his time and to attach less relevance to his social reputation. This chapter analyses the way in which community theatre participants can overcome shame. It describes the theoretical background stemming mostly from social anthropology, presents the context of the ethnographical case study and discusses community theatre as a way to transform shame. The principal conclusion is that collective "exposure" to "shame" is key to its elimination and its transformation into pride, and that shame should always be understood as a cultural construct. This chapter recommends group activities, such as community theatre, that can "protect" individuals from shame and contribute to self-transformation.

Keywords Shame · Activism · Argentina · Theatre · Participation

J. Kunin (✉)
UNSAM/CONICET & EHESS, París, France
e-mail: johanakunin@gmail.com

IDAES, UNSAM, Edificio de Ciencias Sociales UNSAM, Campus Miguelete, 25 de Mayo 1021, B1650HMH San Martín, Provincia de Buenos Aires, Argentina

7.1   Introduction

This chapter deals with vernacular definitions (emic) of "shame", but above all of its "loss"[1] by those who have experienced it and performed (Butler, 2006; Austin, 1975) it, through participation in a social development initiative known as community theatre, presenting insights into and understanding of the loss of social shame and stigma.

Shame is not as an essential, natural feeling, but rather the point from which social relationships unravel within the framework of a political economy of emotions (Scheper-Hughes, 1992) or of emotion as a social practice (Lutz & Abu-Lughod, 1990). As Pita (2010, 80) points out, emotions and feelings are part of what produces subjectivity, thus they are capable of generating emotional communities and moral worlds.

Within the studied context, the vernacular experience of shame could be defined as the fear of dishonour. Feeling "shame" before the possibility of participating in extraordinary or unusual public activities is expected; fear of the perception of others is the hegemonic position in the community where research was conducted. It is the "loss of shame" that locates individuals in an immoral situation or anomie. To experience shame, then, is to be in rhythm with the social context. "Lacking shame" is not knowing how or especially not wishing to prevent disgraceful exposure; it implies breaking the shield of civility provided by shame. Acting or rehearsing in community theatre activities involves exposure to situations of mockery or contempt. Hence, as my field informants assert, their participation has been made possible only by their "loss of shame". Such loss of shame through community theatre participation is a mobilising emotion that allows self-objectification and self-relativisation, deepening a social process of the subject's autonomisation.

Regarding the specific relationship between shame and participation-based development devices like community theatre, Prins (2010) analyzes the unexpected consequences of a participatory photography programme in El Salvador in which peasants were "ashamed" of being involved. Those who managed to "lose their shame" and finally feel pride had successfully overcome the fear of real or potential criticism from their neighbours and were able to "express themselves" and "develop their minds" (438).

The key of this chapter is shame as a morality mark and as a dissuasive element to public participation in uncommon activities. People must lose their shame in order to participate, and it is by means of such participation that they deepen and perform their loss of shame.

---

[1] Words in quotations indicate native expressions of field informants and do not represent categories of the analyst.

7.2 Theoretical Background: From Shame to Pride by Means of Collective Actions

Munt (2008) explains that horizontal bonds can be established through "communities of shame" and that shame can be transfigured into collective desires that fight for a political presence (in a broad sense) and for a legitimate sense of self. In this way, the search for rights and protection can spawn a new sense of identity and self, a self proud of having overcome shame. The author states that finding and participating in an association, club, party, labour union or group with collective and public objectives can be a source of pride and joy to those who have previously felt shame. In the US, the Black Civil Rights Movement, the Gay Liberation Front and the Women's Liberation Movement in the 1970s are just a few historical examples in which, by means of social exposition, shame was transformed into pride.

> Shame has political potential as it can provoke a separation between the social conventions demarcated within hegemonic ideals, enabling a re-inscription of social intelligibility. The outcome of this can be radical, instigating social, political and cultural agency amongst the formerly disenfranchised. When you no longer care that you are being shamed, particularly when horizontal bonds formed through communities of shame can be transmuted into collective desires to claim a political presence and a legitimate self, that new sense of identity can forge ahead and gain rights and protection. (Munt, 2008, p. 4)

Simmel (1938) similarly explains that the actions of the masses are characterised by shamelessness and that shame as embarrassment dilutes in the homogeneity of the mass crowd. Górnicka (2016), on the other hand, studies nudists who lose their shame in a group setting. This author explains that, in order to properly practice nudism and enjoy the activity, participants must not only lose their sense of shame and control their sexual urges, but must also learn to enjoy the activity in spite of such shame and sexual urges (83–84). As a consequence, the individual must continually lose his shame by learning to face it and by finding enjoyment in spite of it on a day-to-day basis.

The next section offers a contextualisation of community theatre and an overview of where the presented study takes place.

7.3   Contextual Description of Community Theatre Activities with a Conservative Town

Ethnographic fieldwork[2] was conducted in La Laguna,[3] a rural agricultural town about 260 km away from Buenos Aires, Argentina's capital city. Numerous factors have played a role in the populating of the outlying neighbourhoods of La Laguna. Over the last 25 years, the exponential growth of soy production based on methods of land concentration and agricultural mechanisation has replaced other traditional productive sectors, such as dairy, and has generated high levels of unemployment or underemployment among agricultural workers (Hernández, 2007, 2009). Additionally, floods at the beginning of the 2000s produced migrations to the town from nearby fields or small villages, while lower and middle-lower class inhabitants originally from town's centre have been pushed to the periphery because of limitations that only extend them access to rentals or to social housing in the outskirts of the town.

The 12,000 inhabitants that populate outlying neighbourhoods of La Laguna live with little or no public infrastructure, no public transportation, no hospitals, no banks and no public administration offices. Men primarily earn their living by working odd jobs in agriculture or construction and women typically work cleaning houses in other, higher-income neighbourhoods of the town. Moreover, the inhabitants of the town centre often stigmatise those who live in the outlying periphery.

The hegemonic sociability both of the town's centre and its periphery are marked by living and working spaces. The metropolitan habits of performing leisure activities outside home or work are not common practice. Nor is it common manifest public protest or dissent.

Within this context, after the nationwide socioeconomic crisis of 2001, a number of initiatives arose that looked to implement symbolic and material strategies for the extension of rights within marginalised sectors of society, of which the theatre group studied is an example.

"The Rail Crossers" is the fictitious name assigned to the community theatre group[4] studied. For nearly 13 years, the group has worked and operated in the outlying neighbourhoods of La Laguna. The members, who range from infants to

---

[2]As part of my doctoral research work in social anthropology, I have conducted participant observation for four years within the group, in addition to formal interviews and registers of informal talks. Within the framework of my research, I participate directly in the group, having been invited to act, travel and participate in national events, negotiations with local public workers, public presentations and rehearsals. I have used fictitious names both for my informants and the town studied.

[3]A note regarding places: the town of La Laguna, with around 36,000 inhabitants, is the head of a county of the same name that consists of twelve other villages and a total population of 47,000. The county of La Laguna is located within the Argentine province of Buenos Aires, which, despite bearing the same name, should not be confused with the city of Buenos Aires, the nation's autonomous capital, a populous urban metropolis. Unless otherwise specified, in this chapter "La Laguna" and "Buenos Aires" refer to the town studied and the national capital respectively.

[4]Other works on community theatre in Argentina are Dubatti and Pansera (2006), Bidegain (2007), Bidegain et al. (2008), Scher (2011) and Elgoyhen (2012).

septuagenarians, create unprecedented dialogues, stories and collective songs from improvisations that are related to their difficulties and life memories. For example, in 2014 and 2015 the group prepared a play that dealt with the history and identity of the marginalised neighbourhoods of La Laguna where many members live and where the community centre in which the Rail Crossers practice and rehearse is located, discussing and denying the stigmas that burden them. Another play referred to a frustrated love between someone from the town's centre and someone from the outskirts, and yet another play questioned gender, education and work. The plays' narrative structures often have a moral component that initially points out the negativities of the present state of things and subsequently proposes other possibilities regarding unity, collectiveness, the breakdown of hegemonic expectations and the possibility of public grievance. Thus, the group sings and plays their dreams for present and future times. Members often express that beyond the content of their plays, the process of group creation is what is most important. Somewhat curiously, in everyday life, little thought is given to the audience or the possible repercussions of their plays; despite the group's declaration that it aims to transform society, those who are most transformed are the members themselves.

The members of the group feel that "they are always the same gang", that they "are few" and that they are perceived as "out of the ordinary", both in the centre and in the outlying neighbourhoods of the La Laguna:

> We are seen as characters. We do not know where to stand. That is why we gather.
>
> Twenty eight-year-old woman, coordinator and member of the theatre group who used to live in a larger metropolis and has returned to La Laguna, her native town. She lives in the town's centre.
>
> In the *barrio* we are branded as crazy. They look at us from the outside and think 'these crazy people feel no shame.' We live in an odd society where people don't take chances. Or they say, 'Since I work in a certain place, they might say that I am crazy.' If you feel shame, forget it. [But] it's good to challenge yourself to do more.
>
> *Thirty five-year-old woman, member of the theatre group who was born in one of the county's small villages and now lives in the outlying neighbourhoods of La Laguna.*

Association with the group can compromise one's reputation, not only individually but also the reputations of his relatives:

> The construction of trust or reputation is put at risk when you do something weird. Something weird is anything that is unusual, right? So it isn't just momentary, but rather all your life that you become 'one of the *jipis*.'[5] Here, you carry all your family history, you are marked by your family lineage. So, to me, the word reputation took shape. Right? Because, given that your reputation is constantly at stake, you are always at risk of being crossed out and disregarded. If you are banished, you have to move at least 200 kilometres away because there is no turning back.
>
> *Sixty-year-old man and member of the theatre group, who is originally from the greater metropolitan area of the Argentine capital city, Buenos Aires.*

---

[5]The Spanish rendition of the English word "hippie"; here it is used for someone who is lazy, dirty and against the established moral order. The members of the Rail Crossers are often referred to as *jipis*, especially those who live in the town's centre.

The community theatre group[6] was created and is coordinated by people who have travelled to Buenos Aires for trips, study sojourns or work, and have acquired knowledge about community theatre and other alternative repertoires. As the coordinators explain, they seek to "improve", "free" and "awaken" the inhabitants of La Laguna's periphery, as well as people from the county in general, by introducing repertoires of feminism, new age movements and the return to "nature" as a redeeming philosophy in response to the advance of "technology", as well as the Argentine "psy-culture" (Visacovsky, 2009). The methodology implemented by the coordinators is based on the notions and practices of the popular education of Paulo Freire that contain the central principals of always being an "active" and not passive receiver of public actions and of horizontality between coordinators and participants. Thus, anyone can be an actor or actress and write plays about his own problems.

The coordinators usually invite out-of-town guests to come to La Laguna to speak or conduct artistic workshops. These activities draw media attention to and, in part, legitimise the work of the Rail Crossers, but at the same time they exacerbate certain ideas about the "oddity" of the group's members. The activities are centred on the native notion of "participation", which implies a corporal presence and a high degree of visibility in public spaces. According to the coordinators, those who experience "participation" inevitably improve their conditions. The coordinators believe not only in positive participation but also in its public visibility in the media and on social networks. Coordinators are often criticised for their lack of "discretion", for "complaining too much", for being "fundamentalists" or for "spreading fear". They are publicly known in the town, potentially stigmatising even further those who are "ashamed" of being linked to group. The members from the town's outlying neighbourhoods understand their participation based on their own perspectives and needs, which are never identical or irreconcilable—but rather are often convergent—with those of the coordinators.

Before rehearsals there is a change in the interpersonal distance between participants; contact between bodies becomes closer and collective massages in a circle are frequent. Additionally, participants create games to somatically instil means of group communication that do not require speech. All these practices are fundamental when understanding the concept of "shamelessness".

To the members of the group, acting is not what is most important; it is meeting each other and connecting through "collective energy circulation". A game always played at the beginning of rehearsal consists of forming a circle in which, one by one, the participants sequentially shout "ia!" as if they were doing a karate manoeuvre. This exclamation is followed by a body movement that enables the next participant to do the same. They repeat this multiple times while increasing both speed and volume until, as the participants say, "the energy rises."

> The 'ia!' is an energy among everybody. Like a collective energy. This is the only place I have ever felt it.

---

[6]Neither the coordinators nor the participants form a homogeneous group, but for reasons of length, I will not enter in detail about the effects of this community experience upon members according to their different trajectories and social statuses.

Twenty-eight-year-old woman who is member of the theatre group and lives in one of the outlying neighbourhoods of the town.

Energy is what I feel. But if I did this alone at home, I wouldn't generate that energy. It's the energy of one plus the energy of another and another and another and other […] and being in a circle makes the energy run. It also has to do with everybody being in unison; there is no possibility to judge. I don't think that anyone in the circle at that moment is watching the way the other is knocking his legs… as if the group allowed free expression.

Forty-one-year-old woman who was born in the county of La Laguna. She is a coordinator and member of the theatre group and lives in one of the outlying neighbourhoods of the town.

It is remarkable how energy is understood to be "collective". So is the association that, when rehearsing, they are not overcome by "shame", which has so much weight over their non-participating neighbours, because of the speed of "circulating energy" or because they feel "protected by the group" when they publicly present their plays.

In public presentations, the participants generally dress alike and usually there are no "leading" roles. In their frequent trips out of La Laguna, the members of the group travel, eat and sleep together, and before acting, they dress and apply make up together. Turner (1969) maintained that in the moment of liminality in the ritual, an intense comradeship and egalitarianism is developed among neophytes, and the secular distinctions of position and status disappear or homogenise (102). In the theatre group formed by people coming from both "central" neighbourhoods and the periphery of La Laguna, such homogenisation seems to occur—at least temporarily—generating a great sense of camaraderie.

The rehearsals include "work" on memories or experienced feelings in moments when the participants were discriminated or when they or their parents arrived to live in the periphery of the town. Such "work" can be executed in three different ways: (1) through spontaneous improvisations acted without much previous reflection, (2) by means of small group debates, or (3) inspired by "research" that members of the group carry out by interviewing their neighbours. Additionally, these methods of gathering information provide data for the composition of song lyrics; the members often change the words of well-known pop songs with their own lyrics and perform their renditions collectively in their plays.

Interestingly enough, acting is considered not merely a reflection of collected or thought-out information, but rather it is a part of a learning process. The idea of "transiting through the body" seems to be essential for members to learn and understand. As Behnke and Ciocan (2012) explain, it could be a "sensual reflectiveness" that must not be ineluctably performed in a retrospective manner (14) because, in this case, the plays are never written down but are "thought out" from working processes based on improvisations of memories. According to my field informants, participation through "*poner el cuerpo*"—which translates literally as "putting the body", and refers to putting one's body on the line—or "putting [problems or memories] into words" is capable of solving some discomfort or difficulty. Such a notion could stem from influences of the "psy" common sense. Just as Visacovsky (2009) holds, psychoanalysis in Argentina exists as practical knowledge, not only in institutionalised forms or as therapeutic practices, but also in the manners of acting and thinking of many Argentines who nourish their social identities and lifestyles. This practical sense helps constitute the everyday ontological reality and also provides solutions to possible setbacks (2009, pp. 57–58). In this context, the idea of "catharsis" has adopted positive value.

The inhabitants of marginalised zones that do participate in the activities of the community theatre group conceive it as a "clearing" that allows them to "feel in another world"; they escape the "reality" that they simultaneously represent, expressing what they wish to say and feel. This is not something that happens to a single individual, but rather is expressed a collective feeling or thought, which is why the members feel they have greater strength.

7.4 Specific Findings Regarding Shame and Its Loss Related to Community Theatre

Those who "lose their sense of shame" give meaning to their feelings and connect to the world as situated subjects. As Scheper-Hughes (1992, 431) explains, we would not know how we feel if not for culture.

Many participants have noticed that their "way of being" has changed since joining the group. They now consider themselves less "ashamed", "timid", "with different ways of feeling" and other desires. They say they can more easily integrate with others and when something bothers them they no longer stay quiet. Thus, it can be affirmed that their participation implies changes in their subjectivity. The subject can only constitute itself as such because it is surrounded by other subjects; it is formed in and by mutual bonds. The constitution of subjectivity consists of incorporating ways of doing and speaking. "It can be understood as a corporeal training, a reproduction of perception, conception and action principles, a system of dispositions or *habitus* with which the self-experience articulates" (Pazos Garciandía, 2005, 8). The analysis of the development of ways of subjectification—of dispositions activated and incorporated by social agent-subjects—is inseparable from the study of social technologies that produce ways of reflection, expression or self-presentation in the heart of historical and culturally specific problems (Pazos Garciandía, 2005, 8).

The group is mainly composed of women[7] who point out that the moments of rehearsal or acting are a time "for them" compared to re st of the day, when they feel that their time belongs to "others". Türken et al. (2016, 11) propose that the neoliberal governmentality refers to the forms in which neoliberalism installs the concept of the human subject as an autonomous, individualised, self-directing, decision-making agent who becomes an entrepreneur of himself. Subjectivity, strengthened by the community theatre, relates to the women's "own" time to self-development, a cornerstone of individual life and well-being. As Rose (1999) states, the individual is morally obliged to engage in a self-realisation project and develop a better version

---

[7]The few men that either coordinate or participate in the theatre group are perceived by others and/or perceive themselves as "feminised".

of himself to manage life. Thus, the "loss of shame" has an ambiguous nature: it exposes those who experience the risk of being classified as anomalous or odd, but at the same time, in relation to neoliberal subjectivity, it enables a space of autonomy, individuality and agency.

If Malinowski poses that religion helps man withstand "situations of emotional stress by providing him a way of escape" (quoted by Geertz 1973, 25), community theatre also poses something close to a way of escape. Nevertheless, Geertz proposes that, paradoxically, the problem of suffering is not its avoidance, but rather knowing how to suffer, how to make suffering bearable (1973, 100). Community theatre provides a language to express unformulated states in other ways, and thus makes personal experience ordered and intelligible.

The director of the theatre group could be compared to the psychoanalyst or the shaman that Lévi-Strauss describes (1958, 222) in conveying to the conscience conflicts and resistances that, up to that moment, had remained in the unconscious, thus "organising" them. Both the psychoanalytic and the shamanic cure (for Lévi-Strauss 1958, 222) seek to provoke an experience that reconstructs a myth that must be lived or relived. In this case, it is about individual and social stories, stories of the neighbours themselves inserted in the history of the outlying neighbourhoods; stories of changes in the agricultural world, housing plans and politics from the 1990s to the present. The psychoanalyst listens, while the shaman speaks. The director of the theatre groups makes the members speak, remember, move, dress, sing, parody or "laugh" at situations of deep inequality, proposing the symbolisation through actions and words of each member's "truth" and "history", generating that—by means of outpouring, losing control and publicly reorganising their emotions—the members lose their sense of shame collectively.

Dias Duarte (1988) talks about the intense, effective and broad-based language of "nerves" in the urban working classes of Brazil, and Lutz (1988) refers to an emotional vocabulary that explains relationships between people. Following these lines of thought, the vocabulary or language of the "loss of shame" can be considered here; it establishes and drives both meanings and subjects in their social practices beginning with the deepening of a self where the individual is positively presented and where the collective weight decreases.

> Thus, the education, the autonomy value, the centrality of an individualistic ideology —stated above all in the psychologised language —would give an account of cultural and distinctive elements that result from a common historical experience. (Viotti, 2011, 8).

Not to say that individualistic ideology did not exist in La Laguna before, but its distribution or differential presence was different to that which is proposed by the moral repertoires presented by the Rail Crossers. In this way, the ideas of Paulo Freire about popular education are compatible with the search of "one's well-being" and of "having one's space". Consideration should be given to the psychologisation and citizenisation processes, together with the different migrations from the countryside to the city and back and forth journeys between La Laguna and Buenos Aires, or La Laguna and a home village, which have differentially modified the population and its repertoires for elucidating personal and social discomfort.

7.5 Some Applied Recommendations to Transform Social Shame Through a Social Development Initiative

1. Develop activities where a whole collective transforms shame within a support group.
2. Implement exercises that focus less on rational sense and more on unplanned improvisations, sensibility and body perceptions.
3. Encourage a sense of pride among participants in order to develop a new sense of identity and self, a self proud of having overcome shame.
4. Remind participants that, while they may be few in number, they form part of a collective and have no reason to care about being regarded as odd or weird.
5. Demystify the participants' position by pointing out that shame is a cultural construct that varies in different contexts and different times, so as to minimise the burden of local social punishment.

7.6 Conclusion

This chapter provides insight into how community theatre participants transform shame and transform themselves as a whole through collective group activities. The transformation of shame can be positively affected by way of collective activities that stimulate not only reasoning but also senses, where a collective struggle, in a broad sense, can exist, causing the participants to feel proud in the face of "shame". Future research should engage in deepening the study of the draw and attraction of community activities, as well as possible obstacles, especially the role shame plays in dissuading or discouraging participation in social development activities, focusing on the collective transformation of shame. As in the fable of the Ugly Duckling, forming part of a group of ugly ducks singing in unison can only bring pride and new selfhoods as beautiful swans, leaving shame in the past.

References

Austin, J. L. (1975). *How to do things with words*. Oxford: Clarendon Press.
Behnke, E. A., & Ciocan, C. (2012). Introduction: Possibilities of embodiment. *Studia Phaenomenologica, 12,* 11–15.
Bidegain, M. (2007). *Teatro comunitario: resistencia y transformación social*. Buenos Aires: Atuel.
Bidegain, M., Marianetti, M., Quain, P., & Cabanchik, A. (2008). *Teatro comunitario: Vecinos al rescate de la memoria olvidada*. Buenos Aires: Ediciones Artes Escénicas.
Butler, J. (2006). Performative acts and gender constitution: An essay in phenomenology and feminist theory. In *The Routledgefalmer reader in gender & education* (pp. 73–83). Routledge.
Dias Duarte, L. F. (1988). *Da vida nervosa nas classes trabalhadoras urbanas*. Brasilia: Zahar.
Dubatti, J., & Pansera, C. (2006). *Cuando el arte da respuestas. 43 proyectos de cultura para el desarrollo social*. Buenos Aires: Artes Escénicas.

Elgoyhen, L. (2012). *Quand les voisins montent sur scène pour chanter le collectif. La mobilisation du théâtre communautaire argentin.* Mémoire de recherche de Master 2 d'Études Latino-Américaines. Mention sociologie. Université Paris 3-Sorbonne Nouvelle. Institut des Hautes Études de l'Amérique Latine.

Geertz, C. (1987 [1973]). *La interpretación de las culturas.* Barcelona: Gedisa.

Górnicka, B. (2016). *Nakedness, shame, and embarrassment: A long-term sociological perspective* (Vol. 12). Wiesbaden: Springer.

Hernández, V. (2007). El fenómeno económico y cultural del boom de la soja y el empresario innovador, En *Desarrollo Económico*, n° 187, vol. 47.

Hernández, V. (2009). La ruralidad globalizada y el paradigma de los agronegocios en las pampas gringas. In C. Gras & V. Hernández (Eds.), *La Argentina rural. De la agricultura familiar a los agronegocios.* Buenos Aires: Biblos.

Lévi-Strauss, C. (1995 [1958]). *Antropología estructural.* Barcelona: Paidós.

Lutz, C. (1988). *Unnatural emotions.* Chicago: University of Chicago Press.

Lutz, C., & Abu-Lughod, L. (1990). *Language and the politics of emotion.* Cambridge [England]: Cambridge University Press.

Munt, S. R. (2008). *Queer attachments: The cultural politics of shame. Queer Interventions.* Surrey: Ashgate Publishers.

Pazos Garciandía, Á. (2005). El otro como sí-mismo. Observaciones antropológicas sobre las tecnologías de la subjetividad. *AIBR. Revista de Antropología Iberoamericana.*

Pita, M. V. (2010). *Formas de vivir y formas de morir: los familiares de víctimas de la violencia policial.* Buenos Aires: del Puerto y CELS.

Prins, E. (2010). Participatory photography: A tool for empowerment or surveillance? *Action Research, 8*(4), 426–443.

Rose, N. (1999). *Governing the soul. The shaping of the private self.* London: Free Association Books.

Scheper-Hughes, N. (1992). *Death without weeping: The violence of everyday life in Brazil.* Berkeley: University of California Press.

Scher, E. (2011). *Teatro de vecinos. De la comunidad para la comunidad.* Buenos Aires: Instituto Nacional del Teatro.

Simmel, G. (1938). *Cultura Femenina.* Buenos Aires: Espasa-Calpe.

Türken, S., Nafstad, H. E., Blakar, R. M., & Roen, K. (2016). Making sense of neoliberal subjectivity: A discourse analysis of media language on self-development. *Globalizations, 13*(1), 32–46.

Turner, V. (1988, [1969]). *El proceso ritual. Estructura y Anti-estructura.* Madrid: Taurus.

Viotti, N. (2011). La literatura sobre las nuevas religiosidades en las clases medias urbanas. Una mirada desde Argentina. *Revista Cultura y Religión, 5*(1).

Visacovsky, S. E. (2009). La constitución de un sentido práctico del malestar cotidiano y el lugar del psicoanálisis en la Argentina. *Cuicuilco, 16*(45), 51–78.

Johana Kunin is a Social Anthropology Ph.D. candidate from Argentina. She writes her dissertation under joint supervision by École des Hautes Études en Sciences Sociales (EHESS, París, France) and IDAES, UNSAM (Buenos Aires, Argentina). She is a CONICET fellow. She researches about the relation of emotions, gender and development activities in an Argentine agro-city. She was a CLACSO fellow and then she studied the relationship of young rappers in Bolivia and development organizations. For her International Studies thesis she conducted fieldwork in 7 countries while studying how the idea of founding a "cardboard picker press" (a development initiative) had been originated in Argentina and had then been appropriated in particular ways in Mexico, Equator, Brazil, Bolivia, Peru and Paraguay. She has an undergraduate degree in Anthropology from Université Paris VIII, Vincennes-Saint-Denis, France.

Part II
Transforming Shame in Society

Chapter 8
A Sociocultural Exploration of Shame and Trauma Among Refugee Victims of Torture

Gail Womersley

Abstract Shame profoundly colours the experiences of the thousands of refugees entering Europe. Not only does the literature attest to the high levels of trauma among this population, research in the past decade has increasingly revealed the hidden yet pervasive role that shame may play in posttraumatic symptomatology. Shame may emerge as a result of the many forms of torture, sexual violence and other atrocities experienced in the country of origin, yet is equally exacerbated by degrading and humiliating asylum procedures, having to accept a new and often devalued social identity of being an asylum seeker, and the embarrassment of not meeting culturally-informed expectations to financially support the family back home. Shame is a complex process affecting core dimensions of the self, identity, ego processes, and personality—and is thus inextricably shaped by culture. It has a detrimental impact on health-seeking behaviour, yet its masked manifestations remain often unnoticed by practitioners. This is a critical consideration for clinicians and researchers working with refugee populations, where the relation is typically marked by power differentials across a matrix of identities informing not only the shame of the refugee but of the clinicians or researchers themselves. As both a researcher and clinical psychologist working with refugee populations, I explore the myriad dimensions of shame within this context based on personal reflections of my time "in the field" as well as the burgeoning literature on this topic. Key implications for techniques and methods which may be drawn upon by both researchers and clinicians are discussed.

Keywords Refugees · Trauma · Culture · Migration · Asylum · Shame

G. Womersley (✉)
Institut de psychologie et éducation, Faculté des Lettres et sciences humaines,
University of Neuchatel, 2000 Neuchâtel, Switzerland
e-mail: gail.womersley@unine.ch

© Springer Nature Switzerland AG 2019
C.-H. Mayer and E. Vanderheiden (eds.), *The Bright Side of Shame*,
https://doi.org/10.1007/978-3-030-13409-9_8

103

8.1 Introduction

The number of refugees seeking asylum across the world is unprecedented. According to the UNHCR,[1] **65.6 million people** around the world have been forced from home. This is a global challenge. Not only does the literature attest to the high levels of trauma among this population, research in the past two decades has increasingly revealed the hidden yet pervasive role that shame may play in posttraumatic symptomatology (Matos & Pinto-Gouveia, 2010; Slewa-Younan et al., 2017; Wilson, Droždek, & Turkovic, 2006; Wong & Tsai, 2007). As defined by Wilson and colleagues, "in the posttraumatic self, shame develops from traumatic experiences that render the victim fearful, powerless, helpless, and unable to act congruently with moral values" (Wilson et al., 2006). In the context of forced migration in particular, both trauma and shame are ubiquitous, pervasive, and contagious.

Shame activates shame. The mystifying dualism of shame is that it is at once an isolating, intimately intra-psychic phenomenon seeking concealment, yet remains deeply embedded in a visual and public interpersonal space where the self is violently and unexpectedly exposed to the critical gaze of the Other (Womersley, Maw, & Swartz, 2011). Unlike guilt (typically related to a particular action or behaviour), shame taints the entire landscape of the individual—colouring the very sense of self. Shame is therefore considered to be a more complex intra-psychic process than guilt because it involves processes concerning attributes about the core dimensions of the self, identity, ego processes, and personality (Wilson et al., 2006). Inasmuch as it lies within the interactional space between self and other, at the divide between the intimate and the public, the individual and society—it tries to hide itself by its very nature. As such, it often remains unnoticed. Its powerful yet seemingly invisible impact may be hidden behind a myriad of emotional cloaks—anger, dissociation, blame, and resentment—even more so in the context of clinicians working with migrant populations, where a plethora of differently nuanced cultural cloaks may further obfuscate this noxious affect (Buggenhagen, 2012; Slewa-Younan et al., 2017; Swartz, 1988; Wong & Tsai, 2007). However, ethically, clinically, professionally, humanly, professionals working with traumatized populations cannot ignore shame. This is particularly true of work within multicultural contexts, where relations are so typically marked by power differentials in terms of race, class, nationality and socio-economic status. It is here, in this "intersectionality" (Grzanka, Santos, & Moradi, 2017; Moradi, 2017) of identities, that shame is located. Therefore, new approaches are needed for clinicians (both researchers and academics) which consider the interactive effects of shame and trauma within sociocultural context among such vulnerable populations. In this chapter, aspects of migration and post-traumatic shame, and implications for professionals, will be discussed. A case study of shame will be presented, taken from a larger study I conducted exploring trauma among this population in Athens, Greece.

---

[1]UNHCR (2017).

8.1.1 Migration and Post-traumatic Shame

Shame significantly shapes the migration experience, linked particularly to extreme feelings of powerlessness, degradation and humiliation. It may emerge as a result of the many forms of torture, sexual violence and other atrocities experienced in the country of origin, yet is equally exacerbated by degrading and humiliating asylum procedures, having to accept a new and often devalued social identity of being an asylum seeker (characterised by a loss of social status, social networks, and employment opportunities), and the embarrassment of not meeting culturally-informed expectations to financially support the family (Buggenhagen, 2012). Shame pervades the experience of no longer being "at home" at home, of being cast out of one's country, of having to metaphorically knock on the door of a potential host country and beg to be accepted, only to be met by significant social discrimination, scrutiny and disbelief at one's claim to asylum (Bhimji, 2015; Goguikian Ratcliff, Bolzman, & Gakuba, 2014; Sanchez-Mazas et al., 2011; Torre, 2016).

The process of migration may therefore be in and of itself a shameful experience, wherein individual and social identities risk being negated through the systemic trauma associated with legal and social practices of exclusion (Goldsmith, Martin, & Smith, 2014). This exclusion serves only to feed monstrous feelings of invisibility and disconnectedness (Bhimji, 2015).

Furthermore, the stressful experiences that many asylum seekers and refugees are exposed to during forced migration, and during the resettlement process, make them vulnerable to mental health conditions. As a consequence, the prevalence of psychological distress and mental disorders in asylum seekers and refugees as reported in the literature appears to be generally high, with significantly elevated rates of post-traumatic stress disorder (PTSD) being found among this population (Li, Liddell, & Nickerson, 2016; Turrini et al., 2017). Research in trauma over the past decade has seen the development of the concept of "posttraumatic shame," with key authors stressing the importance of shame as a social emotion that impacts the severity and course of PTSD symptoms (Hecker, Braitmayer, & van Duijl, 2015; Maercker & Hecker, 2016; Wilson et al., 2006). Indeed, the experience of shame has even been revealed to potentially hold the same properties as traumatic events involving intrusions, flashbacks, strong emotional avoidance, hyper arousal, fragmented states of mind and dissociation (Matos & Pinto-Gouveia, 2010). Shame and trauma are inextricably linked.

Torture in particular represents an extraordinary exception in the psychopathology field—with significant implications for the shame-trauma nexus. The particularity of torture as pathogenic is linked to the fact that the act itself is taught, organized, elaborated, and perpetrated by humans against other humans (Sironi, 1999; Viñar, 2005). Arguably, the aim of the perpetrator is to shame, to disrupt the connection to all that makes us human (Viñar, 2005). As such, torture is not an individual act, but a social one. It is an inherently shameful experience for the tortured, damaging different spheres of an individual including body, personality, hope, aspirations for life, identity, integrity, belief systems, the sense of being grounded and attached to a family and society, autonomy, community relationships, and a sense of safety (Womersley et al., submitted). Humiliation thus arises from torture experiences where the survivor is abused, dehumanized, and made an exhibition for others, essentially representing a profound loss of dignity and power (Wilson et al., 2006; Wilson, Wilson, & Drozdek, 2004). In particular, the dual shame inherent in being both a victim of torture as well a refugee is related to a myriad of losses, human rights violations, shifting power dynamics and other dimensions of suffering linked not only to torture experienced pre-migration, but to different forms of violence experienced during and after migration as well (Hodges-Wu & Zajicek-Farber, 2017).

8.1.2   Cultural Manifestations of Shame and Implications for Clinicians

The source of shame can never be completely in the self or in the Other, but is a rupture of what Kaufman (1989) calls the "interpersonal bridge" binding the two. In thus theorizing shame as being located at this bridge, we understand the important role it plays in community life through promoting socially acceptable or desirable behaviour. It exerts a force that inclines individuals to adapt to socially sanctioned values, rules and beliefs—an integral component of the promotion of cultural ideals (Swartz, 1988). A significant source of shame is the loss of continuity in upholding culturally defined values, norms and respected patterns of behaviour—and the self-consciousness over disappointing others within one's social network and embedded within one's culture (Wilson et al., 2006). We may therefore understand the importance of the sociocultural context in determining its various manifestations. This has been highlighted in the plethora of cross-cultural and anthropological literature paying attention attesting to the variety of culturally diverse forms of shame (Wong & Tsai, 2007).

The model below is used to illustrate the various interrelating levels at which it manifests. When two individuals meet, they also bring with them a specific interpersonal and sociocultural context, all of which inform the interaction. As clinicians and researchers, we come as individuals, yet we come as individuals carrying specific cultural, gender, social and racial identities—and so do the individuals with whom we interact. All of these levels may potentially be sources of shame (Fig. 8.1).

This has significant implications for professionals—both clinicians and researchers—working with populations from a variety of cultural backgrounds. For example, a large potential for misunderstandings between clinicians and traumatized refugees is not only because of a language barrier; very little is known about the concepts of illness and treatment expectations in these patients (Maier & Straub, 2011). Furthermore, shame-related cultural codes of behaviour might prevent migrants from directly reporting earlier traumatic experiences, from trusting the professional or from even attending appointments. As noted by Wilson and colleagues (2006), "the powerful emotions of posttraumatic shame are associated with a broad range of

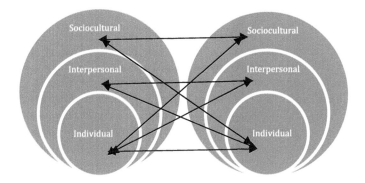

Fig. 8.1 Various interrelating levels at which shame manifests (Womersley)

avoidance behaviours: isolation, detachment, withdrawal, hiding, nonappearance, self-imposed exile, cancellation of appointments, surrender of responsibilities, emotional constriction, psychic numbing, emotional flatness, and non-confrontation with others" (138). These signs are easily misread.

The interpersonal dynamics of this clinical encounter may not be so different from the context of research interviews, similarly marked by power asymmetries (Salazar-Orvig & Grossen, 2008). Here, the individual migrant is placed in the role of a patient-participant object, in the face of an arguably more socially powerful professional subject aiming to scrutinize the most intimate details of their life history. It risks being an inherently shameful encounter, exacerbating extreme feelings of powerlessness, degradation, and humiliation. However, as noted by Wilson and colleagues (2006), shame is a two-way street; it can exist in the patient and therapist at the same time in different intra-psychic configurations. Working with the complexities of shame in the posttraumatic self, both patient and therapist (and arguably, participant and researcher) share a common ground of human vulnerability whose management likely determines the quality of outcome. As we have illustrated elsewhere in the case of research among survivors of sexual abuse (Womersley et al., 2011), shame pervades the entirety of the relationship. It is contagious. All are affected. As much as the identity of a victim, an asylum seeker, an oppressed ethnic minority may be shaming for the migrant, the identity of the oppressor, the colonizer, the privileged ethnic elite, may be shaming for the clinician or researcher.

We need to consider shame in the context of work with vulnerable migrant populations—not only because it may influence our professional work in profound yet often barely perceptible ways, it is our ethical duty as human beings to reflect on these intersubjective encounters. In order to reflect on some concrete case examples of the ways in which shame may manifest in such encounters, and on some applications in dealing with shame constructively, I draw on my work with asylum seekers and refugees in a centre for victims of torture in Athens.

8.2   Contextual Description

As the "reception crisis" continues unabated, Greece remains one of the first ports of sanctuary. While the country is still gripped by one of the worst financial and societal crises of the past 40 years, little attention or funding is available to provide mental health and psychosocial support to refugees (Gkionakis, 2016). Many torture survivors in Greece, only some of whom having been identified as vulnerable, are still trapped on the islands, a context characterized by a lack of specialised medical care and poor living conditions (Farmakopoulou, Triantafyllou, & Kolaitis, 2017; Kadianaki, 2014; Kotsioni, 2016; Maniadaki & Kakouros, 2008). Other torture survivors who have moved to the mainland without permission have also found themselves in limbo, unable to proceed with their asylum claim. The sources of shame within this context are many: from the Greek citizens themselves who may be ashamed of the poor reception conditions, of not being able to do more to help, of the inadequate institutional structures and hostile reactions to foreigners on the part of their compatriots, of not being up to "civilised" Western European standards; to the asylum seekers suddenly finding themselves in an incredibly precarious and vulnerable position, having lost many aspects of their valued social identity linked to their country of origin (Farmakopoulou et al., 2017; Gkionakis, 2016; Kotsioni, 2016).

In this particular context, I conducted participative research in a centre for victims of torture in Athens. Having worked in the humanitarian sector for years, my aim was to study the influence of the sociocultural context on trauma. This involved three months of participative observation with the medical team of the centre: participating in the team's daily morning meetings and group therapy activities, facilitating psycho-education sessions for the beneficiaries of the project, and teaching English in the centre twice a week. My research also involved conducting qualitative interviews with beneficiaries, the health professionals themselves as well as "community representatives"—leaders of the various refugee communities around Athens. It was thus a complex mixture of being both a clinician and a researcher, requiring an on-going negotiation of these multiple identities.

The beneficiaries of this particular project were identified as "vulnerable"—victims of torture in their countries of origin and in particular need of multidisciplinary care. They came from all over the world, notably regions affected by conflict. The team, offering mental health support, physiotherapy, and medical care, worked in collaboration with social workers and lawyers who were assisting the beneficiaries in their request for asylum. The needs were many, varied yet interrelated. An accompanying team of cultural mediators was required—not only for translation but as mediators of this new and complex medico-legal system with which people were confronted.

The use of the term "beneficiaries" to refer to the individuals coming to the clinic, as opposed to others such as "patients" or "asylum seekers" or "victims of torture" was a deliberate one. When the project opened, all individuals would all be presented with a "patient" card, that is until one individual refused to take his. It was, he said, not how he chose to identify. The word "patient" evoked a deep sense of shame. He felt that it implied a victimizing and humiliating identity. He was neither, he had insisted, a patient nor a victim—but an individual in his own right.

It became apparent, during the course of my time as a participant researcher in this context, that it was not only trauma, but also shame, which pervaded the space—with significant and potentially destructive implications for the micro-interactions among the health professionals and the beneficiaries. It was present in the daily meetings, where professionals kept expressing a feeling that they were not "good enough," not doing enough to help the beneficiary find work or shelter, not feeling experienced enough to handle the complexity of the needs of the vulnerable population with whom they were working, ashamed of belonging to a country where the structures supposedly in place to assist the migrants where not meeting their needs. The result appeared to be either an increased or decreased commitment to the work, a feeling of anger which incited a call to action, to respond to the need in front of them—or a resignation, a feeling that they had very little power to effect concrete changes in the lives of the beneficiaries.

As for the beneficiaries of the project, the shame was even more apparent. Finding themselves at the clinic, unable to help themselves and at the mercy of the team of professionals there to help them, ashamed of not being able to support their families financially, of not having met their aspirations of "succeeding" in Europe, ashamed of the humiliating and horrific experiences which they had endured, of how they may have compromised their perceived moral integrity in order to survive, of not being able to fully master the language nor the cultural nuances of their new environment … this was the shame in some way linked to the identity of "victim." The result, often, was a need to hide oneself, to not want to be seen entering the clinic for fear of the stigma attached to being a victim of torture, to mask aspects of their narratives, to not want to answer the professional's questions directly for fear of certain aspects of their lives being exposed or not believed. It resulted in different versions of their life story being told to different professionals. It resulted in many not wanting to see the psychologist as a result of the shame of being identified as "crazy." It resulted in quiet waiting rooms, where the silence among the various beneficiaries may have been out of respect for shame—for not wanting to expose each other as victims.

Shame was similarly present within the intersubjective space between myself, the health professionals, and the beneficiaries/participants. As noted above, I came as both a researcher and a clinician, an active participant in the space. I was both part of the team, yet in many ways a detached third party observer. Other aspects of my identity were similarly present, becoming more or less salient within the micro-interactions. I am South African. Therefore, as so often raised by the beneficiaries of African origin, I am "an African sister." One of "us." Yet, unlike the rest of "us"—I have white skin, I am not subject to the same degrading or humiliating micro-instances of racism so many experience when coming to Europe. Unlike them, I am "legitimized" in my right to be there, to pass unnoticed in the streets, to move freely around Europe. I am in the privileged position of the professional—I have the right to observe, to direct, to interrogate, to pose questions. I am also a woman, like some and not others. As we have explored elsewhere in reflecting on working with South African survivors of rape (Womersley et al., 2011)—the shame linked to the similarities and differences across marks of identity, so boldly and unavoidably expressed through our bodies, is a fundamental part of the interaction between researcher and researched in the context of qualitative interviews being conducted, particularly among vulnerable populations and particularly when exploring the sensitive topic of trauma.

To explore the myriad manifestations of shame—not belonging to the Self or Other but in the intersubjective space between all of these actors—I present a case study of one beneficiary with whom I had multiple interviews over the course of a year. I intend this to be an illustrative case study which may allow us to track the manifestations of shame as it arose in the interactions between us. It is representative of many of the interviews conducted during this period, and, hopefully, representative of so many qualitative interviews being conducted by qualitative interviewers in multicultural settings across the world. Reflecting on these micro-instances of shame, being able to first of all track it and second of all, through this awareness, allow this reflexivity to influence the way in which we interact with the participants whom we interview in qualitative research, is an ethical obligation. It is our responsibility as researchers, and as human beings.

8.3   Applies Approach to Dealing with Shame: The Case of Sylvain

Sylvain is a 35 year old refugee from the Ivory Coast, a beneficiary of the centre for victims of torture in Athens and a participant in my research with whom I conducted five qualitative interviews over the course of the year. Interviews were conducted in French without the use of a translator. However, this is not to say that we were not each interpreting, in our own way, the words of the other. My interpretation and analysis of his words necessarily remain just that—an interpretation necessarily informed by my own culturally determined frames of reference. Our work together is presented as a study on the myriad of ways in which shame was both manifested, and subsequently transformed, during this period. To analyse the case, instances of manifestations of shame in our interaction were identified in the transcripts, and subsequently grouped according to emerging overarching themes. Four identified sources of shame are presented, accompanied by some reflections on implications for transformation.

8.3.1   The Shame of Dependence

During our first interview, Sylvain described his situation as the following:

> Often we are confronted with strangers, and they mistreat us… when he can help you today, it is in two or three weeks that he will help you. They like to play with people, come and go… You go there and you are told to come back where you left first. It is not easy. But we understand them, we have to accept them, otherwise, it's dangerous […] but we have to accept it is life, it hurts, it's stressful, it's hard, but when you're out there, we have to accept.

His shame appeared to have been related to being in the vulnerable position of dependence on the help of others, others who may well "mistreat us." Interestingly enough, the "mistreatment" to which he referred was not related to the many instances of racism he reported, nor to the fact that he was handcuffed by the police and thrown in prison without apparent just cause. Rather, he referred to the people who "play," who "come and go." In other words, the mistreatment he referred to is that which he encountered among those meant to "help"—humanitarian aid workers, state social services, medical professionals etc. This, in turn, evoked in me a sense of shame of being somehow related to those who only help "when they can." Despite my role as an independent researcher, I was still connected to the clinic where he came for assistance. I was aware of this throughout my fieldwork in Athens. In 2015 and 2016, it was a context characterised by a plethora of well-meaning humanitarian workers coming to assist refugees for short periods of time. So many of the asylum seekers with whom I spoke referred to this phenomenon of what I call "trauma tourism"—painting a picture of people arriving, asking questions, offering to help, and then leaving without fulfilling promises of further assistance (Pittaway, Bartolomei, & Hugman, 2010).

8.4 Implications for Transformation

Sylvain's words offer a sobering reminder of the way in which the shame associated with being dependant on the assistance of others may be transformed through simply being (a) attentive to and aware of the possible impact of shame and (b) aware of the responsibility to avoid "playing" with vulnerable populations, to not just "come and go." I would argue that part of the transformation of Sylvain's shame, particularly shame related to this experience of being dependant on external aid, came through the consistent relationships he was able to form with staff at the centre over a period of two years. In our own relationship, it was linked to the fact that I kept to our agreed meeting schedule and consistently returned over the period of a year. It lay in simple details, such as allowing him to choose the time and place of our meetings together—a change compared to the treatment he reported encountering in his dealing with bureaucratic state institutions where he was often left to wait for hours, only to have the appointment delayed by months. Such basic signs of respect seem to have had a transformative impact on his own shame. This allowed for a subtle reshifting of the balance of power in our relationship, allowing my own shame in turn to be transformed in the context of a more equal relationship of mutual respect and "social recognition" (Marková, 2016).

8.4.1 The Shame of Social Discrimination

Throughout our five meetings together, Sylvain reported feeling ashamed at the way in which as an asylum seeker he way he was treated as a "criminal" by a variety of actors, including the police:

> We start from a good one to frustrate you somewhere, and we fled the violence in Africa, arrived in a country where we say there is the human right, you come to sleep in the things that… I am in Greece I have known handcuffs, it is in Greece I have known handcuffs […] Because they say I don't have papers. Is an unregistered person a criminal? […]
>
> it's the things we keep in our hearts, in the prison, the police can hit you…

He also noted facing discrimination by not only local Greek populations, but other migrant communities. In reflecting on this, he highlighted my identity as a white person:

> You're South African, where we are sitting, a lot of people think you're European. So you see, but me seeing myself […] You go to immigration, they say, you wait and give priority to others.

Despite us both being African, a fundamental difference is the colour of our skin. Both physically, and also in terms of cultural identity, I am able to pass as European, he is not. I felt ashamed of this identity: of being unwittingly complicit in my "fellow European's" discrimination against others. I felt the need to apologise on behalf of "Europeans"—regardless of whether or not I identified with this group. His words are testament to the very present psychic consequences of shame and the accompanying feelings of envy seen in the context of deprivation and powerlessness as well as in the ubiquitous (and often unspeakable) presence of racial trauma (Harris, 2000).

8.5 Implications for Transformation

In outlining his experiences of racism and discrimination encountered in Europe, Sylvain stated the following:

> He [a European] does not distinguish you, he says, "The immigrants." But it's not just immigrants.

His words hint at the shame of a loss of individual identity in favour of being seen as "an immigrant." He contested this notion of being "just immigrants," in favour of being "distinguished"—in other words, of being seen and recognised as a complete and complex individual self. I would argue that the implications for transforming shame related to such social discrimination lie in the need for individual aspects of identity to be made visible, recognised, and valued. In exploring this, we similarly cannot ignore our own sense of shame related to being in a position of social privilege. Here, what seemed to have had a transformative impact on Sylvain's shame was my recognition of it. I needed both to be aware of my own shame linked to social privilege, and to recognise and respect his shame related to social discrimination.

8.5.1   The Shame of Being Unemployed

Throughout the year in which we met, Sylvain referred multiple times to the shame he felt at not being able to provide for his family back home who where waiting for his financial assistance. The shame he felt at not being able to meet their expectations eventually got to the point where he stopped answering their phone calls. He did miss them, he explained to me, but he couldn't face the shame of being unemployed (see Ungerer's chapter in this book) and unable to help:

> Tomorrow when you succeed, you will be the pride of the family: the family and the whole village. But when you become a delinquent, it's [a shame for] the father and mother. These are things you don't really want to talk about.

He reported feeling frozen in time, unable to move on with his life and contribute as a productive member of society. Jobless, he felt "worthless," a delinquent who eventually turned to illegal activities in order to make money:

> The situation in Greece here, if you're not morally strong, it can make you do some bad things. It is not easy. We live like we never existed […] I'm starting to do bad things. When you become envious, you're exposed to everything. And the easiest thing in Greece is selling drugs.

The shame of being unemployed (Buggenhagen, 2012, see also Mayer "*Working with Shame through Symbols and Active Imagination: The Case of an unemployed high achiever*" in this book) was therefore double-edged: not only was there shame around being "useless" to society, in other words a "delinquent" family member unable to provide—the situation as an inexistent persona non grata lead him to conduct himself in "shameful" ways which previously would have been unthinkable. The behaviour seems to have been judged as immoral not only by others but by himself, a deep source of shame at the interpersonal bridge between himself and his social world. He was led further and further into the metaphorical shadows of society.

8.6   Implications for Transformation

Sylvain eventually did find legal work, and the transformative effect on his mental health was remarkable. Not only had his material conditions improved, he felt somehow more legitimate in his environment. He had become an active contributor to society, able to take the bus in the morning along with others heading to work, able to share the little that he had with friends and family, able to "show his face" in public. The fact of being employed seemed to lessen his sense of shame more than any other factor. As concisely and poignantly stated by Buggenhagen (2012), "money takes care of shame."

The shame surrounding Sylvain's unemployment serves as important reminder of the embeddedness of this emotion within a socioeconomic context. In my role as researcher, my primary focus was evidently on his psychological state of mind. However, it became abundantly apparent in interviews, with him and other asylum seekers, that this was significantly dependant on his social and economic environment. His sense of self-worth, relationship with family, socioeconomic status and the material conditions in which he found himself, all mutually reinforced the sense of shame about which he spoke so openly. We may not always have the capacity to effect changes in the socioeconomic lives of the people with whom we interact as clinicians and researchers. We can, however, reflect on this shame in our interactions. This could mean, for example, breaking our professional/ethical codes of conduct to accept gifts which we know individuals can ill-afford but for whom it is a point of pride. It means having the courage to address the sensitive topic of money when raised. Practitioners and researchers working with this population cannot ignore this incredibly salient aspect of shame. To do so risks, in many ways, reinforcing a social silence that so often fosters shame.

8.7   Concluding Remarks

Shame is manifest on the micro-level of our daily interactions and cannot be separated from the complex matrix of gender, ethnicity and socio-economic class informing our public identities, which are so boldly reflected through our bodies. What did shame obscure, prevent or facilitate within this space between myself and Sylvain? What are the implications of this noxious affect for reflexive research, particularly with refugee populations? The above reflections intend not only to shed some light on the role of shame in the research relationship which unfolded but to consider the way in which it was intrinsically linked to the representations of our multiple and constantly shifting identities (Burman, 2006; Gray, 2008). It is clear that both the psychologist and the client's individual shame, as well as the shame which they co-construct within the intersubjective space, play an integral part of the therapeutic process. Similarly, reflexive qualitative research should also take into consideration the powerful impact of this affect within the research relationship.

References

Bhimji, F. (2015). Collaborations and performative agency in refugee theater in Germany. *Journal of Immigrant & Refugee Studies*, 1–23.
Buggenhagen, B. A. (2012). *Muslim families in global senegal: Money takes care of shame*. Indiana University Press.
Burman, E. (2006). Emotions and reflexivity in feminised education action research. *Educational Action Research, 14*(3), 315–332.
Farmakopoulou, I., Triantafyllou, K., & Kolaitis, G. (2017). Refugee children and adolescents in Greece: Two case reports. *European Journal of Psychotraumatology, 8*(sup4), 1351179.

Gkionakis, N. (2016). The refugee crisis in Greece: Training border security, police, volunteers and aid workers in psychological first aid. *Intervention, 14*(1), 73–79. Retrieved from https://doi.org/10.1097/wtf.0000000000000104.

Goguikian Ratcliff, B., Bolzman, C., & Gakuba, T. (2014). Déqualification des femmes migrantes en Suisse: mécanismes sous-jacents et effets psychologiques. *Alterstice, 4*(2), 63–76.

Goldsmith, R. E., Martin, C. G., & Smith, C. P. (2014). *Systemic trauma*. Taylor & Francis.

Gray, B. (2008). Putting emotion and reflexivity to work in researching migration. *Sociology, 42*(5), 935–952.

Grzanka, P. R., Santos, C. E., & Moradi, B. (2017). Intersectionality research in counseling psychology. *Journal of Counseling Psychology, 64*(5), 453.

Harris, A. (2000). Haunted talk, healing action: Commentary on paper by Kimberlyn Leary. *Psychoanalytic Dialogues, 10*(4), 655–662.

Hecker, T., Braitmayer, L., & van Duijl, M. (2015). Global mental health and trauma exposure: The current evidence for the relationship between traumatic experiences and spirit possession. *European Journal of Psychotraumatology, 6*.

Hodges-Wu, J., & Zajicek-Farber, M. (2017). Addressing the needs of survivors of torture: A pilot test of the psychosocial well-being index. *Journal of Immigrant & Refugee Studies, 15*(1), 71–89.

Kadianaki, I. (2014). The transformative effects of stigma: Coping strategies as meaning-making efforts for immigrants living in Greece. *Journal of Community & Applied Social Psychology, 24*(2), 125–138.

Kaufman, G. (1989). *The psychology of shame. Theory and treatment of shame-based syndromes.* New York: Springer.

Kotsioni, I. (2016). *Rehabilitation for survivors of torture and other forms of ill-treatment in Athens, Greece—Responding to a protracted refugee crisis.* Paper presented at the 4th MSF Workshop on the thematic of torture: Caring for the human beyond the torture Rome, Italy.

Li, S. S., Liddell, B. J., & Nickerson, A. (2016). The relationship between post-migration stress and psychological disorders in refugees and asylum seekers. *Current Psychiatry Reports, 18*(9), 82.

Maercker, A., & Hecker, T. (2016). Broadening perspectives on trauma and recovery: A socio-interpersonal view of PTSD. *European journal of psychotraumatology, 7*.

Maier, T., & Straub, M. (2011). "My head is like a bag full of rubbish": Concepts of illness and treatment expectations in traumatized migrants. *Qualitative Health Research, 21*(2), 233–248.

Maniadaki, K., & Kakouros, E. (2008). Social and mental health profiles of young male offenders in detention in Greece. *Criminal Behaviour & Mental Health, 18,* 207–215. https://doi.org/10.1002/cbm.698.

Marková, I. (2016). *The dialogical mind: Common sense and ethics.* Cambridge University Press.

Matos, M., & Pinto-Gouveia, J. (2010). Shame as a traumatic memory. *Clinical psychology & psychotherapy, 17*(4), 299–312.

Moradi, B. (2017). *(Re)focusing intersectionality: From social identities back to systems of oppression and privilege.*

Pittaway, E., Bartolomei, L., & Hugman, R. (2010). 'Stop stealing our stories': The ethics of research with vulnerable groups. *Journal of human rights practice, 2*(2), 229–251.

Salazar-Orvig, A., & Grossen, M. (2008). Le dialogisme dans l'entretien clinique. *Langage et société* (1), 37–52.

Sanchez-Mazas, M., Efionayi-Mäder, D., Maggi, J., Achermann, C., Schaer, M., Escoda, R. I., & Coumou-Stants, F. (2011). La construction de l'invisibilité: suppression de l'aide sociale dans le domaine de l'asile.

Sironi, F. (1999). *Bourreaux et victimes: psychologie de la torture.* Odile Jacob.

Slewa-Younan, S., Yaser, A., Guajardo, M. G. U., Mannan, H., Smith, C. A., & Mond, J. M. (2017). The mental health and help-seeking behaviour of resettled Afghan refugees in Australia. *International Journal of Mental Health Systems, 11*(1), 49.

Swartz, M. J. (1988). Shame, culture, and status among the Swahili of Mombasa. *Ethos, 16*(1), 21–51.

Torre, L. D. (2016). The Sans-Papiers. In L. D. Torre (Ed.), *National centre of competence in research—The migration-mobility nexus* (Vol. 2016). Retrieved from http://blog.nccr-onthemove. ch/the-sans-papiers/?lang=fr. NCCR On the Move.

Turrini, G., Purgato, M., Ballette, F., Nosè, M., Ostuzzi, G., & Barbui, C. (2017). Common mental disorders in asylum seekers and refugees: Umbrella review of prevalence and intervention studies. *International Journal of Mental Health Systems, 11*(1), 51.

UNHCR. (2017). *Statistical Yearbooks: Figures at a Glance*. Retrieved from http://www.unhcr.org/ figures-at-a-glance.html on 08/05/2018.

Viñar, M. N. (2005). La spécificité de la torture comme source de trauma. *Revue française de psychanalyse, 69*(4), 1205–1224.

Wilson, J. P., Droždek, B., & Turkovic, S. (2006). Posttraumatic shame and guilt. *Trauma, Violence, & Abuse, 7*(2), 122–141.

Wilson, J. P., Wilson, J. P., & Drozdek, B. (2004). *Broken spirits: The treatment of traumatized asylum seekers, refugees and war and torture victims*. Routledge.

Womersley, G., Kloetzer, L., Van den Bergh, R., Venables, E., Severy, N., Gkionakis, N. … Zamatto, F. (submitted). "My mind is not like before": Psychosocial rehabilitation of victims of torture and other forms of ill-treatment in Athens *Torture Journal*.

Womersley, G., Maw, A., & Swartz, S. (2011). The construction of shame in Feminist reflexive practice and its manifestations in a research relationship. *Qualitative Inquiry, 17*(9), 876–886.

Wong, Y., & Tsai, J. (2007). Cultural models of shame and guilt. In *The self-conscious emotions: Theory and research* (pp. 209–223).

Gail Womersley is based at the University of Neuchâtel, where she is currently engaged in a research project working with refugee victims of torture in Athens, Greece. Before joining the university, she worked with Médecins Sans Frontières as a clinical psychologist in projects assisting refugee and internally displaced populations in South Sudan, the Central African Republic, Ukraine, Zimbabwe and the Democratic Republic of Congo. She has also worked with other nongovernmental organizations in Israel and the United Kingdom, as well as for the Department of Health and the Department of Defense in South Africa. She is particularly interested in cross-cultural manifestations of trauma and its implications for legal and social policy as well as clinical practice.

Chapter 9
Crime and Shame: Reflections and Culture-Specific Insights

Claude-Hélène Mayer

Abstract Shame and shaming are highly important aspects of the study of crime, crime sciences and criminal and restorative justice. This chapter takes selected aspects into account and presents the state-of-the-art in research and practice regarding four questions: (1) How are experiences of shame, crime and criminal behaviour related? (2) What effect does shaming (sanctions) have in criminal law and regulatory systems? (3) What is reintegrative shaming in the context of crime and criminal justice and how does it impact on crime? (4) How does culture impact on the topics of shame and shaming in the context of criminal law, justice and criminal (risky) behaviour? The chapter concludes by presenting questions for reflections on crime and shame with regard to (1) individuals and groups, (2) family members, relatives and friends affected by criminal behaviour/offender behaviour and (3) professionals (such as therapists, psychologists, mediators, lawyers) working with criminals, offenders and lawbreakers in the context of crime and shame.

Keywords Crime science · Criminal justice · Crime · Shame · Shame sentences · Reintegrative shaming · Culture

9.1 Introduction

Many studies have agreed that shame affects emotional and social well-being (Mayer, Viviers, & Tonelli, 2017; Vanderheiden & Mayer, 2017). The experience of shame implies that a person did something bad or wrong and is usually accompanied by feeling worthless and small, powerless and exposed (Tangney, 1993). Shame further impacts on psychological symptoms, the level of self-esteem, predisposition to anger and aggression, and the capacity for empathy (see Tangney, Wagner, Hill-Barlow, Marschall, & Gramzow, 1996).

C.-H. Mayer (✉)
Institut für Therapeutische Kommunikation und Sprachgebrauch, Europa Universität Viadrina, Logenstrasse 11, 15230 Frankfurt (Oder), Germany
e-mail: claudemayer@gmx.net

Department of Management, Rhodes University, Drosdy Road, Grahamstown 6139, South Africa

© Springer Nature Switzerland AG 2019   117
C.-H. Mayer and E. Vanderheiden (eds.), *The Bright Side of Shame*,
https://doi.org/10.1007/978-3-030-13409-9_9

But how do crime and shame relate to each other, if at all? And, if so, in which contexts do crime and shame play a role?

This chapter presents a brief overview of the interconnections of crime and shame in research and practice. The following topics are explored:

1. How are experiences of shame, crime and criminal behaviour related?
   In previous research and studies, it has been argued that crime and shame are interlinked and that certain levels of shame and shame-proneness can even predict tendencies to criminal behaviour. The chapter will present state-of-the art research findings.
2. What effect does shaming (sanctions) have in criminal law and regulatory systems?
   The chapter takes the theory and practice of shaming in the context of crime prevention, criminal law and regulatory systems into account and presents different standpoints.
3. What is "reintegrative shaming" in the context of crime and criminal behaviour and how does it impact on crime?
   In the chapter, the concept of reintegrative shaming (Braithwaite, 1989, expanded in 2001) will be presented and explained.
4. How does culture impact on the topics of shame and shaming in the context of criminal law, justice and criminal (risky) behaviour?
   Examples of culture-specific insights of how to deal with shame and shaming in specific contexts will be presented and discussed.

Generally, research on shame, crime, criminal and risky behaviour, as well as on criminal justice and restorative practice has less frequently been explored than shame and its psychological and/or health-related impact (Stuewig et al., 2015). There is a need for further research, studies and theoretical and practical discourses on these topics (Harris, 2017).

9.2   The Context

This chapter aims to create an awareness of how shame and shaming impacts on the broader context of crime and therefore explores the four selected areas described above. Brief overviews and insights into the topics will be provided, leading to reflexive questions on shame and crime to be used in different situations and within the following specific contextual viewpoints:

1. From an individual intra-psychological viewpoint;
2. From the viewpoint of an affected family member, relative or friend;
3. From the viewpoint of a professional working in the context of shame and crime (for example, in restorative justice, victim-offender mediation, therapeutical practice, or forensic psychology).

The reflective questions posed should create awareness and context-specific, stimulating ideas in order to rethink crime and shame from different perspectives.

In the following, I will now present the theoretical background with regard to the questions posed above.

9.2.1 How Are Experiences of Shame, Crime and Criminal Behaviour Related?

Early research on shame has pointed out that experiences of shame often lead individuals to externalise blame and anger outward, projecting it onto an external source (Tangney, 1993), such as, for example, another person. Shame experiences might even lead to destructive actions, irrational anger and strong aggression (Tangney et al., 1996). This often happens in order for the individual to regain control. Several studies have indicated that it can even strongly interlink with overt physical aggression (Stuewig, Tangney, Heigel, Harty, & McCloskey, 2010).

In a sample of jail inmates, a research study by Dearing, Stuewig and Tangney (2005) showed that shame-proneness is consistently linked to both drug problems and alcohol. This connects to another study which emphasises that experienced levels of shame-proneness in childhood and adolescence predict alcohol and drug misuse later in life; high levels of shame in childhood lead to alcohol, heroine and hallucinogen consumption later in life (Tangney & Dearing, 2002).

Based on previous research focused on shame and criminal behaviour, Tibbetts (1997, 2003) has pointed out that anticipated shame leads students to the intention to drink and drive or shoplift (but shame-proneness does not), while the later study found that an overall shame-proneness does not relate to illegal behaviour.

Tangney and Dearing (2002) point out that shame-proneness does not predict arrests and convictions. However, in a study from 2015, Stuewig, Tangney, Kendall, Folk, Mayer and Dearing highlight that shame-proneneness in childhood is a risk factor for deviant behaviour in later life and, for example, illegal drug use in young adulthood.

Very few studies focus on shame-proneneess and risky sexual behaviour and/or sexual abuse. Shame-proneness seems unrelated to risky sexual behaviour, such as taking risks to contract sexually transmitted diseases (Stuewig, Tangney, Mashek, Forkner, & Dearing, 2009).

Stuewig et al. (2015) emphasise that the empirical data and the relationship of shame and criminal, delinquent and anti-social behaviour are inconsistent, meaning that some studies show relationships whilst others do not show relationships. However, in a long-term study, the authors (Stuewig et al., 2015) found that shame in childhood positively predicts risky behaviour later in young adulthood and is connected to less developed interpersonal problem-solving skills which might lead to increased anti-social behaviour.

As the literature review shows, shame, crime and criminal behaviour still need to be researched further in terms of exploring how shame impacts on criminal and delinquent behaviour, which cultures and societies it affects and how, what the individual and cultural mechanisms on the unconscious levels are to interlink patterns of shame and crime, how do different kinds of shame operate, and how can they be transformed.

In the following, the focus will be on shaming in criminal law.

9.2.2 What Effect Does Shaming (Sanctions) Have in Criminal Law and Regulatory Systems?

Not only have researchers focused on the impact of shame on crime, but they have also evaluated the efficacy of shaming sanctions in criminal law and regulatory systems, particularly in the US from the 1980s and 1990s onwards. The question has been posed how mechanisms of shaming can deter crime and rehabilitate criminals (Harvard Law Review Association, 2003).

Braithwaite (1989: 100) defines shaming as

> all societal processes of expressing social disapproval which have the intention or effect of invoking remorse in the person being shamed and/or condemnation by others who become aware of the shaming.

According to Harris (2017), shaming has a high value in the context of regulatory systems due to its educative approach, the re-affirmation of values and the idea of what is wrong and what is right. At the same time, however, shaming practices and sanctions also raise concerns, particularly when shaming practices are contrary to restorative justice[1] approaches and are used to punish offenders in court through "shame sentences".

Shame sentences have been used in US-systems in which offenders do not spend a long time in jail, but have to take (public) actions in which they are publicly shamed. Particularly during recent years, shaming sentences in which offenders are humiliated publicly are on the rise (Reutter, 2015). Goldman (2015) describes a case in which a mail thief was sentenced to stand in front of a mail office for eight hours holding a sign indicating that he had stolen mail. Goldman (2015) also highlights how shaming punishments are already in print media, publicly listing the names of offenders. Goldman (2015) suggests that it may just be a question of time before shaming sentences include the use of social media to shame offenders through online-systems. According to Goldman (2015), the mail thief stole mail a second time soon after his shaming punishment; it remains an open question how rehabilitation of offenders

---

[1] Restorative justice focuses on crime less as a violation of the law, legal processes, and punishment of the offender, but rather on the emphasis that crime harms individuals as well as the community and therefore needs to include the promotion of accountability and repair (Garland, 2001). The focus is here on the violation of the individual and the community, not as much on the state. Therefore offenders are encouraged to take responsibility and action to repair harm (Braithwaite, 1989).

is best accomplished. Although shaming punishment has a long tradition in the US criminal law and justice system, uncertainty remains concerning the effectiveness of shaming punishments and their particular contribution to rehabilitation.

Arguments which are for public shaming, usually mention the cost-effectiveness, prevention of the indoctrination into a criminal culture, expression of appropriate moral condemnation, and the reflection of accurate societal values. The discourses against shaming sanctions usually include their anticipated failure owing to lack of necessary societal conditions, the inhumanity of shaming punishments, the violation of egalitarian values, the inappropriate inciting of the public, as well as the uncertain psychological effects of public shaming punishments (Goldman, 2015).

The use of shaming punishments and their effects have not been evaluated and cannot be predicted (Condry, 2007). Taking into account research on the effects of experienced shame in childhood and the possible effects on delinquent behaviour later in life, shaming sentences installed by the criminal justice system should be taken into critical consideration and certainly can only be evaluated within the sociocultural contexts of the society.

After having explored shaming sentences as a concept to reach offender rehabilitation, I now focus on other ways of dealing with shame within the context of crime and criminal behaviour.

9.2.3 What Is Reintegrative Shaming in the Context of Crime and Criminal Justice and How Does It Impact?

Braithwaite (1989, 2000) has developed a theory of crime, shame and reintegration, referring to the concept of "reintegrative shaming". This theory reasons that societies have lower crime rates if they communicate shame about crime effectively. At the same time, it has been pointed out that violent behaviour increases if it is not defined as being shameful (Braithwaite, 2000). Braithwaite (2000) emphasises that communicating shamefulness of crime can also contribute to increasing crime when the communication is stigmatising. This would mean that an offender is personally stigmatised in the context of inadequate behaviour, and that the offence is ascribed to the person's personality. In this case, the offence becomes part of the identity and of the person.

Tangney, Stuewig and Hafez (2011) highlight that shame is experienced as a highly disruptive emotion because the self becomes the object of judgement and not the behaviour. A healthy way of communicating shame in the context of crime is, according to Braithwaite (2000), to use a practice of reintegrative shaming which is connected to communicating shame in such a way that it encourages the criminal, offender or delinquent to behave differently. In this case, the disapproval of certain behaviour is communicated, while the delinquent is still respected as a person.

Murphy and Harris (2007) conducted a study on white-collar crime, particularly on tax offenders. Their results concur with Braithwaite's (1989, 2000) theory, supporting the idea that reintegrative shaming leads to lower rates of reoffending, while stigmatisation and stigmatised shaming (as, for example, practised in shaming punishments and sentences) leads to greater rates of reoffending.

Stuewig et al. (2015) reflect on managing shame constructively (within the broader context of reintegrative shaming) to lower the possibility of creating risky behaviour in later young adult life based on childhood shame experiences. Guilt fosters moral behaviour to the benefit of the individual, through the ability to take responsibility for one's own actions. Because there is less likelihood of creating defensiveness, denial and externalisation of blame (in comparison to shame), guilt seems to be the easier emotion to deal with. It appears that the experience of guilt rather leads to adaptive decision-making and problem-solving strategies in interpersonal relationships, and is therefore easier to deal with than shame (Stuewig et al., 2015). The authors suggest that a deeper understanding of the concepts and how they play out across the lifespan is needed to develop an increased knowledge and understanding of pathways to reduce risky behaviour.

Shame represents a critical stepping-stone in the rehabilitation process of offenders in which concepts of reintegrative and disintegrative shaming needs to be differentiated (Tangney et al., 2011). In the interdisciplinary context of criminology, sociology and psychology, discourses on shaming have indicated that restorative justice draws strongly on the concept of reintegrative shaming, while the dangers of reintegrative shaming have been raised and highlighted (Harris, 2017). For Braithwaite (1989), reintegrative shaming includes respectful communication which distinguishes between the action and the person, and which concludes with forgiveness or decertification of deviance to avoid the taking on of a negative master status trait (Harris, 2017, 61).

Reintegrative shaming has, according to Harris (2017), been explored in many regulatory systems such as in school conflicts, workplace bullying, tax evasion, business regulation or sexual offending; however, it has been applied and developed mainly in restorative justice programmes, for example in criminal justice, child protection, prisons or schools. Particularly in restorative justice interventions, it is assumed that an offence creates an obligation for offenders to repair the harm that was caused to others (Zehr, 1990), thereby turning away from the traditional punishment and turning towards a higher degree of reconciliation, reparation and restoration.

But would reintegrative shaming work in different cultural contexts? This will be explored next.

9.2.4 How Does Culture Impact on the Topics of Shame and Shaming in the Context of Criminal Law, Justice and Criminal (Risky) Behaviour?

Braithwaite (1989) has argued with regard to cultural contexts, that in communitarian societies, offenders are easily reintegrated by shaming the offence without stigmatising the offender. Braithwaite (2000) further highlights that in traditional African societies, as well as in First Nations of North American cultures, reintegrative shaming often takes place, while Western societies seem rather to stigmatise offenders or criminals. Baumer, Wright, Kristinsdottir and Gunnlaugsson (2002) point out that Iceland is, to a large degree, a communitarian society which heavily relies on shaming as a method of social control. The authors argue that in terms of recidivism, Iceland should have lower rates than less socially integrated societies, which in fact it does not have. Harris (2017) however points out that healing circles, as often traditionally used by First Nation peoples of North America, as well as family group conferences or victim–offender mediation in Western contexts, are interlinked critically with developing an individual conscience and commitment to law. They represent a cultural concept of dealing with shame on a constructive and healthy level, but focusing on the topic as offending, not on the person.

What kind of crime is viewed as shameful usually relates to the culture, to the definition of power within a society and to value concepts. If, for example, crime hits the powerless individuals of societies, the offending might not be judged as very shameful. In organisations, for example, in which workers do not have a say or a lobby, occupational health crimes might not be defined as shameful (Braithwaite, 2000).

9.3 Managing Shame in a Healthy Way

Ahmed et al. (2001) points out that acknowledged shame which an individual can accept and can take responsibility for, usually reduces negative feelings and supports the individual to manage these accompanying feelings constructively. The awareness of shame is therefore a first step in managing it in a positive way. Further, if shame is managed in a reintegrative way, it usually increases compliance and decreases re-offence (Braithwaite, 1989). Further in the process, shame management stimulates an increase in moral engagement, thereby positively and proactively affecting leading discourses on shame (Harris, 2017). It is therefore more likely that shame can be acknowledged and resolved, leading to promoting empathy, remorse and reparation (Harris, 2017).

In the following section, managing shame constructively in the context of crime will be addressed through questions regarding different viewpoints and perspectives. These questions can be used by individuals, or as reflective questions for group discussions, for example, in educational contexts. They can also be used by professionals working with shame in the context of crime.

9.4 Application: Reflections on Crime, Criminal Behaviour, and Restorative Justice Within the Context of Shame and Shaming

The following questions can be used to guide intrapersonal reflections, interpersonal reflections (such as in the context of affected family members or friends), and in professional contexts, to guide individual and group reflections (intra- and interpersonal) on shame in the context of crime.

9.4.1 From an Individual Intra-Psychological Viewpoint

9.4.1.1 Crime and Shame

- What do you think about the interlinkages of shame and crime?
- Which crimes do you judge as shameful, and which as not shameful?

9.4.1.2 Shaming Sanctions

- What do you think about shaming sanctions?
- How do you feel about them?
- Should they be used, or should they not be used?
- If yes, in which way should they be used (which kind of offenders, which kind of criminal offences)?
- What do you think is the most important argument for or against shaming sanctions?
- In your country of origin—or in the country in which you live—how is shaming used in the context of crime and criminal justice?

9.4.1.3 Reintegrative Shaming and Restorative Justice

- What do you think about the Braithwaite (1989, 2000) model of reintegrative shaming?
- How could you apply it for yourself if you were to experience shame within a criminal context?
- What do you think about the restorative justice approaches existing in the society you were born into, or in which you live? How could they take reintegrative shaming into account?

9.4.1.4   Shame, Shaming and Crime in Cultural Contexts

- How does your culture of origin deal with shame?
- How has it historically dealt with crime? How does it deal with crime currently?
- What would you change in your culture of origin with regard to these two topics (shame and crime) and their interconnections?
- How would an ideal culture manage shame and crime optimally, on an individual, group or national level?

9.4.2   From the Viewpoint of an Affected Family Member, Relative or Friend

9.4.2.1   Crime and Shame

- As an affected family member, relative or friend, how do you see the interlinkages of crime and shame?
- How does the crime and shame affect the family and friendships?
- In what way does the crime and shame affect you personally? Or does the crime and shame stay with the offender?

9.4.2.2   Shaming Sanctions

- What do you think about shaming sanctions with regard to the offence which your family member, relative or friend committed?
- In this case: are you for or against shaming sentences? Why?
- How, in your opinion, should a court or the criminal law system possibly handle the offence?
- What would help you as part of the offender's system (or as part of the criminal system) to deal with the crime or offence, and the shame?
- Who carries the shame mainly within the system? Why?
- If the shame could be transformed within your family or friendship system, who would be able to actively transform it? How?

9.4.2.3   Reintegrative Shaming and Restorative Justice

- How could you, as part of the offender's or the criminal system, help to apply the concept of reintegrative shaming?
- How could restorative justice help to overcome the crime and shame?
- What could you particularly do (describe your detailed actions) to help to apply reintegrative shaming?

- As an affected family member or friend, what might hold you back from applying reintegrative shaming?

9.4.2.4   Shame, Shaming and Crime in Cultural Contexts

- What does your culture of origin say when a member of the family or a friend has committed an offence?
- What does the culture predict in terms of who in the system should mainly carry the shame? (mother, father, friends, offender, community?)
- Which methods, strategies, interventions does your cultural context provide to support the affected family members or friends?

9.4.3   From the Viewpoint of a Professional Working in the Context of Shame and Crime (for Example, in Restorative Justice, Victim–Offender Mediation, Therapeutical Practice, Forensic Psychology)

9.4.3.1   Crime and Shame

- In your professional role as…, when in particular do you come across the topic of crime and shame?
- How do you usually deal with it?
- If it is a new topic for you, why would you like to work with it?
- How do you, as a professional, feel about working with these topics?
- What makes you feel comfortable working in the context of crime and shame; what makes you feel uncomfortable?

9.4.3.2   Shaming Sanctions

- What methods, techniques, strategies, sanctions do you apply in your professional role working with criminals or offenders and shame?
- Why do you exactly apply these?
- Do you or would you work with shaming sanctions? If yes, why? If no, why not?
- What would be the pros and cons for you in your professional role, if you used shaming sanctions?

9.4.3.3 Reintegrative Shaming and Restorative Justice

- What do you think about the Braithwaite (1989, 2000) model of reintegrative shaming with regard to your own professional practice?
- Which professional methods or techniques of communication (such as active listening or reframing) would you use to apply the model of reintegrative shaming? Which techniques would you not use at all?

9.4.3.4 Shame, Shaming and Crime in Cultural Contexts

- In your professional role, what is usually expected from you with regard to your cultural background, in terms of how you should deal with crime and shame?
- Does your cultural background and the cultural values of dealing with shame and crime fit with your personal values?
- Which role does language in your culture play with regard to your professional role and how to address crime and shame correctly and in an acceptable way?
- Which cultural aspects from other cultures are you aware of (when working with, for example, migrants or people from other backgrounds) regarding the management of crime and shame? How do you feel about these?
- What do you think are human universals in dealing professionally with crime and shame?

9.5 Conclusion

Reflecting on shame, shaming and crime is challenging, not least because shame and crime both carry content which is often experienced as part of the shadow (Mayer, 2017; Mayer on dreams in this book). This fact can stimulate heated discourses on values and morals as core aspects of individuals and societies as coherent (or disintegrated) units.

Therefore, the reflection on these topics and the actions taken in the contexts described might evoke reactions of splitting and divisions or defence mechanisms within the self or others. Such reactions need to be dealt with on cognitive, affective and behavioural levels.

First steps to managing shame and crime effectively and constructively might include the following aspects across cultural contexts:

- the openess to look at the topic from cognitive and emotional perspectives,
- the acknowledgement of shame and crime or offence,
- the ability to communicate about it, and
- the will to transform it in the context of human values, humanity and restorative justice.

On this basis, further rehabilitation approaches can be outlined and discussed.

References

Ahmed, E., Harris, N., Braithwaite, J., & Braithwaite, V. (2001). *Shame management through reintegration*. Cambridge, UK: Cambridge University Press.

Baumer, E. P., Wright, R., Kristinsdottir, K., & Gunnlaugsson, H. (2002). Crime, shame, and recidivism. The case of Iceland. *The British Journal of Criminology, 42*(1), 40–59.

Braithwaite, J. (1989). *Crime, shame and reintegration*. Melbourne: Cambridge University Press.

Braithwaite, J. (2000). Shame and criminal justice. *Canadian Journal of Criminology, 42*(3), 281–298.

Condry, R. (2007). *Families shamed: The consequences of crime for relatives of serious offenders*. Cullompton, UK: Willan Publishing.

Dearing, R. L., Stuewig, J., & Tangney, J. P. (2005). On the importance of distinguishing shame from guilt: Relations to problematic alcohol and drug use. *Addictive Behaviors, 30*, 1392–1404.

Garland, D. (2001). *The culture of control: Crime and social order in contemporary society*. Oxford: Oxford University Press.

Goldman, L. M. (2015). Trending now: The use of social media websites in public shaming punishments. *American Criminal Law Review, 52*, 415–451.

Harvard Law Review Association. (2003). Shame, stigma, and crime. Evaluating the efficacy of shaming sanctions. *Harvard Law review, 116*(7), 2186–2207.

Harris, N. (2017). Shame in regulatory systems. In P. Drahos (Ed.), *Regulatory theory. Foundations and applications*. Acton: Australian National University Press.

Mayer, C.-H. (2017). Shame—"A soul feeding emotion": Archetypal work and the transformation of the shadow of shame in a group development process. In E. Vandcrheiden & C.-H. Mayer (Eds.), *The value of shame—Exploring a health resource in cultural contexts* (pp. 277–302). Cham: Springer.

Mayer, C.-H., Viviers, R., & Tonelli, L. (2017). 'The fact that she just looked at me…' Narrations on shame in South African workplaces. *South African Journal of Industrial Psychology* SA Tydskrif vir Bedryfsielkunde, *43*(1), a1385. Retrieved from https://doi.org/10.4102/sajip.v43i0.1385.

Murphy, K., & Harris, N. (2007). Shaming, shame and recidivism. *British Journal of Criminology, 47*, 900–917.

Reutter, D. (2015). For shame! Public shaming sentences on the rise. *Prison Legal News*, February 4, 2015. Retrieved from https://www.prisonlegalnews.org/news/2015/feb/4/shame-public-shaming-sentences-rise/.

Stuewig, J., Tangney, J. P., Kendall, S., Folk, J. B., Reinsmith Meyer, C., & Daring, R. L. (2015). Children's proneness to shame and guilt predict risky and legal behaviours in young adulthood. *Child Psychiatry of Human Development, 46*(2), 217–227.

Stuewig, J., Tangney, J. P., Mashek, D., Forkner, P., & Dearing, R. L. (2009). The moral emotions, alcohol dependence, and HIV risk behavior in an incarcerated sample. *Substance Use and Misuse, 44*(4), 449–471.

Stuewig, J., Tangney, J. P., Heigel, C., Harty, L., & McCloskey, L. (2010). Shaming, blaming, and maiming: Functional links among the moral emotions, externalization of blame, and aggression. *Journal of Research in Personality, 44*, 91–102.

Tangney, J. P. (1993). Shame and guilt. In C. G. Costello (Ed.), *Symptoms of depression* (pp. 161–180). New York: Wiley.

Tangney, J. P., & Dearing, R. (2002). *Shame and guilt*. New York: Guilford.

Tangney, J. P., Stuewig, J., & Hafez, L. (2011). Shame, guilt and remorse: Implications for offender populations. *Journal of Forensic Psychiatry Psychology, 22*(5), 706–723.

Tangney, J. P., Wagner, P. E., Hill-Barlow, D., Marschall, D. E., & Gramzow, R. (1996). Relation of shame and guilt to constructive versus destructive responses to anger across the lifespan. *Journal of Personal Social Psychology, 70*, 797–809.

Tibbetts, S. G. (1997). Shame and rational choice in offending decisions. *Criminal Justice & Behavior, 24*, 234–255.

Tibbetts, S. G. (2003). Self-conscious emotions and criminal offending. *Psychological Reports, 93,* 101–126.

Vanderheiden, E., & Mayer, C.-H. (2017). *The value of shame. Exploring a health resource in cultural contexts.* Cham, Switzerland: Springer.

Zehr, H. (1990). *Changing lenses: A new focus for criminal justice.* Scottsdale, PA: Herald Press.

Claude-Hélène Mayer (Dr. habil., PhD, PhD) is a Professor in Industrial and Organisational Psychology at the Department of Industrial Psychology and People Management at the University of Johannesburg, an Adjunct Professor at the Europa Universität Viadrina in Frankfurt (Oder), Germany and a Senior Research Associate in the Department of Management at Rhodes University, Grahamstown, South Africa. She holds a Ph.D. in psychology (University of Pretoria, South Africa), a Ph.D. in management (Rhodes University, South Africa), a Doctorate in political sciences (Georg-August-Universität, Göttingen, Germany), and a Habilitation with a Venia Legendi (Europa Universität Viadrina, Germany) in psychology with focus on work, organizational, and cultural psychology. She has published numerous monographs, edited text books, accredited journal article, and special issues on transcultural mental health, salutogenesis and sense of coherence, shame, transcultural conflict management and mediation, women in leadership in culturally diverse work contexts, constellation work, coaching, and psychobiography.

Chapter 10
Shame at the Bottom of the Pyramid: Possible Experiences in a Consumer Culture Context

Leona Ungerer

Abstract All people daily consume products and services, irrespective of their income. The millions of people globally who still live in absolute poverty also need to purchase basic necessities for survival. Shame, an emotion that is generated both internally and externally, appears to be a characteristic experience in poverty. The term, Bottom of Pyramid describes the millions of consumers living at the bottom of the global economic pyramid. Estimates of their income vary, but their low-income restrict their consumption capability, generating possible emotional suffering and experiences of ill-being. Consumption plays an essential role in people's participation in society. It provides an indication of their choices and the choices that they cannot make to other people and broader society, including retailers, advertising agencies and the media. Consumer culture is acknowledged as a dominant cultural trend in many societies and this trend may impact on people's perceptions of themselves.

Keywords Bottom of pyramid · Consumer culture · Consumption · Poverty · Shame

10.1 Introduction

All people consume products and services, although they may differ in terms of their income, conditions and abilities (e.g., knowledge and habits) (Ekström & Hjort, 2009). Economic scarcity and its impact on consumption, however, have not yet received in-depth attention in existing consumer research. If they disregard the experiences of people at the lowest income levels, researchers overlook numerous intricacies involved in consumption. Some of the areas investigated in existing research include buyer behaviour (focusing on elements such as decision-making and choice), the symbolic aspect of consumption, the role of consumption in expressing people's

L. Ungerer (✉)
Department of Industrial and Organisational Psychology, University of South Africa (UNISA), AJH vd Walt Building, Pretoria, South Africa
e-mail: ungerlm@unisa.ac.za

© Springer Nature Switzerland AG 2019
C.-H. Mayer and E. Vanderheiden (eds.), *The Bright Side of Shame*,
https://doi.org/10.1007/978-3-030-13409-9_10

131

identity and self-presentation and the culture of consumption. Consumption, however, should be investigated in a variety of socio-economic contextual settings, and not in isolation (Ekström & Hjort, 2009).

Various factors may impact on the quality of life of impoverished people such as being excluded from relationships and communities, suffering physical discomfort and pain, being marginalized and experiencing anxiety and uncertainty about the future (Blocker et al., 2013). Impoverished people are often shamed, experiencing shame in numerous social and institutional contexts (Ali et al., 2018). Living in a consumer culture may add to these experiences. When people, for instance, are unable to participate in consumer culture, they may experience social and psychological risks and stigmas (Hjort & Ekström, as cited in Ekström & Hjort, 2009).

At a concrete level, impoverished people's choices as consumers are restricted and they typically have limited or no access to services such as health care, education and transportation (Fisk et al., 2016). Available insight into impoverished consumers' experiences, however, is incomparable to knowledge about those of non-poor consumers (Singh, 2015). Chakravarti (as cited in Blocker et al., 2013) cautions researchers in this regard not to assume that the priorities and processes underlying consumption in conditions of wealth and poverty correspond.

The largest group of impoverished consumers globally can be found at the Bottom of the Pyramid (BOP). Although opinions about their income levels vary, the term, BOP, describes more than half of the global population surviving on less than nine US Dollars daily (Arnold & Valentin, 2013). Scheff (2003, 255) presents a sociological definition of shame to guide the psychosocial analysis of poverty, namely:

> Shame is the large family of emotions that includes many cognates and variants, most notably embarrassment, guilt, humiliation, and related feelings such as shyness that originate in threats to the social bond. This definition integrates self (emotional reactions) and society (the social bond).

It appears that insight into poverty and possibilities for alleviating this condition globally may be enhanced by considering impoverished people's experiences as consumers (Blocker et al., 2013). A consumption perspective warrants attention, because all consumers have to navigate their way through the marketplace, often involving assumptions about their rank in society based on their consumption practices.

This chapter investigates possible experiences of shame among BOP consumers in a consumer culture context. In the sections that follow the relationships between shame, stigma and poverty are briefly discussed, followed by an exposition of BOP, impoverished consumers' experiences in consumer culture, their strategies for coping with the stigma of poverty and finally, suggestions for addressing shame in terms of impoverished consumers' experiences in the marketplace.

10.2 Poverty, Shame and Stigma

Shame appears to be a universal attribute of poverty (Sen, as cited in Chase & Walker, 2013). The significance of this emotion in conditions of poverty can be attributed to the psychological pain it generates (Hooper, Gorin, Cabral, & Dyson, as cited in Chase & Walker, 2013), and that people experience it in situations beyond their control. Impoverished people experience shame internally because they cannot live up to their own expectations and those of society, but shame is also generated externally during interactions with other people, society at large, and the structures, systems and policies that impoverished people interact with (Chase & Walker, 2013).

Shame involves negatively assessing oneself against personal aspirations and social expectations (Gubrium, Pellissery, & Lødemel, 2013). It is a self-conscious emotion that often negatively impacts on people's self-esteem and dignity (Lister, as cited in Ali et al., 2018).

Stigma involves stereotyping, discrimination, and labeling and occurs in situations where power is imposed on people (Link & Phelan, as cited in Ali et al., 2018). Stigma can take place at various levels, including,

- at institutional level (e.g., components of policies deliberately reflect political ideology),
- at social level (e.g., societal members shame a group for not adhering to societal norms),
- microaggressions, involving covert acts of aggression and/or discrimination.

The above types of stigma typically result in people experiencing shame. The fear of being shamed may cause people to adhere to social norms and societal expectations for suitable behaviour (Walker & Chase, 2014). Shame, as well as people's intent to avoid it, advance socially responsible behaviour and play a vital role in societal progress (Van Vliet, as cited in Roelen, 2017). Walker and Chase (2014) explains that institutions and society externally impose shame on impoverished people through stigma when they do not meet established expectations. Stigma refers to "the active process of external shaming and the psychological emotion of shame as its manifestation and consequence" (Ali et al., 2018, 3).

Walker and Chase (2014) found that impoverished peoples' shame resulted in despair, withdrawal, depression, and even in them considering suicide. People who were not impoverished often imposed shame on impoverished people through their negative attitudes. This may impact on public discussions, policies and the execution of policy programmes. Social welfare policies and programmes are a factor in shaming processes (Gubrium et al., 2013). Although they may reduce the extent of shaming and enhance people's self-respect, they may also add to impoverished people's experiences of shame, when not suitably managed.

10.3   Bottom of Pyramid

A number of complexities are involved in capturing, describing and identifying poverty (Ekström & Hjort, 2009). Poverty may be viewed as something absolute, for instance, how many standard goods and services people can access or possess. It may also be presented as something relative, for example, the extent to which people's standard of living corresponds to the generally expected standard in a particular country. Furthermore, poverty can be measured indirectly by only focusing on income and not taking people's actual living conditions into account. When measured directly, people's living conditions are investigated, without considering their income. Poverty can also be presented as an objective phenomenon (defining it based on certain criteria) or a subjective phenomenon (how people perceive it).

Irrespective of its definition, researchers agree that people do not choose to be poor, characterizing it is an involuntary condition (Lister, as cited in Ekström & Hjort, 2009). The majority of the research on poverty typically involved quantitative matters and focused on identifying the poor, while issues surrounding the implications of living in poverty and people's subjective experiences of living in this condition were neglected. Hamilton and Catterall (2006) advise in this regard that limited research on low-income consumers' experience may result in the continuance of negative stereotypes. Ekström and Hjort (2009) further recommend complementing more established views of poverty by describing the circumstances of consumers from the lowest income groups, facing a constant struggle to cope.

Prahalad and Lieberthal (1998) coined the BOP concept, where after Prahalad and Hart (1999) provided the first complete description of the concept. Prahalad and his colleagues suggested that by doing business with the billions of impoverished people globally, multinational enterprises may generate profits for themselves and contribute to poverty alleviation (Kolk, Rivera-Santos, & Rufín, 2014). Although this suggestion implies a worthy goal, namely contributing to poverty allevation, it may be shameful for multinational enterprises to target impoverished consumers. Jaiswal and Gupta (2015) identify two main views about marketing to BOP consumers, namely those supporting marketing to poor consumers and those who advise against this practice. Researchers who support marketing to the BOP, emphasise the benefits to poor consumers when they are able to choose among products at an affordable price (Prahalad & Hammond, as cited in Jaiswal & Gupta, 2015). Those who are against marketing to the BOP, point out their possible vulnerability as consumers, for instance, that they may be exploited because of limited literacy and product awareness (Karnani, as cited in Jaiswal & Gupta, 2015).

After the foundational work by Prahalad and his colleagues, researchers often used an annual income of about $1500 or $2000 per person to define BOP membership. Another commonly used description of the concept is the poverty threshold of $1 or $2 per day (Kolk et al., 2014). A number of imprecise, implicit definitions can further be found, for instance, the idea that rural populations in general may be considered as being BOP (Zala & Patel, as cited in Kolk et al., 2014), as well as rural women (Schwittay, as cited in Kolk et al., 2014), people living in slums (Whitney &

Kelkar, as cited in Kolk et al., 2014), or merely "the poor" (Heeks, as cited in Kolk et al., 2014). Sheth (as cited in Jaikumar, Singha, & Sarinb, 2017) further points to a distinguishing characteristic of emerging economies, namely the incidence of 'below the poverty line' households, also known as BOP.

Considering the divergent existing definitions of the BOP concept, research in this field often focused on diverse target populations and settings. This lack of conceptual clarity generated criticism of BOP research, for instance, the suggestion that most BOP research do not actually focus on the BOP (Karnani, as cited in Kolk et al., 2014). After a review of three decades of literature on the BOP construct, Kolk et al. (2014) confirm that the term is often used imprecisely and that different researchers investigated quite different "bases" of the pyramid. This lack of clarity highlights the diversity among BOP populations and suggests that a variety of thresholds and dimensions, such as poverty lines or vulnerability, may be suitable to measure poverty (Kolk et al., 2014).

All in all, the term, BOP describes the large group of consumers living at the bottom of the global economic pyramid. Although cut-off points differ, they survive on estimates varying between $1 daily to $9 daily (Arnold & Valentin, 2013), with the accompanying restrictions in consumption capability, possible emotional suffering and experiences of ill-being. These impoverished consumers are not able to access to a number of products or services required for survival, and aspirational products may be completely beyond their reach (Blocker et al., 2013). This points to possible experiences of both internal and social shame because they cannot live up to their own and society's expectations. Low-income consumers often cannot purchase desired items because of their financial restrictions, generating disappointment and aggravating negative emotions (such as shame) (Yurdakul, Atik, & Dholakia, 2017).

Shame essentially is a social emotion and people's levels of shame have social origins, for instance, because of the impact of socio-cultural norms and dominant discourses. The particular social context in which poverty occurs is important in interpreting it fully (Jo, 2013). To truly understand low-income consumers, it is essential to understand their external situation (Darley & Johnson, as cited in Hamilton, 2009). In terms of the impact of broader society, consumer culture often impacts negatively on individuals' and groups' lives, for instance, the effects of materialism and the prevalence of consumption disorders such as compulsive buying (Burroughs & Rindfleisch, as cited in Blocker et al., 2013). Considering the ubiquity of consumer culture in current society, it will now be briefly described.

10.4 Consumer Culture

The importance attached to consumption in people's lives increased to the extent that consumer culture became established in societies (Ekström & Hjort, 2009). Consumer culture originated from the work of Veblen (as cited in Hamilton, 2009) who introduced the term, conspicuous consumption, and established the idea that visible status goods enhance consumers' social identity. Roy Chaudhuri, Mazumdar and Ghoshal (2011, p. 217) define conspicuous consumption as "a deliberate engagement in symbolic and visible purchase, possession and usage of products and services imbued with scarce economic and cultural capital with motivation to communicate a distinctive self-image to others".

In a consumer culture, consumers are expected to respond to the marketplace's temptations (Bauman, as cited in Hamilton, 2009). In a consumer society, consumers experience a sense of empowerment in taking part in the consumption process (Wright, Newman, & Dennis, as cited in Hamilton, 2009). People's sense of self is closely related to their ability to consume in consumer culture (Zukin & Maguire, as cited in Hill & Gaines, 2007). Marketing and advertising constantly contribute to establishing and expanding consumer culture. Omnipresent marketing messages in current consumer societies generate an impression of availability that, however, evades countless people (Chin, as cited in Hill & Gaines, 2007). Consumers at the BOP, however, are not exempt from being exposed to consumer culture, since advertising and marketing messages reach even remote areas of the world and they have to purchase necessities for survival. Designer brand names are sought after in a consumer society and children often show a high level of brand awareness, even at an early stage. Socialisation agents, including the media, peers groups and family members introduce children to consumer society, resulting in an awareness of the image that they project and imbuing status to brand name products (Hamilton & Catterall, 2006).

Ekström and Hjort (2009) further point out how well-established the idea of individual agency is in consumer culture. They, however, explain that because some people may have limited resources (e.g., time, knowledge and money), they may not be able to freely choose the identities and lifestyles they want (Gabriel & Lang, as cited in Ekström & Hjort, 2009). Economic inequalities generate new types of stratification and marginalization (Lodziak, as cited in Ekström & Hjort, 2009), generating possibilities for experiencing shame.

Although consumer culture offers benefits for certain consumers such as an abundance of choice, an enormous group of consumers do not experience these benefits, mainly because of limited funds (Gabriel & Lang, as cited in Hamilton, 2009). Impoverished consumers may be particularly susceptible to the impact of a consumer culture, feeling socially excluded and stigmatised in striving to achieve implicit consumption standards (Bauman, as cited in Blocker et al., 2013). These experiences of social exclusion may be intensified by marketing practices such as relationship marketing and Customer Relationship Management (CRM), encouraging companies to focus on their most profitable consumers (Winnett & Thomas, as cited in Hamilton, 2009).

Although they do not specifically investigate consumers' experiences, Dickerson, Gruenewald and Kemeny's (2004) research may assist in understanding impoverished consumers' experiences of shame in consumer culture. These researchers' research programme focuses on shame as a vital emotional response in conditions where people experience threats to the social self, involving social evaluation or rejection. According to their social self preservation model (Kemeny, Gruenewald, & Dickerson, as cited in Dickerson et al., 2004), certain psychological and physiological responses result when a persons' social self is threatened, including threats to the person's social esteem, status and acceptance.

A number of situations may lead to people potentially experiencing social-evaluative threats. These include contexts where people face the possibility of being rejected, for instance, not being judged worthy of acceptance in a particular group, or contexts where an attribute beyond their control or an unfavourable identity is revealed (Dickerson et al., 2004). Negative self-evaluation plays a fundamental role in shame. Experiences of a devalued self may be evident in behaviour such as submission and withdrawal. Shame consequently results when people convert perceived negative social evaluations into negative self-evaluations.

10.5 Impoverished Consumers' Strategies for Coping with the Stigma of Poverty

Yurdakul et al. (2017) regard the impact of the global consumer culture as a foremost foundation of social deprivation. Jaikumar et al. (2017) suggest that BOP consumers may employ the consumption of products or services to circumvent the shame and humiliation associated with having limited resources. Impoverished people often use the acquisition of material objects to deal with the shame of poverty (Hamilton & Catterall, 2006).

BOP consumers may increase their consumption levels to diminish experiences of estrangement, anger, powerlessness (Sen, as cited in Jaikumar et al., 2017), learned helplessness (Rabow, Berkman, & Kessler, as cited Jaikumar et al., 2017) and a loss of control (Hill & Stephens, as cited in Jaikumar et al., 2017). BOP consumers often make use of conspicuous consumption in such situations to enhance experiences of social inclusion. Jaikumar and Sarin (as cited in Jaikumar et al., 2017) further found that BOP households in emerging societies may employ conspicuous consumption to imply higher levels of status, especially in conditions of considerable income inequality.

Hamilton and Catterall's (2006) research contributed to an understanding of the family dynamics involved in the experiences of consumers that are unable to participate in consumer society at a socially acceptable level of consumption. They found that the social context of poverty may impact on people's choice of coping strategies. The actions that low-income consumers employed in their study for addressing the negative stereotypes of poverty included trying to hide their poverty by reducing the visible signs of being socially different. They applied this masking strategy both outside and inside their families when the family, for instance, limits the visibility of poverty to outsiders and parents protect their children against the effects of poverty (Hamilton & Catterall, 2006). Children especially tried to hide their poverty from outsiders because they did not want to appear different from their peers. Almost all families reflected the impact of peer pressure and feared being socially different, reflecting a strong need for social conformity.

Previous research found that children from impoverished families often own branded clothing, believing that someone could not be poor when wearing these expensive-looking clothing (Elliott & Leonard, as cited in Hamilton & Catterall, 2006). Low-income consumers therefore attempt to reduce the stigma of poverty by means of brand name products that their peer groups perceive as being socially acceptable.

Some parents were concerned that their children may resort to deviant behaviour if they could not obtain brand name clothing, reflecting the ingrained distress about showing visible signs of poverty. Hamilton's (2009) suggestion that consumer culture may generate consumer misbehavior supports these parents' concern. Hamilton (2009) highlights existing research suggesting that impoverished people may misbehave in a consumption context, because they do not have the financial means to meet their desires, such as poor youths committing crime to obtain status-brand sneakers (Goldman & Papson, as cited in Hamilton, 2009). Parents worried about having to make financial provision for expensive, branded clothing (by cutting back on other expenses). Some children even refused to go out if they did not obtain suitable clothing, coercing parents to meet their demands. The stigma involved in poverty therefore has both emotional and behavioural effects. It may, for instance, lead to reduced self-esteem and cause people to overspend or incur debt, in order to avoid others' disapproval.

Jaiswal and Gupta (2015) suggest that the phenomena of compensatory consumption and consumer resistance may particularly assist in understanding BOP consumers' consumption behaviour. Categorised with other types of behaviour such as compulsive buying and addictive consumption, compensatory consumption behaviour is an extreme type of consumption behaviour. It involves reactionary behaviour as a response to people's experiences of lack or deficiencies in their lives (Woodruffe, as cited in Jaiswal & Gupta, 2015). A number of negative emotional states may give rise to compensatory consumption including a lack of self-esteem and factors negatively impacting on people's sense of self-worth and their sense of power (Jaiswal & Gupta, 2015).

Woodruffe-Burton (as cited in Jaiswal & Gupta, 2015, 115) describe compensatory consumption as "when an individual feels a need, lack, or desire which they cannot satisfy with a primary fulfillment, so they use purchasing behavior as an alternative means of fulfillment". Rucker and Galinsky (as cited in Mandel, Rucker, Levav, & Galinsky, 2017) explain that the consumption of products and service embeds psychological value that extends beyond their functional use. Mandel et al. (2017) further investigated how consumption aides people in coping with self-discrepancies. A self-discrepancy refers to an incompatibility between how a person currently views him or herself and how they would like to view themselves (Higgins, as cited in Mandel et al., 2017). Compensatory consumer behaviour may potentially occur when a person perceives a discrepancy between their ideal and actual selves (Higgins, as cited in Mandel et al., 2017).

When people experience a sense of social exclusion, it may result in perceptions of incongruity between their actual and ideal levels of belongingness (Lee & Shrum, as cited in Mandel et al., 2017). If compensatory consumer behaviour alleviates a self-discrepancy, it reduces the psychological discomfort resulting from the discrepancy. Compensatory consumption may result when consumers perceive a discrepancy between their actual self-concept and ideal self-concept (Yurchisin, Yan, Watchravesringkan, & Chen, as cited in Jaiswal & Gupta, 2015). When consumers feel powerless, it may generate cravings for possessing goods, causing them to purchase high-status, luxury items to offset the feelings of powerlessness (Rucker & Galinsky, as cited in Jaiswal & Gupta, 2015). The concept of compensatory consumption may assist in explaining BOP consumers' buying behaviour, when they for instance, disproportionately spend on products implying status and focus on satisfying their aspirational needs rather than their basic needs.

In terms of consumer resistance, Eckhardt and Mahi (as cited in Jaiswal & Gupta, 2015, 116) describe this concept as "consumers' ability to ignore, resist, and adapt market messages and product offerings in the marketplace". To survive in a consumer culture, sophisticated consumers are able to resist some of its temptations. In developing countries, especially in BOP markets consumers may not be as adapt at balancing the scale between temptation and resistance. Considering their high levels of poverty and economic constraints, they may never be able to meet some of their consumption desires. They also may not have extensive experience in circumnavigating the marketplace and do not have sufficient educational levels to choose a suitable model of consumption. Consumers such as these may not have the required skills to resist constant advertising and product releases (Eckhardt & Mahi, as cited in Jaiswal & Gupta, 2015). Consumer resistance or a lack of it may assist in understanding the trend that some BOP consumers first focus on achieving higher-order desires and neglect their basic needs. This results in them spending their limited resources on buying cosmetics, luxury products and status-enhancing items (Subrahmanyan & Gomez-Arias, as cited in Jaiswal & Gupta, 2015).

Hamilton and Catterall (2006) further found that stigma seemed to be less of a concern when impoverished people interacted with their peers or family. Goffman (as cited in Hamilton & Catterall, 2006) suggested that stigma management mainly relates to people's public life and their interactions with strangers or acquaintances. Impoverished consumers and their families often are from low-income areas where they interact with people in similar conditions. It therefore is not that important to mask the visible signs of poverty when interacting with their family and social networks.

Masking poverty within the family is largely aimed at protecting children from the stigma of poverty. Many parents in Hamilton and Catterall's (2006) study suppressed their own needs to provide for their children. All in all, low-income consumers take great effort in minimising the visibility of their poverty. Families' coping strategies mainly focus on reducing disadvantages that children may experience, in order for them to some extent measure up to their peer's consumption practices.

10.6 Addressing Shame in Poverty

The ubiquitous nature of shame and its established relationship with poverty, illustrates the worldwide need to breach existing negative cycles and identify positive approaches for diminishing shame, both to reduce poverty and for its own sake (Roelen, 2017). According to Roelen (2017), reducing multidimensional poverty features as a separate target in the United Nation's Sustainable Development Goal (SDG) #1. The impact of this condition on people's psychosocial, subjective and relational wellbeing is increasingly considered in programme evaluation. Experiences of shame, however, still do not receive sufficient attention (Roelen, 2017). Curtis (as cited in Hamilton, 2009) further points out that despite their high prevalence, low-income consumers often are not considered a priority. This, however, may be changing. Sridharan, Barrington and Saunders (2017) reviewed the theoretical paradigms underlying market research focusing on poverty over four decades and found that market and marketing theory gradually evolved towards regarding impoverished consumers as central figures in the market, shaping it through their involvement.

The World Bank regards empowering impoverished people as a prime poverty reduction strategy, enabling them to negotiate with institutions affecting their lives and holding these institutions accountable (Narayan, as cited in Blocker et al., 2013). When impoverished consumers' marketplace literacy, for instance, is enhanced, it would enhance their consumption decisions, contributing to their individual and collective power (Viswanathan, Sridharan, Gau, & Ritchie, as cited in Blocker et al., 2013), reducing possible experiences of shame. Adkins and Ozanne (2005) recommend a more critical approach to consumer education because it may result in all consumers realising that they have agency. All consumers should also become aware that they are able to participate in market interactions and influence these interactions. Most low-literate adults unfortunately do not seek help to enhance their levels of literacy (Beder, as cited in Adkins & Ozanne, 2005), despite the fact that they may benefit from literacy programmes because it could improve their literacy skills and enhance their choices as consumers. Considering the low uptake of literacy programmes, future educational strategies should include methods that address people's reluctance to enroll for literacy programmes.

Impoverished consumers often attempt to find solutions for consumption situations with the limited resources they have. They may employ a number of power strategies to cope with the stress of consumer culture and experience empowerment, for instance, socialising with consumers who are in the same conditions as them and joining forces as a group to strengthen resistance (Warde, as cited in Blocker et al., 2013).

Despite frequent debate about the moral, social and emotional qualities of shame, the role of shame in poverty reduction policies remains largely unexplored (Roelen, 2017). People experience poverty-related shame personally, but social institutions and people impose their experiences externally by means of external stigma. In terms of social welfare policies, policymakers should look for ways to enhance people's dignity and check language use and practices for whether they may be perceived as shaming. Representatives dealing with impoverished people should also do so with respect.

It is important that future research that aims at breaking negative associations between shame, poverty and related policies do not distinguish between 'shamees' versus 'shamers'. It is essential to investigate impoverished peoples' own experiences and perceptions of their lives in conditions of poverty, compared to their own expectations and other people's experiences, or compared to people who do not live in poverty, and those who advocate for people living in poverty (Roelen, 2017).

Linder and Svensson (2014) further suggest that it is not advisable to regard the BOP as a single consumer market since this approach overlooks the individuality of impoverished consumers. Hamilton et al. (2014) introduce social representation theory (SRT) in this regard. They believe it may assist in addressing one-dimensional views of poverty, encouraging a more subtle understanding of this condition, and reducing the stigma involved. Hamilton et al. (2014) established guidelines for stakeholders dealing with impoverished consumers in marketing and policy contexts, to ensure that they develop empowering representations of impoverished consumers and not marginalising representations. One way to achieve this is not to present impoverished consumers as a homogenous group. People's experience of poverty in consumer culture, for instance, feature in various contexts, including family and individual experiences of poverty; experiencing poverty in rural and urban contexts, hidden poverty and varying degrees of visible poverty.

The different contexts in which people may experience poverty point to its multidimensionality and extensive impact. It also highlights the importance of emic representations of poverty, reflecting the perspectives of poor people themselves (Hamilton et al., 2014). After investigating the influence of marketing on BOP consumers' consumption, Jaiswal and Gupta (2015) concluded that their consumption behaviour is complex and that their cultural norms and social values may limit the impact of marketing influences, generating a degree of resistance to consumption desires and marketing actions.

10.7 Practical Application: Possibilities Offered by Transformative Consumer Research

Existing research on consumer culture typically focuses on the experiences of people in conditions of abundance (Hamilton, 2009). Considering that shame is regarded as the master emotion (Jo, 2013), BOP consumers' experiences of shame in a consumer culture context warrants research attention. Impoverished consumers' experiences in general in a consumption context also deserves attention, for instance, how they choose among limited options, how they experience power imbalances in the marketplace and how consumer education could empower them in their dealings with the marketplace.

A particularly relevant approach in the field of consumer psychology that may enhance an understanding of impoverished consumers' experiences of shame in a consumer culture context is transformative consumer research (TCR). The TCR movement focuses on encouraging, supporting and publicising research that benefits the "quality of life for all beings engaged in or affected by consumption trends and practices across the world" (Mick, Pettigrew, Pechmann, & Ozanne, 2011, 3).

1. Participants to the TCR movement realised that all popular methodological approaches in consumer research may not be suited to investigating TCR issues. Researchers typically are trained in methodologies that are suitable for research among sophisticated consumers, such as focus groups, surveys, and experiments. These techniques may not be effective in research among BOP consumers because of conditions such as low levels of literacy or that these consumers may not be familiar with the required procedures to respond to conventional measuring scales. Which types of research would be suitable for investigating possible experiences of shame among BOP consumers in a consumer culture context?
2. Researchers in the field of TCR examine issues related to the over-consumption of products such as compulsive buying, as well as issues related to the under-consumption of products, as is the case of impoverished consumers. In traditional consumer decision-making models, it is postulated that consumers proceed through a number of stages such as recognising a need for a particular product or service, evaluating alternatives, purchasing the product or service, consuming it and finally disposing of it. These models may not be suitable to explain the behaviour of consumers who have limited or no funds (Ungerer, 2014).
3. Since impoverished consumers constitute such a large part of most societies, it is advisable to investigate how impoverished consumers make purchase decisions in severely restricted conditions and how relevant established models are in explaining their choices. This is an important area to consider for inclusion in consumer psychology curricula because many consumers find themselves in situations of restricted choice and it would guide future scholars in the area of consumption in poverty.
4. Research should also investigate the power strategies impoverished consumers apply to cope with the stress of consumer culture and to feel empowered.
5. "All people, regardless of income or access to other resources, are embedded in the same material world". What types of vulnerability do impoverished consumers experience? How can this be addressed? What types of protection do they need?

10.7.1 Reflective Questions for Consumers Who Are not from Deprived Conditions

1. "It is possible to look at poverty as lack of choices, opportunities and freedom, and as a force that limits life in every possible way" Søiland, (2016, 118). Dis-

cuss this statement. How would you experience these restrictions? How may the restrictions that impoverished people experience contribute to experiences of shame?

2. According to Hill (as cited in Hamilton et al., 2014), poverty can be described as a lack of 'consumer adequacy', referring to 'the continuous availability of a bundle of goods and services that are necessary for survival as well as the attainment of basic human dignity and self-determination'. Which bundle of goods and services do you regard as essential for survival and maintaining human dignity? What do you regard as the minimum daily amount for decent living?

3. Can you think of possible strengths that BOP consumers may have to assist them in dealing with their restricted consumption abilities?

10.8   Conclusion

It is evident that shame plays a central in understanding poverty. At a personal level, people living in poverty experience distress in the form of unpleasant emotions such as shame, anger and frustration. Impoverished consumers may experience feelings of social exclusion and stigmatisation due to consumer culture, because of their inability to attain expected levels of consumption. Not being able to be a part of the consumer society has significant consequences at both individual and societal levels. Low-income consumers adopt a number of coping strategies to deal with the stigma of poverty. Some of their coping strategies involve the consumption of conspicuous products to soothe the distress resulting from consumer culture. Purely financial conceptualisations of poverty appear not to be sufficient in understanding the experiences of consumers at the BOP. Further research into the lived experiences of these consumers may add to knowledge about the psycho-social dimensions of poverty in a consumer culture context.

References

Adkins, N. R., & Ozanne, J. L. (2005). The low literate consumer. *Journal of Consumer Research, 32*(1), 93–105.

Ali, S., Sensoy Bahar, O., Gopalan, P., Lukasiewicz, K., Parker, G., McKay, M., & Walker, R. (2018). "Feeling less than a second class citizen": Examining the emotional consequences of poverty in New York City. *Journal of Family Issues*, 0192513X1876034. Retrieved from https://doi.org/10.1177/0192513x18760348.

Arnold, D., & Valentin, A. (2013). Corporate social responsibility at the base of the pyramid. *Journal of Business Research, 66*(10), 1904–1914. Retrieved from https://doi.org/10.1016/j.jbusres.2013.02.012.

Blocker, C. P., Ruth, J. A., Sridharan, S., Beckwith, C., Ekici, A., Goudie-Hutton, M., et al. (2013). Understanding poverty and promoting poverty alleviation through transformative consumer research. *Journal of Business Research, 66*(8), 1195–1202.

Chase, E., & Walker, R. (2013). The co-construction of shame in the context of poverty: Beyond a threat to the social bond. *Sociology, 47*(4), 739–754.

Dickerson, S. S., Gruenewald, T. L., & Kemeny, M. E. (2004). When the social self is threatened: Shame, physiology, and health. *Journal of personality, 72*(6), 1191–1216.

Ekström, K. M., & Hjort, T. (2009). Hidden consumers in marketing–the neglect of consumers with scarce resources in affluent societies. *Journal of Marketing Management, 25*(7–8), 697–712.

Fisk, R. P. P., Anderson, L., Bowen, D. E., Gruber, T., Ostrom, A., Patrício, L., ... & Sebastiani, R. (2016). Billions of impoverished people deserve to be better served: A call to action for the service research community. *Journal of Service Management, 27*(1), 43–55.

Gubrium, E. K., Pellissery, S., & Lødemel, I. (Eds.). (2013). *The shame of it: Global perspectives on anti-poverty policies*. Bristol, England: Policy Press.

Hamilton, K. (2009). Low-income families: Experiences and responses to consumer exclusion. *International Journal of Sociology and Social Policy, 29*(9/10), 543–557.

Hamilton, K., & Catterall, M. (2006). Keeping up appearances: Low-income consumers' strategies aimed at disguising poverty. In M. C. Lees, T. Davis, & G. Gregory (Eds.), *Asia-Pacific advances in consumer research* (Vol. 7, pp. 184–189). Sydney, Australia: Association for Consumer Research. Retrieved from http://www.acrwebsite.org/volumes/13002/volumes/ap07/AP-07.

Hamilton, K., Piacentini, M. G., Banister, E., Barrios, A., Blocker, C. P., Coleman, C. A., et al. (2014). Poverty in consumer culture: Towards a transformative social representation. *Journal of Marketing Management, 30*(17–18), 1833–1857.

Hill, R. P., & Gaines, J. (2007). The consumer culture of poverty: Behavioral research findings and their implications in an ethnographic context. *The Journal of American Culture, 30*(1), 81–95.

Jaikumar, S., Singh, R., & Sarin, A. (2017). 'I show off, so I am well off': Subjective economic well-being and conspicuous consumption in an emerging economy. *Journal of Business Research, 86*, 386–393.

Jaiswal, A. K., & Gupta, S. (2015). The influence of marketing on consumption behavior at the bottom of the pyramid. *Journal of Consumer Marketing, 32*(2), 113–124.

Jo, Y. N. (2013). Psycho-social dimensions of poverty: When poverty becomes shameful. *Critical Social Policy, 33*(3), 514–531.

Kolk, A., Rivera-Santos, M., & Rufin, C. (2014). Reviewing a decade of research on the "base/bottom of the pyramid" (BOP) concept. *Business and Society, 53*(3), 338–377.

Linder, S., & Svensson, H. (2014). Please, Keep My Secret-How consumer culture influences product-based female empowerment in a specific BOP context. Retrieved from https://gupea.ub.gu.se/bitstream/2077/37682/1/gupea_2077_37682_1.pdf

Mandel, N., Rucker, D. D., Levav, J., & Galinsky, A. D. (2017). The compensatory consumer behavior model: How self-discrepancies drive consumer behavior. *Journal of Consumer Psychology, 27*(1), 133–146.

Mick, D., Pettigrew, S., Pechmann, C., & Ozanne, J. L. (2011). *Transformative consumer research: For personal and collective well-being*. New York: Routledge Publishing.

Prahalad, C. K., & Hart, S. (1999). *Strategies for the bottom of the pyramid: Creating sustainable development*. Working paper. University of Michigan and University of North Carolina. Retrieved from http://www.bus.tu.ac.th/usr/wai/xm622/conclude%620monsanto/strategies.pdf.

Prahalad, C. K., & Lieberthal, K. (1998). The end of corporate imperialism. *Harvard Business Review, 76*(4), 68–79.

Roelen, K. (2017). *Shame, poverty and social protection*. Retrieved from https://opendocs.ids.ac.uk/opendocs/handle/123456789/12998.

Roy Chaudhuri, H., Mazumdar, S., & Ghoshal, A. (2011). Conspicuous consumption orientation: Conceptualisation, scale development and validation. *Journal of Consumer Behaviour, 10*(4), 216–224.

Scheff, T. (2003). Shame in self and society. *Symbolic Interaction, 26*(2), 239–262.

Sridharan, S., Barrington, D. J., & Saunders, S. G. (2017). Markets and marketing research on poverty and its alleviation: Summarizing an evolving logic toward human capabilities, well-being goals and transformation. *Marketing Theory, 17*(3), 323–340.

Singh, R. (2015). Poor markets: Perspectives from the base of the pyramid. *Decision, 42*(4), 463–466.

Søiland, H. (2016). *Experiencing poverty. An interdisciplinary empirical study of poverty in Norway* (Master's thesis).

Ungerer, L. M. (2014). Transformative consumer research: Its origins and possible enrichment of the field of consumer research in South Africa. *SA Journal of Industrial Psychology, 40*(1), 15-pages.

Walker, R., & Chase, E. (2014). Adding to the shame of poverty: the public, politicians and the media. *Poverty, 148*, 9–13. Retrieved from http://www.cpag.org.uk/content/adding-shame-poverty-public-politicians-and-media.

Yurdakul, D., Atik, D., & Dholakia, N. (2017). Redefining the bottom of the pyramid from a marketing perspective. *Marketing Theory, 17*(3), 289–303.

Leona Ungerer (Ph.D.) is an associate professor in the Department of Industrial and Organisational Psychology at the University of South Africa. Her areas of interest are consumer psychology and technology-enhanced teaching and learning.

Part III
Working with Shame and Gender

Chapter 11
Reconstructing Gender to Transcend Shame: Embracing Human Functionality to Enable Agentic and Desexualised Bodies

Sergio A. Silverio

Abstract Now more than ever, our bodies are being used as radical tools with which we negotiate our place and status in society. No longer is it the case that the body is purely a functional, reproductive, machine—passing on genetic information from one generation to the next; but rather they have become a form of language in their own right. Our bodies are increasingly recognised as individual emblems, each with powerful and political meaning. In Western Society in particular, the quest for the "eternal feminine" endures, rendering women passive, sexualised, and objectified; without the opportunity to subvert the shame they are forced to withstand. If women were afforded the opportunity and social standing to overcome the pressures of living in patriarchal and phallogocentric societies; they could instead become members of our civilization who are the *subjects*, allowed to act and experience, rather than be gazed upon, and experienced as the *objects* of hegemonic, heteronormative, and masculinist desire. It is in this regard that we, as a society, must change the entrenched conscious practices of sexualisation, and should expose the unconscious biases towards women's bodies such that women can embrace their bodies, their bodily agency, and the multiple functions of their body (such as athleticism, breastfeeding, childbirth, menstruation, and orgasm) rather than feeling abject shame, which for so long has been the case. It is the aim of this chapter to advocate the reconstruction of gender in society, allowing for an understanding of fluid gender identity and context-specific gender construction to permit the desexualisation of the body and the removal of body-specific shame. It shall further argue for society to instead favour the acceptance of the body as a multi-functional entity, which can be *sexual* without having to be *sexualised*.

S. A. Silverio (✉)
Elizabeth Garrett Anderson Institute for Women's Health, University College London, Medical School Building, 74 Huntley Street, London WC1E 6AU, UK
e-mail: S.Silverio@ucl.ac.uk

© Springer Nature Switzerland AG 2019
C.-H. Mayer and E. Vanderheiden (eds.), *The Bright Side of Shame*,
https://doi.org/10.1007/978-3-030-13409-9_11

Keywords Bodily agency · Femininity · Gender · Lifecourse analysis ·
Sexualisation · Society · Shame

11.1   Introduction to Sexualisation and Shame

The body is arguably the first tool with which human beings began to shape, build, and alter the environment in which they lived. With them, humans have created the world we see today, the different cultures which co-exist, and perhaps most importantly—resulting in a population of over seven billion—humans have created one another. Human bodies have a long history of symbolism and since the dawn of time, human beings have used their bodies as a primary mechanism of communication (Viviani, 2009, 2017). Before humans invented the paintbrush—they used their hands to create magnificent and intricate art, documenting the struggle to survive through migrations, ice ages, plague, and predation. Before humans made instruments—they sang and told tales of their epic battles with beast and man. And before there was written word—there existed a vast array of non-verbal communication; which whilst is not so overt and obvious in exchanges today, still very much exists at the backdrop of every human to human interaction.

11.1.1   Sex, Body Language, Culture, and Shame

When talking about the body as a substitute for verbal speech and, more widely, as a dynamic piece of iconography, it is important to address cultural contexts, within which these exchanges can operate. This chapter shall focus mainly on Western culture and society, unless otherwise mentioned, meaning there is an assumption that the societies and cultures spoken about in this context accept the prevailing biologically dyadic approach to sex—that is that humans can be divided into males and females by definition of their sexual organs. Additionally, it recognises only a minority of individuals do not identify as heterosexual; and that gender is seen as a spectrum dominated by masculine and feminine traits, though these are not rigid, nor the same for everyone. There lies also the suggestion that Western society overall uses speech or the written word as the main forms of communication and is a culture which has an expectation of being clothed, rather than decorating or manipulating one's body to communicate amongst one another. Furthermore, it should be recognised that shame is largely viewed as a negative emotion in the Western cultures mentioned, which has the potential to develop into painful, deep-rooted, and long-lasting psychological damage (Thomason, 2018).

11.1.2 Communicating Sex and Shame

Non-verbal communications are still crucial to our understanding of messages despite speech now being the dominant method of conveying any message and in spite of the fact that humans have developed many different sophisticated languages with which to speak. Body movements and gestures remain universally key to decoding the context in which speech is meant (Ekman, 2016). For example, most cultures on this Earth find it perfectly normal to look one another in the eyes whilst conversing to engage the other in the statement being made. Though it is also common cross-culturally to avert one's eyes—often looking downwards in an insular and introspective posture—should someone be ashamed when speaking to another person perceived as an oppositional character in an argument (Ekman, 1999). The subtleties of communication are important and fundamentally underpin the meaning of any spoken content, though this is somewhat complicated by the fact that men and women interact differently to one another. As Locke (2011) affirms, women do not speak to men in the same way they speak to other women, and nor do men have the same patterns of engaging in conversation if they are speaking with persons of the same, or opposite sex. What we start to see here is that our inter-sex communication is not approached as societal equals by males and females. There is an agenda, even if it is initially or indefinitely unknown and this agenda can be argued as being one of a sexual nature: The ever-present, unconscious, and innate desire to continue one's genetic legacy. To mate and to reproduce in modern society comes with the association of sexual gratification and pleasure, and therefore the speech and non-verbal communications which precede a successful sexual encounter is enacted as an elaborate and somewhat ritualistic display (Toates, 2014). It is at this point where the body, as a sum of its parts, transitions from a private and personal, to a public and political substitute for speech.

11.1.3 Translating Our Bodies

With a societal expectation of a physically smaller and modest postural positioning from women's bodies, we can draw parallels between how women's bodies are seen and the global presentation of the non-verbal communication of shame, whereby the person volitionally wishes to withdraw inside oneself, thus rendering women "*typically more shame-prone than men*" (Bartky, 1990, p. 85). By adhering to Western society's standard of keeping oneself modest, in opposition to the gregarious stances adopted by men, women mirror the non-verbal communications of shame and of an acceptance that there are spaces in conversation and in their society which their bodies cannot or must not occupy (Probyn, 2004). Simultaneously, Western culture also dictates that men cast aside any aspects of femininity in order to not occupy emotional conversation or space in order to maintain a powerful and virile societal position (Kahn, 2009). Here begins the sexualisation of women, as the *objects* of masculinist desire, rather than the *subjects* of their own sexual experiences; causing a power imbalance between *men* and *women*, and what Western society accepts to be *male* and *female*.

Long before we begin to use the body to facilitate sexual messages, human younglings show little by means of gender differentiation for a significant proportion of their early life. Except for obvious external sex organ differences, many babies appear as small, androgynous beings and have a nature which reflects that. What we find in many cultures is that even in the smallest of children, those bold, machismo postures and behaviours are often modelled by young boys, while young girls are much more likely to model behaviours and postural positions of a more contained and demure nature (Kohlberg, 1966; Silverio, 2017a) in a way which perpetuates a hegemonic gender binary presentation in Western society (Budgeon, 2014). It is not simply down to a matter of role modelling however, these actions are conditioned by those significant elders around them—thus maintaining a divide between which behaviours are *appropriate* for boys, and those which are *expected* of girls (Butler, 1990, 2004). With new evidence suggesting children—even before the age of entering primary education—have knowledge and beliefs about their body image, the bodies of those close to them, and wider societal bodies (Liechty et al., 2016), it is fair to claim that the body, its meaning, and how it can be used to convey said meaning is becoming increasingly important at progressively younger ages. Therefore, between role modelling and societal conditioning, young persons have little agency to reject the rigidly adopted phenomenon of how differently gendered bodies are both *presented* and *perceived* in society.

11.2 Theories of Gender, Sexualisation, and Women

Gender is not sex, but a complex and highly individualised part of the human psyche. Sex-organ differentiation between males and females makes biological sex much easier to categorise in accordance with a male-female dyad; but gender does not maintain such similar prescribed and obvious norms. Gender is experienced in many ways and can be affected by the environment in which people are brought up, different cultures, and experiences. It is possibly one of the most debated aspects of human psychology and whilst the discussion around gender continues, there has been some firm and nuanced thought within the academic community, some of which have fed into societal discourse and ideology.

11.2.1 Women's Gender Identity

Whilst for much of the modern-day there had been a stable belief that gender, just like sex, exists as a binary and therefore males and females presented as masculine and feminine—there was a growing movement in the mid-twentieth century, culminating in the idea of a gender spectrum. Spearheading this movement was eminent Stanford University academic Sandra Lipsitz Bem, whose pioneering research on sex roles and psychological androgyny, to this day still shapes our understanding of how gender exists on a spectrum. Her landmark publication was: "The Measurement of Psychological Androgyny"; in which she concluded one main objective: *"In a society where rigid sex-role differentiation has already outlived its utility, perhaps the androgynous person will come to define a more human standard of psychological health."* (Bem, 1974, p. 162). Ahead of contemporary thought, the theory of psychological androgyny put forward by Bem, and her continued work on the gender spectrum and the use and utility of gender as a psychological lens (Bem, 1975, 1977, 1981, 1993) meant that humans could articulate the breadth of experience of gender identity. In a distinct step away from searching for the *eternal feminine* whereby women had to be the object of male (sexual) desire (de Beauvoir, 1949/2011; Mulvey, 1975), or where women were cast in relation to the men who occupied, or governed their lives (Apollon, 1993); gender was now, and continues to be, seen as a spectrum from masculinity to femininity, with those adopting characteristics from both assuming an androgynous identity (Bem, 1974, 1981, 1993). Though modern theorisation suggests a spectrum which continues to respect divisions between gender identities does not go far enough to reflect the performative nature of gender roles in modern—especially Western—society (Butler, 1990, 2004) and does not consider how gender is adapted according to context ("gender fluidity") so therefore can be seen as a *state* and not a *trait* characteristic (Silverio, 2016, 2017a).

11.2.2 The Sexualisation of Women

Despite new understanding allowing for a more individualised and plastic nature of gender identity, women especially, continue to be the target of gender-informed abuse, usually stemming from an omnipresent, yet usually invisible sexualisation of their bodies. As discussed earlier, due to the ability for a body to assume such meaning, women's bodies, in particular, have long been subject to scrutiny, critique, and criticism. The obsession with the female body has traditionally stemmed around virginity, and the symbolism of women and the womb. The Bible depicts perhaps one of the most overt contrasts in that of The *Virgin* Mary and Mary Magdalene, the *prostitute*. It appears, human beings have long been preoccupied with the role of women and the human condition. This, it can be argued, is because there has always been something mystical about women, something which has long been akin to witchcraft: They are the givers of life and with that in mind, can preside over life and death (Ehrenreich & English, 2010; Goldenberg & Roberts, 2011). It is the ability and the power to create life—rather than actually doing so—which has seen women through time subjected to objectification, sexualisation, shaming, shunning, being outcast from or oppressed within society, or even killed (de Beauvoir, 1949/2011; Heinemann, 2000).

Ritual witch-hunts may have been firmly abandoned by Western society, however, the scrutiny which women and their bodies receive lingers on. In social story telling of epic tales, women are oft recounted as using their virginity and ability to have children to torment men, whilst becoming possessive and vengeful through motherhood and old age (King, 2015). This has been found to accurately reflect how women feel they are perceived in society. New research suggests those women who follow a 'normal, but non-normative' lifecourse, such as not marrying and/or not having children feel removed and unlike other women in their society (Silverio & Soulsby, 2020) and therefore struggle to associate with a global womanhood or modern constructions of femininity (Silverio, 2016). With further evidence suggesting women are objectified as beings who can create children, and likewise being ostracised because of the choices or circumstances which lead to them not having them, there is renewed support for the theory of "*the male gaze*" (Mulvey, 1975). The male gaze can manifest as violence and perversion against women and can work independently of visual stimuli (Yahya et al., 2010), suggesting this mechanism is a more deep-rooted psychic reaction, rather than an autonomic, visceral reaction to physical stimuli. It has been rather eloquently articulated by Jacobsson (1999, p. 7) as "*...the idea that the woman is presented as the object of the male gaze and is thereby rendered passive in the frames of the narrative.*" Put simply, the female becomes the *object* of the male sexual desire, while her agency to be the *subject* of her own sexual pleasure is simultaneously removed.

11.3 Sexualisation of 'The Feminine' in Context

Womanhood and femininity have been and continue to be inextricably linked to shame and receive an inordinate amount of public and private scrutiny (Eurich-Rascoe & Vande Kemp, 1997). So far, this chapter has shown how gender is constructed and how gender can be used to frame the differences between *bodily functionality*; and how it can contribute to a reduction of *bodily agency* in women, resulting in sexualisation and shame. It can be argued that women experience far greater bodily changes than men do, and there is a certain fluidity to a woman's body over the lifecourse.

11.3.1 Women, Sexualisation, and Shame

From menstruation and the physical passing of blood each month, to the growing abdominal area when pregnant and the transfer of milk from breast to infant, to the loss of reproductive ability and symptoms associated with the menopause—much of a woman's life is marked by physical changes specific to the female sex. To illustrate the plight of modern-day female sexualisation this debate shall continue by addressing the functionality and cultural values of women's bodies from age of first menarche to widowhood.

11.3.1.1 Virginity and Menstruation

Linking back to the various cultural obsessions with virginity and the ability to bear children, young women are especially sexualised and can experience extreme feelings of shame around the time they first start to menstruate (Lee, 2009; Shaw, 2017). This time is often connected to the hypothetical transition from the preservation of one's virginity, to being able to bear children. With both virginity and childbearing being so highly prized amongst humans, young girls (especially of African, South East Asian, and Middle Eastern origin) are often the subject of physical abuse, such as female genital mutilation and chastity devices, to maintain virginity (Shaw, 2017), but as soon as she is able to produce offspring, there is a social shift into treating women as a commodity for child production (Lee, 2009). Women are expected to respect the taboo rituals surrounding virginity and procreation, and any movement away from what those around them deem proper, is shunned. From this young age, an environment of shame is fostered about the female body, how it should be kept, and for what it should be used—all of which can cause distressing and disturbing mental health outcomes related to shame if these bodily boundaries are confused and disrupted in early life (Talmon & Ginzburg, 2017).

11.3.1.2 Pregnancy and Childbirth

It is not uncommon for women to experience harassment of which the subject of the abuse is the young, sexualised, female body (Gentile, 2017; Ringrose & Harvey, 2015). Should a (Western) woman look to get pregnant, there are again cultural norms imposed to police a woman's pre-pregnancy body. The female body is scrutinised through a sexual lens, whereby society enforces expectations what is desired of modern womanhood. In Epperlein and Anderson's (2016) analysis of men's discourses of the 'perfect' vagina, it was found that young men still hold strong expectations of how a woman should groom *her* genitals for *his* [heteronormative & masculinist] aesthetic preference and sexual satisfaction. This abject sexualisation for male sexual desire leaves women somewhat compromised as should societal ideals of the feminine form change, such is the expectation that women shall adapt to the new norm. However, the functionality of a woman does not change simply because patriarchal societal desires might—the ability to carry a baby to pregnancy remains static. It is therefore the changing of one's form to constantly and consistently meet an ever-changing feminine ideal which can, however, damage psychological health (Smolak & Murnen, 2011), leading to one in three pregnant women flagging body image issues in obstetric and gynaecological consultations (Fuller-Tyszkiewicz, Skouteris, Watson, & Hill, 2012).

11.3.1.3   Breastfeeding

In the immediate postpartum period it is not uncommon for women to at least attempt breastfeeding, although those who have suffered from body-image-related depressive symptomatology are more likely to interrupt their breastfeeding intention or progress (Zanardo et al., 2016). Moreover, this natural act of simply providing one's offspring with nutrition is easily one of the most eroticised aspects of women's bodily functionality (Silverio, 2017b). In Western society, there is a patriarchal expectation of modesty for women, which is challenged when women expose parts of their body. Even though breastfeeding is a perfectly natural way of ensuring a baby's survival, the modesty aspect of the feminine ideal is compromised, and hence in much of the English-speaking world we repeatedly witness events and hear stories of women being harassed and shamed for wanting or attempting to breastfeed publicly. Shame related to breastfeeding is a common occurrence in new, and especially first-time mothers, but as well as having external references, can be internally referenced if a mother feels they are not succeeding (Hanell, 2017).

11.3.1.4   The Changing Feminine Ideal and Athleticism

Not only are women expected to maintain a modest body, capable of producing children before pregnancy, but thereafter having given birth, a woman is expected to return to the current societal feminine ideal. The objectification of women is so ingrained in society that women are conditioned to meet this ideal by *"essentially stripping her of a unique personality and subjectivity so that she exists as merely a body."* (Calogero, 2012, p. 574) and once again appeal to masculinist sexual desire—something which is heavily propagated by modern, (Western) celebrity culture and media publicity of superstar motherhood (Hopper & Aubrey, 2015; Nash, 2015). The feminine ideal is also somewhat challenged by women who maintain particularly athletic body-types, which fail to adhere to the softened appearance of women the patriarchal—particularly Western—society publicises (Tiggemann, 2004). Masculinist sexual desire of our phallogocentric world does not readily accept a woman who is physically strong, nor does it necessarily associate it with motherhood and femininity (Butler, 2013). This scrutiny can lead to psychologically damaging behaviours in a quest to reduce body-size and drop body-weight (Lee, 2013). This is often attempted through disordered eating in the female population, usually resulting in lifelong debilitating physical and mental health conditions (Baldock & Veale, 2017; Weingarden et al., 2016, 2017).

11.3.1.5   Orgasm and Later-Life Sexuality

Unsurprisingly, the most *sexualised* aspect of femininity and the female body is related to the *sexual* self. It has been found that high levels of bodily shame have been intrinsically linked to sexual self-consciousness in both males and females, but this remains more pronounced in women (Sanchez & Kiefer, 2007). Aside from societal obsession with virginity and the ability to create life, the sexual female and the female orgasm ranks highly in human intrigue (Masters, Johnson, & Kolodny, 1994). However, female orgasm remains a taboo topic when it *is* reached, though women report feeling or being made to feel shamed when it *is not* reached during sexual intercourse (Fahs, 2014; Nekoolaltak et al., 2017). Shame has also been found to be experienced when sexual pleasure, gratification, and self-empowerment are achieved by women who achieve orgasm from solitary masturbation without one's partner in the context of heterosexual relationships (Stevenson, 2016). This is despite most women reporting repeated lack of experiencing orgasm and engaging in faking or pretending (Darling & Davdon Sr., 1986; Fahs, 2014). Also, women are less likely to experience orgasm during sexual intercourse, than they are in foreplay and dissociation between a woman experiencing orgasm and engaging in copulatory vocalisations suggests: "*...there is at least an element of these responses that are under conscious control, providing women with an opportunity to manipulate male behavior to their advantage.*" (Brewer & Hendrie, 2011, p. 559). This mechanism of faking the phenomenon of orgasm in women undoubtedly allows women to negotiate the tightrope of female orgasm being at once a *taboo* and a *desire*; but also suggests a greater degree of agency women are experiencing over their *sexual* selves.

Furthermore, later-life female sexuality brings with it both agency over one's sexual self, but also shame. Patriarchal societies, in which the hegemonic, masculinist desire constantly dictates an ever-changing feminine ideal—shifting the male gaze—stigmatize women as they age (Silverio, 2016; Winterich, 2007). The ageing body and a perception that the ageing *female* body does not meet the feminine ideal, can lead to emotional and psychological distress (Rutagumirwa & Bailey, 2017) and render older women "*less sexually objectified and relatively invisible*" (Tiggemann & Lynch, 2001, p. 244). However, when (older) women show agency over their sexuality and seek sexual experience as *subjects* rather than the once-sexualised *objects* of phallogocentric desire, they are often denigrated and shamed for fulfilling their own sexual desire (Fausto-Sterling, 2000; Murray, 2015; Newton-Levinson et al., 2014).

11.4 Approaching and Addressing Shame, Sexualisation, and Bodily Agency in Context

Shame is not easy to transcend and suggesting ways in which a humanity can reconstruct gender, is possibly more difficult still. In imparting knowledge in an attempt to do this there are three ways detailed here: 'Bodily Self-Awareness', 'Visualisation and Empathy', and 'Bodily Empowerment to Normalise Bodies as Bodies'.

11.4.1 Reconstructing Gender

In order to reconstruct gender, we must reflect on how gender is currently constructed. In a Western society, it is done so in a patriarchal setting, thus enforcing a power imbalance between the biological sexes (de Beauvoir, 1949/2011). Whilst there is a general acceptance of gender being more than a binary of masculine and feminine, the spectrum of gender identity respects a clear division between gender identities. Psychological androgyny has helped facilitate gender plurality prevailing over gender polarity, however societal discourse tells us gender identity is still viewed as a scale of broadly two parts. The power imbalance between genders is based on that of the power imbalance between the sexes and facilitates males, and so masculinity, to change cultural norms and societal ideals, whilst females, and those who identify with any identity except masculinity, to be the *object* to which those ideals are applied and scrutinised.

11.4.1.1 'Bodily Self-Awareness'

We should understand better what our bodies do and how they function—further still, how they *should* and *should not* function. Often, especially in illness and ageing, people can dissociate from their bodies—which is more common if one's association was not originally strong. We should all—women especially—engage in self-surveillance of our bodies (McKinley, 2011) and speak out when we feel our bodies are under threat. Higher bodily self-awareness can help us identify feelings of shame and externalise them to the outside source, rather than internalising them (Hadar, 2008). For men, this bodily self-awareness should trigger a meaning that they are responsible for the actions of their bodies and therefore are accountable for the sexualisation they propagate. Bodily self-awareness should make humans of all genders see that we are first humans with different sexes, and gender is simply an overcoat we choose to wear.

Enacting 'Bodily Self-Awareness' as Agents

To achieve 'Bodily Self-Awareness' everybody should engage in spending short periods of time calmly exploring their body and getting to know their bodily rhythms. To do this alone, one can sit quietly and comfortably somewhere free of distractions and disturbances and notice how their body is functioning. It may help to close one's eyes when doing so, and to simply follow the pattern of breathing, slowing it down with increasingly deeper inhalations and controlled exhalations. One can also form mental traces of their bodies, by—again with closed eyes—imagining a line being drawn slowly from the soles of their feet to the tip of their head. Taking as little as twenty minutes per day to do this, can help form stable mental visualisations of our bodies. By forming these mental images and following the functional patterns, one can become more in tune with how one's own body functions and therefore know when it is not functioning as usual or is in danger or under threat.

Enabling 'Bodily Self-Awareness' as Observers

It may not be easy to mentally trace your body and its functionality at first, but with some perseverance, this mentalisation technique can become quite routine. A way to support others to engage in 'Bodily Self-Awareness' is to help them learn this technique, so share with them your best tips for doing so. Additionally, it is important to remember when engaging with others, it is often easy to not realise how our own behaviours can be received and perceived differently to how we had intended them. Therefore, when acting upon another person, first take time to evaluate how your actions may bring another person—or their body—under threat. Thinking about your own mentalisation of your body and its function can help mentally project your actions onto another's body and assess the implications. If it appears that the action you are about to execute may threaten the person for which your action is intended, you can speedily intervene and change or prevent your proposed action.

11.4.1.2 'Visualisation and Empathy'

Shame is a political emotion relying on power being exerted by one counterpart over another (Clare, 2009) and so often hinges on gender imbalance. Too often we are not empathetic to the way in which our words or actions can make someone feel. This has been the case for men in their oppression of women since time immemorial. To transcend shame using this method we should challenge the perpetrator to visualise what it would be like for a person close to them in this situation in a stepped approach. It is best to use a person one step away from the situation (i.e. not the perpetrator themselves) to allow them to engage in reflective empathy, rather than act in defence against the allegation. This deflection in turn, should help to reduce self-objectification (Moradi & Huang, 2008), which could aid transcending shame. To monitor oneself with this technique, practising this visualisation and engagement in reflective empathy is a positive step forward. Seeing whether the behaviour you are about to, or have already, displayed would be acceptable to a person close to you provides an answer as to its appropriateness.

Enacting 'Visualisation and Empathy' as Agents

To enact 'Visualisation and Empathy' one should always bear in mind how their action may affect another. Taking some time to reflect and analyse one's own comments or actions before they are unleashed into the world is never a poor choice to make. It can be likened to the physical equivalent of writing an e-mail in direct response to someone who has angered you, but instead of hitting send, saving it and re-reading it with fresh eyes in the morning. If the e-mail would further inflame a situation then it is better altered before sending or best not sent at all. The same is with actions and commentaries—we are too used to, and expectant of immediacy and instant gratification. One should reflect on their proposed action and evaluate how they would feel if these things were said or done to them or to someone with whom they have a strong personal relationship. If one was to feel negatively about it, the period of reflection offers a chance to augment or extinguish those actions or comments to achieve a more positive outcome for others who would have received them.

Enabling 'Visualisation and Empathy' as Observers

To enable this method among others, say for example you have witnessed a colleague making an overtly sexualised comment about another colleague relating to their appearance or with regard to a real or hypothetical sexual encounter. For this situation, you may—at a later time—wish to ask the perpetrator in conversation what their views were on sexual harassment within a given (work) context. If they disregard it, then illustrate an example from a previous experience in a different context (previous work or education, for example) and see whether they agree that it sounds familiar to the original context. The next step would be to state that you have witnessed this type of behaviour in the original context and calmly explain that it had emanated from *them* on a previous occasion. To diffuse any negative situation which may arise, explain that you do not wish to escalate the matter formally, but invite said person to reflect on how they would feel if they knew someone with whom they had a significant relationship had been spoken to, or about in this way.

11.4.1.3 'Bodily Empowerment to Normalise Bodies as Bodies'

To address sexualisation-based shame, we must reconstruct gender without a power imbalance. Certainly, humans would not be here today if it was not for both biological sexes procreating and so both men and women have an indefinite and indomitable interdependence. To co-exist successfully, we must act to normalise bodies, so they are seen as bodies, capable of being *sexual*, but not incessantly *sexualised* (Silverio, 2017b). In doing so, we could create a society which appreciates the great marvel of creating and sustaining life, without making women the *objects* of sexual desire, but rather *subjects* of their own bodily narratives. In turn, this could empower women to rise-up, demonstrating great bodily agency (Ponterotto, 2016). Being able to choose when they want their bodies to be *sexual* and being truely able to be the *subjects* of their own, and not masculinist, sexual desire means women would experience gender as reconstructed; and sexualisation as the link to shame, would be broken and transcended. Our bodies are our own, whilst they change over the lifecourse in shape and appearance, their function, no matter what our gender, is to exist, house our minds, and enable us to fulfil an agentic life, and no-one—regardless of gender—should have that taken away from them and replaced with shame.

Enacting 'Bodily Empowerment to Normalise Bodies as Bodies' as Agents

For women especially, to accomplish a sense of 'Bodily Empowerment', one should practice recalling one's narrative with themselves as the *subject* of their destinies and desires, rather than as the *object* of the desires and sexualised narratives of others. By placing oneself at the centre of one's own discourse as the heroine or hero enables a person to realise their self-worth, instead of having a valued placed on them by onlookers. To practice reciting our bodily narrative in a practicable manner, as one of being agentic and based on function, one should begin talking about our capabilities and improvements or achievements to affirm how empowering our bodies can be. Furthermore, it is also correct to embrace the extent of functionality whether that be producing offspring, athleticism, orgasm, or how the body ages. By reciting these stories as powerful aspects of ones lifecourse sends a message to others that one is content with their body, and that their body has *experienced* and is the result of *experiences*. In this realisation there is great strength of owning one's own body and using it to its full agentic and functional potential.

Enabling 'Bodily Empowerment to Normalise Bodies as Bodies' as Observers

To do this for others is somewhat more difficult. However, to begin, it is right to see others and their bodies as powerful, individual, and agentic entities; capable of portraying and recounting rich narratives of the struggles people and their bodies have faced, and the accomplishments which they have come to reach. When speaking about others, one should ask about their achievements, difficulties, and experiences—should, of course, others wish to divulge such information. And when viewing others there should be an attempt to see them as human beings capable of being *sexual*, without instantaneously objectifying and *sexualising* them. This is especially true for men interacting with women and can help to further empower women in any patriarchal setting, where women have traditionally been ill-treated and continue to be maligned in society.

11.5   Conclusions

The point of this argument has been to demonstrate how our (Western) hegemonic, heteronormative, patriarchal, masculinist, and phallogocentric ideals are perpetuated resulting in women and their bodies being sexualised, leading to experiences of shame in various contexts. In doing so, there was an objective to make readers take time to pause and reflect on current societal situations, and to address incidences of abject sexualisation and shaming of women when they happen, or whenever possible, before they even occur, using constructions of gender as a guiding principle to enable bodily agency. Whilst this debate has discussed how we can reconstruct gender and focus on agentic human functionality with a view to transcend shame, it was by no means the intention of this chapter to exclude those who are differently abled, those who have disabilities, or those who identify with a bodily abnormality or deformity. Sexualisation and shame are not discriminatory facets of the human condition, or our psychosocial behaviour, and nor should the ability to be agentic. If this chapter was to achieve any mark on society, it is hoped it would be to trigger the debate on how we understand the relationship between gender and sexualisation to accept our bodies being *sexual* without having to be *sexualised*, meaning we can afford women the same opportunity as men to be the agentic *subjects* of sexual experiences, rather than the experienced *objects* of sexual desire.

References

Apollon, W. (1993). Four seasons in femininity or four men in a woman's life. *Topoi, 12,* 101–115.
Baldock, E., & Veale, D. (2017). The self as an aesthetic object: Body image, beliefs about the self, and shame in a cognitive-behavioral model of body dysmorphic disorder. In K. A. Phillips (Ed.), *Body dysmorphic disorder: Advances in research and clinical practice* (pp. 299–312). New York, NY: Oxford University Press.
Bartky, S. L. (1990). *Femininity and domination: Studies in the phenomenology of oppression.* New York, NY: Routledge.
Bem, S. L. (1974). The measurement of psychological androgyny. *Journal of Consulting and Clinical Psychology, 42*(2), 155–162.
Bem, S. L. (1975). Sex role adaptability: One consequence of psychological androgyny. *Journal of Personality and Social Psychology, 31*(4), 634–643.
Bem, S. L. (1977). On the utility of alternative procedures for assessing psychological androgyny. *Journal of Consulting and Clinical Psychology, 45*(2), 196–205.
Bem, S. L. (1981). Gender schema theory: A cognitive account of sex typing. *Psychological Review, 88*(4), 354–364.
Bem, S. L. (1993). *The lenses of gender: Transforming the debate on sexual inequality.* New Haven, CT: Yale University Press.
de Beauvoir, S. (1949/2011). *The second sex* (C. Borde & S. Malovany-Chevallier, Trans.). London: Vintage—The Random House Company (Original work published 1949).
Brewer, G., & Hendric, C. A. (2011). Evidence to suggest that copulatory vocalizations in women are not a reflexive consequence of orgasm. *Archives of Sexual Behavior, 40,* 559–564.
Budgeon, S. (2014). The dynamics of gender hegemony: Femininities, masculinities and social change. *Sociology, 48*(2), 317–334.
Butler, D. (2013). Not a job for 'girly-girls': Horseracing, gender and work identities. *Sport in Society, 16*(10), 1309–1325.
Butler, J. (1990). *Gender trouble.* London: Routledge.
Butler, J. (2004). *Undoing gender.* London: Routledge.
Calogero, R. M. (2012). Objectification theory, self-objectification, and body image. In T. F. Cash (Ed.), *Encyclopedia of body image and human appearance* (pp. 574–580). San Diego, CA: Elsevier Academic Press.
Clare, E. (2009). Resisting shame: Making our bodies home. *Seattle Journal for Social Justice, 8*(2), 455–465.

Darling, C., & Davdon Sr., J. K. (1986). Enhancing relationships: Understanding the feminine mystique of pretending orgasm. *Journal of Sex and Marital Therapy, 12*(3), 182–196.

Ehrenreich, B., & English, D. (2010). *Witches, midwives & nurses: A history of women healers* (2nd ed.). New York, NY: The Feminist Press.

Ekman, P. (1999). Basic emotions. In T. Dalgleish & M. Power (Eds.), *Handbook of cognition and emotion* (pp. 45–60). Hoboken, NJ: Wiley-Blackwell.

Ekman, P. (2016). *Nonverbal messages: Cracking the code*. San Francisco, CA: Paul Ekman Group.

Epperlein, E., & Anderson, I. (2016). Man vs. Vagina—A Foucauldian analysis of men's discourses about the perfect vagina and female genital grooming. *Psychology of Women Section Review, 18*(1), 5–12.

Eurich-Rascoe, B. L., & Vande Kemp, H. (1997). *Femininity and shame: Women, men, and giving voice to the feminine*. Lanham, MD: University Press of America.

Fahs, B. (2014). Coming to power: Women's fake orgasms and best orgasm experiences illuminate the failures of (hetero)sex and the pleasures of connection. *Culture, Health & Sexuality, 16*(8), 974–988.

Fausto-Sterling, A. (2000). *Sexing the body: Gender politics and the construction of sexuality*. New York, NY: Basic Books.

Fuller-Tyszkiewicz, M., Skouteris, H., Watson, B., & Hill, B. (2012). Body image during pregnancy: An evaluation of the suitability of the body attitudes questionnaire. *BMC Pregnancy and Childbirth, 12*(91), 1–11.

Gentile, K. (2017). Playing with shame: The temporal work of rape jokes for the cultural body. *Studies in Gender and Sexuality, 18*(4), 287–293.

Goldenberg, J. L., & Roberts, T.-A. (2011). The birthmark: An existential account of why women are objectified. In R. M. Calogero, S. Tantleff-Dunn, & K. J. Thompson (Eds.), *Self-objectification in women: Causes, consequences, and counteractions* (pp. 77–99). Washington, DC: American Psychological Association.

Hadar, B. (2008). The body of shame in the circle of the group. *Group Analysis, 41*(2), 163–179.

Hanell, L. (2017). The failing body: Narratives of breastfeeding troubles and shame. *Journal of Linguistic Anthropology, 27*(2), 232–251.

Heinemann, E. (2000). *Witches: A psychoanalytical exploration of the killing of women*. London: Free Association Books.

Hopper, K. M., & Aubrey, J. S. (2015). Bodies after babies: The impact of depictions of recently post-partum celebrities on non-pregnant women's body image. *Sex Roles, 74*(1–2), 24–34.

Jacobsson, E.-M. (1999). *A female gaze?* Stockholm, Sweden: Centre for User Oriented IT Design, KTH Royal Institute of Technology, Numerical Analysis and Computing Science.

Kahn, J. S. (2009). *An introduction to masculinities*. Oxford: Wiley-Blackwell.

King, R. (2015). A regiment of monstrous women: Female horror archetypes and life history theory. *Evolutionary Behavioral Sciences, 9*(3), 170–185.

Kohlberg, L. (1966). A cognitive-developmental analysis of children's sex-role concepts and attitudes. In E. E. Maccoby (Ed.), *The development of sex differences* (pp. 82–172). Stanford, CA: Stanford University Press.

Lee, J. (2009). Bodies at menarche: Stories of shame, concealment, and sexual maturation. *Sex Roles, 60*(9–10), 615–627.

Lee, M. S., (2013). *Women's body image throughout the adult life span: Latent growth modeling and qualitative approaches* (Unpublished doctoral dissertation). Iowa State University, Ames, IA.

Liechty, J. M., Clarke, S., Birky, J. P., Harrison, K., & STRONG Kids Team (2016). Perceptions of early body image socialization in families: Exploring knowledge, beliefs, and strategies among mothers of preschoolers. *Body Image, 19*, 68–78.

Locke, J. L. (2011). *Duels and duets. Why do men and women talk so differently?* Cambridge: Cambridge University Press.

Masters, W. H., Johnson, V. E., & Kolodny, R. C. (1994). *Heterosexuality*. New York, NY: Thorsons.

McKinley, N. M. (2011). Continuity and change in self-objectification: Taking a life-span approach to women's experiences of objectified body consciousness. In R. M. Calogero, S. Tantleff-Dunn, & K. J. Thompson (Eds.), *Self-objectification in women: Causes, consequences, and counteractions* (pp. 101–115). Washington, DC: American Psychological Association.

Moradi, B., & Huang, Y. (2008). Objectification theory and psychology of women: A decade of advances and future directions. *Psychology of Women Quarterly, 32*(4), 377–398.

Mulvey, L. (1975). Visual pleasure and narrative cinema. *Screen, 16*(3), 6–18.

Murray, J. (2015). "It left shame in me, lodged in my body": Representations of shame, gender, and female bodies in selected contemporary South African short stories. *Journal of Commonwealth Literature, 50*(2), 216–230.

Nash, M. (2015). Shapes of motherhood: Exploring postnatal body image through photographs. *Journal of Gender Studies, 24*(1), 18–37.

Nekoolaltak, M., Keshavarz, Z., Simbar, M., Nazari, A. M., & Baghestani, A. R. (2017). Women's orgasm obstacles: A qualitative study. *International Journal of Reproductive Biomedicine, 15*(8), 479–490.

Newton-Levinson, A., Winskell, K., Abdela, B., Rubardt, M., & Stephenson, R. (2014). 'People insult her as a sexy woman': Sexuality, stigma and vulnerability among widowed and divorced women in Oromiya, Ethiopia. *Culture, Health and Sexuality, 16*(8), 916–930.

Ponterotto, D. (2016). Resisting the Male Gaze: Feminist responses to the "normatization" of the female body in western culture. *Journal of International Women's Studies, 17*(1), 133.

Probyn, E. (2004). Everyday shame. *Cultural Studies, 18*(2–3), 328–349.

Ringrose, J., & Harvey, L. (2015). Boobs, back-off, six packs and bits: Mediated body parts, gendered reward, and sexual shame in teens' sexting images. *Continuum: Journal of Media & Cultural Studies, 29*(2), 205–217.

Rutagumirwa, S. K., & Bailey, A. (2017). "I have to listen to this old body": Femininity and the aging body. *The Gerontologist*, 1–10.

Sanchez, D. T., & Kiefer, A. K. (2007). Body concerns in and out of the bedroom: Implications for sexual pleasure and problems. *Archives of Sexual Behavior, 36*(6), 808–820.

Shaw, S. (2017). The case of the Arab woman. *British Mensa's: ANDROGYNY, 1*(2), 11–14.

Silverio, S. A. (2016). *Not a princess in a fairy-tale, but a female of society: A qualitative examination of gender identity in the never married older woman* (Unpublished master's dissertation). University of Liverpool, Liverpool.

Silverio, S. A. (2017a). Down the rabbit-hole of modern-day Androgyny studies: How far have we come, and how far have we left to go?. *British Mensa's: ANDROGYNY, 1*(1), 17–22.

Silverio, S. A. (2017b). Why breast is best, but boobs are banned: From sustenance to sexualisation and shame. *British Mensa's: ANDROGYNY, 1*(2), 15–20.

Silverio, S. A., & Soulsby, L. K. (2020). Turning that shawl into a cape: Older never married women in their own words—The "Spinsters", the "Singletons", and the "Superheroes". *Critical Discourse Studies*, in press.

Smolak, L., & Murnen, S. K. (2011). The sexualization of girls and women as a primary antecedent of self-objectification. In R. M. Calogero, S. Tantleff-Dunn, & K. J. Thompson (Eds.), *Self-objectification in women: Causes, consequences, and counteractions* (pp. 53–75). Washington, DC: American Psychological Association.

Stevenson, J. H. (2016). *"You start to think you're the only woman that must do it": An interpretive phenomenological analysis of female pornography use within a heterosexual relationship.* (Unpublished dissertation). Nottingham Trent University, Nottingham.

Talmon, A., & Ginzburg, K. (2017). Between childhood maltreatment and shame: The roles of self-objectification and disrupted body boundaries. *Psychology of Women Quarterly, 41*(3), 325–337.

Thomason, K. K. (2018). *Naked: The dark side of shame and moral life*. Oxford: Oxford University Press.

Tiggemann, M. (2004). Body image across the adult life span: Stability and change. *Body Image, 1*(1), 29–41.

Tiggemann, M., & Lynch, J. E. (2001). Body image across the life span in adult women: The role of self-objectification. *Developmental Psychology, 37*(2), 243–253.

Toates, F. (2014). *How sexual desire works: The enigmatic urge.* Cambridge: Cambridge University Press.

Viviani, F. (2009). Body studies: Issues and trends. *International Journal of Body Composition Research, 7,* 11–22.

Viviani, F. (2017). When concepts trump percepts: How our visions on the body are changing in the transition from the analogic/televised to the digital/reticular era. *Antrocom Journal of Anthropology, 13*(1), 5–19.

Weingarden, H., Renshaw, K. D., Davidson, E., & Wilhelm, S. (2017). Relative relationships of general shame and body shame with body dysmorphic phenomenology and psychosocial outcomes. *Journal of Obsessive-Compulsive and Related Disorders, 14,* 1–6.

Weingarden, H., Renshaw, K. D., Wilhelm, S., Tangney, J. P., & DiMauro, J. (2016). Anxiety and shame as risk factors for depression, suicidality, and functional impairment in body dysmorphic disorder and obsessive-compulsive disorder. *Journal of Nervous & Mental Disease, 204*(11), 832–839.

Winterich, J. A. (2007). Aging, femininity, and the body: What appearance changes mean to women with age. *Gender Issues, 24*(3), 51–69.

Yahya, W. W., Rahman, E. A., & Zainal, Z. I. (2010). Male gaze, pornography and the fetishised female. *International Journal of Interdisciplinary Social Sciences, 5*(1), 25.

Zanardo, V., Volpe, F., Giustardi, A., Canella, A., Straface, G., & Soldera, G. (2016). Body image in breastfeeding women with depressive symptoms: A prospective study. *Journal of Maternal-Fetal and Neonatal Medicine, 29*(5), 836–840.

Sergio A. Silverio is an academic Psychologist and Registered Scientist of The Science Council. His primary research interest lies in the 'Female Psychology' branch of 'The Psychology of Women' and he adopts a lifecourse analysis approach, using qualitative methodologies to examine women's mental health and social wellbeing outcomes in relation to changes in gender identity, across the lifespan. Having graduated from the University of Liverpool in 2016, his Master's research into older never married women, later-life femininity, and ageing social networks attracted critical acclaim from his learned academy: The British Psychological Society. Since moving to the University College London in 2018, and assuming the role of Research Assistant in Qualitative Methods within the Elizabeth Garrett Anderson Institute for Women's Health, where he is now an Honorary Research Fellow, he has been able to further pursue his wider interests into women's experiences of motherhood and bereavement. This has only supported his endeavours to bring women's health to the forefront of academic debate, whilst continuing to strive for better provisions of psychological health and greater female empowerment.

Chapter 12
Interventions for Shame and Guilt Experienced by Battered Women

Kathryn A. Nel and Sarawathie Govender

Abstract In both developed and developing countries worldwide abuse of women is rife thus interventions are needed which are practical and have a broad application. Battered Woman Syndrome (BWS) represents a specific set of psychological and behavioural symptoms that result from prolonged exposure to physical, sexual and/or psychological abuse. In most cases, the woman develops a sense of Learned Helplessness and feels the abuse is deserved which reinforces the power and control of her male partner. In sub-Saharan Africa, which is dominated by patriarchy, woman abuse is associated with traditions such as Lobola (bride price). This practice is meant to bring families together but in contemporary sub-Saharan society it is often distorted. Poor rural women are frequently unable to leave their abusive partners as their families compel them to remain because of the 'shame' attached to parting from their spouse. This chapter focuses on interventions which help women deal with feelings of guilt and shame related to their abuse. These have proven effective in a poor, rural sub-Saharan socio-economic context. The authors suggest that these can be used in similar contexts globally. The specific interventions found most effective are religious practices linked to Person Centred Therapy, Narrative Therapy and Brain Working Recursive Therapy (BWRT). The purpose of these interventions is to enable women to gain enough self-esteem to change their circumstances.

Keywords Battered woman syndrome · Religion · Brain working recursive therapy (BWRT) · Shame · Lobola

12.1 Introduction

Interventions for women experiencing shame and guilt as a result of physical, sexual and/or psychological in a sub-Saharan Africa are explicated in this chapter. Although used successfully in a South African arena these interventions can be used successfully in a global arena. According to the World Health Organisation [WHO] (2013)

K. A. Nel (✉) · S. Govender
University of Limpopo, Private Bag X1106, Sovenga 0127, South Africa
e-mail: kathynel53@gmail.com

© Springer Nature Switzerland AG 2019
C.-H. Mayer and E. Vanderheiden (eds.), *The Bright Side of Shame*,
https://doi.org/10.1007/978-3-030-13409-9_12

Africa has one of the highest frequencies of lifetime woman abuse (by male partners) in the world (±37%). This is reflected in a large scale survey in South Africa
(SA) in 2016 with 13,000 participants where it was reported that 21% of women had
suffered physical abuse and 6% had experienced sexual violence (Statistics South
Africa, 2018). It was also stated that women are more likely to experience physical violence if they are divorced or separated from their male partners. Professional
woman are also victims of psychological, sexual and physical abuse in the country (Barkhuizen, 2004) thus the problem is not only amongst the working classes.
Naidoo (2013) states that in 2009 over 68,000 of cases of rape were reported (and
probably just as many un-reported) to the South African Police Services (SAPS) furthermore, he suggests that a woman is raped every 35 seconds in SA. This, in spite
of far reaching laws aimed at protecting women from domestic abuse. These include
the Domestic Violence Act No 116 of 1998 and Criminal Law (Sexual Offence and
Related Matters) Act No 32 of 2007 (Mogale, Burns, & Richt, 2012). Women who
are the victims of abuse (including psychological abuse) can also experience mental
health problems (Moultrie & Kleintjes, 2006) these range from for instance, shame
and guilt which result in anxiety and depression to Post Traumatic Stress Disorder (PTSD) and suicidal ideation (Shivambu, 2015). Interventions to help battered
women deal with domestic abuse are documented to help clinicians review their own
practices and also to understand that the authors do not adhere to the 'one size fits
all' approach to therapy, which can (and should) be tailored to individual clients.
This does not mean that a clinician has every single therapy in his or her repertoire
but has several therapeutic tools which can be tailored to work in various situations.
We acknowledge that this is not the standpoint of many clinicians but it is ours and
underpins an eclectic approach to counselling and therapy. It must also be stated that
women who experience random acts of violence (RAOV) will also benefit from the
documented interventions which can be transferred to other contexts successfully
(for instance, in developed countries with middle class clients).

12.2 Theoretical Approaches

12.2.1 Battered Woman Syndrome (BWS)

The theoretical approach underpinning the chapter is Battered Women Syndrome
(BWS) which is a pattern of psychological and behavioural symptomology which
occurs when a woman is abused over a long period of time. Walker (2009) first coined
the term when she became aware of the similarity and signs women recounted when
detailing physical and psychological abuse. In this syndrome women are often not
able to help themselves and develop Learned Helplessness which means they believe
the abuse is justified and their partners are right to psychologically, physically and/or
sexually abuse them (Renzetti, Edleson, & Bergen, 2001) and feel shame and guilt
as a result of their perceived poor behaviour (Shivambu, 2015). According to Walker

(2009) BWS has a distinct set of characteristics and before it is diagnosed there must have been two sets of battering with three distinct phases in each separate incident. Firstly, a tension building phase occurs where the male partner is edgy and angry and where he verbally insults his partner and begins to physically abuse her. In the second phase he 'explodes,' during this period he physically and sometimes sexually assaults his partner (during this phase he can cause her grievous injury and sometimes death). The last phase is when he feels 'sorry' for his behaviour and often states that it will 'never happen again.' The woman, wants to believe the man who was kind and good to her before marriage (or long term relationship) is still 'inside' this 'monster' forgives him—and so the cycle continues. Some women are unable to break the relationship and remain in the abusive partnership until either they, (or their) partner, either dies or leaves them and a few manage to 'get out.' The latter often takes much time and occurs because women either see the effect of the abuse on their children or leave because their children are also abused.

12.2.2 Patriarchy as a Contributor to Woman Abuse

Renzetti et al. (2001), report that patriarchal practices are linked to historical rules which dictate family roles such as males being head of households and in charge of all things pertaining to the family. In much of Africa and sub-Saharan Africa conservative cultural and traditional norms feed into patriarchy and facilitate physical, sexual and verbal abuse against women (and often children). The South African constitution and judicial laws are wide-ranging and do not condone abusive practice however, historical practices which deem physical punishment the prerogative of the head of the household (Finley, 2013) still prevail. The authors assert that many of these traditions are bound to cultural values which are often unstated but mean that men must live up to their role as the dominant person in any relationship. In many instances in patriarchal countries like South Africa this leads to the physical, verbal and psychological abuse of women who 'need to know their place' (Shivambu, 2015). According to Shivambu (2015) in traditional societies many women who are abused do not see their own identity they only exist through their male partner. Wadensgo, Rembe and Chabaya (2011) link abuse of women to practices such as lobola (bride price) and polygamy as they become chattels or possessions of their husband (or partner). Lobola is the so-called 'gift' or payment to the parents of the bride for keeping her virtuous and bringing her up well by the bride's fiancé and his parents (Khomari, Tebele, & Nel, 2012). If this payment is given in full the pair can be married however, as it is often expensive lobola can be paid off (lobola price can be anything from R 40.000 upwards even for the poor). This means the couple often live together and have children but cannot marry. Divorce or leaving a long-term partner (when the payment of lobola is not yet complete and/or paid) is seen as shameful and both the woman and her family feel anxiety and guilt as the community avoids them (Shivambu, 2015).

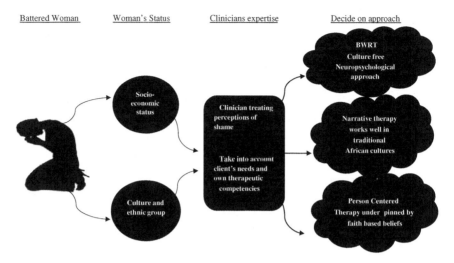

Fig. 12.1 Interventions for dealing with shame experienced by battered women

12.2.3 Theory Behind the Psychological Interventions Used to Help Battered Women Overcome Shame and Guilt

The interventions use different theoretical approaches which have proven useful in helping women who experience shame and guilt resulting in psychological problems as a result of abuse and RAOV. Firstly, religion (broad based not a specific faith) secondly, narrative therapy and thirdly BWRT. The first two interventions cannot be objectively (scientifically) proven as beneficial thus have many detractors however, in practice they are used widely and are useful and effective. The third intervention is relatively new, it was developed by Watts (2011) and fine-tuned in South Africa by Lockhat (2015) and as yet has little research in terms of its efficacy. However, papers presented at the first Pan African Psychology Conference (PAPU) in 2017 held in Durban, South Africa suggest it is a ground breaking therapy that cannot be ignored (Fig. 12.1).

12.3 Religion and Person Centred Therapy

Religious/spiritual beliefs and practices constitute an important part of culture clients use to shape judgement and process information (Delaney, Miller, & Bisonó, 2007). Many would say that religion per se is not a theoretical approach however, the authors look at followers of a specific faith and use religion (belief in a specific set of values related to divinity) in terms of the psychology of religion as used by Spilka, Hood, Hunsberger and Gorusch (2003) who interpret faith within different philosophical options. The religious faith and beliefs of the woman involved in the case study are thus reported within the context of the framework of helping her as a victim and survivor of physical, sexual and psychological abuse.

According to Okun (2002) Person Centred Therapy has the notion that people have the ability to make good choices and self-actualise (become the best person they can be). It does as a theory and practice recognise that negative emotions and behaviours exist however, this is as a result of their unfulfilled needs (for love and safety). Its stress on the social and individual environment and perceptions of self and interactions with family and others in the community makes it an appropriate therapy for individuals who have had poor life experiences. These individuals have distorted perceptions of their own reality which impacts on their ability to self-actualise and recognise new ways to deal with challenges in their lives. The therapy uses active listening and the therapist being 'open' with a positive attitude towards the client and uses their "frame of reference," to develop both the clinician's and client's self-awareness to "facilitate growth and responsibility in clients" (Okun, 2002, 129).

12.3.1 Narrative Therapy

Narrative therapy stems from social constructionism and deals with how people think, feel and interpret their unique subjective experiences (Crossley, 2000). It was first suggested as a therapy by D. Epston and M. White in the latter part of the 20th century. Fundamentally, it allows clients to tell stories about or which illustrate their understanding of their lives. The clinician is able to visualise the client's experiences through what is told and what may be left out (Epston & White, 1990). It allows a client to re-examine their life through storytelling which is an intrinsic part of African culture thus suited to therapy on the continent. The clinician helps the client to filter their narratives and essentially helps them re-define (co-discover) their lives in a way which helps them overcome challenging events which facilitates emotional growth. This type of therapy does not allow for one unambiguous 'truth' and is contextually bound within the social reality of both the client and clinician. Woman abuse is a severe challenge and it may take some time before the client is able to regain self-esteem and understand her own situation. In South Africa storytelling is a traditional way of passing on knowledge amongst the indigenous population groups and is thus non-threatening and non-invasive (Deacon, 2012) which makes narrative therapy appropriate therapy for many clients (Yule, 1993). Women find looking at events related to physical, psychological and sexual abuse extremely challenging because of the mental anguish, shame and guilt that are involved. Nonetheless, if they tell their own stories they take possession (and are thus in charge) of them which makes narrative therapy a powerful tool in the context of an abusive relationship particularly, a long-term one.

Narrative therapy is essentially a co-collaboration with the clinician. The client narrates the story and the therapist shows interest and helps the person see that they have the knowledge to help themselves (Winslade & Monk, 1999). The client thus looks at their lives with the help of an interested and empathic 'observer' who is able to help them 'see' through a different lens by the use of probing and appropriate comments. In this manner the client is able to discern different ways of doing and is able to reflect on 'how' and 'why' they are embedded in their present situation. From this they are able to develop resilience (through understanding how they have lived and coped with challenges in their lives) and comprehend that their lives can take a different path to the one they have followed thus far. It must be noted that after some time with gentle probing they are able to understand the difference between coping mechanisms that are negative and essentially just add to the challenge (which is always cyclical in nature) and those that are positive (that can help them deal with issues in a constructive manner). In many instances the clinician helps the client remember things long forgotten which assists them in recalling positive skill sets that they have not used for many years.

12.3.2 Brain Working Recursive Therapy (BWRT)

BWRT is a new approach or model of psychology that fits within the broad framework of neuroscience (Watts, 2017) and Libet's (1985) work which critically examined perceptions of so-called free-will and demonstrated through experiments that there is actually no such thing. Watts (2017) hypothesises:

> … what we usually consider as subconscious process is actually all to do with the speed of the physical brain. The 'Pattern Recognition Matrix' of the physical brain simply recognises input patterns, or creates new patterns if something new is encountered. (Watts, 2017, p. 1)

The therapy is built around the Watt's model and has several distinct steps which are summarised briefly (Watts, 2017). Briefly, the client is asked how they would prefer to respond to a specific situation but it has to be 'Plausible, Possible and Fair,' it cannot be unrealistic or impossible. Next the client has to remember when they experienced the worst symptoms which must be a valid and real memory. After this the client must tell the clinician their Perceived Arousal Level (PAL) which must be very high (on a scale of 1–10 should be an 8–10). In other words, they will feel very agitated and emotional (lower scores mean they are not aroused or emotional). Following steps allow the client to 'see' a different or new reality which is not threatening to them. They recognise that they had been distressed about an incident (ranging from fear of dogs to rape) and can tell the therapist about that memory but do not feel the intense, anxiety, fear and/or depression they had previously experienced.

The authors assert a very important issue in that this therapy is it is contextually bound (to the client) and thus more culture free than any other psychological therapy. It is situated within neuroscience and underpinned by how the brain works which, although some will argue this is not so, is factual not culture bound. This is really important when working in multi-cultural contexts as every therapy that clinicians use to-date has its roots in western—social culture (either European or American). When working with perceptions and concepts of shame BWRT is extremely useful to the clinician, in the opinion of the authors, as therapists often work without in-depth knowledge of cultural behaviours. This therapy allows cross-cultural practice without risk of offending people in dealing with shame (or guilt).

12.3.3   The Neuroscience Behind BWRT

Brain Working Recursive Therapy (Watts, 2017) uses the way the brain processes information to change unwanted habits, urges and behaviours into more resourceful and healthier ways of being. It is based on the principle that we learn something new by practising it over and over again until it becomes second nature to us. BWRT has been designed to remove emotive responses from memories that are deeply troubling and creates, new adaptive neural pathways which do not have the undesirable emotional responses attached to them. The therapy extends the neural pathways in that the client's brain is able to understand the new (desirable) patterns to use in future. Every new experience creates a new template. Immediately after the therapy is finished, the client can no longer feel any negative response to the usual triggers for their presenting symptomology, no matter how hard the neurons try to 'fire it up.' BWRT is different from other therapies in neuroscience which work directly with the amygdala and limbic systems of the brain. BWRT works with brain stem structures that receive information and that are responsible for consciousness.

12.4   Background Descriptions of the Clients and Context for the Interventions

The clients were seen at different times and provinces in South Africa. Their initials, names, identities and area where they live is not provided for the sake of confidentiality and ethical practice. Their stories are similar to many others in the country and illustrate the challenges pertaining to woman abuse.

Mrs M is a 25-year-old married woman with 2 children living in a peri-urban area. She has been hospitalised several times because of violent assaults from her husband but 'only when he is drunk.' Ms M was very depressed and suicidal during her last hospitalisation and did not know how she could carry on. She had been diagnosed with Post-Traumatic-Stress Disorder (PTSD) as she constantly re-lived her beatings. Her mother and father had paid lobola and did not want to 'interfere' in the relationship between their daughter and her husband. Mrs M's husband's family felt the same way and her mother-in-law had admonished her to be a 'better wife' so the beatings would not be so often.

Mrs R is a 46-year-old woman who had been traditionally married when she was 19 years old and later married in a church (when lobola had been paid). Her husband had been a 'family' choice and not her own. He is relatively successful and works away from home in a city while she resides in a rural area. Mrs R had been abused all her married life but was relieved that her husband didn't live with her all the time. She suspected 'girlfriends,' but didn't care. Her 4 children lived with her and were also subject to beatings and psychological abuse when her husband returned home.

Mrs P is a 65-year-old woman who was married at 20 years old. Her husband had always verbally abused her and, in the past, sexually assaulted her. Fundamentally, when he demanded sex he insisted even if she did not want it, which is synonymous with rape (sexual abuse). He had not 'hit' her however, which she felt was a 'good thing.' Mrs P was tired of the ongoing verbal insults and was depressed and felt hopeless as she did not see her 2 children very often as they lived in the 'big city.' She is very religious and involved in her church but had never revealed her 'home life' to her pastor as she was ashamed of it. Mrs P said she felt guilty when everyone commented how wonderful it was to have had a long and happy marriage (which they often did). Mrs P stated that she just smiled and nodded because it would have been shameful to do otherwise.

12.5 Interventions Used to Help Battered Women Overcome Shame and Guilt

12.5.1 Case Study 1

The clinician recognised that before she could make informed choices she needed to be treated for PTSD as she was not being physically abused at the time and was feeling stronger emotionally. Together with the clinician it was decided treatment could begin. She had tried Cognitive Behavioural Therapy (CBT) and Narrative Therapy with another therapist but these had not worked well. Mrs M was desperate for help thus it was decided that she would be an appropriate case with which to use Brain Working Recursive Therapy (BWRT).

> I don't feel comfortable thinking about being beaten or dreaming about it…I feel scared and my heart beats fast. I want help. I am ashamed of my life and I don't know how I will go on…. I also fear that everyone will call me names and talk about me if I leave my husband.

In her intake session she spoke about how guilty she felt about letting her children see her abused. However, she also noted that she was ashamed she could not make the marriage 'work' and was apprehensive about the community and both families reaction to any separation or divorce. Mrs M stated she felt shame and sadness about not being a 'good wife.' The first thing however, was to treat the symptomology for the PTSD before she could look to the future.

> I feel scared and worried when I think about going to sleep because I think it's torture to remember such things [being beaten and abused]. I want not to suffer so I can think of the future.

BWRT therapy is brief and can have good results in three sessions. In this instance, during session 1 background and intake information (the intake session is exactly the same as a clinician would usually follow) was gleaned from the client. In the second session BWRT therapy took place. BWRT was used first used to treat the clients PTSD and later repeated to treat other symptomology related to her experience of shame. After the initial PTSD session she said:

> But how does this work? It's like…I don't know. I remember but when I think about sleeping I don't feel scared. It seems like not clear but there.

Mrs M was sent away and told to come back for another session the following week to see if all the PTSD symptoms had alleviated. The first words she stated in her this session were:

> But you know I feel fine…it's like a relief…I know what happened it is there I remember everything but it doesn't make me scared [thinking about it or going to sleep]. It is just a magic thing. I don't feel sad or unhappy anymore. I want to go on with my life.

After this session several others were undertaken to help her plan her future and overcome feelings of shame and guilt related to her feelings of being a 'bad wife.' BWRT has a 'knock on' effect and, although other symptomology can be treated it is often not necessary as the initial BWRT has an holistic effect on the overall emotional and behavioural reactions of the client. Whenever it is necessary it can be used for specific sets of symptoms related to for instance, phobias and even personality disorders and other mental illnesses.

After the initial BWRT and other therapy sessions Mrs M regained self-esteem and confidence and eventually separated from her husband who she 'allowed' to divorce her (thus mitigating community and familial shame). She felt it was the most pragmatic option as her family did not have to repay lobola. She negotiated this with him and told him they could divorce because of irreconcilable differences (which she said could be 'her fault') so that no one would question him (or make him feel ashamed or guilty) as he was a man (patriarchy in play). At present BWRT training is given by Watts (2017) and Lockhat (2015) and readers should access their websites for further information as a detailed explanation is beyond the scope of this chapter.

Fundamentally, BWRT uses a recursive feedback loop (utilising neural responses) and these complex interactions, which are continuous, address any irrational or embedded negative behaviours or beliefs (which prevent the client from engaging in typical day-to-day behaviours) by overriding existing responses. In BWRT situations which provoke reactions of shame (or guilt) are dealt with through addressing these responses at a neuropsychological level. This is underpinned by (Watts, 2017, 10) who states that BWRT therapy uses:

> a motor action, an understanding or recognition that has become a part of the information [in our brain – neural pathways]. It feeds back into the network along with our conscious response and is added to the rest of the information stream that is still being received.

12.5.2   Case Study 2

In the first session Mrs R gave lengthy, detailed descriptions when answering the clinician's questions which indicated that Narrative Therapy would be an appropriate treatment. As part of her story she told the clinician that her husband rarely came home and she thought he had a 'girlfriend' or 'girlfriends.' He always verbally and sometimes physically abused her.

> He hit me before we lived together, before we were married…I thought it is because he just wants to show me he is boss and it will stop. He said it would when lobola was paid and we were properly married.
>
> I didn't know him properly my family and his arranged the marriage. He insisted on sex and it wasn't pleasant, I was a virgin.
>
> I told my mother I didn't want to marry him she said that arrangements had been made and I must not bring shame onto the family. I couldn't see how I could escape.

However, the last time he had attempted to beat their eldest daughter with a sjambok (large stick) she told him that 'this was the last time,' and that she would call the police. He had stopped the assault and left the house immediately. She said she felt 'so sad' and 'ashamed' she had let him 'beat' her children.

> I had the phone in my hand and said the police are coming you are going to jail. I shouted after him [as he was leaving], if you come back you will be arrested.

She wanted to move on and tell him never to come back but was not sure how. Mrs R was surprised that he had not come back to beat her but she thought that he was scared that she and her children (no longer very young) would attack him. Mrs R had been working for a number of years at a local retail outlet and had been supporting herself and her children (one of whom now had a job) and was thus able to support her family.

As the therapeutic process continued she told her 'truth' through the stories or narrations at first retrospectively through remembered memories and then present day narrations about her day-to-day life. She was asked questions in a respectful non-threatening manner for instance, 'Can you tell me what you remember about your childhood?" This was followed up with, 'Is this interesting you?' and, 'Can you keep this conversation (or story) going?' The conversation or storytelling in a therapeutic setting is always collaborative in nature. Mrs R was then encouraged to tell her present story which was much more difficult for her. The clinician asked her to tell her story 'as if' she was looking through a mirror saying, 'I would like you to tell me the story about you and your husband.' Mrs R stated this made her 'heart very sore' and 'this part of my story makes me feel ashamed.' She looked close to tears. The clinician then said, ' Please tell me your story as if you were looking at yourself and your husband through a mirror.' This technique is used by one of the authors who is a psychologist as she has found that clients are able to tell their painful stories as they 'watch' themselves through their 'inner-lenses or mirrors,' which allows them to narrate agonising details without breaking down. She calls it the 'Alice through the Looking Glass' technique' as it separates clients from their problems and helps them understand their true skills and capacities (sometimes a small hand mirror is used as it helps the client 'see.' The clinician has observed that clients appear to be looking 'through' not 'at' the mirror). When Mrs R had finished the disturbing story about her physical, sexual and psychological abuse she stated that, 'much has been [lifted] gone from my shoulders.' At this point it was clear to the clinician that Mrs R's self-esteem was much higher as she stated she was 'so happy now.' When the session ended she was asked to go and write a story about herself in the future (as homework from the session). At the next session her story started with the following line.

> My story, Me, I want a proper house, I have applied [Government housing]. I will live there with my family and never see him again or if I see him I won't be scared. It will be a good future.

Her husband did come to the area but stayed with family and didn't have contact with his wife or children as none of them wanted to see him. The families were not happy initially and tried to get them to reconcile but she told them an emphatic 'No.' As the husband lived away most of the time and she intended moving to a new house when it became available they decided they would deal with the 'shame' their daughter and daughter in law had brought on them for the sake of the children. A truce, albeit an uneasy one exists but as the client stated:

> Everything is much better and if people say bad things about me well, it doesn't matter it is just jealousy. There is no shame in what happened.

During Narrative Therapy Mrs R was able to tell her story in the way she had heard stories told to her as a child. She had loved listening to these stories and was always curious about them and where they came from. This 'curiosity' helped her explore her own narration in an inquisitive manner while looking at her story through a 'looking glass.' She achieved this in collaboration with the therapist who helped direct and focus the conversation. Mrs R was able to understand that shame had no place in her story. She was able to tell the therapist of her 'struggles' and said that she hoped her story would have a 'better ending,' because she had 'no place for yesterdays and shamefulness.' Reminiscent of a quote from Lewis Carroll's wonderful story, Alice's Adventures in Wonderland (1895, Chap. 10):

> But It's no use going back to yesterday, because I was a different person then.

12.5.3   Case Study 3

Mrs P referred to her faith many times during the first session. Mrs P told the clinician that she felt really old and that she knew that she looked much older than her actual age (65 years). She ascribed this to her unhappy life with her husband who she had stayed with because it was not acceptable in her culture for a woman to leave. Moving away from her husband would have brought shame and condemnation on to both her and her family, resulting in her community shunning her. It would have also meant that Mrs P would have been 'allowed' to attend her church but would not have been welcome and she would not have been invited to church activities. As she reported that her church was her only source of 'hope,' she did not feel that she could ever do this. Mrs P stated that:

> I have been married for 45 years and it has been bad. He still talks badly to me but he no longer wants that thing [sex]. I am too tired of all the bad words – it is too much. Sometimes I dream of him dead and am happy.

Her eldest daughter had offered to have her mother come and live with her in the city but she did not want to because she went to church and her daughter did not. Mrs P told the clinician that the church had changed a lot and supported women who had 'a hard time' with their husbands. She had never told a pastor about her 'troubles' as she thought he might look at her in a 'different way [negative way].' She had heard that there was a group which many women had joined so that they could support one and other but had not joined as she felt her standing in the community would be diminished.

> If they know what he says and how badly he has treated me then he would not be so respected so I wouldn't be either.

The clinician probed this remark as it was apparent that Mrs P's self-identity as a woman, at that point, was subsumed under her husband's identity. This is not related to the African philosophy of Ubuntu, where indigenous communities see themselves through one and other as a collective rather than individually, but through being subjected to long-term abuse (on an individual basis) and Learned Helplessness (where an individual believes the situation cannot change because to an extent they believe their partner and social mores are right).

Mrs P talked about herself with her main point of reference as the church and her Christian beliefs. She had a clear vision and coherent understanding of the abuse she had suffered over the years but did not recognise that the shame (and guilt) she felt about leaving her husband or trying to change the situation (becoming a partner who was equal in the relationship) was mistaken. Person Centred Therapy utilising Mrs P's religious beliefs as a focus for her healing process was thus seen as appropriate for this client

This approach is linked to pastoral counselling which is embedded in Rogerian Person Centred Therapy (Capps, 1985). It is useful for clinicians who understand that clients lives and behaviours are embedded within their every-day behaviours and beliefs (strong faith based beliefs in particular). Person Centred Therapy highlights trustworthiness and honesty between client and clinician and is based on "congruence, unconditional positive regard and empathic understanding," (Bartley, nd, 3). Fundamentally, it supports the clients existing faith-based beliefs and has a sound psychotherapeutic base.

Mrs P was encouraged to tell her husband that the verbal abuse must stop and bring it to his attention how it had hurt her, and continued to do so over the years. As he was no longer sexually active Mrs P did not want to raise what she termed 'old demons' and felt she could come to terms with and deal with those memories.

The clinician considered the context and Mrs P's personality, age and present context and adhered to her wishes in that regard. It was an act that required the clinician to recognise what was best for the client which, to be open and authentic, was discussed with Mrs P.

During therapy Mrs P was encouraged to discuss her Christian faith and beliefs and how these had helped her through the years. She often quoted the Christian Bible about forgiveness and helping those in need. Mrs P was encouraged to take part in more activities at the Church and to join the group where women spoke about their abuse with a Christian lay pastor and counsellor. After research she found out that the group had strict rules about confidentiality and decided to go. This was the first decision she had made in her life in which she could be authentic about her true life and self. Mrs P was really saddened to find that the abuse she had suffered through the years was commonplace in her congregation and she said:

> It is even much worse than what happened to me if I can say that so much worst.

The lay pastor was open to speaking to her husband which at first she didn't want because she felt 'he' might feel too much shame. At this point she had still not separated her self-identity from that of her husband. However, after a period of time she allowed this and although she had no idea what was said in the meeting her husband stopped verbally abusing her. Mrs P felt he was 'shamed' into it as someone else knew but it was never mentioned or discussed with her. The last time the clinician saw her she way buoyant and self-assured and reported that she was helping out in a shelter for abused women that the church regularly gave services at. Mrs P said her husband was old and ailing and that she had forgiven him and, as he no longer abused her in any way she had decided to look after him. She did state that forgiveness does not mean forgetting but that it was her Christian duty to care for him. Her self-actualisation was still in progress however, she saw herself as a Christian woman who did her duty to God and as she stated:

> My God forgives and so do I.
>
> I don't feel ashamed to tell people as it is not my shame.

It must be re-iterated that the individual, social and community context of Mrs P was taken into account and that therapy is about effective helping not necessarily text book outcomes where all ends are 'neatly tied.'

12.6 Transforming Shame Through Using Narrative, BWRT and Religion and Person Centred Therapy

No therapy stands alone in treating shame or guilt (or any other trauma or psychological need) however, the use of BWRT in treating shame on a neurological level using what can best be described as a 'culture free' neuropsychological treatment has had excellent results. It is a new therapy and may well revolutionise psychological interventions in the future. Narrative therapy has been utilised for decades and, in South Africa, it has great efficacy as people from traditional societies have an oral story-telling culture. This type of therapy allows clients to look at their own stories and reflect on them. This allows them to build a clear understanding that shame, when it is mistakenly attributed, may have occurred (in their yesterdays) but that their stories can be re-written with the knowledge that shame will not be present in their future narratives (about specific events). Person Centred Therapy is useful when treating clients with deep-rooted faith based belief systems as its principles echo those found in pastoral therapy. The religion in the case study presented in the chapter was Christianity however, most mainstream faith-based belief systems can be used with Person Centred Therapy. In the existing study the client was able to reconcile her faith with the realisation that she had no need to feel shame as her 'God' forgives her. This, in terms of her cultural and social contexts which support her belief system allowed the client to realise that she could have a better future without feeling shame.

12.7   Conclusion

Battered women come from a wide-range of backgrounds and have different life-experiences and experience many different mental health problems and challenges which means that there is no single intervention model (magic bullet) that will fit the needs of all. The specific interventions found most effective in helping women, from deprived backgrounds deal with shame and guilt in a South African context are described in this chapter. These are related to religious practices and Person Centred Therapy underpinned by faith-based beliefs, Narrative Therapy and Brain Working Recursive Therapy. As 'no one size fits all,' more research is needed to find out if these interventions would be effective in a global context.

Glossary 1: Questions for Person-Centered Therapy and Narrative Therapy

In Person Centered Therapy the clinician must always think about their understanding of the client's meaning and if necessary ask a 'probing' question to clarify meaning and then give a summary of what s/he understands back to the client (to verify). When doing this the clinician helps the client understand their own 'thoughts' and cognitive processes. Active, empathic listening that is non-judgemental in nature underpins this type of therapy. Examples of questions are: How are you feeling today? What is your experience of—whatever the situation is that is being explored? (if the answer needs clarification) Please explain you answer to me in more detail? How did you deal with the situation you described to me? What did you hope to achieve by dealing with the situation in that way? As a result of what you described what happened? (If the answer needs clarification). Please explain in more detail? Did you feel listened to? (Probe) Can you explain your answer to me in more detail?

Probing, Clarification and verification occur throughout the process which is non-judgemental questions beginning with Why should not be used for instance, "Why did you do that?" This makes the client defensive as s/he waits for 'judgement.' The clinician can nod his or her head, lean forward attentively and keep an empathic non-judgemental expression on his or her face (useful to practice this in the mirror—clinicians can benefit by practicing through their own 'looking glass.'

Examples of Questions for Narrative Therapy

In this type of therapy, the clinician enables the client to tell his or her story however, as the therapist is a 'listener' she or he becomes a part of the story as a co-collaborator (if you like a ghost writer—as the clinician is the one recording/transcribing/writing down the story through field notes). The therapist engages in active listening and encourages the client to focus on the narrative that the client wants to discuss. Sometimes this might mean listening to a narrative or story from the past that has a bearing on the present (and most do). If for instance, a client is mild-to moderately depressed about an issue questions such as: Can you tell me a story about a time in your life when you felt very happy? (This does not work with severely depressed clients who always need a psychotherapeutic intervention which needs time to work before therapy begins). The next question could be: Would you like to feel like this more often? The next question could be: So, tell me how you were feeling when you told me that story? Follow up with questions like: If I had seen you then what do you think I would have thought about you (answer given). Please tell me a story why you think that is? (or why I would have thought about you like that?).

This type of question picks up the client's beliefs, attitudes and behaviours and includes the clinician or co-collaborator in the story. You can explore further with questions such as:

- In the story you told me can you tell me what you understood (know, learned, recognised) about yourself?
- Look in the mirror (not on the wall hand held and brought out) and tell me a story about the person you see? (This works very well as they see their mirror image and engage in reflexion about who they are and what they 'think' or 'want' or 'believe' their story is).

References

Barkhuizen, M. (2004). *Professional women as victims of emotional abuse within marriage or cohabiting relationships: a victimological study.* Retrieved from https://repository.up.ac.za/dspace/bitstream/handle/2263/23512/dissertation.pdf?sequence=1.

Capps, D. (1985). Pastoral counselling for middle adults: A Levinsonian perspective. In R. J. Wicks, et al. (Eds.), *Handbook of pastoral counselling.* New York, NY: Paulist Press.

Bartley, J. B. (n.d.). *The pastoral applicability of Person Centred Therapy.* Retrieved from http://www.nvo.com/bartley/nss-folder/termpapers/Pastoral%20-%20Person-Centred%20Therapy.pdf.

Carroll, L. (1895). *Alice's adventures in Wonderland.* Retrieved from https://www.adobe.com/be_en/active-use/pdf/Alice_in_Wonderland.pdf.

Crossley, M. (2000). Narrative psychology, trauma and the study of self-identity. *Theory & Psychology, 10*(4), 527–546.

Deacon, H. (2012). *Rediscovering our stories: Intangible cultural heritage in South Africa.* Retrieved from http://www.goethe.de/ins/za/prj/wom/inw/enindex.htm.

Delaney, H. D., Miller, W. R., & Bisonó, A. M. (2007). Religiosity and spirituality among psychologists: a survey of clinician members of the American Psychological Association. *Professional Psychology, 38*(5), 538–546.

Epston, D., & White, M. (1990). *Narrative ends to therapeutic ends.* New York, NY: Norton.

Finley, L. (2013). *Encyclopaedia of domestic violence and abuse [2 volumes].* Santa Barbara, USA: ABC-CLIO.

Khomari, D., Tebele, C., & Nel, K. (2012). The social value of lobola: Perceptions of South African college students. *JPA, 22*(1), 143–145.

Libet, B. (1985). Unconscious cerebral initiative and the role of conscious will in voluntary action. *The Behavioral and Brain Sciences, 8,* 529–566.

Lockhat, R. (2015). *BWRT Professionals.* Retrieved from https://bwrtsa.co.za/presenter.

Mogale, R. S., Kovacs-Burns, K., & Richt, S. (2012). Violence against women in South Africa: policy position and recommendations. *Violence Against Women, 18*(5), 580–594.

Moultrie, A., & Kleintjes, S. (2006). Women's mental health in South Africa: women's health. *South African Health Review, 1,* 347–366.

Naidoo, K. (2013). Rape in South Africa—A call to action. *South African Medical Journal, 103*(4), 209–2011.

Okun, B. F. (2002). *Effective helping* (6th ed.). Pacific Grove, CA: Brooks/Cole.

Renzetti, C. M., Edleson, J. L., & Bergen, R. K. (2001). *Sourcebook on violence against women.* Thousand Oaks, CA: Sage.

Shivambu, D. (2015). *An investigation into psychological factors that compel battered women to remain in abusive relationships in Vhembe District, Limpopo Province.* Retrieved from http://ulspace.ul.ac.za/handle/10386/1311.

Spilka, B., Hood, R., Hunsberger, B., & Gorusch, R. (2003). *The psychology of religion: an empirical approach.* New York, NY: Guilford Press.

Statistics South Africa. (2018). *Crime against women in South Africa.* Retrieved from http://www.statssa.gov.za/publications/Report-03-40-05/Report-03-40-05June2018.pdf.

Wadesango, N., Rembe, R., & Chabaya, O. (2011). Violation of women's rights by harmful traditional practices. *Anthropologist, 13*(2), 121–129.

Walker, L. E. (2009). *The battered woman syndrome.* New York, NY: Springer.

Watts, T. (2017). Institute of Brain Working Recursive Therapy (BWRT). *The professional practitioner's manual.* Retrieved from https://www.bwrt.org/.

Winslade, J., & Monk, G. (1999). *Narrative counseling in schools: Powerful and brief.* Thousand Oaks, CA: Corwin Press.

WHO. (2013). *Global and regional estimates of violence against women: Prevalence and health effects of intimate partner violence and non-partner sexual violence.* Retrieved from http://apps.who.int/iris/bitstream/handle/10665/85239/9789241564625_eng.pdf;jsessionid.

Yule, H. (1993). *Narrative therapy in the South African context: a case study.* Retrieved from https://open.uct.ac.za/bitstream/handle/11427/14249/thesis_hum_1993_yule_heather.pdf?sequence=1.

Kathryn A. Nel (Prof. Ph.D.), University of Limpopo (Turfloop Campus), Sovenga, Limpopo Province South Africa. She acted as HOD Industrial Psychology at the University of Zululand for a period of 3 years before moving to the University of Limpopo in 2009. She has a National Research Foundation (South Africa) rating and broad research interests including gender issues, neuropsychology, social psychology, sport psychology and community psychology.

Associate Professor Saraswathie Govender University of Limpopo (Turfloop Campus), Sovenga, Limpopo Province, South Africa. She has acted as HOD Psychology in the Department of Psychology at the University of Limpopo (Turfloop Campus). She is Head of Research in the Department and serves on many of the institutions research committees. Her main areas of interest are neuropsychology, social psychology and Indigenous Knowledge Systems (IKS).

Part IV
Managing Shame in Spiritual and Religious Perspectives

Chapter 13
Transforming Shame: Strategies in Spirituality and Prayer

Thomas Ryan

Abstract This chapter draws on two sources, first, the religious/theological and, second, psychology. Building on an inclusive approach to spirituality, our discussion's context is the christian tradition. Understanding prayer as a personal relationship, we explain the role of emotional transparency (with special reference to shame) needed for a life-giving spiritual relationship with a divine Other (and with oneself and others). Again, psychology offers significant points of convergence with spirituality and prayer. Shame's transformative potential can be viewed in the light of socio-phenomenological theory with its focus on the meaning people attach to events and their impact on a person's life. On these foundations, we offer specific practices, biblical texts and strategies in prayer to explore meaning in shame-laden events in two life-contexts. Greater transparency brings insight, greater acceptance (of oneself, by others and by God), an acknowledged vulnerability and growing empathy for others. Painful shame, then, when named, accepted and shared (in prayer and inter-personally), can become life-giving at the human and spiritual levels and offer deeper meaning—in increased self-awareness, self-transcendence and love.

Keywords Shame · Healing · Transparency · Insight · Life-giving

13.1 Introduction

The above abstract can serve as a suitable introduction since it distils the key elements and basic structure of this chapter. The theoretical foundations to the applied approaches and exercises are first outlined (Sect. 13.2). There follows an explanation of the context, applied approach, strategies, and exercises (reflective and in prayer) in Sects. 13.3–13.5 with a brief conclusion.

T. Ryan (✉)
3 Mary St., Hunters Hill, NSW 2110, Australia
e-mail: tryansm@bigpond.net.au

13.2   Theoretical Perspectives

This section considers four aspects underling the practical methods outlined later.

13.2.1   Spirituality and Its Christian Expression

First, 'spiritual', used in an inclusive sense, is captured in Schneiders' definition of spirituality as

> the experience of conscious involvement in the project of life integration through self-transcendence toward the ultimate value one perceives. (Schneiders, 2005, 1)

The definition has four elements: it concerns something or someone ultimate; it involves a conscious decision about the direction of one's life; 'one perceives' suggests a person who is living according to their 'lights', sincerely doing their best. Finally, such a life is measured in terms of a reaching out beyond oneself in response to the needs of others as an ongoing life-project, namely, as a moral quest ('value') in a relational context.

Our context is the christian tradition of spirituality and prayer. Central here is the person of Jesus Christ, a community of faith (Church) and the Bible. Scriptural texts offer helpful resources in elaborating strategies to facilitate shame's transforming potential.

13.2.2   Spirituality and Prayer

Second, prayer is a conscious relationship with God who sustains everyone and everything in being. For christians, the Bible offers a record of the varied ways in which God tries to arouse human beings to awareness of the divine presence. Further, this text calls us to appreciate that the world and all humankind are God's 'beloved', particularly as revealed in the person of Jesus Christ, the divine Word Incarnate.

God, then, wants us to have a conscious relationship with him that is mutual. God will not force us but invites us, using life and ordinary experiences to arouse our awareness of the divine presence. These can range from watching the beauty of a sunset to holding a new born baby or being overwhelmed with gratitude for a gesture of love. It can be the unexpected sense of God present in a moment of suffering or of crisis. When we pay attention to these and become conscious of God's presence and action, this is prayer. As William Barry notes:

> Finally, if prayer is just conscious relationship, it is not something esoteric, for saints and mystics. It is open to anyone, including the likes of us. (Barry, 1987, 15)

With prayer as a relationship, two things are crucial. If I want to get to know someone better, I have to spend time with that person. So too with God. Further, it means that I believe God

> …cares how I feel and whether I am willing to let him know what I feel and desire, that is, to reveal myself. (Barry, 1987, 15)

As with any relationship, one involving God develops when there is mutual and increasing trust and transparency. This is easy when there are warm and 'positive' emotions. It is more difficult when we feel angry, afraid, hurt, ashamed, even with God. We can't just will those feelings to go away. We can only be honest with God and ourselves. If not, prayer will become boring with, often, a barrier between God and myself. Hence,

> …our relationship with (God) will develop the more that we can just admit who we are even if we wish we were different. (Barry, 1987, 31)

These considerations highlight the role desires and emotions play as points of convergence of the psychological and spiritual aspects of our human experience. A healthy, harmonious relationship with God manifests itself at the emotional level: peace, tranquillity, harmony joy, even when there may be experiences of darkness. Persistent flatness in our relationship with God is generally related to a painful emotion that is unacknowledged, e.g., anger, shame. Only when this feeling is recognised and engaged will the sense of God's presence and associated harmony and peace return (Barry, 1987, 47–55).

13.2.3 Prayer, Psychology and Growth

Third, engaging an emotion such as shame will, normally, entail particular situations. More broadly, it involves ongoing growth (psychological and spiritual)—an aspect aligned with the 'practical applications' and 'exercises' in this present volume.

Relevant here is the generalised character of structural theories of development (e.g., Erikson, Erikson, & Kivnick, 1986; Fowler, 1984; Kegan, 1982). In these approaches, stages of development are viewed as linear, namely, universal, invariant and hierarchical. Criticism of these theories concerns the interruptions that often happen in the adults' lives. Through such events, personal development can also be charted in non-linear terms as unique, adaptive re-integrations. This distinction between logical progression and adaptability enables a more adequate approach to adulthood, and especially aging, in a developmental model (Labouvie-Vief, 1982, 161–191).

Of particular relevance is socio-phenomenological theory which refers to the meaning or the critical importance people attach to events (here critical life events) and the impact they have on a person's life (Block, 1982; Labouvie-Vief, 1982, 2008).[1]

Events happen for adults that can disrupt, even shatter, the continuity of an individual's life. Their impact depends on the individual's ability or inability to negotiate these events; for instance, illness, accidents, loss of a job, divorce, death of loved ones, or actions of a family member leading to public humiliation. Such events can be traumatic and have profound effects for the person and other family members.

According to socio-phenomenological theory explained above, the crucial factor in understanding how adults grow or regress psychologically hinges on the meaning adults attach to the experiences they undergo in life, most particularly to these *critical life events*. 'People are disturbed, not by things, but by the views they take of them' (Epictetus).

What happens when an event occurs which contradicts or disrupts one's assumptions and beliefs (the frame of reference) through which I find meaning in my life? It can bring, at times, indescribable emotional suffering and pain.

It brings both uncertainty but also a challenge to grow and broaden one's horizons of meaning, truth and love (with their psychological and spiritual implications). Growth depends on the two strategies invoked to cope with the event. The individual may continue to try to *assimilate* the experience of the event to previous constructs and ways of making meaning. Or he/she may *accommodate*, i.e., feel constrained to modify his/her assumptions or behaviour in the light of that experience so that growth is likely to occur (Block, 1982, 281–295).

Finally, for an individual to negotiate such critical events successfully, certain qualities are required: a leap of faith; ego strength; a surrendering to uncertainty, and most especially 'an open orientation toward complexity' that is needed for 'positive development and well-being along the total life span' (Labouvie-Vief, 2008, 265).

13.2.4 Psychology and Spirituality in Relationship

Fourth, psychology offers valuable resources for engaging in, and understanding, the spiritual quest, and specifically, in developing prayer as a personal relationship. One must beware, however, of reducing spirituality to psychology or prayer to human effort and techniques. Christian spiritual growth is measured by the standard set by Jesus, namely, 'a movement into a deeper and more comprehensive love'. Further, 'the same movement from self-centredness to self-transcendence is the criterion of growth in developmental psychology' (Conn & Conn, 1990, 3–4). Because both the spiritual tradition and development psychology 'describe the goal of life as intimacy,

---

[1] In the approach adopted here, there is clearly an overlap with Rational Emotive Behaviour Therapy elaborated by Ellis (1975), particularly in interplay of the affective and the cognitive that is the concern of Labouvie-Vief.

as authentically mutual relationship, the latter's clarification of human relationship can be profoundly helpful for understanding and promoting mature relationships of religious experience (i.e., to God, others, self, the cosmos)' (Conn & Conn 1990, 3–4).

Two caveats follow. First, a 'more advanced stage of psychological development is not necessarily holier' since holiness is not a measure of one's abilities but of how well one uses these abilities, especially from the benchmark of love (Conn & Conn, 1990, 12). Second, both christian spiritual direction and psychotherapy help in providing space for individuals to explore their personal journey. But there are crucial differences. As Peter Tyler notes:

> Christian spiritual direction presupposes a whole hinterland of faith development, prayer and the *ecclesia* that is not necessary for psychotherapy. (Tyler, 2012, 211)

Again, Tyler counsels 'caution' about a trend in recent times to 'equate the action of the Holy Spirit with good mental health.' The realm of spirituality and prayer is animated by the Holy Spirit (the primary spiritual guide) 'who blows where it will' (Jn. 3:8) (Tyler, 2012, 211). Alternatively, spiritual direction itself should acknowledge its limits and, when indicated, refer a person to those with appropriate medical or psychological expertise.

Spiritual direction or guidance is, perhaps, best seen as a form of 'befriending' which at times, will 'transcend or transgress' the boundaries of therapy or counselling (Tyler, 2012, 211). It may also mean that psychological impairment is not, in itself, an obstacle to a deep relationship with God, namely, holiness. As St Paul reminds us, God's power and love, paradigmatically embodied in Jesus Christ, are at their best in weakness and limitation (2 Cor. 12:9). This brings us to the next stage of our discussion.

13.3   Contextual Description

The specific context in dealing with the transformation of shame is personal spirituality and prayer; here the applied approaches (reflection methods and prayer exercises) focus on two specific issues.

The first concerns the influence of adolescent 'shame experiences' on an adult's prayer and relationship with God, oneself and others. The second issue is familial (broadly understood)—concerning its individual members. The specific focus is a representative life-situation in a catholic family or religious order: 'John'—a male member of the 'family' (a father, or religious brother or priest), is charged, found guilty and imprisoned for sexual abuse of a minor. Other 'family' members' relationship with God and others is affected through their share in the humiliation and shame of John's crime and any public proceedings. This example is representative of recent events in Australia following the Royal Commission into Institutional Responses to Child Sexual Abuse.

13.4 Applied Approach

To engage painful emotions such as shame, it is crucial to be attentive so that we can discern that something or someone is beckoning us to something 'more'. Shame as a health resource is extensively discussed in a companion volume to this present study (Vanderheiden & Mayer, 2017). It suffices here to note that shame provides both the internal guardian of our moral standards ('discretionary shame') and the response when we have failed to be our best selves ('disgrace shame').[2]

Helpful, given the practical focus of this chapter, is the recourse of Whitehead & Whitehead (1994) to James Zullo's three 'critical elements in emotional life' (the A-I-M of emotions). Arousal reminds us that feelings happen in our bodies but need to be named for us to know what we are feeling. In so doing, we start to make sense of what's happening, namely, the work of Interpretation. From there, we are Moved, namely, impelled to respond, and, at times, to act, e.g., fight in anger (Whitehead and Whitehead, 1994, 10–13). Let's tease this out.

13.4.1 A Four—Step Strategy

'Transforming shame' suggests engaging shame in a healing process so that it becomes a constructive influence in a person's life. It is a movement from shame as 'disgrace' to shame as 'grace' (Whitehead and Whitehead, 1994, 93–99). Adapting the A-I-M framework noted above, we apply a four-step process to shame. The destructive face of shame feeds on silence and secrecy. Its healing starts, therefore, from within a person. Our approach will be framed primarily in the setting of prayer, aided by writing and growing transparency with God and a spiritual guide.

Name We may need time to put a name to what and how we are feeling; to distinguish 'it's shame' from other lingering feelings (e.g., guilt or fear).

Claim Perhaps simultaneously, the shame can be owned or claimed as mine (not anyone else's): 'I feel ashamed'; 'I feel dirty and worthless'.

Tame Name/Claim are the first steps whereby shame lessens its hold. While the pain may not recede immediately, it now 'serves more as a stimulus to change than simply as self-punishment' (Whitehead and Whitehead, 1994, 99). One gradually realises that shame is a response that is learned, an 'interpretation' from within a 'damaging environment' (Whitehead and Whitehead, 1994, 100). It can be 'unlearned' and healed through adjusting or adapting the interpretative window through which shame's meaning is understood. Again, these three steps, when combined with sharing and self-disclosure, not only help the healing process but enhance a sense of safety for intimacy (Whitehead and Whitehead, 1994, 100).

---

[2]This terminology is indebted to Schneider (1992).

Aim This final stage makes explicit the 'stimulus to change' triggered earlier. Self-awareness, renewed by healed shame, helps us recognise (and accept) our limits and vulnerabilities. One is more realistic, less in the grip of 'distorted ideals and compulsions that feed on them' (Whitehead and Whitehead, 1994, 1000). Healthy shame is a corrective to self-deception. Further, it brings not only a re-connection with one's true self but also an accompanying compassion for the self and, especially, for the vulnerabilities and limitations of others. Shame named, embraced and shared leads to greater empathy.

13.4.2   Two Written Reflection Exercises Using the FOUR STEP Strategy[3]

This exercise is applied to (a) the generic issue of adolescence and its influence on adult life; (b) a specific context, here, of criminal proceedings concerning sexual abuse against an individual ('John'—lay person, priest or religious brother) and its impact on other 'family' members.

Adolescence is often a time when many people had experiences of being embarrassed or self-conscious. Take a few minutes and go back to that period of your life.

Name/Claim Think of an instance during adolescence when you felt somehow ashamed or embarrassed. It may have been to do with your family, religious or racial background, your body, appearance, a physical characteristic or manner of behaviour.

Let that incident come to the forefront of your awareness. Allow yourself to feel again what you felt when it happened. Can you put words to it? Can you describe how it affected your attitude to yourself, to others and their attitude to you?

Tame What did the feeling of shame mean for you at that time? What triggered your feelings of embarrassment? When you re-enter that sense of shame, can you see any links between yourself now and your adolescent self? What sort of things trigger similar feelings of shame and embarrassment?

Aim In doing these steps, is there a change of perspective? Do you see the shame differently? Do you feel more understanding and accepting about yourself?

---

[3] Adapted from Whitehead and Whitehead (1994, 100–1).

Criminal proceedings of John—a family member or fellow priest or religious

Name/Claim Think back to when you were first told the news about John. Can you put words to your first reactions and the feelings you experienced?

When John's photo and the charges were on the front page of the paper and a leading item on TV news, how did that affect you? What about when you went to work the next day or involved in public liturgy as a priest? Can you pin point what was happening for you and inside you? Was embarrassment and shame part of it all? What about when you passed your neighbours in the street?
Then, there were the court appearances, the media, the crowd, especially the first day. Many days later the final verdict and jail sentence. What toll did that take on you, on other family or community members?
Let all that float back into your awareness. Allow yourself to feel again what you felt when it happened. Can you put words to it? How did it affect your attitude to yourself, to others and to John and their attitude to you (and to him)?

Tame What did the feelings of shame and humiliation, the desire to just hide, all mean for you at that time? After allowing yourself to re-enter those feelings, especially the sense of shame and embarrassment, do they still have the same hold on you or have they eased?

Aim In doing these steps, you may detect a change of perspective and perhaps see the shame differently. It may be you feel more understanding and accepting about yourself. Can you name your attitude and feelings now about John?

Let's move to approaching the two specific issues of these reflection exercises but now using a method based on a passage from Scripture.

13.4.3 Prayer Exercise with a Scripture Passage 1

Background Comments on Jesus Heals a Leper (Mark 1: 40–45)

In Jesus' time, leprosy covered a range of skin diseases and triggered an understandable fear of contagion. There was also the overlay of religious 'uncleanness'; it was seen as associated with sin and a form of punishment from God. The person, then, was subject to quarantine—no social contact, no sharing in common worship. Imagine it: the person could not be touched or hugged. Jesus can't help himself. He touches the leper who begs to be cured. From that spontaneous action, Jesus is seen a health risk (physically and spiritually).

Adapted Guide to Praying with Scripture[4]

Below, are some helpful steps for praying with Scripture using the imagination. Our focus is the Healing of the Leper in Mark's Gospel in the context of adulthood and residual effects of shame from adolescence.

My adult self engaging my adolescent self

1. Begin with an opening prayer: ask the Holy Spirit to be with you, to guide you, to give you the desire to be open and transparent. Ask the Lord to reveal himself.
2. I read the text slowly the first time then ponder it for a few minutes. I read the text (perhaps aloud) a second time. What words stand out? What phrases appeal to you? What aspect draws you further to sit still and reflect on it?
3. In my imagination, I construct what the scene was like. I become aware of the characters, their feelings, the overall mood of the scene.
4. I allow my personal feelings, memories etc. to become part of the meditation. Where am I in this story?
5. I place myself next to the leper and pray his words with him. Can I name what I am ashamed of? Can I point to a part of me that feels its energy (a specific memory, an incident from adolescence, a particular relationship, in a specific part of my body)? Has this been with me a long time?
6. Focus on the final verse 42. Jesus is not able to 'go openly into any town', he has to stay outside where nobody lived yet 'people from all around would come to him'. I sit with Jesus for a while. What's it like? Ask for help to capture some sense of being excluded, a non-person.
7. I reflect on the statement, 'Lord, what I hear you saying to me is…'
8. I notice what I am feeling when I hear the Lord speak to me this way. What do I say to the Lord in return? I continue my dialogue with the Lord. I ask for the courage to keep going and let Jesus transform my shame.
9. I close my prayer by asking again for the grace I am seeking: 'Lord, my greatest desire now is…'

Review of Prayer Time

After a few hours, take a few minutes to jot down what happened in your prayer session on the Mark passage:

- What insights did I gain?
- What feelings, desires, reactions arose for me?
- What was the prevailing mood of my prayer: peaceful, agitated, excited, confused, bored, calm?
- What word, image or memory meant most to me during prayer?
- How is Jesus for me now? Can I describe how my relationship with God may have changed?
- Looking back on praying this text of Mark, can I detect any shift in how I understand or feel my shame?

---

[4]Gula, (1984, 8–9).

- It may be there is a change in how I see myself (and God). Can I say that I now have some sense of a constructive role for shame looking ahead in my life, especially concerning other people?
- Do I feel drawn by God to repeat the prayer session with this text: there may be 'unfinished business'?

13.4.4 Prayer Exercise with a Scripture Passage 2

Background to Jesus' Agonizing Prayer in Gethsemane Mark 14: 32–42

This scene is graphic in its emotional intensity. It provides a most suitable setting for anyone wishing to share with, and gain insight into, the love of God in Jesus and the extent to which it will go for humanity and the world.

Relevant, here, is the interplay of the two faces of shame: Jesus' is willing to enter the suffering and humiliation of 'disgrace shame'. He does so out of convictions and ideals animated by self-giving love, namely, 'discretionary shame'. Within this dynamic, family and religious community members can undertake prayerful reflection on their situation concerning one of their own, namely, John and his conviction for child sexual abuse.

1. Begin with an opening prayer: ask the Holy Spirit to be with you, to give you the desire to be with Jesus in his emotional turmoil, to be open and transparent. Ask the Lord to reveal himself,
2. I read the text slowly the first time and ponder it for a few minutes. I read the text (perhaps aloud) a second time. What words stand out? What phrases appeal or draw you to sit still with them?
3. Imaginatively, I construct the environment of the scene. I become aware of the feelings of the characters, the mood, the atmosphere of the setting, etc.
4. I notice how Jesus is overwhelmed by fear, distress, confusion. I pray for the grace to stay with Him.
5. I allow my personal feelings, memories etc. to become part of the meditation. Where am I in this story? It may be like the disciples, it is all too much. I sense resistance within me. I pray for courage to keep going.
6. I place myself beside Jesus and pray his words with him. Part of him feels terrified repulsion about where his Father is calling him to go: to unimaginable suffering, humiliation, shame, loneliness and death.
7. I try to focus on what Jesus was feeling. Can I identify in me something of what Jesus was feeling over the situation with John?
8. I now pray with Jesus: 'let it be as you, not I would have it': that my Abba/Father will give me the strength and resolve to walk with Jesus (and John). I ask God to feel shame at what Jesus endures for me.
9. I pray to share in Jesus' love and his resolve to be faithful—to his Father, to John—even for the grace to share in the shame and humiliation, to go where I 'would rather not go'.

10. I ponder: 'Lord, what I hear you saying to me is…'
11. I notice what I am feeling when I hear the Lord speak to me this way. What do I say to the Lord in return? I continue my dialogue with the Lord. I ask for the courage to keep going and let Jesus transform my shame so that it can be a grace to accompany John.
12. I close my prayer by asking once more for the grace I am seeking: 'Lord, my greatest desire now is…'

Review of Prayer Time (as described above)

13.5 Ritualization

After the reflection and prayer strategies outlined above, it can be helpful to ritualize what has happened: lighting a candle as a sign of renewed life; writing a brief letter of reassurance to someone we love; look at photo albums as reminders of past joys and 'graces' that are part of our lives (Rupp, 1993, 90).

13.6 Conclusion

This chapter considered transformative strategies for shame in the context of christian spirituality and prayer. Acknowledging the relationship between psychology and spirituality, practical strategies were suggested for engaging the painful emotion of shame. With hopeful perseverance, such processes lead to increasing transparency with others, oneself and with God. While shame can be an episodic factor in the spiritual domain, attention to, and engagement with, this specific emergency emotion is also needed as part of a life-long developmental process. Shame's energy, if tapped and guided, contributes to the healing and integration of the person (in wholeness and holiness) and in heightened emotional sensitivity (whether interpersonally, inter-personally or trans- personally). Shame's inbuilt trajectory, then, is towards healing, growth in empathy, and, ultimately, in love of God and of others.

References

Barry, W. A. (1987). *God and you: Prayer as a personal relationship*. New York/Mahwah: Paulist Press.

Block, J. (1982). Assimilation, accommodation and the dynamics of personality development. *Child Development, 53*(1), 281–295.

Conn, J. W., & Conn, W. E. (1990). Christian spiritual growth and developmental psychology. *The Way Supplement, 69*, 3–14.

Ellis, A. (1975). *A new guide to rational living*. Chatsworth, CA: Wilshire Book Company.

Erikson, E. H., Erikson, J. M., & Kivnick, H. Q. (1986). *Vital involvement in old age*. New York: W.W. Norton & Co.

Fowler, J. W. (1984). *Becoming adult, becoming christian: adult development and christian faith*. San Francisco: Harper & Row.

Gula, R. M. (1984). Using scripture in prayer and spiritual direction. *Spirituality Today, 36*(4), 292–306.

Kegan, R. (1982). *The evolving self: Problem and process in human development*. Cambridge, MA: Harvard University Press.

Labouvie-Vief, G. (1982). Dynamic and mature autonomy: A theoretical prologue. *Human Development, 25*(3), 161–191.

Labouvie-Vief, G. (2008). When differentiation and negative affect lead to integration and growth. *American Psychologist, 63*(6), 564–565.

Rupp, J. (1993). *Praying our goodbyes*. Notre Dame, IN: Ave Maria Press.

Schneider, C. (1992). *Shame, exposure, and privacy*. New York: W.W. Norton.

Schneiders, S. M. (2005). Christian spirituality: definitions, methods and types. In P. Sheldrake (Ed.), *The new westminster dictionary of christian spirituality*. Louisville, KY: Westminster John Knox Press.

Tyler, P. (2012). Christian spiritual direction. In R. Woods & P. Tyler (Eds.), *The bloomsbury guide to christian spirituality* (pp. 200–213). London, UK: Bloomsbury.

Vanderheiden, E., & Mayer, C.-H. (Eds.). (2017). *The Value of shame: Exploring a health resource in cultural contexts*. Cham: Springer.

Whitehead, J. D., & Whitehead, E. E. (1994). *Shadows of the heart: A spirituality of the negative emotions*. New York: Crossroad.

Thomas Ryan (Ph.D.) is a Marist priest based in Sydney, Australia. He is an Honorary Fellow of the Faculty of Theology and Philosophy of the Australian Catholic University and an Adjunct Associate Professor of the School of Philosophy and Theology of the University of Notre Dame Australia. Apart from chapters in books, he has published numerous articles in theological journals both nationally and internationally.

Chapter 14
Shame Transformation Using an Islamic Psycho-Spiritual Approach for Malay Muslims Recovering from Substance Dependence

Dini Farhana Baharudin, Melati Sumari and Suhailiza Md. Hamdani

Abstract Previous literature has reported the relationship between shame and substance dependence. Some studies suggested that experiencing shame is a risk factor for relapse. Negative feelings of shame are temporarily relieved using substances therefore reinforcing use and maintaining addictive behavior. Consequently, learning how to cope with shame without the use of substances may improve recovery. In contrast, other evidences found that addressing shame may be helpful for developing reasons for stopping use and as a protective factor that helps prevent relapse. This paper describes some Islamic psycho-spiritual approaches and practices for transformation and alleviation of shame for Malay Muslims recovering from substance dependence. These include healing through the process of self-audit (*muhasabah*), repentance and forgiveness (*tawbah*), constructing new narrative of the self, and developing a stronger relationship with Allah (*hablum min Allah*) and other humans (*hablum min annas*) as the foundation for healthy recovery. It also covers the main areas of definition and prevalence of substance dependence in the Malaysian context as well as literature on shame from the perspectives of the Malaysian Muslim culture.

Keywords Shame · Substance dependence · Recovery · Muslim · Malaysia

D. F. Baharudin (✉)
Counseling Program, Faculty of Leadership and Management, Universiti Sains Islam Malaysia, Bandar Baru Nilai, 71800 Nilai, Negeri Sembilan, Malaysia
e-mail: dini@usim.edu.my

M. Sumari
Department of Educational Psychology and Counseling, Faculty of Education, University of Malaya, Jalan Universiti, 50603 Wilayah Persekutuan, Kuala Lumpur, Malaysia
e-mail: melati2112@gmail.com

S. Md. Hamdani
Da'wah Program, Faculty of Leadership and Management, Universiti Sains Islam Malaysia, Bandar Baru Nilai, 71800 Nilai, Negeri Sembilan, Malaysia
e-mail: suhailiza@usim.edu.my

© Springer Nature Switzerland AG 2019
C.-H. Mayer and E. Vanderheiden (eds.), *The Bright Side of Shame*,
https://doi.org/10.1007/978-3-030-13409-9_14

14.1 Introduction to Shame in the Described Context

Malaysia is a multicultural country. It is situated in the Southeast Asia, in which the cultures adhere to the collectivistic values. From the total population of 31.7 million, the largest population is the Bumiputra comprising the Malays and the native ethnics (68.6%), followed by the Chinese (23.4%), Indians (7.0%), and others (1.0%) (Department of Statistics Malaysia, 2016). In the Malaysian Constitution, Article 160(2) 'Malay' is defined as a person who professes the Muslim religion, habitually speaks the Malay language, and conforms to Malay customs (Burhanudeen, 2006). As Islam influences almost every aspect of the life of the Malays and is central to the Malay identity, is it not surprising that their concept of shame is similar to Islam; thus, upholding Islam as their religion and at the same time maintaining their cultural values (Ismail, Stapa, Othman, & Yacob, 2012; Burhanudeen, 2006).

A deeper understanding of this particular group in terms of their cultural and religious values, relevant characteristics, and challenges are important aspects for culturally competent intervention for recovery from substance dependence. The development of effective intervention tools which consider the integration of Islamic framework of values with existing conventional models is crucial as it supports the norms and expectations of the people. This also allows new alternatives for Malay Muslims experiencing distress due to shame-related issues. Shame within the Malay Muslim group relates to many situations, including substance abuse and dependency (Ali-Northcott, 2012).

The socio-cultural system of the Malays is basically hierarchical and relationship-oriented. Class-based social structure continues even in the face of modernization and industrialization, in the way Malays express the values of respect for elders and fulfil mutual obligations. The Malays also have specific ways of communicating these values in communication, whether verbal or non-verbal such as the use of honorifics for elders and appropriate body postures when walking or sitting in front of them as a sign of respect (Abdullah & Pederson, 2003; Mohamad, Mokhtar, & Abu Samah, 2011).

Another important characteristic of the Malays is their value of *budi bahasa* (courtesy). For the Malays, *budi bahasa* is considered as the key ingredient for harmonious living in a collectivistic society as it guides appropriate conduct, politeness and good manners. Inherited from previous generations, this ethical system (*budi*) is used to guide their everyday life in terms of the way they relate with others (Baharudin, Mahmud, & Amat, 2013, 2014; Musa, Sheik Said, Che Rodi, & Ab Karim, 2012; Noor & Azham 2000; Mohamad, Mokhtar, & Abu Samah, 2011; Wan Husin, 2012; Ibrahim & NoorShah, 2012). Therefore, *budi* governs the code of personal and social conduct of most Malays; reflected in their refined behavior (*halus*) and good manners (*akhlak mulia*).

Not so different from other collectivistic culture, one of the values that the Malays have is shame or '*malu*' in Malay language. Members in the collectivistic culture are expected to behave appropriately to preserve one another's good name and reputation. Members must conform to a set of agreed norms and display them when they interact with others to be part of a group. Thus, behaviour has to be framed in a social context as one is a member of a family, community, and organization. Often it is the family who defines how members should play their roles (Abdullah & Pedersen, 2003). Those who experience shame are often under pressure from their group to act on their behalf and maintain their good name. The key motivation to prevent a person from being shamed is to safeguard his interpersonal relationships with other members of the group.

In the Malay culture, the concept of shame (*malu*) shapes the Malays' character of *budi bahasa*. A person who has no shame (*malu*) means he or she no longer has that special Malay quality of refined behaviour and good manners. As shame (*malu*) is considered important, the Malays tend to avoid disgracing others or being disgraced by them. Those who understand shame (*malu*) are those considered to be well-bred and of high moral character (*akhlak tinggi*) (Abdullah & Pedersen, 2003). This concept of shame (*malu*) in the Malay culture is also in line with Islamic teachings.

This chapter aims to describe selected Islamic psycho-spiritual approaches and practices for transformation of shame for Malay Muslims recovering in substance dependence. It is divided into a discussion of shame from the Malay culture and followed by shame from the Islamic perspective. The chapter continues by describing psycho-spiritual approaches which help Malay Muslims in dealing with shame in the recovery of substance dependence. This chapter ends with a summary and suggestions for future studies.

14.2 Theoretical Framework Anchoring the Chapter

Collectivistic cultures are usually contrasted with individualistic cultures. There are several characteristics that people from collectivistic cultures mostly have in common. People of collectivistic cultures are interdependent and strongly value harmonious relations with their groups such as families. Therefore, they are likely to give priority to group goals (Gorodnichenko & Roland, 2012). This explains why people in collectivistic cultures tend to be concerned with the consequences of a person's actions as they relate to their group or society as a whole. Collectivistic culture concepts of shame include giving high regard to personal and family reputations. As discussed before, this relates to the concept of losing or maintaining face in front of group members (Abdullah & Pedersen, 2003). Therefore, one's behavior is considered as reflecting his or her entire family and extended group reputation (Kobeisy, 2004). Shameful behavior involves violating collectively held understanding of moral conduct and family boundaries (Abudabbeh, 2005). Families experiencing a loss of face in front of their particular group may feel trapped and without resources to regain their sense of dignity.

Muslims in general have a collectivist family structure (Abdullah & Pedersen, 2003; Al-Krenawi & Graham, 2005), especially if roots in traditional culture are retained by the family where family relationships are interdependent. For example, adult children may not leave home until marriage and rather than through asserting personal and financial independence, young adults may reach adulthood by assuming more responsibility within the family collective (Gerson, 1995). Families have a patriarchal structure, gender roles, and hierarchies (Helms, 2015). They highly give importance on respect and authority of elders which influence communication and decision-making processes between family members (Daneshpour, 2012; Hodge & Nadir, 2008). Decisions of those in higher ranking (such as father) are expected to be followed by the wives and children. Any discussions to explore feelings and options may be interpreted as disrespectful (Abudabbeh, 2005). Hence, the extended family plays an important role in exerting influence on the family unit (Al-Krenawi & Graham, 2005; Schlosser, Ali, Ackerman, & Dewet, 2009). Maintaining harmony and stability is preferred over attaining progress or achievement in the family (Daneshpour, 1998). At times, difficult family patterns and interactions may be left unaddressed to preserve family harmony (Daneshpour, 1998; Hodge & Nadir, 2008). Therefore, family members may come to seek help for somatic symptoms instead of discussing problematic relationships.

From the Islamic perspective, shame plays the role of a shield from bad and blasphemous acts, thereby preventing a person from committing sin as well as from neglecting the rights of others (Maskawaih, 2011). Shame is also described as a basic human characteristic as it is a part of an innate affective system. In other words, shame is a self-conscious emotion. While the conventional definition of shame is perceived as a product of dishonour or disgrace, Islam sees shame through a different light by having a preventive stance. Ibnu Qayyim Al Jauziyah (n.d.) said, "Shame is one of the most important, highest, most glorious, and most beneficial traits". Shame is a priority for every Muslim as a proof of obedience to Allah, as described in the Hadith of Prophet Muhammad: "Every religion has its distinct characteristic, and the distinct characteristic of Islam is modesty" (Ibn Majah, 4332).

Many Islamic scholars discuss the priorities and advantages of shame. Among the advantages of shame is that it creates the nature of *'iffah* (guarding honour) because anyone who has shame in his daily living will produce *'iffah* and *'iffah* will produce *wafa'* (faithful belief). This is because not feeling shameful to Allah and human beings will cause a person to be easily caught up in bad things. If shame exists therefore good behaviour will become stronger and bad behaviour will be weaker. On the same note, when shame weakens, bad behaviour will soon dominate. As such, shame from the Islamic understanding covers a broader perspective as it acts as a sanction in preventing one from getting involved in wrongdoings as compared to shame experienced after the events that include the element of guilt.

For Muslims, honor in front of Allah is contrasted against honor based on social approval. The Quran in Surah Ali-Imran, 3: 26 shows that honor and dishonor come only from Allah: "(Allah) Thou (honours) whom Thou willest, and (dishonors) whom Thou willest. In Thy hand is all good. Verily, Thou hast the power to will anything" (Asad, 1980, 70). Additionally, Islam also promotes taking responsibility for one's action, and in the context of this chapter, addressing the experience of shame with inner spiritual effort. This is stated in the Quran, Surah ar-Ra'd, 13: 11: "Verily Allah does not change (a people's) condition unless they change their inner selves" (Asad,

1980, 360). Islam also encourages Muslims to be patient, deterring one from using coercion or violence (Asad, 1980, 32). "Seek aid in steadfast patience and prayer: for behold, Allah is with those who are patient in adversity" (Quran, Surah al-Baqarah, 2: 153).

14.3 Contextual Descriptions

Substance dependence in Malaysia has become a serious problem like many other countries in the world. Despite the declaration of 'War Against Drug' by the country government, the number of relapsing and new cases of substance dependence keep increasing every year (National Anti-Drugs Agency, 2016). Statistics from the Malaysia National Anti-Drug Agency show the involvement of Malay Muslims as the highest in substance dependency. Out of 30844 cases in 2016, 24901 are Malays, followed by 2428 Indian, and 2182 Chinese (National Anti-Drugs Agency, 2016). The numbers are rising rapidly and this illustrates the need for a more comprehensive treatment that includes the elements of culture, religion and spirituality.

However, one of the challenges in providing treatment for people involved in substance dependence in this context is shame. The high number of relapse cases suggests that relapse endorses feelings of failure and shame (Saunders, Zygowicz, & D'Angelo, 2006). On one hand, shame can be negative because it delays or hinders someone from getting treatment because of the value of saving face in the society. It may also reinforce usage and maintain addictive behavior by using substances to eliminate the feelings of shame itself (Wiechelt & Sales, 2001). But on the other hand, shame can be a protective factor because addressing shame may be helpful for developing reasons for stopping use and preventing relapse (Luoma, Kohlenberg, Hayes, & Fletcher, 2012).

In the Malay Muslim culture, having a son or daughter who is involved in substance dependence (addiction) or any other social illnesses can bring shame (*malu*) to the bigger family. This concept of bringing shame (*malu*) to the family is often observed among the more wealthy and respectable families. It is important that the good name of the family and their status are being preserved at all times in order to save face (*jaga air muka*). Family members may hide the problem in order to preserve their good name (*jaga nama baik*). Sometimes, by so doing they are indirectly enabling their son or daughter to continue with the addiction. However, at a later stage, this action may no longer be possible to be covered.

Additionally, many Malay Muslims understand addiction from the perspective of the Moral Model of Addiction. This model sees addiction as a result of human weakness or a defect in one's character. People who subscribe to this model offer little sympathy for those who display addictive behaviors. In their mind, addiction is the result of poor choices by the addicts caused by lack of moral strength or will power. Addicts are stigmatized as they are also associated with other negative behaviours including sin, crime, and domestic violence. Because society had little sympathy towards them, addicts and their family experience shame and become reluctant to acknowledge their problem (Cook, 1987). This may also reinforce further dependency on the part of the addicts because it is a self-medicating method to cope with negative emotions (West & Brown, 2013). In addition, feelings of inadequacy may be triggered by relapse and intensify shame allowing it to evolve into a vicious cycle (Wiechelt, 2007).

Both the concept of saving face from shame and the Moral Model have affected Malay Muslims' help-seeking behaviour, because they are led to believe that this indicates deficiency in faith or family relationships (Kobeisy, 2004). Seeking counseling, admitting problems, or revealing family secrets may also be considered shameful (Abugeideiri, 2012; Scorzelli, 1987).

On the other hand, even though evidences show that shame seems to be a hindrance to recovery, recent discoveries suggest that shame may have positive impact on recovery and this calls for further exploration (Gilbert, 2003, 2006). From the Islamic perspective, shame can be helpful to the internal self—to rectify wrongdoings—and this relates to one's realization, seeking for forgiveness, and connection to Allah and others. Compared to the earlier perspective of defect, this perspective is closer to the Medical or Disease Model of Addiction (Miller, 2014). The Disease Model of Addiction looks at substance dependence as an affliction of the brain resulting in uncontrollable and chronic use, despite negative outcomes for the individual and those around them. This model is seen as an attempt to move away from value laden language inherent in the Moral Model. Addiction as a disease appreciates the vulnerability and fragility of the individual working to reduce stigma and shame of addiction (Miller, 2014).

14.4   Applied Approach

General and specific approaches focusing specifically on the Muslim community have been addressed in multicultural literature for providing a framework in understanding an Islamic worldview as well as suggesting relevant techniques. Significant points in understanding issues and vital elements to be considered when dealing with Muslim clients have been highlighted in these studies. General approaches involve enhancing counselor awareness on the Muslim population, creating therapeutic working alliance and utilizing culture-infused counseling framework (Collins & Arthur, 2010). While specific approaches include explanation of Islamic beliefs and practices, views in mental health and healing, as well as impact of religious factors on treatment planning (Ahmed & Amer, 2012; Hamdan, 2007; Haque & Kamil, 2012; Helms, 2015; Hodge & Nadir, 2008; Ibrahim & Dykeman, 2011; Padela, Killawi, Forman, Demonner, & Heisler, 2012; Skinner, 2010). Previous studies have also found that attention needs to be given to the importance of moral values (Testa, 2012), patriarchal family structures, gender roles, and the role of extended family (Al-Krenawi & Graham, 2005; Deneshpour, 2012; Schlosser et al., 2009) and religious leaders and community in promoting and supporting psychological well-being (Ansary & Salloum, 2012). Extended family, for example, will support in terms of providing comfort and unconditional acceptance while religious leaders help by guiding and teaching. In addition, the act of performing daily prayers together at a mosque and giving charity as encouraged by Islam provide a sense of community or integration among Muslims which also help increase one's well-being (Stack & Kposowa, 2011).

Previous studies have also found positive therapeutic effects when integrating Islamic concepts into the treatment of Muslim clients regardless whether issues of faith are directly or not directly related to the presenting problems (Daneshpour, 2012; Haque & Kamil, 2012). In some cases, studies have also found that religion is a protective factor for the Muslim youth (Abu Raiya & Pergament, 2010). Islamic religious practices and rituals, for example the daily five times compulsory prayer and religious invocations (*zikr*), provide a way to feel closeness to Allah (Abou-Allaban, 2004). Additionally, activities that may lead to harming oneself or others such as taking drugs and gambling is considered forbidden in Islam. These facilitate positive outcomes by buffering individuals from constructs that place them at risk of engaging in addictive substances and practices (Coceran & Nichols Casebot, 2004).

Several studies have shown an emerging trend of integration of religion and spirituality, especially Islam, in mental health counseling in Malaysia (Mat Akhir & Sabjan, 2004; Ahmad, Mustaffa, & Ramli, 2005; Hamjah & Mat Akhir, 2007; Sarmani & Ninggal, 2008; Mohamed, 2009). By integrating religion and spirituality in counseling, a counselor would be utilizing a holistic approach when providing treatment to clients and this will improve the outcome.

Other studies look at the techniques and process of counseling and religious practices used (Azimullah & Muhammad, 2011; Abdul Razak et al., 2011; Koding, 2010; Ahmad Ibrahim, Wan Razali, & Othman, 2006; Kamis, 2010; Nik Yaakob & Mohd. Yusof, 2009; Amat & Hamjah, 2014; Ghazali, Chin, & Jayos, 2009; Hamjah, 2010a, 2010b; Sipon & Ramli, 2011; Hassan, 2015; Ismail, Wan Ahmad, & Ab Rahman, 2014).

In the treatment of substance dependence, many rehabilitation and treatment institutions in Malaysia have incorporated Islamic psycho-spiritual approaches such as understanding the five pillars of Islam, performing prayers and religious invocations (*zikr*), and developing the sense of piety (*taqwa*) into their framework (Seghatoleslam et al., 2015). Some examples include the Malaysian Cure and Care Rehabilitation Centers (CCRC), Pondok Remaja Inabah (1) Malaysia, and some private drug rehabilitation centers. Previous studies that can be found in Ghani et al. (2017), Dara Aisyah et al. (2013), Khalid (2008), Mohamed and Marican (2017), and Muhamad et al. (2015), show positive results when Islamic psycho-spiritual approaches are implemented at these institutions. The Islamic psycho-spiritual approach support addicts in recovery, guided by Islamic principles (Rozeeda et al., 2017) which encourage a person to resubmit themselves to their Creator, Allah and acknowledge that as human beings, they are weak. In this approach, feelings of shame are encouraged to be expressed in the form of religious and spiritual practices in order to make amends. Shame is acknowledged and reframed into the positive, motivating the people in recovery to change. They are given insight that despite of their wrongdoings, shame is an acceptable feeling to start moving towards the right path and reconnect with

Allah, the Most Forgiving and One who will accept their repentance. This removes blame and consequently, shame. By acknowledging the experience of shame in a safe and supportive space allows them to construct an understanding of shame and subsequently heal them.

14.4.1 Applied Method/Techniques Dealing with Shame Constructively

The Islamic resources supported by previous studies provided sufficient information to emerge as an approach to be integrated and expanded into a psycho-spiritual intervention for addressing issues of shame in substance dependence recovery for the Malay Muslims. This model would comprise healing through the process of *muhasabah* (self-audit), *tawbah* (repentance and forgiveness), constructing new narrative of the self, and developing a stronger relationship with Allah (*hablum min Allah*) and other humans (*hablum min annas*) as the foundation for healthy recovery.

14.4.2 Muhasabah *(Self-audit)*

Muhasabah or self-audit is the state of awakening, where the person in recovery is encouraged to become aware of the need for change and the problem that must be solved (Rassool, 2016). Discussion of how shame influences the taking of substances will help in developing an insight of how his/her past sin is part of his/her nature as a human being who is created weak. And understanding that the behavior of taking substance was an act of negligence of his/her duty as a servant of Allah allows for a sense of shame on oneself. Reflecting on one's past sins allow for self-consciousness to the extent that one may be able to become aware that Allah is watching and monitoring him/her (*muraqabah al-nafs*) and this is important in changing any thought or behavior (Al-Ghazali, 1991). In many cases, *muhasabah* will lead to *tawbah* (repentance and forgiveness).

14.4.3 Tawbah *(Repentance and Forgiveness)*

Tawbah is based on the belief that humans are not perfect and by nature is weak and that Allah is the Most Forgiving. *Tawbah* literally means to turn back toward something (in this case to turn back toward Allah). The act of *tawbah* is to repent or seek forgiveness sincerely for sins and mistakes that have been committed (Al-Makki, 1997). It is the hallmark of *tazkiyyatun nafs* (purification of the heart). Realising that one regrets for not being shameful in the past by letting oneself be tempted to substances, he/she must now clean or purifies himself/herself from the sins that he/she has committed in life. He/she must also have the believe and hope that Allah will accept his/her repentance similar to the story of Adam and Eve in the Quran whereby when they committed their mistake, they realised their mistake then repented and prayed sincerely to Allah who forgave both of them (Quran, Surah al-Baqarah, 2: 37).

Tawbah can be divided into two stages. Firstly, a person must repent his sins and promise not to repeat the sin, grieving over the sin committed, and continuously (*istiqamah*) follow Allah's commands and avoiding what is prohibited. This is followed by the second stage that focuses on striving to correct the sin by replacing bad deeds with good ones, as well as being sad and remorseful of the past sins (Al-Makki, 1997).

In terms of experience of shame in the recovery of substance dependence, repentance and forgiveness enable Muslims to admit their mistakes and the weaknesses and to re-connect and further re-build their relationship with Allah. Additionally, by repenting, they are also resubmitting their will to the will of Allah and admitting that they are totally reliant upon Allah for sustenance (Rassool, 2016).

Besides seeking forgiveness from Allah, self-forgiveness is also important in accepting shame and preventing relapse. By providing a safe and supportive setting in treatment where shame can be explored and revealed, healing can occur through acceptance of the person. Once the feeling of shame is accepted, recovery can happen In summary, *muhasabah* (self-audit) and *tawbah* (repentance) are two important elements in the process of healing and recovery. The next element is constructing new narrative of the self.

14.4.4 Constructing New Narrative of the Self

Having the opportunity to acknowledge and accept shame as part of being human allows one to develop a new narrative about the self during recovery process. This involves believing in the power of Allah to guide oneself towards the right path and restore shame and honour in one's life.

The process of constructing new narrative of the self also includes *raja'* (hope) and *khauf* (fear). *Raja'* or hope is a strong desire when seeking help from Allah that shows the dependence of human being to Allah (Al-Makki, 1997). As servants of Allah, it is important to go back to Allah who decrees what may befall him even though one has a sense of motivation or goal-oriented purpose and perception of his ability to initiate and maintain goal-directed behaviors (Snyder, Lopez, Shorey, Rand, & Feldman, 2003). At the same time, one needs to think well of Allah (*husnus zhan*) that the goal or request that one has will be fulfilled by only Him. The feelings of hope should be balanced. If it gets better than our judgment and make us complacent, there is a need to cultivate *khawf* (fear) (Rassool, 2016). *Khawf* or fear of Allah helps one to regain the sense of shame (for fear of not being able to perform or fulfil the duties of a good Muslim).

14.5 Developing a Stronger Relationship with Allah (*Hablum Min Allah*) and Other Humans (*Hablum Min Annas*)

After constructing their story of shame and moving toward a new story of hope and possibilities, Malay Muslims in recovery, whether individuals or family, will be encouraged to develop a stronger relationship with Allah and reconnect them into their communities. These are the two major relationships emphasized in Islam. A Muslim's relationship with Allah is central to their belief. The Quran constantly reminded that Allah is closer to the human being than a vital vein (Quran, Surah al Qaf, 50: 16); therefore, He knows the human soul and the struggles that it faces (Rassool, 2016). Religious practices such as reading Quranic scriptures, performing daily prayer and supplications (*do'a*), as well as religious invocations (*zikr*), along with fasting, and works of charity are generally recommended for the purpose of becoming closer to Alllah (Ali & Aboul-Fotouh, 2012; Padela et al., 2012; Utz, 2012).

Having a good relationship with other humans is also highlighted by the Quran as good manners and proper way of dealing with other people (*adab/akhlak*) are emphasized in the teachings of Islam (Rassool, 2016). Community resources such as mosques, associations, governmental or non-profit rehabilitation and treatment agencies can be utilized to facilitate an environment of acceptance and responsibility for previously shamed person in recovery from substance dependence and the family affected as they regain their face in front of their community and proceed with their journey towards a renewed honour and dignity.

The following case presents the narration of self of Ahmad and his transformation through psycho-spiritual development.

14.6 Case Study

Ahmad is 29 years old, Malay Muslim male, and is 8 months in recovery from alcohol and poly-drug addiction. As a child he was an introvert and a shy child. He began taking substances at the age of 11 and described the transforming effect it had on his confidence. Ahmad acknowledged that he was addicted to substances by the age of 16 causing out-of-control behavior which effected his school performance. He dropped out of school and later got into a pattern of getting in and out of jobs. He got married and had one child, but his marriage broke down as a result of his addiction. Many of the events in Ahmad's past were shameful and he was still struggling to overcome these. His recovery was part of a rehabilitation program that integrates psycho-spiritual components.

At the early stages of treatment, Ahmad was asked to audit (*muhasabah*) himself of past experiences that led to shame. He shared how the feelings of not being worthy and inferior led him to take substances. Discussions on human being created weak and his disconnect from Allah helped Ahmad develop a sense of shame on himself for not fulfilling his duty as a servant of Allah. By acknowledging Ahmad's shame and explaining how Allah is the Most Forgiving, Ahmad was encouraged to accept his mistakes and weaknesses by repentance and seeking forgiveness (*tawbah*) from Allah. The process of *tawbah* was explained. Ahmad was taught a specific prayer known as the *tawbah* prayer and religious invocations for example "*Astaghfirullah*" to practice. Ahmad was also encouraged to re-connect and re-build his relationship with Allah through performing daily prayer, reading Quranic scriptures, supplications (*do'a*), other religious invocations (*zikr*), and fasting. Homework were given during this stage to ensure that Ahmad was able to apply what was learnt.

Treatment continued with Ahmad constructing a new narrative of self, of his hope and how he sees himself in the future. This was followed by discussions on relapse and the believe in the power of Allah to guide him towards the right path as well as accepting shame and restore honour in his life. The intention here was to assess progression in Ahmad's story - moving from a place of failure and blame towards acceptance, positive self-regard, and dependence to Allah. Finally, Ahmad was re-connected to the community with the support and involvement of Ahmad's family and religious leaders at the place they live. He is now working with his brother in a family business and goes to mosque for his daily prayers. Follow-up sessions found that even though Ahmad still faces daily battles in maintaining his recovery, he was also reflective of the positive changes he has made.

14.7 Conclusion

Understanding shame in the context of Malay Muslims and its role in recovery would help support those with issues of substance dependency. More work needs to be done to provide mental health practitioners in Malaysia with specific therapeutic tools to counsel Malay Muslims. It is hoped that the psycho-spiritual approach shared in this paper provides valuable information that can be used by mental health practitioners in a practical form. One limitation is the lack of research studies documenting outcome measures when implementing the psycho-spiritual or intervention tools. Research in other areas that are related to shame in the Malay Muslim community such as sexual relations outside of marriage, infidelity, teen pregnancies, abuse/domestic violence, and other behaviors or conditions that are socially unacceptable could also be addressed as those would also help explore fundamental factors and develop more alternative strategies regarding this issue.

References

Abdul Razak, A. L., Mohamed, M., Alias, A., Wan Adam, K., Mohd Kasim, N., & Mutiu, S. (2011). Iman restoration therapy (IRT): *A new counseling approach and its usefulness in developing personal growth of Malay adolescent clients.* Paper presented at the 3rd conference of the international association of muslim psychologists. International Islamic University of Malaysia. Gombak, December 6–8, 2011.

Abdullah, A., & Pedersen, P. B. (2003). *Understanding multicultural Malaysia: Delights, puzzles, & irritations.* Petaling Jaya: Pearson Prentice Hall.

Abou-Allaban, Y. (2004). Muslims. In A. M. Josephson & J. R. Peteet (Eds.), *Handbook of spirituality and worldview in clinical practice* (pp. 111–123). Arlington, VA: American Psychiatric Publishing Inc.

Abu Raiya, H., & Pargament, K. (2010). Religiously integrated psychotherapy with Muslim clients: From research to practice. *Professional Psychology: Research and Practice, 41*(2), 181–188. Retrieved from https://doi.org/10.1037/a0017988.

Abudabbeh, N. (2005). Arab families: An overview. In M. McGoldrick, J. Giordano, & I. Gracia Preto (Eds.), *Ethnicity and family therapy* (3rd ed., pp. 423–436). New York, NY: Guilford Press.

Abugeideiri, S. (2012). Domestic violence. In S. Ahmed & M. Amer (Eds.), *Counseling muslims: Handbook of mental health issues and interventions* (pp. 309–328). New York, NY: Routledge Press.

Ahmad Ibrahim, M. A., Wan Razali, W. M. F. A., & Othman, H. (2006). *Kaunseling dalam Islam.* Nilai: Fakulti Kepimpinan dan Pengurusan.

Ahmad, R., Mustaffa, M. S., & Ramli, J. (2005). *Kesihatan mental rakyat Malaysia masa kini. Suatu pendekatan kaunseling berdasarkan nilai-nilai Islam.* Paper presented at the Persidangan Kaunseling Universiti Malaya 2005. Universiti Malaya. Kuala Lumpur, November 29–29, 2005.

Ahmed, S., & Amer, M. (2012). *Counseling Muslims: Handbook of mental health issues and interventions.* New York, NY: Routledge Press.

Al-Ghazali. (1991). *Ihya' 'Ulum al-Din.* Misr: Maktabat al-Tijariyah al-Kubra.

Ali, O., & Aboul-Fotouh, F. (2012). Traditional mental health coping and help-seeking. In S. Ahmed & M. Amer (Eds.), *Counseling Muslims: Handbook of mental health issues and interventions* (pp. 33–55). New York, NY: Routledge Press.

Ali-Northcott, L. (2012). Substance abuse. In S. Ahmed & M. Amer (Eds.), *Counseling Muslims: Handbook of mental health issues and interventions* (pp. 355–382). New York, NY: Routledge Press.

Al-Jauziyyah, I. Q. (n.d.). *Madaarij-Salikin fi Manaazilis-Saa'ireen* (trans Talib Ibn Tyson al-Britaanee).

Al-Krenawi, A., & Graham, J. (2005). Marital therapy for Arab Muslim Palestinian couples in the context of reacculturation. *Family Journal, 13,* 300–310. Retrieved from http://dx.doi.org/10.1177/1066480704273640.

Al-Makki, A. T. (1997). *Qut al-Qulub* (Vol. 1). Beirut: Dar al-Kitab al-Ilmiyah.

Amat, N., & Hamjah, S. H. (2014). Asas pembinaan kelaurga sejahtera menurut Islam. In Z. Ismail, S. H. Hamjah, & R. M. Rasit, (Eds.), *Isu Dakwah Masa Kini: Keluarga, Komuniti Marginal dan Pendidikan* (pp. 15–26). Bangi: Penerbit Universiti Kebangsaan Malaysia.

Ansary, N., & Salloum, R. (2012). Community-based prevention and intervention. In S. Ahmed & M. Amer (Eds.), *Counseling Muslims: Handbook of mental health issues and interventions* (pp. 1461–182). New York, NY: Routledge Press.

Asad, M. (1980). *The message of the Qur'an.* London, UK: E. J. Brill.

Azimullah, A. Z., & Muhammad, (2011). *Islamic solution for 21st century societal problems: Transcendent integrative psychology based on the Khalifah method.* Paper presented at the 3rd conference of the international association of muslim psychologists. International Islamic University of Malaysia. Gombak, December 6–8, 2011.

Baharudin, D. F., Mahmud, Z., & Amat, S. (2013). *Pandangan golongan Melayu dewasa tentang kesejahteraan: Satu penerokaan awal*. Paper presented at the PERKAMA counseling convention 2013. Persatuan Kaunseling Malaysia. Kuala Lumpur, June 9–11, 2013.

Baharudin, D. F., Mahmud, Z., & Amat, S. (2014). *Definition of wellness among diverse groups of adults in Malaysia*. 2014 Asian Congress of Applied Psychology Proceeding, pp. 320–335. Retrieved from http://academy.edu.sg/ACAP-Conference-Proceedings.pdf (May 7–8, 2014).

Burhanudeen, H. (2006). *Language & social behaviour. Voices from the Malay World*. Malaysia, Bangi: Penerbit Universiti Kebangsaan.

Coceran, J., & Nichols Casebot, A. (2004). Risk and resilience ecological framework for assessment and goal formulation. *Journal of Child Adolescent Psychotherapy, 21*, 211–235.

Collins, S., & Arthur, N. (2010). Culturally sensitive working alliance. In N. Arthur & S. Collins (Eds.), *Culture-infused counselling* (2nd ed., pp. 103–138). Calgary, AB: Counselling Concepts.

Cook, D. R. (1987). Measuring shame: The internalized shame scale. *Alcoholism Treatment Quarterly, 4*(2), 197–215.

Daneshpour, M. (1998). Muslim families and family therapy. *Journal of Marital and Family Therapy, 24*(3), 355–390.

Daneshpour, M. (2012). Family systems therapy and postmodern approaches. In S. Ahmed & M. Amer (Eds.), *Counseling Muslims: Handbook of mental health issues and interventions* (pp. 119–134). New York, NY: Routledge Press.

Dara Aisyah, H. M., Ali Puteh, Ibrahim M., Norizan A. G., et al. (2013) Drug addict treatment and rehabilitation programme at Pondok Inabah, Kuala Terengganu, Terengganu, Malaysia (1998–2011). *British Journal of Social Sciences, 1*(5), 37–46.

Department of Statistics Malaysia. (2016). *Current population estimates, Malaysia 2014–2016*. Retrieved on January 30, 2018 from https://www.dosm.gov.my/v1/index.php?r=column/cthemeByCat&cat=155&bul_id=OWlxdEVoYlJCS0hUZzJyRUcvZEYxZz09&menu_id=L0pheU43NWJwRWVSZklWdzQ4TlhUUT09.

Gerson, R. (1995). The family life cycle: Phases, stages, and crises. In R. H. Mikesell, D. D. Lusterman, & S. H. McDaniel (Eds.), *Integrating family therapy: Handbook of family psychology and systems therapy*. (pp. 91–111). Washington DC: American Psychological Association.

Ghani, A. A., Maamor, S., Ali, A. B., Razimi, M. S. A., Wahab, N. A., Abdullah, N. S. N., et al. (2017). Kaedah rawatan penagih tegar dadah melalui pendekatan kerohanian: Kajian kes di Pondok Inabah (1) Malaysia Pri(1) M, Kedah. *Journal of Advanced Research in Business and Management Studies, 7*(1), 39–50.

Ghazali, N. M., Chin, K. S., & Jayos, S. (2009). *Spirituality approach and narrative therapy as post-structuralist approach in counselling practice*. Paper presented at the Seminar Kebangsaan PERKAMA Kali Ke-14: Kepelbagaian dan Kesejagatan dalam Kaunseling 2009. Anjuran Persatuan Kaunseling Malaysia dan Universiti Putra Malaysia. Serdang, June 2–3, 2009.

Gilbert, P. (2003). Evolution, social roles, and differences in shame and guilt. *Social Research, 70*, 1205–1230.

Gilbert, P. (2006). A biopsychosocial and evolutionary approach to formulation with a special focus on shame. In N. Tarrier (Ed.), *Case formulation in CBT: The treatment of challenging and complex cases* (pp. 81–112). East Sussex: Routledge.

Gorodnichenko, Y., & Roland, G. (2012). Understanding the individualism-collectivism cleavage and its effects: Lessons from cultural psychology. In M. Aoki, T. Kuran, G. Roland (Eds.), *Institutions and comparative economic development. International Economic Association Series* (pp. 213–236). Palgrave MacMillan: London.

Hamdan, A. (2007). A case study of a Muslim client: Incorporating religious belief and practices. *Journal of Multicultural Counseling and Development, 35*, 92–100.

Hamjah, S. H. (2010a). Bimbingan spiritual menurut al-Ghazali dan hubungannya dengan keberkesanan kaunseling: Satu kajian di Pusat Kaunseling Majlis Agama Islam Negeri Sembilan (PK MAINS). *Islamiyyat, 32*, 41–61.

Hamjah, S. H. (2010b). Kaedah mengatasi kebimbangan dalam kaunseling. *Analisis dari perspektif al-Ghazali. Jurnal Hadhari, 3*(1), 41–57.

Hamjah, S. H., & Mat Akhir, N. S. (2007). Riyadah al-Nafs menurut Al-Ghazali dan aplikasinya dalam kaunseling di PK MAINS. *Jurnal Usuluddin*, 26, 45–62.

Haque, A., & Kamil, N. (2012). Islam, Muslims, and mental health. In S. Ahmed & M. Amer (Eds.), *Counseling Muslims: Handbook of mental health issues and interventions* (pp. 3–14). New York, NY: Routledge Press.

Hassan, S. A. (2015). Islamic transcendental wellbeing model for Malaysian Muslim women: Implication on counseling. *Asian Social Science, 11*(21), 331–341.

Helms, B. L. (2015). Honour and shame in the Canadian Muslim community: Developing culturally sensitive counseling interventions. *Canadian Journal of Counselling and Psychotherapy, 49*(2), 163–184.

Hodge, D., & Nadir, A. (2008). Moving toward culturally competent practice with Muslims: Modifying cognitive therapy with Islamic tenets. *Social Work, 53*(1), 31–41.

Ibrahim, F., & Dykeman, C. (2011). Counseling Muslim Americans: Cultural and spiritual assessments. *Journal of Counseling and Development, 89*, 387–396.

Ibrahim, Z., & NoorShah, M. S. (2012). Indigenising knowledge and social science discources in the periphery: Decolonising Malayness and Malay Underdevelopment. In Z. Ibrahim (Ed.), *Social Science and knowledge in a globalising world* (pp. 1–35). Kajang: Persatuan Sains Sosial Malaysia.

Ismail, A. M., Stapa, Z., Othman, M. Y., & Yacob, M. (2012). Islam dalam pendidikan dan hubungannya dengan pembangunan jati diri bangsa Melayu di Malaysia. *Jurnal Hadhari*, Special Edition, 37–50.

Ismail, Z., Wan Ahmad, W. I., & Ab Rahman, A. (2014). Counseling services in Muslim communal life in Malaysia. *Middle-East Journal of Scientific Research, 20*(11), 1445–1448.

Kamis, M. S. (2010). *Kaunseling Islam: Soalan-soalan untuk klien semasa sesi kaunseling.* Paper presented at the Seminar Kaunseling Silang Budaya 2010. Anjuran Persatuan Kaunseling Malaysia. Serdang, March 20, 2010.

Khalid, Muhammad Yusuf. (2008). Psycho-spiritual therapy approach for drug addiction rehabilitation. *Malaysian Anti-Drug Journal, 3 & 4*, 143–151.

Kobeisy, A. (2004). *Counseling American Muslims: Understanding the faith and helping the people.* Westport, CT: Praeger.

Koding, A. (2010). *Penjernihan hati: Penyelesaian masalah secara kaunseling peribadi.* Paper presented at the seminar Kaunseling Silang Budaya 2010. Persatuan Kaunseling Malaysia. Serdang, Mac 20, 2010.

Luoma, J. B., Kohlenberg, B. S., Hayes, S. C., & Fletcher, L. (2012). Slow and steady wins the race: A randomized clinical trial of acceptance and commitment therapy targeting shame in substance use disorders. *Journal of Consulting and Clinical Psychology, 80*(1), 43–53.

Maskawaih, I. (2011). *Tahdzib Al Akhlaq fii At Tarbiyah.* Beirut: Mansyurat al-Jamal.

Mat Akhir, N. S., & Sabjan, M. A. (2004). The spiritual dynamic elements in Al-Ghazali's theory of soul. In Long, A. S., Awang, J., & Salleh K. (Eds.), *Islam: Past, present, future* (pp. 565–569). Bangi: Department of Theology and Philosophy, Faculty of Islamic Studies, Universiti Kebangsaan Malaysia.

Miller, G. (2014). *Learning the language of addiction counseling.* (4th ed., pp. 6–8). Hoboken, NJ: Wiley.

Mohamad, M., Mokhtar, H. H., & Abu Samah, A. (2011). Person-centered counseling with Malay clients: Spirituality as an indicator of personal growth. *Procedia Social and Behavioral Sciences, 30*, 2117–2123.

Mohamed, O. (2009). Counseling and the spiritual context of harmony and peace. *International Counseling and Social Work Symposium Proceeding, Penang, 2009, 332*–335.

Mohamed, M. N., & Marican, S. (2017). Incorporating Islam in the therapeutic community modality for rehabilitation of substance and drug users. A Malaysian experience. International *Journal of Human and Health Sciences, 1*(1), 7–17.

Muhamad, S. N., Yusof, F. M., Nizar, T. J., Ghazali, M. A., Abdullah, A., & Mamat, A. (2015). Keberkesanan rawatan pemulihan dadah menggunakan pendekatan keagamaan: Kajian dalam kalangan pelatih wanita di CCRC Bachok (Kelantan), AADK Besut, AADK Kemaman, dan CCSC Kuala Terengganu (Terengganu). *Jurnal Antidadah Malaysia, 9*(1), 50–63.

Musa, H., Sheik Said, N., Che Rodi, R., & Ab Karim, S. S. (2012). Hati budi Melayu: Kajian keperibadian sosial Melayu ke arah penjanaan Melayu gemilang. *GEMA Online Journal of Language Studies 12*(1), 163–182.

National Anti-Drugs Agency. (2016). Drugs Statistics 2010–2016. Retrieved on January 30, 2018 from https://www.adk.gov.my/en/public/drugs-statistics/.

Nik Yaakob, N. R., & Mohd. Yusof, N. (2009). Integrating spirituality and religion in counselling practice from Islamic perspective. In *International counseling and social work symposium 2009 Proceeding* (pp. 173–181).

Noor, I., & Azham, M. (2000). *The Malays par excellence… warts and all. An introspection.* Subang Jaya: Pelanduk Publications.

Padela, A., Killawi, A., Forman, J., Demonner, S., & Heisler, M. (2012). American Muslim perceptions of healing: Key agents in healing and their roles. *Qualitative Health Research, 22,* 847–858.

Rassool, H. G. (2016). *Islamic counselling: An introduction to theory and practice.* New York: Routledge.

Rozeeda, K., Nasir, M., Rohayah, H., Khairi, C. M., Syed Hadzrullathfi, S. O., & Syed Mohd Hafiz, S. O. (2017). Addiction and Islamic based therapy in Malaysia. *Man in India, 97*(26), 233–239.

Sarmani, Y. & Ninggal, M. T. (2008). *Teori Kaunseling al-Ghazali.* Selangor: PTS Publications.

Saunders, S. M., Zygowicz, K. M., & D'Angelo, B. R. (2006). Person-related and treatment-related barriers to alcoholtreatment. *Journal of Substance Abuse Treatment, 30,* 261–270.

Schlosser, L., Ali, S., Ackerman, S., & Dewey, J. (2009). Religion, ethnicity, culture, way of life: Jew, Muslims, and multicultural counseling. *Counseling and Values, 54,* 48–64.

Scorzelli, J. F. (1987). Counseling in Malaysia: An emerging profession. *Journal of Counseling & Development, 65,* 238–240.

Seghatoleslam, T., Habil, H., Hatim, A., Rashid, R., Ardakan, A., & Esmaeili Motlaq, F. (2015). Achieving a spiritual therapy standard for drug dependency in Malaysia, from an Islamic perspective: Brief Review Article. *Iran J Public Health, 44*(1), 22–27.

Sipon, S., & Ramli, R. M. (2011). *Strategi berdaya tindak kaedah keagamaan terhadap masalah pelajar: Strategi memperkasakan kaunseling melalui kaunseling berkualiti.* Paper presented at the PERKAMA International Convention 2011. PERKAMA International. Kuala Lumpur, June 21–22, 2011.

Skinner, R. (2010). An Islamic approach to psychology and mental health. *Mental Health, Religion & Culture, 13*(6), 547–551.

Snyder, C. R., Lopez, S. J., Shorey, H. S., Rand, K. L., & Feldman, D. B. (2003). Hope theory, measurements and applications to school psychology. *School Psychology Quarterly,* 18(2), 122–139.

Stack, S., & Kposowa, A. J. (2011). Religion and suicide acceptability: A cross-national analysis. *Journal for the Scientific Study of Religion, 50*(2), 289–306.

Testa, G. (2012). Intergenerational issues with the Muslim community. *Research Ethics, 8,* 15–146.

Utz, A. (2012). Conceptualizations of mental health, illness, and healing. In S. Ahmed & M. Amer (Eds.), *Counseling Muslims: Handbook of mental health issues and interventions* (pp. 15–32). New York, NY: Routledge Press.

Wan Husin, W. N. (2012). *Peradaban dan Perkauman di Malaysia.* Kuala Lumpur: Penerbit Universiti Malaya.

West, R., & Brown, J. (2013). *Theory of addiction* (2nd ed.). Hoboken, NJ: Wiley.

Wiechelt, S. A. (2007). The spectre of shame in substance misuse. *Substance Use and Abuse, 42*(2–3), 399–409.

Wiechelt, S. A., & Sales, E. (2001). The role of shame in women's recovery from alcoholism: The impact of childhood sexual abuse. *Journal of Social Work Practice in the Addictions, 1*(14), 101–116.

Dini Farhana Baharudin (Ph.D.) is a lecturer at the Faculty of Leadership and Management, Universiti Sains Islam Malaysia, Nilai, Malaysia. She holds a degree in Law, Master degrees in Community Counseling (M.A.) and in Education (M.Ed.), and a Ph.D. in Counseling. She is also a Registered and Licensed Counselor in Malaysia. Besides teaching, she is actively involved in research and publications on multiculturalism and diversity in counseling, marriage and family counseling, addiction counseling, and holistic wellness.

Melati Sumari (Dr.) is a Senior Lecturer at the University of Malaya, Kuala Lumpur, Malaysia. She has been working at the university since 1997. She obtained a Bachelor and Master degrees in Education (Counseling), both from the University of Malaya, and a doctoral degree in Counselor Education and Supervision from Western Michigan University, USA. She has published two academic books in counseling, more than 10 book chapters and journal articles in counseling. She has also been awarded a number of research grants. Her research and writing focus mainly on marriage, family, and addiction counseling in cultural context. She also presented in local and international conferences.

Suhailiza Md. Hamdani is lecturer at the Faculty of Leadership and Management, Universiti Sains Islam Malaysia, Nilai, Malaysia. She has a Bachelor degree in Usuluddin from the University of Malaya, Malaysia, a Master degree in 'Aqeedah from the University of al Al Bayt, Jordan. She currently finishes her Ph.D. in Islamic Revealed Knowledge from the Islamic International University of Malaysia. Her interests are in da'wah, psycho-spiritual therapy, and 'aqeedah.

Part V
Transforming Shame in Organisational Contexts

Chapter 15
Managing Shame in Organisations: Don't Let Shame Become a Self-destructive Spiral

Rudolf M. Oosthuizen

Abstract After a major mistake, it is natural to feel ashamed. Nevertheless, shame is also a powerfully destructive feeling. Left to fester, it can have a profound effect on psychological well-being (Mayer, Viviers, & Tonelli, in SA J Ind Psychol/SA Tydskrif vir Bedryfsielkunde 43(0):a1385, 2017). It is concealed behind guilt, it lurks behind anger, and it can be disguised as despair and depression. The question as to how employees can cope with shame in organisations can be asked. Here are two maladaptive strategies: attacking the self or attacking other employees. Initially, hostility is directed inward ("I'm worthless," "I've never been any good"). In an attempt to feel better, some employees will lash out in defensiveness and denial. Others may try to compensate by being exceptionally nice or by pleasing other employees in the hopes of improving their feelings of self-worth (Velotti, Garofalo, Bottazzi, & Caretti, in J Psychol 151(2):171–184, 2017). An improved approach is to discover the true source of shame, and then practice self-compassion (Irons & Lad, in Aust Clin Psychol 3(1):47–54, 2017).

Keywords Shame · Self-compassion · Mindfulness · Common humanity · Self-kindness · Organisational psychology

15.1 Introduction

Employees who feel shame tend to internalise and over personalise everything that happens to them. They cannot see things in perspective. When something goes wrong, they say to themselves, "I'm to blame for what happened. It's entirely my fault." Not only do they demean themselves, but they also feel helpless, and do not think that there is anything they can do to change the situation. The internal critic in their heads

R. M. Oosthuizen (✉)
Department of Industrial and Organisational Psychology, School of Management Sciences, College of Economic and Management Sciences, AJH van der Walt Building, 03-77, Pretoria, South Africa
e-mail: oosthrm@unisa.ac.za

© Springer Nature Switzerland AG 2019
C.-H. Mayer and E. Vanderheiden (eds.), *The Bright Side of Shame*,
https://doi.org/10.1007/978-3-030-13409-9_15

continually judges and criticises them, telling them that they are inadequate, inferior, or worthless (Kets de Vries, 2017).

At work, anxiety, suffering, disaffection—and, sometimes, emotional exhaustion or burnout—can be precipitated by a single event. Just as harmfully, they can also arise from incremental or longer-term experiences or as a result of progressive mental injury or maladaptation over time. These conditions are related to the chronic symptoms occasioned by acute mental health and post-traumatic stress disorder (PTSD) related traumas and appear in addition to them (Devenish-Meares, 2015). Any of these conditions or symptoms can have a profound effect on an employee's psychological well-being.

Excessive feelings of shame are at the heart of much psychopathology. Shame is concealed behind guilt; it lurks behind anger; it can be disguised as despair and depression. As employees rarely talk about experiences involving shame, it is a difficult emotion to detect, especially as it hides behind so many disguises (Ludwiga, Fellner-Röhlinga, & Thomab, 2017).

15.2   Theoretical Background of Shame in Organisations

Shame is an overwhelming and unpleasant emotion, for example, as a typically discrete and intense but short-lived affective experience in reaction to a stimulus (Elfenbein, 2007; Smith & Ellsworth, 1985) that occurs in response to a self-attributed failure in meeting the expectations of others in the organisation (Bagozzi, Verbeke, & Gavino, 2003; Brown, González, Zagefka, Manzi, & Čehajić, 2008). In other words, shame arises when employees encounter differences between what they actually do (actual self) and what they are expected to do (ought self) (Ghorbani, Liao, Çayköylü, & Chand, 2013). In organisational settings, experiences of shame may be triggered by failure to meet obligations, making a mistake in a report or presentation, being criticised by a peer or supervisor or failing to meet performance standards. Shame experiences make individuals feel and fear negative evaluations from others (Agrawal, Han, & Duhachek, 2013), and it is this social scrutiny that motivates them to protect the self from further damage (De Hooge, Zeelenberg, &, Breugelmans, 2010, 2011; Ferguson, 2005). As such, coping with a damaged self-image is a central concern for ashamed employees (González-Gómez, & Richter, 2015).

In order to elude negative evaluations from others, employees typically express shame in the form of withdrawal and avoidance tendencies, including avoidance of eye contact, a hunched posture, and withdrawing from contact with others by hiding in their offices or remaining silent in meetings (Bagozzi et al., 2003; Fischer & Tangney, 1995). By means of withdrawal from, or avoidance of situations related to the shame experience, employees aim to protect the self from further damage. In the light of the unpleasantness of shame experiences, it is not surprising that prior research has predominantly examined their negative effects, including low self-efficacy and self-esteem, social anxiety, and depression (Lazarus & Folkman, 1984; Leary & Kowalsky, 1995; Tangney, Miller, Flicker, & Barrow, 1996; González-Gómez & Richter, 2015).

15.2.1 The Origins of Shame in Organisations

Given the pervasiveness of this emotion across ages and cultures, what is the adaptive purpose of shame? From an evolutionary point of view, we could hypothesise that shame evolved under organisational conditions where survival depended on employees abiding by certain norms. They needed to stand together to operate effectively as a group in order to better deal with complex situations. Interestingly, these behaviour patterns can still be observed today when employees tend to take a compliant posture out of shame, when they subject themselves to the power and judgment of other employees (Kets de Vries, 2017).

From a systems psychodynamic perspective (Tonelli, in this book), shame can be seen as a complex emotional response that employees acquire during the early phases of their careers in their organisations and when they are completely dependent on the bond with their supervisors. It is a very basic emotion: employees seek to live up to their supervisor's expectations and, failing to do so, experience shame. Employees exhibit early feelings of embarrassment that can turn into full-blown shame within the early stages of their careers (Kets de Vries, 2017).

While it may seem that shame can ultimately serve a purpose, perhaps in the example of an employee feeling ashamed after being scolded by a supervisor, such shameful experiences may damage the roots from which self-esteem grows. Dysfunctional organisational parenting styles can make employees shame-bound and this kind of shame is very difficult to overcome. The formative wounds of new employees—scars from being bullied (Merkin, in this book) or ostracised by supervisors, peers, and other colleagues—can become fixed in their identity (Kets de Vries, 2017; Mayer, Viviers, & Tonelli, 2017).

15.2.2 Managing Shame in Organisations

The more powerful the experience of shame is for employees, the more they feel compelled to hide those aspects from others, and even from themselves. The first step is thus to bring to light whatever is seen as shameful. After all, a wound that is never exposed will never heal. If the wound is deep enough, employees may need to ask a counsellor or therapist for help. Being able to discover the origins of shame-like experiences will set the stage for having greater control over their lives as they become attuned to what triggers these shame reactions (Kets de Vries, 2017).

A second step is for employees to cultivate self-compassion—to embrace who they are and to treat themselves in the same respectful, empathetic way they would treat others. For example, if one of Steven's colleagues or direct supervisors had gone badly wrong in making a presentation, he would have been supportive. "You tried hard, but you let your nerves get the better of you," he might have said, or "You'll get better with more practice. Let's hire a consultant." When you are feeling shame, ask yourself: Would I talk to a colleague the way I am talking to myself right now?

This question can help you recognise when a negative thought spiral is getting the upper hand and can challenge your shame-based thinking (Kets de Vries, 2017).

Engaging in these corrective emotional actions can assist employees to improve their sense of self-esteem, increase their feelings of worthiness and belonging, foster greater self-acceptance, and reduce unhealthy reactions to shame, such as withdrawal and counterattack. Shame is part of the human experience. Keeping their feelings of shame in perspective can relieve them of a harmful tendency to self-blame, and, eventually, make peace with their shadow side. Knowing that they are good enough, worthwhile, and deserving of love and acceptance is essential for building resilience and living their most authentic lives (Kets de Vries, 2017; López, 2017).

15.3   Self-compassion

15.3.1   What Is Self-compassion?

Self-compassion (Gilbert Vanderheiden and Merkin, in this book) is simply compassion directed inward (Neff, 2003a, 2003b). Self-compassion is relevant when employees consider personal inadequacies, mistakes, and failures, as well as when they confront painful life and work situations that are outside of their control (Barnard & Curry, 2011; MacBeth & Gumley, 2012). For example, if a colleague tells you about an ordeal, they are facing or a mistake they have made, how do you typically respond? In all likelihood, you offer kindness and comfort, perhaps speaking in a warm and soothing tone, and possibly offering a hug to show how much you care. When your colleague recovers, and the conversation continues, chances are that you will expand your support by encouraging your colleague to take any necessary action or to try to discover how to avoid similar difficulties. Now, reflect for a moment on how you treat yourself when you make a big mistake or experience a setback. It is likely that you are much tougher on yourself—that you spring to self-criticism ("I am such an idiot!"), hide in embarrassment or shame ("Ugh!"), or ruminate for a long time on your perceived shortcomings or bad luck ("Why did this happen to me?"). When things go wrong in our lives, we tend to become our own worst enemies.

Self compassion is a powerful resource that helps employees to stay present and focused on their tasks. Mindfulness is also often overlooked as essential for emotional resilience (Neff, Hseih, & Dejitterat, 2005). In particular, when employees fail in a big way, they are likely to become engulfed in shame, and their sense of self is likely to be dismantled. Employees may be unable to think straight, finding themselves suspended in time and place, dislocated from their bodies, and uncertain who they really are. Shame has a way of wiping out the very observer who is needed to be mindful of his or her own situation. What does it take to rescue yourself and begin to address the situation effectively? You need to treat yourself with the same kindness and support that you would provide for a colleague or friend (Germer & Neff, 2013).

While self-compassion helps employees deal with life struggles, it is important to remember that it does not push negative emotions away in an aversive manner. With self-compassion, instead of replacing negative feelings with positive ones, positive emotions are generated by embracing the negative ones. In fact, self-compassion is associated with numerous psychological strengths, such as happiness, optimism, wisdom, curiosity and exploration, personal initiative, and emotional intelligence (Heffernan, Griffin, McNulty, & Fitzpatrick, 2010; Hollis-Walker & Colosimo, 2011; Neff, Rude, & Kirkpatrick, 2007).

Furthermore, there is a substantial and growing body of research that shows that self-compassion is closely associated with emotional resilience, including the ability to soothe ourselves, recognise our mistakes, learn from them, and motivate ourselves to succeed. Self-compassion is consistently correlated with a wide range of measures of emotional well-being, such as optimism, life satisfaction, autonomy, and wisdom, as well as with reduced levels of anxiety, depression, stress, and shame. To achieve self-compassion, it must include three components.

15.3.1.1 Mindfulness

Mindfulness (Gilbert and Vanderheiden, in this book) refers to an awareness of what is going on in the present moment. Employees need to be kind to themselves, they need to know that they are struggling while they are struggling. It helps them to name the emotions they are feeling in tricky situations and to ground themselves in the here and now (sensations, sounds, sights). These are all skills associated with mindfulness and that make space for a compassionate response (Germer, 2017). Mindfulness and self-compassion have both been associated with various aspects of well-being and are considered buffers against psychopathology (Beshai, Prentice, & Huang, 2017).

For employees, mindfulness involves their turning toward their painful thoughts and emotions and seeing them as they are—without suppression or avoidance (Neff, 2003b). Employees cannot ignore or deny their pain and feel compassion for it at the same time. Suffering might seem blindingly obvious, but how many employees, when they look in a mirror and do not like what they see, remember that this is a moment of suffering worthy of a compassionate response? Similarly, when work life goes awry, they often go into problem-solving mode immediately, without even knowing they are in pain or recognising the need to comfort themselves for the difficulties they are facing. Being mindful of their suffering is therefore necessary for self-compassion (Germer, 2017).

Mindfulness also requires that employees not be overly identified with negative thoughts or feelings, something that brings the risk of being caught up in and swept away by their aversive reactions (Bishop et al., 2004). This type of rumination on our negative feelings narrows their focus (Fredrickson, 1998) and creates an overly negative self-concept (Nolen-Hoeksema, 1991). The mental space provided by taking a mindful approach to their difficult feelings, however, allows for greater clarity, perspective, and equanimity (Baer, 2003; Choi, Lee, & No, 2016; Germer & Neff, 2013).

15.3.1.2 Common Humanity

The term "common humanity" refers to people knowing that they are not alone. Most employees tend to hide in shame when things go wrong in their work lives, or to hide from themselves through distraction or substance abuse. The antidote is recognising their common humanity, understanding that many other employees would feel the same way in similar work situations, and that they are not the only ones who suffer in life (Germer, 2017).

Thus, common humanity involves recognising that the human condition is imperfect, and that the person concerned is not alone in their suffering. This is part of the human experience, a basic fact shared with everyone else on the planet. Individuals are not alone in their imperfection—rather, their imperfections make them card-carrying members of the human race. Often, however, employees feel isolated and cut off from others when considering their struggles and failures, irrationally feeling that it is only "them" having such a hard time of it. They think that, somehow, they are abnormal, that something has gone wrong. This sort of tunnel vision makes them feel alone and isolated, making their suffering even worse. They forget that failure and imperfection are actually normal (Germer, 2017; Tóth-Király, Bőthe, & Orosz, 2017).

With self-compassion, however, employees could take the stance of a compassionate "other" toward themselves, allowing them to adopt a broader perspective on themselves and their work lives. By remembering the shared human experience, they may be able to feel less isolated when they are in pain. For this reason, self-compassion is quite distinct from self-pity. Self-pity is a "woe is me" attitude in which employees become immersed in their own problems and forget that other employees have similar problems. Self-compassion recognises that everyone suffers, and it therefore fosters a connected mind-set that is inclusive of other employees (Germer, 2017).

15.3.1.3 Self-kindness

Self-kindness entails being warm and understanding toward yourself when you suffer, fail, or feel inadequate, rather than flagellating yourself with self-criticism. Sadly, however, many employees tend to use harsh, critical language with themselves—"You are so stupid and lazy, I am ashamed of you!" They would be unlikely to say such things to a close colleague, or even a fellow employee. When asked directly, most employees report that they are kinder to other employees than to themselves (Neff, 2003a), and it is not unusual to encounter extremely kind and compassionate employees who continually beat themselves up. In addition, when your problems stem from forces beyond your control, such as losing your job or being involved in a car accident, they often do not give themselves the sympathy they would give to a colleague in the same situation. With self-kindness, however, they soothe and nurture themselves when confronting their pain rather than getting angry when life falls short of their ideals. The inner conversation is gentle and encouraging rather than harsh and belittling. They clearly acknowledge their problems and shortcomings, but do so without judgment, so they can do what is necessary to help themselves (Germer, 2017).

Thus, self-kindness is a kind and warm-hearted response to yourself. This can take many forms, such as a gentle hand over the heart, validating how you feel, talking to yourself in an encouraging manner, or a simple act of self-kindness such as drinking a cup of tea or listening to music. Ask yourself: "Would I talk to a friend or colleague the way I am talking to myself right now?" Keeping your feelings of shame in perspective is essential for building resilience and living your most authentic life (Elices et al., 2017).

15.3.2 Sources of Self-compassion

Gilbert (in this book) and Proctor (2006) suggest that self-compassion provides emotional resilience because it deactivates the threat system (associated with feelings of insecure attachment, defensiveness, and autonomic arousal) and activates the caregiving system (associated with feelings of secure attachment, safety, and the oxytocin-opiate system). In support of this proposition, Rockcliff, Gilbert, McEwan, Lightman, and Glover (2008) found that giving employees a brief self-compassion exercise lowered their levels of the stress hormone cortisol. It also increased heart rate variability, which is associated with a greater ability to self-soothe when stressed (Germer & Neff, 2013).

Other findings support the idea that self-compassion is linked to the attachment system. For instance, employees who lack self-compassion are more likely to have critical mothers, come from dysfunctional families, and display insecure attachment patterns than self-compassionate employees are (Neff & McGeehee, 2010; Wei). Childhood emotional abuse is also associated with lower levels of self-compassion. Self-compassion appears to mediate the relationship between childhood maltreatment and later emotional dysregulation, meaning that abused employees with higher levels of self-compassion are better able to cope with upsetting work events (Vettese, Dyer, Li, & Wekerle, 2011). This relationship holds even after accounting for history of maltreatment, current distress level, or substance abuse, suggesting that self-compassion is an important resiliency factor for those seeking treatment for past trauma (Germer & Neff, 2013).

15.4 Practical Application of Self-compassion in the Organisational Context

This self-compassion approach outlines ways in which Industrial psychologists can coach employees to reduce shame and self-criticism by developing a compassionate understanding of themselves in relation to their work experiences. It is a constructive practical application that allows employees to work with shame in different social and cultural contexts. Furthermore, it can be applied on a professional level in terms both of the self and of learning contexts. Industrial psychologists could unlock the growth potential of individuals, teams, groups, and organisations to develop constructively and positively by adopting this approach, which counters shame with self-compassion.

15.4.1 Self-compassion on Individual Level

Self-compassion on the individual level could be fostered by the following techniques:

15.4.1.1 Self-compassion Break

Consider the following practical example of a self-compassion break in action. You, as employee, were given a difficult assignment by your supervisor to lead a critical project. The project was a great success, due in large part to your skilful leadership, and you believe you demonstrated that you are ready for a promotion. However, when you raise the idea with your supervisor, she laughs dismissively and changes the subject. Livid with anger, you retreat from the conversation, asking yourself why you bothered to work so hard in the first place since you were never going to be recognised for it. Of course, your supervisor was not going to support you, or even notice. Perhaps all she wanted was for someone to do the difficult work to promote her own selfish agenda, or possibly you are hopelessly out of touch and your performance really was not as good as you thought it was. When employees are in the grip of strong emotions, their minds run wild (Germer, 2017).

A well-informed employee might think that this would be the perfect moment to advocate for him or herself if it were only possible to make a balanced, compelling case for their promotion. Nevertheless, without a moment of self-compassion, their emotional reactivity is likely to stand in their way (Barnard & Curry, 2011). They have put their anger on display instead of showing off their leadership skills to see the discussion through to an acceptable conclusion (Germer, 2017).

How do you activate self-compassion in the heat of the moment? Begin by acknowledging how you feel. For example, recognising that you might still feel angry ("She's terrible and I hate her"); victimised ("She made me go through all of that – for what?!"), or doubt ("Maybe she's right that I don't deserve a promotion – I didn't do that great a job after all"). Next, acknowledge that others would probably have similar feelings in this situation. Requesting a promotion after you have expanded your skills and taken on more responsibility is a reasonable thing to do, and your emotional reaction to the rejection of that request is not out of line. Consider any examples you know of others in similar situations. Perhaps Anika in the finance department told you last year that her promotion was denied, and perhaps then, you noticed how angry she was and how she doubted her own worth. You are not alone (Germer, 2017; Sharma & Davidson, 2015).

Finally, express kindness to yourself. What would you say to a friend in your shoes? Perhaps you would say: "It is rough being taken for granted," or "Whatever comes of it, that project was a huge success – look at the numbers." Also, think about how you care for yourself already. Do you go for a run, pet your dog, and call a friend? If you do that when you are suffering, that is self-compassion (Elices et al., 2017). Once you've shifted your frame of mind from a threat state to self-compassion, you're likely find yourself calmer and able to sit down and write a thoughtful and persuasive proposal about your promotion, one that builds on the success of your project and exhibits your leadership potential under stress (Germer, 2017).

In closing, employees may dismiss self-compassion because they think it flies in the face of their ambition or hard-driving attitude—qualities that they think have made them successful. However, being self-compassionate does not imply that you should not be ambitious or push yourself to succeed (Lenz, 2017). It is about how you motivate yourself; instead of doing it with blame and self-criticism, self-compassion motivates like a good coach, with encouragement, kindness, and support. It is a simple reversal of the Golden Rule: Learning to treat ourselves as we naturally treat others in need—with kindness, warmth, and respect (Germer, 2017).

The following exercise could be used by employees when they notice that they are under stress or are emotionally upset. They can locate where the emotional discomfort resides in their body. Where do they feel it the most? They can then say to them self slowly:

"This is a moment of struggle"

That's mindfulness. Employees can find their own words, such as:

"This hurts"

"This is tough"

"Ouch!"

"Struggle is a part of work life"

That's common humanity. Other options include:

"Other employees feel this way"

"I'm not alone"

"We all struggle in our work life"

Employees can put their hands over their heart, or wherever it feels soothing, sensing the warmth and gentle touch of their hands, and say to them self:

"May I be kind to myself." "May I give myself what I need."

Perhaps there are more specific words that they might need to hear right then, such as:

"May I accept myself as I am."

"May I learn to accept myself as I am."

"May I be safe."
"May I be strong."
"May I forgive myself."

If they are having trouble finding the right language, it can help to imagine what they might say to a close employee struggling with that same difficulty. Can they say something similar to them self, letting the words roll gently through their mind? (Germer, 2017).

15.4.1.2 The Compassionate Image

Organisational applications of the compassionate image ask employees to visualise the "perfect nurturer", in instances such as these, a colleague who can offer them unquestioning warmth, nonjudgment, and acceptance (Gilbert & Irons, 2004, 2005; Lee, 2005). Every time the employee engages in self-judgment, they are to call upon their perfect nurturer (Gilbert & Procter, 2006). Although the image starts as something external, the goal is for it to become internalised (Barnard & Curry, 2011).

The following exercise can help employees to build up a compassionate image for them to work with and develop (they can have more than one if they wish, and they can change over time). Whatever image comes to mind, or they choose to work with, note that it is their creation and therefore their own personal ideal what they would really like from feeling cared for and cared about.

However, in this exercise it is important that employees try to give their image certain qualities. These will include wisdom, strength, warmth and non-judgement. Employees should think of these qualities and imagine what they would look, sound or feel like. If possible, they should begin by focusing on their breathing, finding their calming rhythm and making a half smile. Then they can let images emerge in their mind—as best as they can—they do not have too try to hard if nothing comes to the mind, or the minds wanders, just gently bring it back to the breathing and practice compassionately accepting.

Here are some questions that might help them build an image: would they want their caring/nurturing image to feel/look/seem old or young; male or female (or non-human looking e.g., an animal, sea or light). Would their 'image' have gone through similar experiences as them? Would they be like a colleague or even part of a team that welcomes them to belong? What colours and sounds are associated with the qualities of wisdom, strength, warmth and non judgement. Employees must remember that their image brings full compassion to them and for them.

Also consider the following questions: How would they like their ideal caring-compassionate image to look—visual qualities? How would they like their ideal caring-compassionate image to sound (e.g., voice tone)? What other sensory qualities can they give to it? How would they like their ideal caring-compassionate image to relate to them? How would they like to relate to their ideal caring compassionate image? (Gilbert, 2018).

15.4.1.3 Gestalt Two-Chair

The Gestalt two-chair intervention—designed to help employees extend empathy to self and to challenge their self-judgmental, maladaptive beliefs—may raise self-compassion (Gilbert & Irons, 2005; Greenberg, Watson, & Goldman, 1998; Whelton & Greenberg, 2005). Employees are asked to think of themselves as having two "selves" that relate to one another: a judgmental self and a self that experiences the judgment. They are then asked to move between two chairs, acting and speaking like the judgmental self in one chair and the "experiencing self" in the other (Neff et al., 2007). Coaches note both the content of the self-judgments and how the employees respond to their self-judgments (Brown, 1952; McKay & Fanning, 2000). Coaches train employees in compassionately defending themselves and in recognising the cost of listening to or submitting to their self-judgmental side (Barnard & Curry, 2011).

15.4.2 Self-compassion on Group Level

Self-compassion on the group level could be explained by a study conducted by Horan and Taylor (2017) that introduces mindfulness and self-compassion as potential tools to strengthen health behaviour change interventions in organisations. The following practical example of a 10-week health behaviour change programme was offered through the employee wellness programming office of a Midwestern university in the United States of America. Participants were 24 university faculty and staff (M age = 51.8, SD age = 12.2, 79.2% female). The weekly meetings featured the following components: thirty minutes of didactic psycho-education, thirty minutes of guided group exercise, and guided at-home workbook activities. Participants were also offered optional health coaching meetings.

Participants completed a number of pre-test and post-test measures. First, participants completed an objective fitness assessment that was supervised by a certified personal trainer. The assessment contained measures of body composition (for example, body fat percentage as measured by a handheld bioelectrical impedance device) and physical fitness (for example, cardiovascular and muscular endurance as measured by a three-minute step test, push-up test, and abdominal crunch test). Second, the participants completed an online survey that contained measures of mindfulness, self-compassion, self-reported participation in health behaviours, self-reported participation in mindful health behaviours, measures of well-being, and variables related to job attitudes and their work environment (Horan & Taylor, 2017).

Findings from the fitness assessment analysis revealed that there was a significant reduction in abdominal circumference and a significant increase in thigh circumference from pre-test to post-test. Muscular endurance significantly increased, as measured by both abdominal crunches and push-ups. Although the pattern of means for the remaining variables in the fitness assessment was in the expected direction, no other significant changes were observed. The small sample size may have reduced the ability to uncover significant effects (Horan & Taylor, 2017).

Findings from the survey data analysis revealed that mindfulness and self-compassion increased from pre-test to post-test, as well as participation in mindful eating and mindful exercise. Diet quality improved in terms of consumption of dietary fat, although no other dietary quality variables changed significantly. Participation in leisure time physical activity increased. The analysis of well-being variables revealed that life satisfaction and energy improved. The analysis of work-related variables revealed that perceived climate for healthy weight maintenance improved, but other work-related variables such as perceived organisational support did not change significantly.

15.4.3 Self-compassion on Organisational Level

Self-compassion on organisational level could be cultivated by the following interventions:

15.4.3.1 Self-compassion Induction Studies

In an induction study, participants were asked to recall a failure, rejection, or loss that elicited negative self-evaluative emotions (for example humiliation or shame; Leary, Tate, Adams, Batts Allen, & Hancock, 2007). There were four conditions. In the self-compassion induction, condition subjects were asked to write down ways in which others had experienced similar events, how they would express understanding to a friend if they had experienced the event, and to list their emotions about the event in an objective and unemotional fashion. In the self-esteem induction, condition participants were instructed to write about their own positive characteristics, why they believed that the event had not been their fault, and why the event did not indicate anything about the type of person they are. The third condition was a writing control condition in which subjects were simply instructed to write about the event. The last condition was a true control in which participants filled out the dependent measures immediately after recalling the negative event, but without any writing. Subjects in all conditions were asked to rate their feelings and the extent to which they believed the negative event had been their own fault.

The self-compassion group differed statistically from all the others in that they reported the lowest negative affect and the greatest perception of being similar to others. They also were the most likely to say that the event had been their fault but not to exhibit corresponding negative affect ($r = -0.03$), whereas internal attributions in other conditions were positively correlated with negative affect. These results suggest that self-compassion may help employees take responsibility and may decouple the association between taking responsibility and experiencing negative affect. This provides further evidence that self-compassion does not lead to self-complacency (Barnard & Curry, 2011).

15.4.3.2 Compassionate Mind Training

Compassionate mind training (CMT) could be developed for employees with high levels of self-criticism and shame to teach them how to produce self-soothing and self-reassuring thoughts (Gilbert [see his contribution to this book] & Irons, 2005; Gilbert & Procter, 2006). Employees could therefore be trained how to respond with assertiveness rather than appeasement. Employees could, in addition, be taught to think about self-compassion as a skill that can be learned and self-judgment as a habit that can be overcome. CMT aims to help employees develop a compassionate understanding of their distress and a concern for their well-being, and to mindfully tolerate feelings and thoughts (Barnard & Curry, 2011).

15.4.3.3 Mindfulness-Based Stress Reduction

A further way to raise self-compassion is to raise mindfulness. Raising mindfulness should raise overall self-compassion. Mindfulness-based stress reduction (MBSR) is designed to enhance present moment awareness through disengaging from rumination and intrusive self-judgment (Kabat-Zinn, 2003; Leary, 2004). In MBSR, employees could be coached to tolerate, acknowledge, label, and embrace thoughts and feelings rather than reacting to or avoiding those (Shapiro, Astin, Bishop, & Cordova, 2005). Three MBSR treatment studies (Moore, 2008; Shapiro et al., 2005; Shapiro, Brown, & Biegel, 2007) have found robust relationships among self-compassion, mindfulness, and meditation (Barnard & Curry, 2011).

15.4.3.4 Acceptance and Commitment Therapy

Acceptance and commitment therapy (ACT) aims to help employees live according to their values by expanding their behavioural flexibility and effectiveness (Hayes et al., 2004). ACT's six core processes are cognitive diffusion, acceptance, present-moment focus, self as context, values, and committed action (Hayes, Luoma, Bond, Masuda, & Lillis, 2006). The first three core processes are elements of mindfulness (Forman, Herbert, Moitra, Yeomans, & Geller, 2007; Kocovski, Fleming, & Rector, 2009). The fourth core process, self as context, involves exploring how the self-judgmental side of self relates to the experiencing side (Hayes et al., 2006). ACT focuses on increasing employees' ability to recognise that self-judgments are not necessarily realities. This may promote self-compassion by softening judgments. The fourth and fifth processes of ACT coach employees how to take action that is directed toward values (Hayes et al., 2004). ACT may also foster self-compassion as employees envision the type of employee they want to be rather than berate themselves for their failures (Barnard & Curry, 2011).

With ACT, metaphors, paradoxes, and experiential exercises are frequently used. Many interventions are playful, creative, and clever. ACT protocols can vary from short interventions done in minutes to those that extend over many sessions. There are myriad techniques categorised under the following protocols (Gifford, Hayes, & Stroshal, 2005):

Facing the current situation ("creative hopelessness") encourages employees to draw out what they have tried to make better, examine whether they have truly worked, and create space for something new to happen. Confronting the unworkable reality of their multiple experiences often leaves the employee not knowing what to do next, in a state of "creative hopelessness." The state is creative because entirely new strategies can be developed without using the previous rules governing their behaviour.

Acceptance techniques are geared toward reducing the motivation to avoid certain situations. An emphasis is given to "unhooking"— realising that thoughts and feelings do not always lead to actions. Often these techniques are done "in vivo," structuring experiences in session. Discriminating between thoughts, feelings, and experiences is a salient focus.

Cognitive defusion (deliteralisation) redefines thinking and experiencing as an ongoing behavioural process, not an outcome. Techniques are designed to demonstrate that thoughts are just thoughts and not necessarily realities (Blackledge, 2007). It can involve sitting next to the employee and putting each thought and experience out in front as an object in an effort to "defuse and deliteralise."

Valuing as a choice clarifies what the client values for his or her own sake: What gives life meaning? The goal is to help employees understand the distinction between a value and a goal, choose and declare their values, and set behavioural tasks linked to these values.

Self as context teaches the employee to view his or her identity as separate from the content of his or her experience (Dewane, 2008).

15.5   Chapter Summary

This chapter focused on managing shame in organisations by proposing a self-compassionate approach in which industrial psychologists can coach employees to reduce shame and self-criticism by developing a compassionate understanding of themselves in relation to their work experiences. It is a constructive practical application intended to work with shame in different social and cultural contexts. Furthermore, it can be applied on a professional level in terms of the self and learning contexts. A number of techniques, and interventions were explained which could unlock the growth potential of individuals groups, and organisations.

References

Agrawal, N., Han, D., & Duhachek, A. (2013). Emotional agency appraisals influence responses to preference inconsistent information. *Organizational Behavior and Human Decision Processes, 1,* 87–97.

Baer, R. A. (2003). Mindfulness training as a clinical intervention: A conceptual and empirical review. *Clinical Psychology: Science and Practice, 10*(2), 125–143.

Bagozzi, R. P., Verbeke, W., & Gavino, J. C. J. (2003). Culture moderates the self-regulation of shame and its effects on performance: The case of salespersons in the Netherlands and the Philippines. *Journal of Applied Psychology, 88,* 219–233.

Barnard, L. K., & Curry, J. F. (2011). Self-compassion: Conceptualizations, correlates, & interventions. *Review of General Psychology, 15*(4), 289–303. https://doi.org/10.1037/a0025754.

Beshai, S., Prentice, J. L., & Huang, V. (2017). Building blocks of emotional flexibility: Trait mindfulness and self-compassion are associated with positive and negative mood shifts. *Mindfulness.* Retrieved from https://doi.org/10.1007/s12671-017-0833-8.

Bishop, S. R., Lau, M., Shapiro, S., Carlson, L., Anderson, N. D., Carmody, J., & Devins, G. (2004). Mindfulness: A proposed operational definition. *Clinical Psychology: Science and Practice, 11*(3), 230–241.

Blackledge, J. T. (2007). Disrupting verbal processes: Cognitive defusion in acceptance and commitment therapy and other mindfulness-based psychotherapies. *The Psychological Record, 57,* 555–576.

Brown, B. (1952). *Soul without shame: A guide to liberating yourself from the judge within.* Shambhala Publications.

Brown, R., González, R., Zagefka, H., Manzi, J., & Čehajić, S. (2008). Nuestra culpa: Collective guilt and shame as predictors of reparation for historical wrongdoing. *Journal of Applied Psychology, 94,* 75–90.

Choi, H. J., Lee, S., & No, S.-R. (2016). Effects of compassion on employees self-regulation. *Social Behavior and Personality, 44*(7), 1173–1190.

De Hooge, I. E., Zeelenberg, M., & Breugelmans, S. M. (2010). Restore and protect motivations following shame. *Cognition and Emotion, 24,* 111–127.

De Hooge, I. E., Zeelenberg, M., & Breugelmans, S. M. (2011). A functionalist account of shame-induced behaviour. *Cognition and Emotion, 25,* 939–946.

Devenish-Meares, P. (2015). Call to compassionate self-care: Introducing self-compassion into the workplace treatment process. *Journal of Spirituality in Mental Health, 17*(1), 75–87. Retrieved from https://doi.org/10.1080/19349637.2015.985579.

Dewane, C. (2008). The ABCs of ACT—Acceptance and commitment therapy. *Social Work Today, 8*(5), 34.

Elfenbein, H. A. (2007). Emotion in organizations: A review and theoretical integration. *Academy of Management Annals, 1,* 315–386.

Elices, M., Carmona, C., Pascual, J. C., Feliu-Soler, A., Martin-Blanco, A., & Soler, J. (2017). Compassion and self-compassion: Construct and measurement. *Mindfulness & Compassion, 2,* 34–40.

Ferguson, T. J. (2005). Mapping shame and its functions in relationships. *Child Maltreatment, 10,* 377–386.

Fischer, K. W., & Tangney, J. P. (1995). Self-conscious emotions and the affect revolution: Framework and overview. In J. P. Tangney & K. W. Fischer (Eds.), *Self-conscious emotions* (pp. 3–24). New York: Guilford Press.

Forman, E. M., Herbert, J. D., Moitra, E., Yeomans, P. D., & Geller, P. A. (2007). A randomized controlled effectiveness trial of acceptance and commitment therapy and cognitive therapy for anxiety and depression. *Behavior Modification, 31,* 772–799. Retrieved from https://doi.org/10.1177/0145445507302202.

Fredrickson, B. L. (1998). What good are positive emotions? *Review of General Psychology, 2,* 300–319. Retrieved from http://doi.org/bkc3tg.

Germer, C. K. (2017). To recover from failure, try some self-compassion. *Harvard Business Review*. Retrieved on January 5, 2017. Retrieved from https://hbr.org/2017/01/to-recover-from-failure-try-some-self-compassion.

Germer, C. K., & Neff, K. D. (2013). Self-compassion in clinical practice. *Journal of Clinical Psychology, 69*(8), 856–867.

Ghorbani, M., Liao, Y., Çayköylü, S., & Chand, M. (2013). Guilt, shame, and reparative behavior: The effect of psychological proximity. *Journal of Business Ethics, 114*, 311–324.

Gifford, E., Hayes, S., & Stroshal, K. (2005). *Acceptance and Commitment Therapy*. Retrieved from 9/20/2005. www.acceptanceandcommitmenttherapy.com.

Gilbert, P. (2018). Handout compiled by Teresa Kleffner, MSW, LCSW. St. Louis Counseling and Wellness. www.stlcw.com. Exercise created by Paul Gilbert Retrieved from http://www.stlcw.com/Handouts/Building_a_Compassionate_Image.pdf on February 21, 2018.

Gilbert, P., & Irons, C. (2004). A pilot exploration of the use of compassionate images in a group of self-critical people. *Memory, 12*, 507–516. Retrieved from https://doi.org/10.1080/09658210444000115.

Gilbert, P., & Irons, C. (2005). Focused therapies and compassionate mind training for shame and self-attacking. In P. Gilbert (Ed.), *Compassion: Conceptualisations, research and use in psychotherapy* (pp. 263–325). New York, NY: Routledge.

Gilbert, P., & Procter, S. (2006). Compassionate mind training for people with high shame and self-criticism: Overview and pilot study of a group therapy approach. *Clinical Psychology & Psychotherapy, 13*, 353–379. Retrieved from https://doi.org/10.1002/cpp.507.

González-Gómez, H. V., & Richter, A. W. (2015). Turning shame into creativity: The importance of exposure to creative team environments. *Organizational Behavior and Human Decision Processes, 126*, 142–161.

Greenberg, L., Watson, J., & Goldman, R. (1998). Process-experiential therapy of depression. In L. Greenberg, J. Watson, & G. Lietaer (Eds.), *Handbook of experiential psychotherapy* (pp. 227–248). New York, NY: The Guilford Press.

Hayes, S. C., Bissett, R., Roget, N., Padilla, M., Kohlenberg, B. S., Fisher, G., & Niccolls, R. (2004). The impact of acceptance and commitment training and multicultural training on the stigmatizing attitudes and professional burnout of substance abuse counsellors. *Behavior Therapy, 35*, 821–835. Retrieved from https://doi.org/10.1016/s0005-7894(04)80022-4.

Hayes, S. C., Luoma, J., Bond, F., Masuda, A., & Lillis, J. (2006). Acceptance and commitment therapy: Model, processes, and outcomes. *Behavior Research and Therapy, 44*, 1–25. https://doi.org/10.1016/j.brat.2005.06.006.

Heffernan, M., Griffin, M. T. Q., McNulty, S. R., & Fitzpatrick, J. J. (2010). Self-compassion and emotional intelligence in nurses. *International Journal of Nursing Practice, 16*, 366–373.

Hollis-Walker, L., & Colosimo, K. (2011). Mindfulness, self-compassion, and happiness in non-meditators: A theoretical and empirical examination. *Personality and Individual Differences, 50*, 222–227.

Horan, K. A., & Taylor, M. B. (2017). *Mindfulness and self-compassion as tools in health behaviour change: A workplace intervention case study*. USA: Department of Psychology, Bowling Green State University.

Irons, C., & Lad, S. (2017). Using compassion-focused therapy to work with shame and self-criticism in complex trauma. *Australian Clinical Psychologist, 3*(1), 47–54. ISSN 2204-4981.

Kabat-Zinn, J. (2003). Mindfulness-based interventions in context: Past, present, and future. *Clinical Psychology Science and Practice, 10*, 144–156. Retrieved from https://doi.org/10.1093/clipsy.bpg016.

Kets de Vries, M. F. R. (2017). Don't let shame become a self-destructive spiral. *Harvard Business Review*. Retrieved on September 5, 2017. Retrieved from https://hbr.org/2017/06/dont-let-shame-become-a-self-destructive-spiral.

Kocovski, N. L., Fleming, J. E., & Rector, N. A. (2009). Mindfulness and acceptance-based group therapy for social anxiety disorder: An open trial. *Cognitive and Behavioral Practice, 16*, 276–289. Retrieved from https://doi.org/10.1016/j.cbpra.2008.12.004.

Lazarus, R. S., & Folkman, S. (1984). *Stress, appraisal, and coping*. New York: Springer.

Leary, M. R., & Kowalsky, R. M. (1995). *Social anxiety*. New York: Guilford Press.

Leary, T. (2004). *Interpersonal diagnoses of personality: A functional theory and methodology for personality evaluation*. Wipf and Stock Publishers.

Leary, M. R., Tate, E. B., Adams, C. E., Batts Allen, A., & Hancock, J. (2007). Self-compassion and reactions to unpleasant self-relevant events: The implications of treating oneself kindly. *Journal of Personality and Social Psychology, 92*, 887–904. Retrieved from https://doi.org/10.1037/0022-3514.92.5.887.

Lee, D. (2005). The perfect nurturer: A model to develop a compassionate mind within the context of cognitive therapy. In P. Gilbert (Ed.), *Compassion: Conceptualisations, research and use in psychotherapy* (pp. 326–351). New York, NY: Routledge.

Lenz, D. S. (2017). *Understanding the relationship between compassion and employee engagement* (Master of Science dissertation). Pepperdine University.

López, R. G. (2017). The heteronomous moral value of shame. *South African Journal of Philosophy, 36*(3), 393–409. Retrieved from https://doi.org/10.1080/02580136.2017.1317565.

Ludwiga, S., Fellner-Röhlinga, G., & Thomab, C. (2017). Do women have more shame than men? An experiment on self-assessment and the shame of overestimating oneself. *European Economic Review, 92*, 31–46.

MacBeth, A., & Gumley, A. (2012). Exploring compassion: A meta-analysis of the association between self-compassion & psychopathology. *Clinical Psychology Review, 32*, 545–552.

Mayer, C.-H., Viviers, R., & Tonelli, L. (2017). 'The fact that she just looked at me…'—Narrations on shame in South African workplaces. *SA Journal of Industrial Psychology/SA Tydskrif vir Bedryfsielkunde, 43*(0), a1385. Retrieved from https://doi.org/10.4102/sajip.v43i0.1385.

McKay, M., & Fanning, P. (2000). *Self-esteem: A proven program of cognitive techniques for assessing, improving, and maintaining your self-esteem*. Oakland, CA: New Harbinger Publications.

Moore, P. (2008). Introducing mindfulness to clinical psychologists in training: An experiential course of brief exercises. *Journal of Clinical Psychology in Medical Settings, 15*, 331–337. https://doi.org/10.1007/s10880-008-9134-7.

Neff, K. D. (2003a). Development and validation of a scale to measure self-compassion. *Self and Identity, 2*, 223–250.

Neff, K. D. (2003b). Self-compassion: An alternative conceptualization of a healthy attitude toward oneself. *Self and Identity, 2*, 85–102.

Neff, K. D., Hsieh, Y.-P., & Dejitterat, K. (2005). Self-compassion, achievement goals, and coping with academic failure. *Self and Identity, 4*, 263–287.

Neff, K. D., & McGeehee, P. (2010). Self-compassion and psychological resilience among adolescents and young adults. *Self and Identity, 9*, 225–240.

Neff, K. D., Rude, S. S., & Kirkpatrick, K. (2007). An examination of self-compassion in relation to positive psychological functioning and personality traits. *Journal of Research in Personality, 41*, 908–916.

Nolen-Hoeksema, S. (1991). Responses to depression and their effects on the duration of depressive episode. *Journal of Abnormal Psychology, 100*(4), 569–582.

Rockcliff, H., Gilbert, P., McEwan, K., Lightman, S., & Glover, D. (2008). A pilot exploration of heart rate variability and salivary cortisol responses to compassion-focused imagery. *Clinical Neuropsychiatry, 5*, 132–139.

Sharma, M., & Davidson, C. (2015). Self-compassion in relation to personal initiativeness, curiosity and exploration among young adults. *Indian Journal of Health and Wellbeing, 6*(2), 185–187.

Shapiro, S. L., Astin, J. A., Bishop, S. R., & Cordova, M. (2005). Mindfulness-based stress reduction for health care professionals: Results from a randomized trial. *International Journal of Stress Management, 12*, 164–176. Retrieved from https://doi.org/10.1037/1072-5245.12.2.164.

Shapiro, S. L., Brown, K. W., & Biegel, G. M. (2007). Teaching self-care to caregivers: Effects of mindfulness-based stress reduction on the mental health of therapists in training. *Training and Education in Professional Psychology, 1*, 105–115. https://doi.org/10.1037/1931-3918.1.2.105.

Smith, C. A., & Ellsworth, P. C. (1985). Patterns of cognitive appraisal in emotion. *Journal of Personality and Social Psychology, 48,* 813–838.

Tangney, J. P., Miller, R. S., Flicker, L., & Barrow, D. H. (1996). Are shame, guilt, and embarrassment distinct emotions? *Journal of Personality and Social Psychology, 70,* 1256–1269.

Tóth-Király, I., Bőthe, B., & Orosz, G. (2017). Exploratory structural equation modelling analysis of the self-compassion scale. *Mindfulness, 8,* 881–892. Retrieved from https://doi.org/10.1007/s12671-016-0662-1.

Velotti, P., Garofalo, C., Bottazzi, F., & Caretti, V. (2017). Faces of shame: Implications for self-esteem, emotion regulation, aggression, and well-being. *The Journal of Psychology, 151*(2), 171–184. https://doi.org/10.1080/00223980.2016.1248809.

Vettese, L. C., Dyer, C. E., Li, W. L. & Wekerle, C. (2011). Does self-compassion mitigate the association between childhood maltreatment and later emotional regulation difficulties? *International Journal of Mental Health and Addiction, 9,* 480–491. Retrieved from https://doi.org/10.1007/s11469-011-9340-7.

Whelton, W., & Greenberg, L. (2005). Emotion in self-criticism. *Personality and Individual Differences, 38,* 1583–1595.

Rudolf M. Oosthuizen, D.Litt. and Phil. received a B.A. degree (Cum Laude) from the University of Pretoria in 1992 and obtained a B.A. (Honours) in Psychology at the same university in 1993. In 1999, he received an M.A. degree in Industrial and Personnel Psychology from the Potchefstroom University for Christian Higher Education. In 1999, he registered as Industrial Psychologist with the Health Professions Council of South Africa. In 2005, he completed a D.Litt. and Phil. in Industrial and Organisational Psychology at the University of South Africa (Unisa). Currently Rudolf Oosthuizen is an associate professor in the Department of Industrial and Organisational Psychology at the University of South Africa. Rudolf is the manager for the MComIOP programme, and he is responsible for the lecturing of honours subjects and the supervision of master's and doctoral students. He has presented conference papers at national and international conferences, and published articles in accredited scientific journals. His fields of interests are (1) career psychology, career development and management from an individual and organisational perspective in the 21st century world of work; (2) positive psychology, with the focus on salutogenesis, sense of coherence, locus of control, self-efficacy, the hardy personality and learned resourcefulness; and (3) employment relations and the improvement of the quality of employment relations in organisations and in society in general.

Chapter 16
Shame! Whose Shame, Is It? A Systems Psychodynamic Perspective on Shame in Organisations: A Case Study

Louise Tonelli

Abstract The focus of this chapter is on shame from a systems psychodynamic perspective. An experience of shame in the form of a case study, conducted by Mayer and Tonelli (The value of shame: exploring a health resource in cultural contexts. Springer, Cham, pp. 110–135, 2017) is presented. The case study forms part of a larger research project on shame in South African organisations and serves as an example of how shame may be experienced by an individual and a system. A coaching model is applied to the case study as a possible method of transforming shame in an organisational and professional context. Presented from a view that individuals and organisations operate on both conscious and unconscious levels as part of larger groups, systems and networks.

Keywords Coaching · Defences · Military power · Shame · Systems psychodynamics

16.1 Introduction

From the perspective of an individual, the literature disputes a common definition for shame. Shame is often closely linked to humiliation, embarrassment and guilt (Leask, 2013; Zavaleta Reyles, 2007). Shame seems to indicate a painful discord between the self and a specific recognised norm or failure of own standards (Mayer, Viviers, & Tonelli, 2017; Wüschner, 2017; Zavaleta Reyles, 2007). When the self, splits into observed and observing parts, the personal judgement of shame may lead the person to believe they were somehow deserving of the feelings of shame (Zavaleta Reyles, 2007). Imposed or self-imposed withdrawal behaviour may follow as attention is focused inwardly. Wüschner (2017) states that excessive shame experienced in situations of high visibility rests heavily on an individual because of the intensity of the feeling and loss of agency often expressed in the lowering of the gaze or covering the

L. Tonelli (✉)
Department of Industrial and Organisational Psychology, University of South Africa (UNISA), AJH vd Walt Building Room 3-108, Pretoria, South Africa
e-mail: leyl@unisa.ac.za

© Springer Nature Switzerland AG 2019
C.-H. Mayer and E. Vanderheiden (eds.), *The Bright Side of Shame*,
https://doi.org/10.1007/978-3-030-13409-9_16

face. In effect, an individual trying to hide from the situation from which they may not be able to remove themselves physically, remaining in a position of discomfort in the presence of others. Shaming an individual in this manner leaves no room for the individual's subjectivity, but rather seeks to destroy the person, not physically but socially. A power relationship which involves dominance over the shamed according to Long (2008) by the proud, the social character of shame. Through exclusion in the form of inclusion, the odd one and the unwelcomed, according to Wüschner (2017).

From a systems psychodynamic perspective, shame intersects with the manifestation of envy (May, 2017), a defence which serves as a mask to hide anxiety within a system which results in envious attacks on individuals and groups within social and organisational systems. When envy manifests as a negative emotion malicious pleasure may be taken at others' misfortune, enticing aggressive behaviour and conflict in groups, and trying to bring down the other (Tai, Narayanan, & Mcallister, 2012).

Strong emotional reactions of anger, anxiety, shame, envy or idealisation are clues to underlying dynamics such as transferences and projective identification dynamics in systems (Cilliers & Smit, 2006). The underlying behavioural dynamics of experiencing the idealised parts of the self as unattainable and, unwanted parts such as shame as denigrating, the system splits of those parts and projects them onto others where the others contain the unwanted or idealised parts on behalf of the system (Cilliers & Smit, 2006). In a perverse form of defensiveness against shame those who wish to distance themselves from shame lest their own shame be exposed need to see the other shamed so that they might see that which they are afraid of in the other and deny the shame in themselves (Long, 2008). In this manner, members of organisations, through unconscious processes of splitting and projection, covertly mobilise individuals and sub-groups to hold and express intolerable emotions such as shame and envy on their behalf (Newton & Goodman, 2009).

16.1.1 Systems Psychodynamics a Composite of Three Distinct but Related Theories

The concept of an organisation as a system originates from Open Systems Theory (Rice, 1953), which is the study of organisations as any open living entity. The primary task of an organisation is to transform inputs to outputs; a task the system must carry out to survive and to which all sub systems must be aligned. Transferring inputs to outputs requires permeable boundary regions around the system. These open systems are comparatively independent of individuals. However, individuals are affected by the system both psychologically and emotionally (Eloquin, 2016). More recently, the permeability of the boundaries of systems have been extended to include the realities of the internet, technology and social media which operate without boundaries where an organisation is no longer just a whole made up of parts, but an ever-changing network (Western, 2012).

Psychoanalytic perspectives on individual experiences and mental processes within systems or networks, such as transference resistance, objects relations and phantasy, are considered as the psychodynamics of individuals in organisations and organisations themselves. These include unconscious group and social processes, which are simultaneously both a source and a consequence of unresolved and unrecognised organisational difficulties. The central view is the existence of primitive anxieties of a persecutory and depressive nature and the mobilisation of social defences against them. Which would either impede or facilitate task performance (Cilliers & Africa, 2012).

The fundamental principle of psychoanalysis in systems psychodynamics considers that individuals have an unconscious mind that shapes their behaviour to a greater or lesser extent (Eloquin, 2016). The task of psychoanalysis is to identify hidden patterns of past experiences and relieve the individual from their power. Often by confronting painful emotional "truths" which trigger anxiety, an individual can defend against by resorting to defence mechanisms in order not to become overwhelmed with feelings of anxiety. Understanding anxiety is therefore a key part of psychoanalysis and systems psychodynamics, as are the defence mechanisms mobilised to manage anxiety (Eloquin, 2016).

Group relations is the third distinct theory within systems psychodynamics, which was largely the work of Bion (1961). In this theory, Bion (1961) postulates basic assumptions as the cornerstones for studying relationships in organisational systems (Cilliers & Africa, 2012; Eloquin, 2016):

- Dependency, which is the groups' unconscious projection for attention and help onto an authority figure as if a parent object
- Fight/flight a defence mechanism to try to cope with discomfort involving an authority figure, that is, management or leadership
- Pairing with perceived powerful others, such as a manager or leader, splitting the authority figure as an individual or pair in order to be able to identify with one part as a saviour.

Basic assumptions are never exhausted. It is not imperative that groups rid themselves of these characteristics either (Hayden & Molenkamp, 2002). For example, the military and industry capitalise on fight/flight needs, all strong primitive feelings channelled in the service of the work task. However, when individuals or sub-groups become stuck or over-reliant on these basic assumptions, defence mechanisms are employed (Cilliers & Africa, 2012; Hayden & Molenkamp, 2002). Rationalisation, intellectualisation, regression and denial are used unconsciously by the system to act against anxiety to remain in control and to stay emotionally uninvolved to avoid pain and anxiety.

Defence mechanisms such as splitting, and projection does not change the behaviour of the receiver of the projection necessarily. If, however, the receiver of the projection identifies, with the projection, and takes it onto himself or herself, or the system, projection identification occurs (Bartle, 2015). Identifying with the projection could be because of the systems tendency or unconscious vulnerability or predisposition to being drawn into a basic assumption type of functioning such as feelings of anger, guilt, shame and envy; where an individual or system has a valence for regularly receiving these projections and act out a role accordingly. Counter transference, on the other hand, is a state of mind where other people's feelings are experienced as one's own. The projective identification could lead to the recipient acting out the projected feelings (Cilliers & Africa, 2012; Handy & Rowlands 2017; Motsoaledi & Cilliers, 2012).

Basic group functioning means becoming stuck in these basic assumptions and defence mechanisms at the expense of transferring inputs to outputs. When there is insight into and taking responsibility for own relationships, the work group functions towards the primary task of the system (Cilliers & Africa, 2012). However, the work group with the underlying elements of maturity and reflective processes combined with well-structured agreement to work on a clearly defined primary task may be rare (Allcorn, 2015).

A case study, part of a larger research project on shame in South African organisations by Mayer and Tonelli (2017) is presented next. Considering the lens of systems psychodynamics, the case study is an example of a system experiencing anxiety over its own performance and the resulting projection of shame (attack on an individual) onto and into the individual. This military setting serves as an example of a system which has an over reliance on the basic assumption fight/flight in the service of its task. From this example coaches, consultants and other professionals working with individuals and organisations might consider the unconscious dynamics at play in systems, which may have ramifications for transforming shame if unconscious behaviour remains unknown, as it will influence relationships mostly negatively and possibly even destructively according to Cilliers (2006) and highlighted in the case study.

16.2   War and Peace—A Case Study

The South African military had undergone a change process from a military power towards a peacekeeping force. This was during a time after 1994 when the South African Defence Force, which was known as a formidable force on the African continent while upholding the apartheid regime, transformed by integrating previously combatant forces into one national peacekeeping force. In this setting, an Industrial and Organisational (IO) psychologist shares his experience of shame.

He was attached to a battalion as part of the executive team and was invited by the commanding officer and senior personnel to different platoons in the area to address these troops. On one specific day, the commanding officer could not accompany the team to address the troops, at which time the commanding officer instructed the team to address the troops on his behalf. When the time came for the IO psychologist to address the troops he mentioned to them, that as a psychologist he noticed a certain amount of tentative behaviour from the troops when they had to engage "the enemy" in their training. He suggested to the troops that it might be difficult to engage and diffuse a situation if they were tentative. In his mind he was aware that the soldiers were moving away from the role of combatent soldier to peacekeeping force and that this process was difficult for them. What he was not aware of was that the troops did not take his observation positively but perceived it as negative feedback.

He recalls that some of the troops then complained to the platoon officer and the news was communicated to the commanding officer. The next morning, the commanding officer called him over within listening distance of others, where people could hear that he was being scolded. The commanding officer said: "How dare you break the morale of the soldiers!" He then told the IO psychologist that he was there to motivate people, but he was actually destroying the morale of the troops. The IO psychologist felt shocked at the statement as well as being attacked in public. He recalls that he felt his shoulders go down and head drop until he felt himself being filled with rage, at which time he responded by telling the commanding officer: "How dare you speak to me like that!" He told the commanding officer that he would go and talk to the troops, not to apologise as the commanding officer expected from him, but to explain why he said what he had said. The commanding officer then walked away from him, which the IO psychologist found strange, as that was not the ordinary way such an altercation with a commanding officer would have ended. Usually, the commanding officer "was supposed to thrash him further", the IO psychologist remarked as he was attacking the commanding officer in the presence of the troops. However, at that time, the commanding officer just returned to his tent. From that day onwards, the commanding officer excused the IO psychologist from his order group and said that he was no longer welcome to attend those meetings. The IO psychologist recalled that "The exercise was still going on for three weeks; I was lying there in my tent not doing anything."

He communicated the situation to his peers who told him to ignore the situation and write a report. He recalls that he often thinks of this experience, and how it made him feel. He worked with many of the soldiers' present, which made him think of his own credibility and reputation after the incident. He had feelings of humiliation and embarrassment about it. He recalls that to this day he has not spoken to his wife about the incident. Other than the "very cold clinical" report he had to write about the incident, he has never spoken about his feelings and emotions around the incident to anyone. He does recall that it was very difficult. When he thinks back on the incident, he is aware that it has so many layers.

16.3   Connecting the Inner, Personal World to Outer Work

A possible working hypothesis may be that, the possible shame the troops felt at having to become a peacekeeping force, and their struggle with the new identity, resulted in anxiety. An anxiety, which manifested in experiences of shame in the system. In defending against feelings of shame, shame was projected onto the IO psychologist to rid themselves of these feelings as "how dare he" call them tentative. The IO psychologist then introjected the shame to carry on behalf of the system. The introjection of the shame seems to be held in the expression of "how dare he" which the IO Psychologist projected back at the Commanding Officer.

The hypothesis as a tentative reflection, from a meta-position, has interpretive value for an individual and a system, about what may be happening in the system. There seems to be acknowledgement of the emotional task of the system in creating a new identity. Which according to Cilliers (2006) provides evidence for recognising the psychodynamic evidence, of basic assumptions. One such basic assumption would be fight/flight where the troops flight from the anxiety of what it would mean to be tentative in their role as troops while creating their new identity, which manifests as shame. The troops then fight the IO Psychologist for daring such an observation and report him to the leadership to be dealt with. A familiar defence in the military which harnesses the basic assumption dependency towards its task. What needs to be explored though is how these basic assumptions, core anxieties and social defense patterns influenced task performance, Cilliers (2006). Mobilising thinking processes in this manner then creates potential space for linking where new meanings and insights can be formed (Rao, 2013) towards transforming shame in a space which is often confronting and uncomfortable as it may challenge habitual ways of thinking and doing things (Nossal, 2007).

16.3.1 Transforming Shame a Coaching Model

At the time of the case study the military's task was to transform towards a peace-keeping force. Addressing the personal shame experienced by the IO Psychologist alone, without making the connections between the individual and the system would not lead to sustainable changes for both the individual and/or the system. Sustainable changes can only be brought about if connections are made between the individual and the system. A coaching model by Dr. Simon Western is presented which considers relationships, teamwork and leadership capabilities, towards sustainable changes, developed from a rigorous theoretical base and extensive practice (Western, 2012).

By applying the Analytic-Network Coaching (A-N coaching) model, to the case study, there is an acknowledgement that, the individual has an unconscious mind that shapes behaviour and understanding, in terms of past experiences which may assist the coach when it comes to transforming the experienced shame in the system (Eloquin, 2016). From a systems perspective there is acknowledgement that destructive forces of shame may be used to maintain the status quo. Nossal (2007), states that both the individual and the system may defend against feelings of shame in possibly destructive ways in avoiding the task as evident in the case study.

The A-N coaching model could assist an individual to process feeling of shame through five frames. The first of these are depth analysis, the search for the authentic self, identifying defences and patterns of defences against shame. Relational analysis goes beyond intra-personal dynamics focused on by many coaching models by taking account of inter-personal relationships and their influences on feelings of shame. Leadership analysis enables the individual to discover the "unique leader within and

Fig. 16.1 ANC coaching
frames Western (2012)

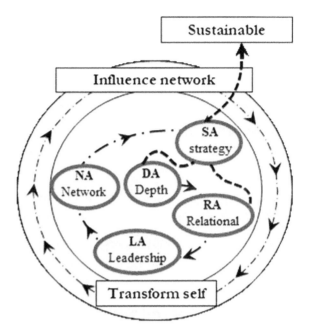

"challenge and disrupt the individual's ideas of what leadership is. Network analysis
not only focuses on the system in which the individual operates but extends to the
concept of a network society taking in the new realities of the internet, technology
and social media into account where boundaries and hierarchical structures are not
that clear (Western, 2012). Finally, the frame strategic analysis works on two levels
connecting and learning from the previous frames where individuals develop a personal strategy to maximise their potential and an organisational-networked strategy
which focuses on where the individual can influence the strategic direction of the
organisation most effectively. Analysing and connecting the learning in the previous
frames makes the whole greater than the sum of the parts (Western, 2012).

In the section to follow the frames are applied to the case study however, it must
be noted that applying the full coaching frame is out of the scope of this chapter. For
further reading, the literature on the topic by Dr. Simon Western could be consulted.

16.3.2   Steps in Analytic Network Coaching

See Fig. 16.1.

16.3.2.1 Depth Analysis

Depth analysis is the foundation stone on which this coaching system rests. It helps people to understand who they really are and to discover and re-discover themselves. Within the context of experiencing shame, it is important to explore the emotions that were provoked by questioning meaning, identity, authenticity and engagement.

It is important to create a space where the individual can take a step back and explore the inner self. As the frame suggests this is a depth analysis, the mundane needs to be set aside to focus on emotions, the unconscious and the human spirit. The aim is to ground the individual about their feelings of shame with courage and authenticity.

In this stance, reflection is encouraged towards exploration of defence patterns. The IO psychologist could be encouraged to play with ideas creatively to disrupt normative thinking about the shame he experienced. Free associations in an environment such as an art gallery, museum or the use of materials such as photos or drawings to open a space for new reflections of shame experiences could be encouraged, to view the environment in a new way. The individual is coached to make links between shame and the space or materials. The IO Psychologist did allude to a pattern when he stated that he had a strong valence for competence, a "need" in almost everything he does, and when his competence is questioned, he reacts "forcefully" as he did to the commanding officer. The IO psychologist could be asked to consider a question such as this in terms of his cultural self, to identify important cultural themes that is a vital part of himself such as "how does he perceive his age, ethnicity, place, family history, religion, gender and economic back ground shape what he thinks and feels are normal feelings of shame"?

Working through these reflections in a deeply personal manner could bring about understanding and insight of where the feelings of shame come from. Recognising patterns would enable the IO psychologist to identify where these may play out in the future.

16.3.2.2 Relational Analysis

Moving from the inner self towards the outer self, the focus shifts to an individual's team or group, family and friends to gain an understanding of the relational dynamics that exist between themselves and others. The aim is to gain insight to these dynamics and to realise that an individual does not need to be at the mercy of past patterns of shame he may have identified in the previous frame. Inter-personal dynamics are real and powerful. In terms of the IO Psychologist, inter personal relationships such as those with family, authority figures, groups and social roles are explored, gaining insight to these relationships. Coaching the individual to recognise how they are caught up in roles, where they carry their own and other emotions can open new perspectives of feelings of shame together with what the individual contains on behalf of others. In terms of the case study the IO Psychologist would consider the shame he carried on behalf of the troops and their need to see him shamed by the

Commanding Officer, thereby reinstating their "morale" a common sub-task of the military and a rational argument from the Commanding officer which allows them to maintain the status quo and flight away from the experiences of shame held for them by the IO Psychologist.

In this method the coaching process itself becomes the approach to explore inter-relationships. The coaching-client relationship is not unique or different from other relationships. In exploring the feelings of shame, the coach would use the coaching relationship as live data, by becoming aware of transference, counter-transference and projections that take place between the coach and individual. Providing hypotheses to the individual of what the coach had become aware of during their interactions. In this manner the individual often gains tremendous insight into their own inter-relationships with others.

16.3.2.3 Leadership Analysis

Western (2012) views leadership as a "complex process and distributed phenomenon" where leadership transcends one individual. A-N coaching uses a framework of leadership to explore an individual's unique leadership and followership potential. The central idea being that leadership is both within and beyond the individual and distributed throughout the organisation. In this phase, through reflecting back on the previous two phases of the coaching, the IO psychologist would discover his unique "leader within" towards developing personal leadership and follower potential. Acknowledging the valence for shame, he would explore how he takes up his own authority and reacts to authority and power, while working constructively with the defence mechanism of shame. Normative ideas of what leadership is may be disrupted which may promote insights concerning the de-authorisation he experienced from the commanding officer and expand possibilities of his own and others leadership and followership role and how it affects his own leadership position past, present and future. The focus here is to explore how he conceives leadership itself. Understanding how he takes up his own leadership role and how he can develop greater leadership capacity in the system, through considering formally invested leadership, and the enactment of leadership both covertly and overtly within a system (Cilliers, 2006). He would then work with how he can play a part in influencing the organisational system and wider networks and external influences where feelings of shame may manifest.

16.3.2.4 Network Analysis (NA)

As a coping strategy, the IO psychologist contacted his peers in his home unit for advice. This phase of the coaching model guides individuals in identifying and recognising where the power and resources lie within their networks and which are accessible to them, while situating themselves within their own network.

The approach here is often to have the individual draw their network as a conceptual map, which includes work and the broader society. Seeing where the power and resources lie, who the strong and weak connections are, and how change takes place over time. In terms of the IO Psychologist he would then be able to identify the connections he needs to make and the nodal points of power he would need to influence, should he find himself in a similar position in the future. The future being a concern for the IO Psychologist, as he stated he would work again with some of the people he had the altercation with. Feelings of disempowerment could be transformed to empowerment, as possible opportunities for influence and change. Working within this phase of the coaching model he would become aware of options, and not only rely on one node of influence such as the home unit he had innitially identified.

He would be encouraged to think spatially and connectedly. A conceptual map drawn by the IO psychologist would allow himself to re-think many assumptions of the military system and extend the assumptions to include how social defence patterns of relationships and collaboration, influence task performance. The conceptual map would allow for external factors such as a social change the military was undergoing at that time and to identify sensitive patterns, relationships and connections, which would be key to understanding change. Nodes of power or areas of resistance could be identified and their influence on change. The IO psychologist would then be able to locate himself in his network, re-imagine how it really works and learn how to take a more strategic, systemic, ethical and connected approach to his work.

16.3.2.5 Strategic Analysis (SA)

The holistic approach of the model enables individuals to see connections between inner and relational selves; how their emotions and behaviours play out in their various roles, and how strengths and challenges enable them to influence change in the organisation and other networks applying future thinking and action (Western, 2012).

To this end, the previous four frames are reviewed enabling the individual to evaluate, consolidate and innovate by evaluating what is working or not working and then identifying strategies to consolidate, doing more of the same or building on success; identifying where personal strategic changes need to be made for sustainable changes to recurring patterns of shame. This is not a quick fix phase to jump in and leap into action, but rather to reflect and revaluate by revisiting the previous four frames.

In reflecting, the individual would consider both the conscious and unconscious dynamics concerning the challenges, their purpose and an outcome that is desired authentically while questioning its meaning. As the individual works through the phases they may find themselves returning to this phase and others periodically as this process is dynamic where insights in other phases may result in questioning meaning and the outcome from time to time.

The A-N coaching model is not about leaping into action with five steps to transforming shame in organisations it needs to be considered as a process. Western (2012) states that each frame is an important piece of coaching on its own however used together the A-N coaching process becomes more than the sum of its parts. It provides a conceptual framework for coaches and clients to internalise the process of how they think and work creating sustainable change, as individuals work and move across networks, acknowledging personal patterns, how these patterns are used by systems and influence systems. Leadership as a concept of the mind and its distributive qualities are acknowledged by considering how it influences systems and how these need to be adapted towards influencing a network. While continuously building on a strategy towards evaluation, consolidation and innovation towards sustainable change.

16.3.3 Transforming Shame in Organisations

The systems psychodynamic lens and a coaching model has been applied to a case study which highlights the manifestation of shame in a system. How these two methods can be applied in other systems is explored next.

As previously indicated the case study formed part of a larger study on shame within the South African context, with its own unique multi-culture society (Mayer & Tonelli, 2017). When considering how the systems psychodynamic lens and the A-N coaching frame as methods to transforming shame, could be applied in different organisations, systems and networks, it may be useful to take note of the findings of the study. Comparisons can then be made to different organisations and how shame may be influencing individuals and the system at large.

Findings from the study seemed to indicate that experiences, triggers and, the results of shame come from deep personal feelings of not being good enough where personal errors in judgement often leave individuals exposed to shameful experiences. Feelings that could resurface later with negative connotations. Triggers for a shameful situation at work seem to be activated when there are attacks on employee's competence and not being supportive to others or not receiving support from the system they operate within. Exclusion from, or voluntary removal from the situation, seems to reinforce shameful experiences as Wüschner (2017) and Mayer and Tonelli (2017) found while at the same time shame is seen as a coping strategy.

From a systemic perspective, leadership was repeatedly emphasised during the study when it came to dealing with shame. First leadership was seen to be shying away from dealing with issues of shame and not being supportive enough, and on the other hand, leadership was encouraged to use shame to enforce the morals and principles of the organisation. These contradicting views could be evidence for Long (2008) statement that in a perverse form of defence against shame, there is a need to see others shamed, to defend against own experiences of shame.

16.3.3.1 Practical Application for Working with Shame in Organisations

Bearing in mind findings of studies conducted on shame accross different contexts and organisations such as just described coaches would hold the five coaching frames in mind while considering both the conscious and unconscious dynamics at play within the individual and the system they operate within, as it relates to the shame experiences. However, how the process unfolds would be dependent on the individuals own process and insight, which means different frames may be visited at different times and reflected upon based on the insights the individual gains. The coach does allow the process to unfold as such; however, it is also important that the individual does not become stuck in a specific frame. This is where the coach's knowledge of the unconscious dynamics at play in the individual, the system and the coaching relationship, helps maintain a constructive flow as seen in Table 16.1. The framework is not exhaustive but provides an example of what the aims are in each of the five frames of A-N coaching, possible influences in the system from a systems psychodynamic perspective and, possible reflections for the coach and individual.

It must be stressed that there are no neat and tidy conclusions in coaching practices nor should there be (Western, 2012). In this chapter the focus is on shame a so-called destructive emotion (May, 2017). It consists of a devaluation element in the confront of others, embarrassment, humiliation and guilt whether imagined or real. On an unconscious level and at its most unbearable shame signals social annihilation (May, 2017). Guiding an individual through the process and learning how we experience each other, even through what might be considered a destructive force, such as shame, it is important to gain an understanding and awareness of how we relate to one another through these experiences. Working constructively with experiences of shame, and not from a defended position allows individuals to be more confident in their interactions with others. Understanding how shame could possibly shape working relationships, a clearer sense of self and purpose emerges, as individuals see themselves in the confront of others and how they may be "persuaded" by a system to act out expressions of shame.

16.3.4 Conclusion

Working with the individual from a systems psychodynamic stance considering both the conscious and unconscious processes of groups and individuals would enable the individual to understand where they fit into their system. He or she should identify their own key values; work with their authentic self; consider their own conscious and unconscious patterns relating to their needs and purpose in order to dismiss feelings of powerlessness; become more grounded; and learn how to influence the system for sustainable change (Western, 2012). The individual would then be able to monitor the system and evaluate how an emotion such as shame may move the individual and the system. In this way, individuals see connections between their inner selves and

Table 16.1 A framework for holding the individual and the system in the mind

A-N coaching frame	A-N coaching (Western, 2012)	Systems psychodynamics (SP)—task performance (Cilliers & Smit, 2006)	Possible questions for reflection
DA	Authentic self Values Purpose	Basic assumptions: Dependency Fight/Flight Pairing and splitting Attitudes Beliefs Core anxieties patterns defences	A-N: What brings meaning and contentment? SP: Reflect on past experiences of shame
RA	Self and others Group dynamics	Relationships and relatedness between subsystems Containment and boundaries Roles and de-authorisation of roles Loss of control	A-N: Identify an important relationship that triggers shame SP: Explore the relatedness of shame in the system/coaching relationship
LA	Unique leadership approach Distributive leadership	How is leadership and authority psychologically distributed Overt and covert leadership	A-N: What is leadership? SP: How is leadership enacted when confronted with shame?
NA	Connections Influencing networks	Inter-relationships between technical and social aspects of the group Structures Organisational design Work culture	A-N: Conceptual map of the organisation SP: Role configurations/where is shame perceived to emerge?
SA	Evaluate Consolidate	Emotional system task of the system Chaos Difficult experiences Envy Shame	A-N: Where can the individual influence the system to address shame in the system SP: Reflect on the emotional task of shame in the system

relational selves; and how emotions such as shame and behaviour play out in their roles and in the system as a whole to achieve system goals.

In sum: people relate to one another based on the very real and powerful impact families, authority figures, groups and social roles have on the sense of self and our way of being with others. In this manner, people may be caught up in roles where they carry their own emotions and can become carriers of others anxieties and emotions (Western, 2012).

References

Allcorn, S. (2015). Understanding organisational dynamics and leadership: A comparison of four perspectives. *Organisational & Social Dynamics, 15*(2), 181–209.

Bartle, D. (2015). *An exploration of trainee educational psychologists experience of attending a group relations conference using Interpretive Phenomenological Analysis*. Thesis submitted for Doctorate in Child and Educational Psychology at the University of Essex, United Kingdom.

Bion, W. R. (1961). *Experiences in groups and other papers*. London: Tavistock Publications.

Cilliers, F. (2006). A systems psychodynamic interpretation of South African diversity dynamics: A comparative study. *South African Journal of Labour Relations, 30*(2), 5–18.

Cilliers, F., & Africa, S. (2012). A systems psychodynamic description of organisational bullying experiences. *SA Journal of Industrial Psychology, 38*(2), 1–11. Retrieved from https://doi.org/10.4102/sajip.v38i2.994.

Cilliers, F., & Smit, B. (2006). A systems psychodynamic interpretation of South African diversity dynamics: A comparative study. *South African Journal of Labour, 30*(2), 18 p. Retrieved from http://reference.sabinet.co.za/sa_epublication_article/labour_V30_n2_a2.

Eloquin, X. (2016). Systems-psychodynamics in schools: A framework for EPs undertaking organisational consultancy. *Educational Psychology in Practice, 32*(2), 163–179. Retrieved from https://doi.org/10.1080/02667363.2016.1139545.

Handy, J., & Rowlands, L. (2017). The systems psychodynamics of gendered hiring: Personal anxieties and defensive organizational practices within the New Zealand film industry. *Human Relations, 70*(3), 312–338. Retrieved from https://doi.org/10.1177/0018726716651690.

Hayden, C., & Molenkamp, R. J. (2002). *Tavistock primer II*. Jupiter, FL: A. K. Rice Institute.

Leask, P. (2013). Losing trust in the world: Humiliation and its consequences. *Psychodynamic Practice, 19*(2), 129–142. Retrieved from https://doi.org/10.1080/14753634.2013.778485.

Long, S. (2008). *The perverse organisation and its deadly sins*. London: Karnac Books.

May. (2017). Shame! A system psychodynamic perspective. In E. Vanderheiden & C. Mayer (Eds.), *The Value of Shame: Exploring a Health Resource in cultural contexts* (pp. 110–135). Cham: Springer.

Mayer, C., & Tonelli, L. (2017). "Dream on-There is no Salvation!": Transforming shame in the South African workplace through personal and organisational strategies. In E. Vanderheiden & C. Mayer (Eds.), *The value of shame: Exploring a health resource in cultural contexts* (pp. 110–135). Cham: Springer.

Mayer, C. H., Viviers, R., & Tonelli, L. (2017). "The fact that she just looked at me…"—Narrations on shame in South African workplaces. *SAJIP: South African Journal of Industrial Psychology, 43*, 1–10. Retrieved from https://doi.org/10.4102/sajip.v43i0.1385.

Motsoaledi, L., & Cilliers, F. (2012). Executive coaching in diversity from the systems psychodynamic perspective: Original research. *SA Journal of Industrial Psychology, 38*(2), 11 p. Retrieved from http://reference.sabinet.co.za/sa_epublication_article/psyc_v38_n2_a6.

Newton, J., & Goodman, H. (2009). Only to connect: Systems psychodynamics and communicative space. *Action Research, 7*(3), 291–312. Retrieved from https://doi.org/10.1177/1476750309336719.

Nossal, B. S. (2007). *Systems psychodynamics and consulting to organisations in Australia.* A thesis in Philosophy (doctoral thesis). Australia: RMIT University.

Rao, A. (2013). Taming resistance to thinking: Place of containment in organisational work. *Organisational & Social Dynamics, 13*(1), 1–21.

Rice, A. K. (1953). Productivity and social organization in an Indian weaving shed: An examination of some aspects of the socio-technical system of an experimental automatic loom shed. *Human Relations, 6,* 297–329.

Tai, K., Narayanan, J., & McAllister, D. J. (2012). Envy as pain: Rethinking the nature of envy and its implications for employees and organizations. *Academy of Management Review, 37*(1), 107–129. Retrieved from https://doi.org/10.5465/amr.2009.0484.

Western, S. (2012). *Coaching and mentoring. A critical text.* London: Sage Publications.

Wüschner, P. (2017). Shame, guilt, and punishment. *Foucault Studies*, (23), 86–107. Retrieved from http://dx.doi.org/10.22439/fs.v0i0.5343.

Zavaleta Reyles, D. (2007). The ability to go about without Shame: A proposal for internationally comparable indicators of shame and humiliation. *Oxford Development Studies, 35*(4), 405–430. Retrieved from https://doi.org/10.1080/13600810701701905.

Louise Tonelli is an industrial and organizational psychologist and lecturer within the Department of Industrial and Organizational Psychology at the University of South Africa (UNISA) one of the largest distance education institutions in the world. As a member of the Society of Industrial and Organizational Psychology of South Africa's (SIOPSA) Interest Group in Systems Psychodynamics of Organizations (IGSPO), her research interests lie in the unconscious/conscious processes within individuals, organizations, and society as a whole.

Chapter 17
Transforming Shame in the Workplace: A Brainfit Approach

Dirk Geldenhuys

Abstract Although the study of wellness from an applied neuroscientific perspective is already acknowledged in the literature, the role of shame and addressing shame in organisations from an applied neuroscientific perspective is still neglected by scholars and practitioners in the field. The purpose of this theoretical chapter is to discuss the role of shame in the workplace from an organisational neuroscientific perspective. It is argued that viewing shame from this perspective may add a unique contribution to the development and implementation of interventions to prevent and even address toxic shame, and hence contribute to organisational wellness. It may also assist in offering a form of triangulation to the study of other interventions developed for overcoming shame in the workplace. The author firstly provides insights into the development of the human brain as a social organ, followed by discussions on the role of the brain as a survival mechanism and the formation of memory systems. The author then proceeds to a discussion of the basic human needs according to Grawe's neuropsychotherapy model, as adapted by Rossouw, to serve as the foundation for arguing that shame can be conceptualised as a survival strategy to overcome the pressures experienced in today's volatile, uncertain, complex and ambiguous (VUCA) world of work. Following these discussions, the author introduces the concept of brain fit as an approach for leaders in organisations to prevent and deal with shame. Based on this discussion, implications for addressing shame are provided.

Keywords Triune brain · HPA-axis · Neuropsychotherapy · Basic needs · Motivational schemata · Memory systems · Brain fit · Resilience · Shame

D. Geldenhuys (✉)
Department of Industrial and Organisational Psychology, University of South Africa (UNISA), AJH vd Walt Building, Pretoria, South Africa
e-mail: geldedj@unisa.ac.za

© Springer Nature Switzerland AG 2019
C.-H. Mayer and E. Vanderheiden (eds.), *The Bright Side of Shame*,
https://doi.org/10.1007/978-3-030-13409-9_17

17.1 Introduction

Although there is no agreement on the definition of shame, Gilbert and Procter (2006) identified two components of the concept, namely external shame and internal shame. External shame refers to feelings and thoughts about the perceptions of others, while internal shame starts with the development of self-awareness, devaluations of the self and self-criticism (Gilbert & Procter, 2006) (Gilbert, in this book). However, the authors also reason that the two components can be fused, resulting in the experience that the outside world is turning against the person and that self-evaluations also become hostile. The fusion of the dimensions is also evident from an empirical study done among women, defining shame as "an intense feeling or experience of believing we are flawed and therefore unworthy of acceptance and belonging", with the main concerns of the participants, a combination of feelings of being trapped, powerless and isolated (Brown, 2006) (Silverio, in this book). Based on this study, Brown (2006) concludes that the shame construct is not exclusively psychological, social or cultural but comprises components of each.

In line with the above reasoning, the author argues that neuroscience adds a further dimension to the study of shame. According to Cozolino (2017, p. 216), "shame is represented physiologically by a rapid transition from a positive to a negative state and from sympathetic to parasympathetic dominance". However, viewing shame from an applied neuroscientific perspective also includes psychological, social and cultural components, and more specifically, for the purpose of this chapter, components of neuropsychotherapy (Cozolino, 2017; Rossouw, 2014; Schore & Schore, 2007; Siegel, 2012). This integrative nature of shame is evident in Cozolino's (2017, 217) definition of shame as "the emotional reflection of a lost attunement with the caretaker, drawing its power from the child's primal need to stay connected for survival".

The purpose of this theoretical chapter is to discuss the role of shame in the workplace from an organisational neuroscientific perspective (Oosthuizen, in this book). Organisational neuroscience as a recent development in organisational studies can be viewed as "a paradigm or interpretative framework that sheds new light on existing problems as well as highlighting problems that might not otherwise have been considered" (Becker, Cropanzano, & Sanfey, 2011). Although studying wellness from an applied neuroscientific perspective is already acknowledged in organisational literature, the role of shame and addressing shame as a wellness construct in organisations from an organisational neuroscientific perspective is still neglected by scholars and practitioners in the field. It is argued that viewing shame from this perspective may shed new light on the concept of shame and assist in the development and implementation of interventions to prevent and address toxic shame, and hence contribute to organisational wellness. It may also assist in offering triangulation for other interventions developed for overcoming shame in the workplace.

17.2 The Brain as a Social Organ

The idea of the human brain as a social organ started in the 1970s as scholars started realising that neuroanatomy, neurochemistry and social relationships are intrinsically related (Cozolino, 2017). This relationship is evident, for instance, in the slow maturation process of the human brain. Although the human nervous system is functional at birth, the motor, perceptual and cognitive abilities develop much slower in comparison with other species. This delayed maturation process offers time needed to develop the specialised functions of the human brain, through interaction with the environment (Cozolino, 2017). This implies that human beings depend largely on experience, not only to survive, but also to develop and thrive. The role of interpersonal relationships is vital to this process. People are born into relationships, develop their identity through relationships and are influenced throughout their lives by social interactions. According to Hanna (2014, 2), the nervous system and all the other systems, including interpersonal systems form a network or "ecology of survival" that reveals the biological impact of interpersonal processes on brain development.

MacLean (1990) offered a more elaborate theory, based on evolution, to describe the development of the human brain. According to MacLean's (1990) triune theory, the human brain developed through evolution in a sequence, starting with the Reptilian Complex (the most primitive structure that we share with all animals), followed by the Paleomammalian Complex (that we share with mammals) and thirdly the Neomammalian Complex as the most recent step in the evolution of the brain. This development, from the most primitive to the most advanced structures, can be recognised in human beings. Although some scholars today challenge certain aspects of MacLean's theory, the division of the brain in three distinguishable but interrelated parts and communication between these parts, is still recognised in the neurosciences with important implications for neuropsychotherapy and for shame (Cozolino, 2017; Rossouw, 2014).

Based on the triune theory, the human brain comprises three interconnected brain systems or regions within the primitive brain including the brainstem, pons and medulla, as the first system. This system is fully developed and fully functional at birth and is responsible for physical survival as it regulates breathing, heart rate, motor planning and the physiological aspects of basic affect such as aggression and anxiety (Henson & Rossouw, 2013; Rossouw, 2014). This is the most protected system of the brain and in need of constant blood flow (Henson & Rossouw, 2013).

Next is the limbic region, also known as the emotional or impulsive brain. The limbic region comprises the thalamus, hypothalamus, amygdala, hippocampus, basal ganglia and nucleus accumbens (Henson & Rossouw, 2013). At birth, this system is fully developed but not fully functional. In order to develop in functionality, it needs to interact with the physical and social environment. At times, however, it also has to protect itself from a hostile environment. The limbic region enables emotions, learning, memory, social behaviour and the ability to refine basic affect (aggression and anxiety) that originate in the primitive brain (Henson & Rossouw, 2013). The amygdala and hippocampus are regarded as two very important structures of the limbic region for the purpose of neuropsychotherapy and hence for this chapter. The amygdala is a key component in neural networks that are involved in attachment, the appraisal and expression of emotion, while the hippocampus plays a major role in consolidating explicit memory and in contextualising emotion (Cozolino, 2017).

The development of the limbic region is followed by the development of the cortical systems or outer layer of the brain (especially the left and right prefrontal systems), also known as the smart brain (Rossouw, 2014). The cortex comprises the left and right hemispheres that are connected by the corpus callosum and is subdivided into four lobes, known as the frontal lobe, parietal lobe, occipital lobe and the temporal lobe. This system is mostly underdeveloped at birth and develops until early adulthood. Through its networking with the limbic region, its development depends on experience and hence it is shaped by interactions with the environment (Cozolino, 2017). The frontal parts of the cortex are responsible for execution control, namely language, abstract cognition, sequential planning and perception abilities. It allows mental representations of the self, others and the environment (Cozolino, 2017). An important function of this system is that it serves to down-regulate the limbic region (Dahlitz & Rossouw, 2014). It is first organised and then serves to organise experiences and interactions with the outside world (Cozolino, 2017). Other than in the case of the primitive systems (such as the brainstem region and the limbic system), damage in the cortical areas of the brain is in most instances not life threatening.

The implication of viewing the brain as a social organ is that, although shame is a highly personalised experience, it originates as a social phenomenon when the cortical areas of the brain are not yet fully functional. It develops when the expectation of positive interactions with the caregiver is met with expressions of anger or disapproval (Cozolino, 2017). As the child depends on the attunement of a caretaker to survive, shame is an attempt to get acceptance and approval from the caretaker. Shame is therefore a reaction on the influence of the social environment and is motivated by the need for survival.

Before exploring shame as a strategy for survival and presenting an approach to deal with shame in organisations, one needs to understand first how the brain functions under stress, how memory systems develop and how the satisfaction of basic human needs influences the functioning of the brain.

17.3   The Brain and Survival

Considering the sequence of development from the most protected brainstem to the most advanced cortical areas (from the bottom to the top and from the inside to the outside) such as the prefrontal cortex, it is apparent that the brain is primarily wired for survival (Dahlitz & Rossouw, 2014; Cozolino, 2017). To regulate our responses in dealing with survival threats, two separate but interconnected neural circuits have been identified (Cozolino, 2017; LeDoux, 1994). The first system, a primitive reflexive system, sends cues from the sensory organs through the thalamus to the amygdala where it is, based on crude experiences, appraised for potential threats or danger. The amygdala, through its connections with the autonomic nervous system, translates the input into a stress response. During the stress response, the hypothalamus-pituitary-adrenal axis (HPA axis) is activated, shutting down systems such as the immune and digestion systems. The stress response therefore, is a survival response of fight, flight or freeze.

The second system involved in regulating fear is a much slower system, involving the hippocampus and prefrontal cortex in the evaluation process (Dahlitz & Rossouw, 2014; Cozolino, 2017). In this instance, the information is carefully appraised and contextualised in time and space by comparing the information with memories of similar situations. This system also has the role of making sense and downregulating the behavioural and visceral reaction of the impulsive system. As the primitive systems are better developed than the cortical systems, the primitive systems take precedence in activation in situations when danger or threat is perceived. The implication for shame is that if the primitive, reactive system is activated by negative social experiences, such as a performance review a person will immediately react, for instance by becoming defensive without reflecting on the possible value of the feedback. However, if the slower system is intact, it will be easier to recover, to reflect and to make sense of social experiences before reacting in a thoughtful manner.

The function of the fast, reactive system is important in times of danger when quick action is called for. However, extensive or prolonged activation of this primitive system leads to even stronger wiring in this area, the strengthening of neural connections due to the ongoing firing between neurons, the activation of stress chemicals such as CRF, ACTH, adrenalin and cortisol, and the inhibition of serotonin, which is associated with smart brain development (Dahlitz & Rossouw, 2014). This in turn leads to compromised neural proliferation in the frontal systems, resulting in the development of the "anxious brain" where any stimulus, even positive ones, are paired with fear (Cozolino, 2017). The stress response is thus not only a neurochemical reaction, but also changes the neural networks and even structures of the brain, signifying a change from an anxious state to a trait characterised by anxiety. In the long term, it may even lead to cell death and a decrease in brain volume (Henson & Rossouw, 2013). This explains why stress can lead to physical illness as well as psychological pathology (Cozolino, 2017; Dahlitz & Rossouw, 2014). It is therefore reasoned that the prolonged experience of shame can have the same detrimental effects as stress on the wellness and wellbeing of the worker and thus not only the emotional disengagement of employees, but also their physical absenteeism from the workplace.

17.4   Memory Systems

In line with the development of the human brain, a distinction is made between the development of implicit and explicit memory networks as two broad categories of long-term memory. Systems of implicit memory are unconscious and include instinctual memories and memories responsible for controlling reflexes and inner bodily functions, as well as memories that are primarily related to emotional and conditioned learning (Cozolino, 2017) with little conscious processing involved (Schacter & Wagner, 2013). Thus, most of our emotional and interpersonal memories are formed early in our life when our primitive brains are still in control. Explicit memory is classified as semantic memory (memory of facts) and episodic memory (autobiographical memory or memory of personal experiences) (Schacter & Wagner, 2013). Explicit memory is especially important for the formation and maintenance of emotional regulation, self-identity, and the transmission of culture (Cozolino, 2017). As explicit memory systems mature later than implicit memory systems, the early memories can intrude into adult consciousness. Early trauma in the absence of the explicit memory is then not experienced as a reaction to a hostile environment, but as an affirmation of inner feelings of essential badness (Cozolino, 2017). Thus, when shame is experienced in a prolonged or traumatic manner during early life, for instance due to the attunement of a caretaker, the child does not have the capacity to make an accurate assessment of the situation and as the experience is stored in the implicit memory system, it might lead to the development of a trait of not being good enough or toxic shame (Bradshaw, 1990) or a shame-based personality (Kaufman, 1985). In order to maintain consistency, experiences later in life will only serve to confirm the negative self-image.

17.5 Basic Human Needs

Due to the principles of neuroplasticity, the function and even the structure of the brain are modified by the influence of the environment. Experiencing a compromised environment constantly activates the protective patterns that surface in the stress response, leading to the development of motivational schemata of avoidance. However, if the environment is experienced as physically and emotionally safe, the over-activation of these systems will be downregulated, leading to the development of approach motivational schemata (Dahlitz & Rossouw, 2014). According to Grawe (2007), motivational schemata of "approach" and "avoidance" operate on different neural pathways and change throughout life to satisfy basic human needs and to protect human beings from the violation of these needs. These schemata form the basis of Grawe's consistency model (2007). The model is presented in Fig. 17.1 and should be read from the bottom to the top.

Grawe (2007) identified neural correlates for the basic human needs of Seymour Epstein's "cognitive-experiential self-theory" (Epstein, 1990) and postulates that the need for attachment (Ainsworth, Blehar, Waters & Wall, 1978; Bowlby, 1969, 1973) is one of the most fundamental needs for an infant's psychological wellbeing and development. This is the first survival need that needs to be fulfilled, as infants are not able to ensure their own survival (Hanna, 2014). As the infant's neocortex is still underdeveloped at this stage, the attachment processes entail more reactive responses than responses that are cognitively controlled. The development of secure or insecure attachment patterns therefore depends on the consistency of the caregiver's

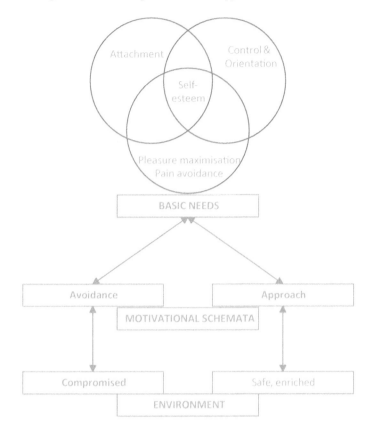

Fig. 17.1 Consistency model. Adapted from Rossouw (2014, p. 57)

availability, proximity and sensitivity (Bowlby, 1969, Henson & Rossouw, 2013) or attunement with the needs of the baby (Cozolino, 2017). If the basic need for attachment is met in a consistent manner, the infant feels safe to explore the environment further. This facilitates learning, resulting in optimal stimulation and neural growth (Grawe, 2007; Henson & Rossouw, 2013).

Another crucial fundamental need for human functioning is the pervasive need for control and orientation (Epstein, 1990; Grawe, 2007). The need for control begins when an infant needs to respond to the environment in order to survive. As the mother is instrumental in satisfying the need for control, there is a clear relation between the need for control and the need for attachment. If the need for control is not met, the infant experiences incongruence between its goals and its perception of the extent to which the environment can satisfy these goals and hence a violation of this need. However, if the need is met, congruence is experienced and neural proliferations are enhanced. Shame in the workplace is thus also related to the experience of control and orientation. It is reasoned that knowing expectations, having clear goals, and experiencing a sense of autonomy for example, will assist in preventing shameful situations.

Human beings need to experience that their environment, or their perceptions of their environment, are congruent with their activated goals. They therefore need to experience a sense of control and orientation over their environment. However, for growth to happen, incongruence is needed, but to such an extent, that control is still experienced (Grawe, 2007). Past life experiences influence the perception of controllability and predictability, of the extent to which life makes sense in general, and about whether investing resources and approaching life is likely to be rewarding (Henson & Rossouw, 2013). The need for control does not only refer to control over the current situation but also to the maximum number of options available to act upon (Grawe, 2007). If there are options available for the future, a sense of control is thus experienced.

The need for orientation is regarded as a component of the need for control (Grawe, 2007) or even as a need on its own (Habermacher, Ghadiri & Peters, 2014). Orientation refers to the ability to form an accurate appraisal of a situation and to make sense of what is happening (Dahlitz & Rossouw, 2014). If a situation is understood clearly, it will in most instances result in the experience of a greater sense of control.

According to Epstein (1998), another crucial need is the need for pleasure maximisation (good, beautiful, etc.) or distress avoidance. Experiences are neurologically evaluated as either good or bad, with the motivation to maximise good experiences and minimise bad experiences. The motivation for pleasure maximisation might be so strong that people are even prepared to suffer for the greater good, or to deny some short-term pleasure to obtain something better in the future (Dahlitz & Rossouw, 2014) with the release of dopamine in the reward system in the brain. However, dopamine is not only released when a sense of pleasure is expected, but also when people are successful in avoiding pain or discomfort. In this sense, avoiding shame, for instance by avoiding a meeting where a worker's shortcomings could be exposed in public, could also be experienced as successful. This explains why people can experience comfort within their discomfort, making it difficult to transform shame.

The evaluation of what is good or bad is subjective and influenced by the individual's activated goals and how the experience of the environment is consistent with satisfying the individual's other basic needs (Rossouw, 2014). According to Grawe (2007, p. 244), we are in a maximal state of pleasure when our "current perceptions and goals are completely congruent with one another, and the transpiring mental activity is not disturbed by any competing intentions." This maximum state is similar to the concept of "flow" (Csikszentmihalyi, 1991), with its focus on intrinsic motivation and the alignment of perception of experience with intentions. It is also congruent with happiness as described by Seligman (2002) to be the meaningful life where people use their strengths in pursuit of a purpose higher than they are.

Furthermore, the need for pleasure maximisation provides substantiation for Frederickson's research whereby the experience of positive emotions broadens and builds the mind (Frederickson, 2009). Positive experiences in the workplace, such as receiving recognition for and celebrating accomplishments can therefore serve as powerful mechanisms in transforming shame.

The fourth basic need, the need for self-esteem enhancement or protection differs from the other needs in the sense that it is distinctly human (Grawe, 2007), probably because the neural circuits associated with this need seem to be more complex and perhaps more extensive than those associated with the other needs (Henson & Rossouw, 2013; Rossouw, 2014). Self-esteem is defined as an individual's subjective self-evaluation of his or her worth as a person. As a basic need, it is secure and congruent, as opposed to unstable, narcissistic or discrepant (Grawe, 2007; Henson & Rossouw, 2013). Conscious self-awareness and the capacity for reflective thinking are required for the regulation of self-esteem and probably evolved as result of the survival value of social relationships. As these qualities are primarily facilitated by the cortical areas, they are still absent in young humans, and thus the last to mature. However, life experiences that occur before the development of these qualities already influence the self-image and self-esteem of the individual. According to Grawe (2007), the tendency to enhance self-esteem can be related to approach motivational schemata, whereas self-esteem protection can be related to avoidance schemata. As the development of toxic shame relates to traumatic or prolonged negative experiences of the social environment, it is motivated by schemata of avoidance; hence the tendency to avoid social engagement in an attempt to protect self-esteem from harm. This motivation to avoid can become visible for instance in withdrawal (flight reaction) or aggression (fight reaction) or submission (freeze).

Grawe's consistency model (2007) was refined by Rossouw (2014) who suggests that the need for self-esteem is an emerging property of the other basic needs and that the "condition of safety is essential for the satisfaction of those *needs*" (Dahlitz & Rossouw, 2014, p. 32). Furthermore, it is argued that the self-esteem concept does not seem to have an approach/avoidance reflex in relation to the environment. It should rather be seen as an emerging property of the other needs, "an *emergent* sense of *self* – shaped by basic need satisfaction and the motivational schemata that serve those needs – as a neural meta-structure that influences our approach/avoid violation" (Dahlitz & Rossouw, 2014, 32).

With self-esteem as an emerging property of the other needs, it is reasoned that shame relates not only to self-esteem, but also to compromising the other basic needs. Shame therefore relates also to the experience of not having trusting, supportive relationships, not being in control of the demands life throws at you, and not experiencing a sense of purpose in life.

17.6   Shame as a Survival Strategy

Based on the work of Grawe (2007), as adapted by Rossouw (2014), it is argued that shame can be regarded as a survival strategy, related to the violation of the basic need for self-esteem when experiencing an unsafe, hostile social environment. It is already established that the environment, more specifically the social environment, plays a major role in the development of shame (Cozolino, 2017). If the environment is experienced as dangerous or hostile, patterns of avoidance are activated as a protective mechanism to avoid damage to self-esteem.

As shame is related to the protection of the self, it is motivated by avoidance schemata. Although these motivational schemata develop early in life, relationships in the workplace reshape these patterns and mould the underlying neural substrate throughout life (Henson & Rossouw, 2013). Instead of approaching life by engaging in relationships, taking on risks and new challenges that could have enhanced their self-esteem, people in a state of shame would rather avoid the risk in order to preserve their self-esteem. In this manner, they would survive without losing face. If employees expect that their self-esteem will be threatened, they might for instance avoid engagement and risk-taking, keeping valuable contributions to themselves, doing only the necessary to keep out of trouble, and even covering up mistakes (Henson & Rossouw, 2013).

With self-esteem as an emergent property of the other basic needs, a state of shame can also be experienced when the satisfaction of one or more of the other basic needs are compromised. Shame, for example, can be related to the experience of exclusion from a task team (need for attachment), the experience of not knowing rules or policies (control and orientation) or being overlooked for promotion (pleasure/pain).

The different needs are also related to each other. For instance, negative self-images can be interpreted as an indication of the effects of fulfilling the need for control (Henson & Rossouw, 2013). It is argued that young people who are still dependent on their caretaker (need for attachment) for survival, would blame themselves, rather than the wrongful party, if their basic need of attachment is not met. They perceive themselves as not worth taken care of and consider the ill-treatment as justified (Henson & Rossouw, 2013). Similarly, it is reasoned that employees could for instance blame themselves for being overlooked for promotion, even if this was due to unfair labour practice. By blaming themselves, they can experience a sense of control by adapting to the need of the manager, hence enhancing their ability to cope.

Furthermore, similar to the development of the anxious brain as discussed earlier, a "shameful" brain or toxic shame (Bradshaw, 1990) can develop under repeated or prolonged states of shame. If not downregulated by the prefrontal cortex, shame becomes part of the implicit memory system that unconsciously distort current perceptions and influence appropriate reactions. According to Cozolino (2017, p. 90), these individuals "can find criticism and rejection in every interaction, resulting in a life of anxiety, a struggle for perfection, and depression".

It seems clear that transforming shame in the workplace could be challenging (Rossouw & Rossouw, 2018). It is therefore more conducive to be proactive and prevent shame from becoming toxic, than to intervene in an attempt to transform shame. However, due to neuroplasticity and the dynamic nature of memory (Alberini, 2013), brain networks could be transformed from survival to thriving by transforming leadership, organisational culture and climate.

17.7 Brainfitness

Brainfitness is an approach to working with shame from an organisational neuro-scientific perspective in the work context. Similar to the requirements for training the body to become physically fit for performance as an athlete, what is required to transform the brain to be fit for managing shameful experiences in the workplace can be described by the concept of brainfitness. Brainfitness is defined by the author as the capacity of transforming neural networks that are primarily wired for survival, to thriving, even in the VUCA (volatile, uncertain, complex and ambiguous) world of work. The need for brainfit employees to use shame as a survival strategy will become less prominent and even diminish, allowing the employees to fully engage and use their strengths to make a difference for themselves and their place of work. Similar to physical fitness, brainfitness requires effort and persistence. Instilling resilience therefore, is a key component of the transformation process (Davidson & Begley, 2012; Henson & Rossouw, 2013; Rossouw & Rossouw, 2018). It is not about pre-venting shameful experiences from happening, it is about the capacity to bounce back with vigour and resourcefulness. This view is congruent with Cozolino (2017, 217) stating, "Repeated and rapid return from shame to attuned states also consoli-dates into an expectation of positive outcomes during difficult social interactions". It "creates a kind of body memory that becomes an expectation of a positive outcome for relationships and life".

Rossouw and Rossouw (2018) identified six domains that comprise the concept of resilience, of which five pertain to mental constructs with neural structures associated with them. Brainfit people are characterised by optimal functioning in each of these domains.

The domains are

- vision (a sense of purpose and direction that drives us)
- composure (the ability to effectively downregulate emotions during stressful situations)
- reasoning (the ability to screen out emotional distractions in order to effectively solve problems)
- tenacity (the ability to persevere through difficulty and quickly get back on track)
- collaboration (having close and secure connections and support networks)
- physical health (regular exercise, healthy nutrition and quality sleep).

All these domains have identified neural networks and are related to the basic needs of Grawe's consistency model (Rossouw & Rossouw, 2018).

17.8 Implications for Organisations, Leaders and Employees

To become brainfit has certain implications for organisations, their leaders and employees.

On an organisational level, it implies that organisations have to create an environment conducive to the satisfaction of the basic needs of their employees, also known as an enriched environment, characterised as safe, nurturing and stimulating (Rossouw, 2014). The establishment of a safe organisational climate and culture is thus the first and foremost intervention in transforming shame. This, for instance, implies a culture of trust and mutual support, characterised by benevolence between leaders and followers and followers among themselves. It also implies a clear vision, shared by all. Furthermore, it implies the implementation of a learning organisation where employees are cognitively stimulated, encouraged to take risks, obtain positive feedback and learn from mistakes. It is only when people feel safe that they will consider strategies to enhance the sense of self (Cozolino, 2017; Henson & Rossouw, 2013) and learn to overcome the experience of shame.

Brainfitness requires from leaders to ensure that the abovementioned requirements are facilitated for their team members. In order to instill brainfitness in team members, leaders have to practice brainfitness themselves. The first requirement for leaders is to become knowledgeable about the basic principles related to the development and functioning of the human brain as discussed in this chapter, known as neuro-education (Miller, 2016). Leaders and followers need to learn to differentiate between themselves and shame as a function of the brain (Siegel, 2007). This will assist them with objectifying shame as a phenomenon thereby instilling the experience of a sense of control and orientation (Badenoch, 2008; Henson & Rossouw, 2013).

Secondly, brainfitness also requires self-awareness (Henson & Rossouw, 2013). When leaders know how the brain develops and operates, they need to reflect on the functioning of their own brains. They have to be aware of their own motivational schemata, the importance of and the extent to which their own basic needs are satisfied. They also need insight into their own implicit memory systems, learn what triggers them and how they respond towards their team members when their own PFC, as well as those of their team members have gone "off-line" (Henson & Rossouw, 2013, 23). Conscious self-awareness and the capacity for reflective thinking is regarded as a requirement for self-esteem regulation (Grawe, 2007). Practicing mindfulness can significantly contribute to the development of self-awareness (Cozolino, 2017).

Although the importance of safety should not be underestimated, leaders also need to provide their team members with cognitive stimulation to enhance their self-esteem. Stability needs to be integrated with sufficient levels of stimulation in order to enable curiosity, learning, creativity and risk-taking. Stimulation should, however, be to such an extent that the employee still experiences control, referred to as controlled incongruence, controlled disruption or inconsistency in neuropsychotherapeutic literature (Dahlitz & Rossouw, 2014; Grawe, 2007; Henson & Rossouw,

2013). One way of accomplishing this is by gradually introducing mechanisms to transform shame.

Only once leaders start practicing brainfitness themselves, can brainfitness be facilitated for employees per se in a similar manner as for leaders. However, the mere practice of brainfitness by leaders will already influence the experience of employees. When leaders experience that they are helping their employees to make a positive contribution to their organisation, it will enhance not only the self-esteem of the team members, but also the self-esteem of the leaders.

17.8.1 Case Study

The following case study will help you to apply the theory of brainfitness. You will get the opportunity to reflect on motivational schemata, see how basic needs can be compromised in a typical work setting, read about implicit and explicit memory systems and explore how movement from incorporating experiences of shame and attunement can be used to develop resilience, hence becoming brainfit.

Read through the case and reflect on the questions that follow.

Anne is appointed in the role of risk manager in a manufacturing company, comprising a number of departments. One of her objectives was to create an awareness of the possible risks they were facing in the different departments. After a successful engagement with the HR department, which made her feel very proud, she went to the engineering department, who were, coincidently, all males. It came to her attention that there were a number of safety issues in this department. For instance, she realised that, due to a shortage of engineers, some of them work such long hours overtime that their safety, and the safety of their colleagues are compromised. Anne thoroughly prepared for providing feedback at her first meeting. At a departmental meeting the head of the department who chaired the meeting, asked section heads to report on reaching their targets. After they did, Anne, who wants to sell herself and wants to make a difference, was also offered an opportunity to speak. She started her presentation: "As you all know, part of my task is to ensure compliance with safety regulations. I want to bring some safety issues to your attention, in particular the risks you are running in driving so much overtime due to being short staffed. The way that you are achieving your productivity targets is putting yourselves and your colleagues at serious risk." As she started, the manager looked at his watch and some members started preparing to leave. One of the members though, made a sarcastic remark by stating that if it wasn't for their productivity, they wouldn't have had a job, herself included. Then another person jokingly added, "Maybe you should rather study engineering so that you can assist them!" The chair reprimanded him, thanked her for her contribution and adjourned the meeting without further discussion. Anne left the room with mixed feelings. She felt upset at the rude manner in which the men treated her, but she decided to say nothing. She also felt ashamed and blamed herself for not preparing well enough. She left the room.

It is easy to see how Anne's safety needs were compromised during this meeting and the impact thereof on her self-esteem. She surely did not feel that she belonged to the team or that she was supported by them and even by the manager (attachment need); she might feel hopeless without future direction as no feedback was provided, except for the negative remarks (need for control/orientation); the experience was painful—meaningless (pleasure maximisation/pain avoidance) and eventually she lost face since she did not experience that she had made any contribution (self-esteem needs).

From the scenario, it seems clear that Anne applied her approach motivational schemata when she approached the meeting (probably motivated by her previous success with the HR department).

- Reflect on how the motivational schemata of avoidance could become operational if she is confronted with similar negative situations in future. This could also influence her willingness to work with engineers, or even with men.
- Reflect on how it could have assisted Anne if she interpreted (made sense of) the engineers' behaviour from a brainfit perspective. Remember that they were confronted with changing their behaviour.
- What implicit memory could she possible have triggered with them?
- Reflect on the relevancy of the different domains of resilience needed for her future in the company.
- Now, reflect on any emotions, or bodily experiences, if any, that were triggered in you as you read the scenario. If any, what triggered this?
- Did you also consider the positive experience with the HR department? We all tend to first focus on the negative as our brains are wired for survival. It could be helpful to take stock consciously of your strengths, to share those and think about ways to apply your strengths to the benefit of your colleagues and your work. This is what brainfitness is about!

17.9   Conclusion

The purpose of this theoretical chapter was to discuss the role of shame in the workplace from an organisational neuroscientific perspective. The authors conclude that shame is a multidisciplinary concept and that an organisational neuroscientific perspective offers a valuable contribution to the study and practice of shame. As the literature on shame in the workplace is still very limited, and even lacking in the literature on organisational neuroscience, the implications identified are, to a large extent, based on hypotheses derived from neuropsychotherapy. Much more research, especially empirical research, on shame is thus needed to augment, test and refine the conceptualisation of shame and interventions to prevent shame.

References

Ainsworth, M. D. S., Blehar, M. C., Waters, E., & Wall, S. (1978). *Patterns of attachment*. Hillsdale, NJ: Erlbaum.

Alberini, C. M. (Ed.). (2013). *Memory reconsolidation*. San Diego, CA: Academic Press.

Badenoch, B. (2008). *Being a brain-wise therapist: A practical guide to interpersonal neurobiology*. New York, NY: W. W. Norton & Co.

Becker, W. J., Cropanzano, R., & Sanfey, A. D. (2011). Organizational neuroscience: Taking organizational theory inside the neural black box. *Journal of Management, 37*(4), 933–961. Retrieved from https://doi.org/10.1177/0149206311398955.

Bowlby, J. (1969). Attachment and loss. *Vol. 1. Attachment*. New York: Basic Books.

Bradshaw, J. (1990). *Homecoming: Reclaiming and championing your inner child*. New York: Bantam.

Brown, B. (2006). Shame resilience theory: A grounded theory study on women and shame. *Families in Society, 87*(1), 43–52.

Cozolino, L. (2017). *The neuroscience of psychotherapy: Healing the social brain*. New York: Norton & Company.

Csikszentmihalyi, M. (1991). *Flow: The psychology of optimal experience*. New York: Harper Perennial.

Dahlitz, M. J., & Rossouw, P. J. (2014). The consistency-theoretical model of mental functioning: Towards a refined perspective. In P. J. Rossouw (Ed.), *Neuropsychotherapy: Theoretical underpinnings and Clinical applications* (pp. 21–41). Mediros: Brisbane.

Davidson, R. J., & Begley, S. (2012). *The emotional life of your brain*. London: Hodder & Stoughton.

Epstein, S. (1990). Cognitive-experiential self-theory. In L. A. Pervin (Ed.), *Handbook of personality: Theory and research* (pp. 165–192). New York.

Epstein, S. (1998). Cognitive-experiential self-theory. In D. F. Barone, M. Hersen, & V. B. van Hasselt (Eds.), *Advance personality* (pp. 212–238). New York: Springer Science & Business Media New York.

Frederickson, B. L. (2009). *Positivity*. New York: Crown.

Gilbert, P., & Procter, S. (2006). Compassionate mind training for people with high shame and self-criticism: Overview and pilot study of a group therapy approach. *Clinical Psychology and Psychotherapy, 13*, 353–379.

Grawe, K. (2007). *Neuropsychotherapy: How the neurosciences inform effective psychotherapy*. New York: Psychology Press.

Habermacher, A., Ghadiri, A., & Peters, T. (2014). The case for basic human needs in coaching: A neuroscientific perspective—The SCOAP coach theory. *The Coaching Psychologist, 10*(1). ISSN 1748-1104.

Hanna, S. M. (2014). *The transparent brain in couple and family therapy: Mindful integrations with neuroscience*. New York: Routledge.

Henson, C., & Rossouw, P. (2013). *Brainwise leadership: Practical neuroscience to survive and thrive at work*. Sydney: Learning Quest.

Kaufman, G. (1985). *Shame: The power of caring*. Cambridge: Schenkman.

LeDoux, J. E. (1994). Emotion, memory and the brain. *Scientific American, 270*(6), 32–39.

MacLean, P. D. (1990). *The triune brain in evolution: Role in paleocerebral functions*. New York: Plenum Press.

Miller, R. M. (2016). Neuroeducation: Integrating brain-based psychoeducation into clinical practice. *Journal of Mental Health Counseling, 38*, 103–115.

Rossouw. P. J. (Ed.). (2014). *Neuropsychotherapy: Theoretical underpinnings and Clinical applications* (pp. 1–20). Brisbane: Mediros.

Rossouw, P. J., & Rossouw, J. G. (2018). *The predictive 6-factor resilience scale: Clinical guidelines and applications* (2nd ed.). Melbourne: RForce.

Schacter, D. L., & Wagner, A. D. (2013). Learning and memory. In E. R. Kandel, J. H. Schwartz, T. M. Jessel, S. A. Siegelbaum, & A. J. Hudspeth (Eds.), *Principles of neural science* (5th ed., pp. 1441–1460). New York: Mc Graw-Hill.

Schore, J. R., & Schore, A. N. (2007). Modern attachment theory: The central role of affect regulation in development and treatment. *Clinical Social Work Journal, 36*(1), 9–20. Retrieved from https://doi.org/10.1007/s10615-007-0111-7.

Seligman, E. P. (2002). *Authentic happiness: Using the new Positive Psychology to realize your potential for lasting fulfillment.* New York: Free Press.

Siegel, D. J. (2007). *The mindful brain: Reflections and attunement in the cultivation of well-being.* New York, NY: W.W. Norton & Co.

Siegel, D. J. (2012). *The developing mind: How relationships and the brain interact to shape who we are* (2nd ed.). New York: Guilford Press.

Dirk Geldenhuys, DAdmin (IOP) holds a B.A., B.D. and a P.G.D. form the University of Pretoria and a DAdmin in industrial and organisational psychology from the University of South Africa. He is registered as an industrial psychologist with the health professions council of South Africa (HPCSA) and as a master practitioner with the South African Board of People Practices (SABPP). He is a lifelong honorary member of the Society of Industrial and Organisational Psychology of South Africa (SIOPSA) and was responsible for the establishment of an interest group in organisational neuroscience for SIOPSA. Currently, he is a full professor at the University of South Africa, teaching and researching in the field of organisation development, change management and executive coaching. He published scientific articles and books, supervised master and doctoral students and presented papers at local and international conferences. He is Director and co-founder of BrainFit partners and is involved in leadership assessment and development, executive coaching, interpersonal relations and group dynamic interventions. His major fields of interest include organisational neuroscience, systems psychodynamics, appreciative inquiry, social constructionism and the use of relational practices as approaches to study and facilitate change. He is also interested in interdisciplinary studies in the applied fields of economic and management sciences such as risk management.

Chapter 18
Transforming Shame to Collective Pride and Social Equity in Bicultural Organizations in Japan

Clifford H. Clarke and Naomi Takashiro

Abstract There are increasing intercultural misunderstandings between Japanese and American managers in their bicultural organizations in Japan. The intercultural misunderstandings are often caused by feelings of shame that are based upon perceived inadequacies in adjusting to a new workplace. These issues cause companies to lower productivity, managers to make bad decisions based on inaccurate information, employees to make stereotypic negative attributions, and everyone to display attitudes of disrespect and distrust. In order to solve these issues, we developed a bicultural organization development model based on our extensive experiences in working with several dozen U.S. subsidiaries in Japan. The purpose of this chapter is to present a practical intercultural developmental model that transforms shame through respect, empathy, trust, and social equity to a collective pride in bicultural organizations in Japan. We first describe the common issues related to shame in the bicultural workplace and then present the developmental model that we have found effective in building integrated corporate cultures in Japan. The model has four key elements: the program model design, intercultural facilitation skills, the transformative intercultural identity development stages, and the implementation of the model. Each element is described in detail. Successful interventions of the model require skillful intercultural communication facilitators, top management and employees' cooperation, and shared commitments from all parties to work collaboratively through the issues that arise.

Keywords Bicultural organization model · Japan–U.S. business · Bicultural identity development stages · Intercultural facilitation training · Intercultural management development

C. H. Clarke (✉)
24-801 Saiin Higashi Kaigawa-cho, Ukyu-ku, Kyoto-shi 615-0057, Japan
e-mail: chclarke@me.com

N. Takashiro
Kyoto, Japan
e-mail: takashiron@me.com

18.1   Introduction

There are today increasing intercultural misunderstandings between Japanese and American managers in their bicultural organizations in Japan. These can cause serious consequences. These are often caused by feelings of shame that are based upon perceived inadequacies in adjusting to a bicultural bilingual workplace. Inappropriate behaviors lead to bad judgments that often lead to lower productivity due to decisions made without accurate information in an environment of defensive accusations or attributions of negative stereotypes, and attitudes of disrespect and distrust that are demonstrated by members of each culture without empathy toward the strange other.

We introduce herein an intercultural intervention model that enables constructive client discussion of the conflicting cultural values, attitudes, and communication norms that fester discontent in intercultural intergroup interactions, with a focus on the role and function of shame in the Japanese organizational culture and its impact on a bicultural workplace. We describe this bicultural organization development model for facilitating the building of respect and trust in such an organization that increases group productivity, collective pride in achievements, career satisfaction, and enduring intercultural competencies in bicultural organizations in Japan, possibly by encouraging some transformative intercultural identity development.

18.2   Shame in the Bicultural Businesses in Japan

Shame (or *haji* in Japanese) is prevalent in the Japanese culture. Lebra (1983) explained that what differentiates Japanese from Westerners seems to be that Japanese are more sensitive to shame affecting their private as well as public self; whereas Westerns are more sensitive to public shame which is more like embarrassment.

Naturally, when business people from Japanese and the U.S. cultures encounter in the workplace different values and norms, stress and conflicts tend to arise. The common context of a U.S. bicultural business project in Japan consists of social status inequities and social justice issues, which are associated with shame due to the mutual perceptions of the parent company members as management and the new hires as trainees.

The Americans are usually in roles of trainer or manager, but in whatever role, most feel an obligation to adjust their assumptions, expectations, and communication styles in facing the different values and norms of a new culture. Their job is to perform effectively in their respective roles and not to lose face or be embarrassed. Japanese usually reach this conclusion earlier than their American counterparts, however, when the Americans discover their potential of failure by not adapting, they soon discover their own needs for modifications. Due to the parent company's 'privilege-of-rank' perceptions and the local new hires' realization that they signed on to a 'foreign' company in Japan, as subordinates they usually accept this condition for success earlier than their managers.

Notwithstanding many management teams in U.S. company subsidiaries in Japan initially will not recognize this requirement for assignment success. U.S. managers often rely on their perception of the universality of English while many Japanese may refuse to learn English and choose to just avoid the foreigner in the building. This creates a feeling of social injustice among the Japanese because after all they are in Japan. But, without English, Japanese may develop feelings of unfairness. They will not have equal opportunities for promotion. This is especially the case when the Americans give more respect to the Japanese English speakers who other Japanese perceive as trying to 'sell' their English skills to their advantage. In any case, Japanese and Americans feel shame or embarrassment in high-pressured bicultural business situations and some feel degrees of frustration upon their first efforts after the honeymoon stage of excitement passes.

The Americans' pride and confidence can cause a chafing at their perceived condition of being compelled to hide their individuality and demonstrate more sensitivity and effort to conform to the Japanese. The Japanese' pride often reaches a point of collective frustration with what they perceive to be conditions lacking common sense or appreciation for the local values and social norms. This causes a chafing in response to such imposed unreasonableness. These Japanese and American difficulties in adapting to unfamiliar working conditions can produce a sense of shame or embarrassment felt by both. In these conditions, how can building a shared collective pride eliminate any shame in a bicultural workforce?

Without any interventions inevitably confrontations will increase and workplace productivity will rapidly decline. This phenomenon would seldom occur in Japanese companies in Japan because of the effects of the positive role of shaming that encourages group harmony. Yamazaki (2005) suggests that shaming processes depend heavily on an intense consciousness about surrounding audiences and environments, which explains why shame is associated with saving face and avoiding shame. Japanese people tend to avoid public confrontations because their cultural norm is to maintain harmony with others, hence they are often interpreted as shy, hesitant, courteous, and conforming by American business persons.

By *shaming* we mean the effort to shame another by public judgments rendered in negative attributions and stereotypes in public, or by transferring blame to the other in public for creating an unfortunate situation. The Japanese recipient of shaming suffers the pain of shame, gets the message, and quickly complies with the known social norms and values. Americans in business leadership roles are not known in Japan to demonstrate much hesitation. However, there are some who try very hard to soften their more natural individual assertiveness in their management roles.

Members of both cultures feel shame even though at different levels of their psyche when they become aware that they have violated values and behavioral norms of the group (Lebra, 1983). When Japanese demonstrate shameful behavior the result can be social ostracism from the Japanese group, which can be devastating since the group is the source of one's public identity. With both cultures it can lead to altercations with negative consequences for the work team. While such shaming behavior can have a positive effect that motivates a change in behavior, the more effective intrinsic motivation factor in business is a fear of professional failure and loss of face. Shaming could actually be constructive in terms of admonishing one to conform to group norms (Hornsey, 2016), such as maintaining a group's core value of harmony.

There are three ways to work toward reducing status inequity consequences. First, an initial structural approach to jump-start the learning process is to assign all employees to bicultural partnerships in order to develop two-way mentoring relationships. This method establishes equity in the learning process (Woods, Poropat, Barker, Hills, Hibbins, & Borbasi, 2013). Such one-on-one relationships also facilitate the reduction of shame and shaming moments through personal discussions about their causes and consequences. Such collaborative dialogues also contribute to the development of mutual respect and trust (Williams, 2007). The Japanese member of each pair focuses on learning the U.S. company culture and communication style while the U.S. company member focuses on learning the Japanese cultural values, norms, and communication styles in Japan. All managers thereby play roles of teacher and student as each other's mentor. Second, the company can create conditions for learning together that build equal status among the members by holding hierarchical role assignments until an organizational structure is formed. Third, a process of validating the equal value of every member's contribution is another way to reduce status differentiations and its consequences. The group's manager can support this method as Cohen (1982, 1998) and Cohen and Lotan (1995) have done in their status equalization research in educational settings.

Regarding the creation of social justice with equal access to opportunities, Sandage and Jankowski (2013) found a strong association between intercultural competence and commitment to social justice. This finding supports the assumptions and purposes for this program and the role modeling of Ruben's (2015) intercultural communication competencies for the participants.

On-site in the company's workplace, intercultural interventions can assist a bicultural company in finding resolutions to these issues. Based on 30 years of experiences in working with both American and Japanese in U.S. subsidiaries in Japan, we have created a method for developing a bicultural organization through which participants transform their shame into pride. In sequence below, we present our program model overview, the Intercultural Communication Facilitation (ICF) skills, the transformative intercultural identity development (TIID) stages, and the generic instructions for implementing the ten-step bicultural management development (BMD) model for an organization. The process skills and the implementation methods enable the participants to progress through the intercultural identity transformation.

Feeling shame or embarrassment is an uncomfortable emotion for anyone. Managers can escape these feelings by striving to learn new ways through facilitated learning. They feel a powerful motivation to avoid loss of face in a professional failure in their personal careers. A commitment to company goals and effective bicultural teamwork will assure them of success.

18.3 Program Overview of the Bicultural Management Development (BMD) Model

1. **The program purpose** of this model is to transform shame into a collective pride by focusing on integrating each culture's managerial system. It is further to create a smoothly operating organization reflecting the equitable integration of two cultures' communicating and managing styles that is developed by synergistic and bilingual consensus. The consulting team's underlying goal is to create a pathway for participants through initial feelings of shame toward collective pride in a record-setting level of organizational productivity by inspiring status equity, mutual respect, empathy, and trust between its bicultural members. With these ingredients we have demonstrated that this model leads to success.

2. **The program conditions** include the group manager setting the integrated team's goal and asking for positive attitudes toward each other from the start. The group manager must require members' total commitment to the project's goals with a strong incentive of success. The members then begin their learning experiences with all of the supportive conditions of equal status housing that their families are enjoying, assigned bicultural mentors, emergent leadership potential, and ICFs that the company provides. Amir (1969) has identified the necessary positive conditions and Ruben and Kealey (1979) have identified the intercultural competencies that lead to success. Amir's six favorable conditions are: equal status, common goals, interaction intensity, cooperative-pleasurable activities, a supportive organization, and facilitative leadership.

3. **A counseling approach** is taken to recognize everyone's anxiety and fears of losing face by being inappropriate or ineffective in managing their perceived differences. Feelings of shame that can evolve into defensive behavior in cross-cultural situations must be responded to at first notice by an ICF. The ICFs can lead them to an understanding of the natural consequences of any two cultures interacting in a workplace with hidden assumptions. Values and communication norms will be violated to the point of natural friction, but the participants can see those as learning opportunities. The anxiety and shame that may be felt by both culture's members require joint understanding, empathy, and action planning to initiate the development activities. The ICFs can facilitate mutual learning among members about their strengths in their diverse values and norms of behavior in the BMD workshops.

4. **The workshop design** of this model requires the integration of company management, the ICFs, and the bicultural team members. Personal experiences, company culture factors, intervention design content, and prior knowledge and skills of all participants are drawn together in a design that builds upon the collaborative dialogues within the bicultural mentor pairs. The program is entirely and jointly custom designed. Before they begin work together comprehensive introductions are necessary because they give insights not previously known about each other. The workshop design alternates working with two separated cultural teams and one integrated bicultural team throughout the ten-steps in the BMD

process below. Each session lasts four hours in duration, and teams can be given as many sessions as they need to complete each task. The workshop frequency depends on the schedule demands of the company. The location is inside the company without any intrusions due to the intensity of the BMD workshop. Ideally there would be an equal number of Japanese and Americans assigned to the project to allow for one-to-one bicultural mentoring relationships to develop. An imbalanced number could be accommodated but too much change from an equal number of each might negatively impact efforts to create social equity. It is the social equity that facilitates feelings of collective pride in a sense of ownership of their achievements (Cohen, 1998; Cohen & Lotan, 1995).

5. **The group process** is an intercultural communication workshop (ICW) approach, facilitated by the ICFs, that increases intercultural competencies for bicultural teamwork in two languages, i.e., with skills for maintaining balanced conversations that incorporate appropriate turn taking, supportive listening, and adjusting or compromising in ways that avoid face-loss and shame. These skills encourage group learning and productive intercultural teamwork and are role modeled by two trained ICFs, Japanese and American. The ICFs work with two separate cultural membership groups with distinctly conflicting languages and cultures, as they begin forming one productive new synergistic corporate membership group with which they all ultimately identify proudly because they have jointly created its values and norms. Members enable their own changes when they begin seeking out other group members regardless of culture 'for evaluating their personal situation and for influencing their feelings,' which is the definition of a reference group. Hence, their development is from two distinct membership groups into a new reference group that eventually becomes their new membership group (Hyman, 1960).

6. **The role functions** of ICFs are to facilitate the group's communication in the workshops and in actual workplaces as intercultural coaches. They may also be called upon as interpreters. Along with the tasks in the ten-step BMD program, ICFs take adequate time to work through interpersonal and intercultural issues in a manner explained in our next section on intercultural communication facilitation skills. There is no company-assigned leader in any of the groups, except for the project's group manager. The bicultural group members have multiple roles in the workplace as organization developers, technology and language trainers and trainees, mentors for assigned partners, and heads of families outside the project facilities.

7. **The scope of the program** elements represented in this chapter are limited to the development of the managerial functions. Many other aspects of a broader scope of organizational development activities are not engaged herein.

18.4 Intercultural Communication Facilitation (ICF) Skills

The ICFs roles must be clearly explained to all members in both languages before the first few meetings get underway. Japanese have little to no experience with processing communication orally in a workplace. ICFs encourage discussion of role functions because intercultural communication processes are not understood very well in businesses by Americans either. The group members require assurance that the purpose of monitoring communication processes is not an evaluation process. Bicultural meetings are conducted largely in English with pauses for Japanese interpretations that must be permitted in order to achieve clarity. ICFs often check if translations of expressions are needed. ICFs may be required to serve as interpreters.

The ICFs functions focus primarily on the process of interactions in the following ways:

- Facilitators attend to ways people managed their interactions, i.e., turn taking, interrupting, and nonverbal signaling that need support. They demonstrate abilities to read indicators provided by word choices, implied feelings, and nonverbal expressions, such as the readiness to take a turn.
- Facilitators invite members to speak from their own experiences and from their cultural perspectives. They should take opportunities to share their assumptions, interpretations and values underlying their experiences. The BMD model provides this opportunity.
- Facilitators throughout the discussions explore any manifestation of cultural differences and encourage members to consciously look for differences in behaviors or feelings that might point to cultural differences in perception, value orientations, communication and learning styles. Yamazaki (2005) discusses differences in learning styles of Japanese and Americans and suggests that Japanese learn more through concrete experiences emotionally while Americans learn more through abstract conceptualizations.
- Facilitators discourage interruptions when someone else is talking and encourage talk story time, a process familiar to traditional cultures.
- Facilitators maintain interactions that focus on learning across cultures utilizing the intercultural communication competencies identified by Ruben and Kealey (1979) as: displaying respect, being nonjudgmental, personalizing your view of knowledge, displaying empathy, demonstrating role flexibility, displaying reciprocal concern, and tolerating ambiguity. They demonstrate these skills as role models in a way that is supportive of all members helping other participants learn about each other's culture.
- Facilitators question cross-cultural judgments and encourage members to explore diverse cultural premises unknown to some before making any judgments.
- Facilitators demonstrate communicative responsiveness, to both expressed thoughts and feelings, and encourage others to be similarly attentive and responsive.
- Facilitators seek clarification, offer supportive comments, and encourage members to explore each other's opinions and feelings, especially when they are confusing.

- Facilitators offer possible feelings and opinions from group members' unexpressed assumptions or expectations attempting to clarify each unexpressed premise that may be at the root of misunderstanding. This trains members in utilizing the descriptive, interpretive, and evaluative functions of communication (Barnlund, 1976) that help reduce judgments.
- Facilitators seek harmony and encourage honesty indirectly by asking more questions than giving statements or opinions, while being aware that both harmony and honesty are paths to integrity in their respective cultures. Nuance, indirectness, active and passive voices are all supported as a means of communicating without being forced to articulate exactly what one feels. Facilitators encourage others to listen to these clues by role modeling.
- Facilitators establish a low-risk and comfortable environment in which to explore differences in how people interact in everyday life and business without making judgments and by collaborating in discussions that show respect and understanding.
- Facilitators communicate their sensitivity to each member's value system, communication style, and perception orientation, based upon knowledge from research in these areas. For example, they frequently are requested to clarify definitions of concepts like 'trust', which are perceived differently by Japanese and Americans. Nishishiba and Richie (2000) inform us that trustworthiness to Japanese is commitment to the common good while Americans show it by commitment to personal integrity.
- Facilitators encourage learning about one's self. This is usually the result of seeing ourselves as others see us and of learning about others through affirmative inquiry, balanced interaction and empathic listening. Others rarely see us as we see ourselves.
- Facilitators maintain mindfulness in the room with a degree of objectivity about personal feelings, one's own as well as those of others, expressed or not.
- Facilitators demonstrate awareness of each participant's pace along Clarke's TIID stages (Clarke, 1971, 2017) and respond appropriately and affirmatively to each person's stage at any appropriate time inside or outside of the workshop time.

18.5 Transformative Intercultural Identity Development (TIID) Stages

Note that these six stages of development (Clarke, 1971, 2008, 2017) are interspersed in the implementation of the BMD model below, but are never described as a purpose of the BMD. Throughout the workshop the ICFs' monitor the members' progress in personally growing through the six stages of expanding one's self-perception toward a synergistic transcultural identity. Moran, Harris, and Moran's (2011) definition of cultural synergy "implies a belief that we can learn from others and others can learn from us" (p. 232).

The first stage of *awareness* begins with bowling-ball type introductions that are distinguished from the ping-pong types that limit introductions to one minute each. Through storytelling of everyone's experiences participants enter into discussion and soon discover insights never before imagined about their cultural differences in perceptions, values and feelings about them. The introductions are about common subjects that encourage sharing and curiosity.

The second stage of *mutual respect* begins when participants express their commitment to support the diversity within the group. Respect for the other is demonstrated by a member expressing support for another to express perspectives without being judged because perceptions are relative. Members express their increasing interest and curiosity in exploring each other's experiences.

The third stage of *understanding* occurs when participants express their new insight into each other's perspectives, values, and feelings because of their willingness to respect differences, while beginning to feel pleasure in developing friendships in the group. A growing comfort reduces any shame of inappropriateness or of being misjudged. As a result, confidence in offering one's own experiences, thoughts, and feelings increases as status equalization begins to develop among group members (Cohen, 1998; Cohen & Lotan, 1995).

The fourth stage of *appreciation* evolves when group members offer others their expressions of appreciation for learning from each other. Such appreciation can be characterized as the attribution of value to or admiration of another's perspective. A growing in-group becomes obvious when members begin enjoying each other's stories and become considerably more spontaneous (Triandis, Villareal, Asai, & Lucca, 1988).

The fifth stage of *adaptation* is marked by curiosity and interest in adopting different values or norms into their own feelings and behaviors, to see what it feels like by trying it out. Some members may begin role-playing unfamiliar behaviors within the group. The in-group laughter continues to strengthen the group's interpersonal relationships.

The sixth stage of *integration* is manifested when participants share their sense of integrating two or more cultures within themselves. Not everyone reaches this stage. They have resolved what Festinger (1957) called cognitive dissonance and practice a balanced centeredness, not unlike how Japanese integrate both a public and a private self (Barnlund, 1989) without any cognitive dissonance. These persons express a fulfillment in the capability of integrating cultural differences in cognition, affection, and behavior within themselves. They may feel increasingly like the Useem and Downie's (1976) Third Culture Kid (TCK). As West, Zhang, Yampolski, and Sasaki (2017) suggest, a transformative bicultural identity is more than the sum of its parts. Bonebright (2010) reviewed the TCK literature and explores the opportunities and challenges of the TCK for human resource development to become *cultural bridges* in businesses.

Those who have integrated multiple cultural perceptions into themselves have the highest potential of becoming cultural *bridge persons* that this world sorely needs to work toward peace. Many serve happily as bridges between cultures in a way that uniquely expresses their own integrated identity and often have deeply shared feelings much like cousins. Their intercultural competencies serve in career-fulfilling roles such as intercultural facilitation specialists in multinational businesses organizations (Clarke, 2016). As Abe (2018) found, "... the ATCKs [Adult TCK] showed normative changes in personality and well-being in the direction of greater maturity and adjustment during adulthood, with those reporting higher levels of multicultural engagement generally exhibiting a more resilient personality profile, higher levels of well-being, and more adaptive cognitive and affective styles" (p. 811).

18.6   Implementation of the Bicultural Management Development (BMD) Model

We describe this model in a descriptive manner that explains the process of developing only one managerial function out of the eleven or more that each new management team usually has full responsibility to develop. In addition to decision making (D-M), the focus of this model, there are functions of motivating, evaluating, leadership, teamwork, problem solving, negotiating, conflict resolving, training, and managing and participating in bicultural meetings to which this program model can be applied.

The following steps are facilitated with patience and awareness that some the members are second language speakers and therefore are allowed to express themselves in their first language whenever necessary. The ICF team of two, one Japanese and one American, are both bilingual and bicultural. They demonstrate intercultural sensitivity and mindfulness in utilizing the necessary intercultural competencies in their roles.

Following are the 10-steps of the model that begins after the first intercultural group has met for extensive personal introductions. This model's design requires weaving together four separate cultural team meetings and four integrated integrated group meetings in this sequence.

1. In the first separate cultural team meetings held simultaneously in separate rooms, ICFs ask team members in each group in their first language to write a one page Critical Incident (CI) (Flanagan, 1954) from their experiences by which they learned each of the key steps in their D-M process. They create the number of key steps themselves. Each step may have its own CI or may combine several steps into one. There are to write four parts for each CI: (a) a behavioral description of the incident, (b) an interpretation of the incident, (c) a conclusion on how the incident is resolved, and (d) what assumption and values does the solution reflect. This is their individual homework. Upon completion these incidents are collected and distributed respectively to members of each cultural team that wrote them for their analyses.

2. In the second separated cultural team meetings, each team in their first language identifies the essential critical steps that they can all agree upon that comprise their best D-M process. Each team creates by consensus a list of steps of their

D-M process after explaining and discussing their respective CIs. They then work to determine the best CI to represent each step. Each cultural team combines similar steps of their individual CIs until the team has one CI per step. They will use these to explain to the other cultural team the importance of each step within their culturally appropriate D-M process.

3. As preparation for the next step, the ICFs alone create a Cultural Assimilator (CA) (Fiedler, Mitchell, & Triandis, 1971) tool for each culture that comprises a step-by-step sequence of each team's chosen CIs for their ideal D-M process. The ICFs create four interpretations for each CI's fourth part of each story, the assumptions and values that the resolution reflects. Only one of these four interpretations represents the original assumptions and values chosen by each cultural team. Two others are only partially appropriate and the fourth is not appropriate but resembles a meaningful choice from the other culture's point of view. In each CI these four multiple choice responses are scrambled. The purpose for this pair of CAs is for each cultural team to discuss and verify their consensus on each of their CI's assumptions and values when faced with four choices. Every member's contribution is respected and understood throughout this process. The resulting CAs are prepared to be returned to their CIs originators.

4. In the third separate cultural team meetings, the ICFs return each CA to its cultural team by which to examine their abilities to identify which of the four options on their team's CI's is accurate from their four alternative responses. The purpose of this exercise is to develop a final team consensus on each of the CI's values and prepare to use the CA to teach the other cultural team about their prefered steps in the D-M process. After the CA administrations, each team's consensual cultural assumptions and values of each CI are compared to the individual responses from each team member. Where there are differences in responses, the team works together to correct them and reach consensus again. Also in preparation, they identify and discuss the choice that reflects the other team's possible interpretations with the objective of understanding their perspectives.

5. In this first integrated bicultural team meeting, each cultural team presents to the other team their summaries of their essential steps in their D-M process and then explains each of their CIs. The objective is to educate each other on their respective cultural perspectives on D-M to increase respect and understanding of the differences and the similarities, and attribute positive value toward each. These objectives are achieved with the ICFs' assistance to the point of members understanding, respect, and appreciation of the other team's perspectives. This process is designed also to develop a sense of cultural equity with the shared knowledge that the other team feels the same way about them.

6. In the fourth separate cultural team meetings, the team members rank order the relative importance of their decision making process, without regard to their sequence. Those at the top of the list are labeled as the must haves and those lower in the list can be integrated. This decision may take a significant amount of time due to each member's preferences brought from former places

of employment. In this meeting they also chose who will advocate for each step of the five or six steps at the top of their list for presenting to the other team.

7. In the second integrated bicultural team meeting, each cultural team writes their rank-ordered list of steps on the board according to their importance. This process should reveal that the two groups agree on 75% of the two cultural teams' proposed steps. The ICFs can take at least a moment or a lunch break together to celebrate this finding that will contribute to relationship and bicultural team building. But, important to the task is that 25% of the steps for each function on which the two teams disagree are at the top of each list. They are the must haves. In other words, the 5 or 6 steps that each team cares about the most are in conflict and require considerable effort and flexibility to integrate or synergize. Through this exercise the value of this developmental process becomes clearer to everyone. They must resolve these differences to avoid conflicts in developing their new management culture. In this meeting they also chose who will advocate for each of the five or six steps at the top of their list for leading negotiations with the other team in step 9 of this BMD.

8. In the third integrated bicultural team meeting, the ICFs prepare to utilize the two CAs again by administering them across cultures: American CA to the Japanese and Japanese CA to Americans. The purpose of this CA application is to assess their perceptions of each step (CI) of their counterparts' CAs and hopefully identify the same interpretations of assumptions and values of the CIs as the authoring group decided. The results should provide confidence and inspiration in entering the next bicultural meeting's negotiations. The Japanese teams on average identified 72% and the American teams on average identified 76% of the other's interpretations, which are both about three times higher than an untrained person's chance of scoring 25%. This enables the discussion of the day to focus on reviewing those inaccurate responses toward reaching a better understanding of the other team's own interpretations and values in order to negotiate fairly from similar understandings of cultural assumptions.

9. In the fourth integrated bicultural team meeting, their objective is to create a synergistic decision for each step of their D-M process. The ICFs assist in working through these differences with respect, understanding, and appreciation of all members in such a way that continues building trust across cultures and challenges the members to create adaptations with mindfulness of their intercultural process norms. In this case trust means to commit to negotiate for the best interest of the new bicultural company and to do so in a way that is true to oneself (Yamazaki, 2005). They proceed through the give and take, the fun and frustration, of resolving their differences for each step by consensus, keeping in mind that they all have the same goals and commitments to depend upon their cooperative collaboration. Utilizing the ICFs' skills in this step are critical for reaching their goal.

10. A very important final step in such an intense intercultural process of resolving differences and creating synergies is to celebrate their accomplishments. Rewards of different types can be both intrinsic and extrinsic. The intrinsic rewards may be such as the feeling of confidence and friendships that develop

through this process, as well as the self-confidence and pride. Such rewards assure all that there is no shaming or feelings of shame in this bicultural organization. An extrinsic reward that is an effective motivator is a sponsored-by-the-company party or field trip at the conclusion of the program. It is important in integrating these two cultures to publicly announce team rewards to the whole team, not to single out individuals. The standards that bicultural teams develop for their synergistic managerial system can become a model for wider utilization within a global company. The processes that they develop will be useful to them for a lifetime. And, so will their collective pride.

In summary, this process and its outcomes are effective in reducing initial feelings of shame that members working in such a bicultural team often feel. The process itself values each member for the contributions they bring to it. Through developing mutual respect, empathy, and trust they will surpass their company's productivity goals (Clarke, 2017; Lewis, 1999; Wiley & Kowske, 2012; Williams, 2007) and recognize the futility of shaming others and feeling shame themselves. Shaming may serve a vital function of maintaining harmony in Japan, but in a bicultural organization it serves no purpose. It rather has a destructive consequence of diminishing individual contributions by devaluing diversities, creating in-groups and out-groups, maintaining status quo with status inequality, and festering hostilities that destroy all efforts to unite in the interest of shared goals.

Trained ICF led discussions yield much deeper understandings across cultures because of the respectful listening that the facilitators inspire and the empathy they have for all members. The facilitators encourage members to share their mutual understandings and appreciation of the other member's thoughts and feelings. Members express these feelings within the group in their own way, some directly, indirectly, or with nonverbal behaviors. These feelings lead to mutual trust, adaptation, and integration. Thereby a new reference group with greater and deeper importance has grown into their new membership group.

At the end of the program, the members celebrate and share their commitment to their new organization's managerial role functions. With their new intercultural communication competencies they have created new managerial style synergies that have greater appeal than each of their former styles of managing. Their commitment to continue building a synergistic corporate culture, a third culture organization following this process assures their success in the future and their friendships will sustain them (Fig. 18.1).

18.7 Conclusion

We have discussed this practical workshop module for transforming shame into pride, through building respect, empathy, and trust in bicultural organizations in the context of businesses in Japan. The key elements in the bicultural management development model are the program model design, the transformative intercultural identify devel-

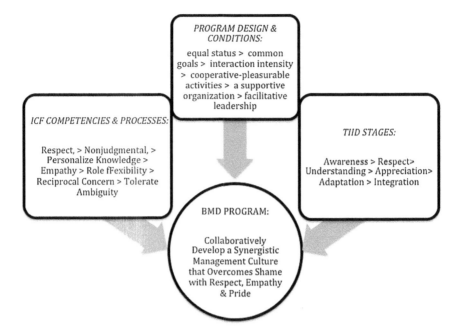

Fig. 18.1 Inputs and outcomes of the model

opment process with the intercultural facilitation skills, and the implementation of the model's ten steps. Successful interventions of the model require top management commitments, skillful intercultural facilitators, and the employees' willingness and cooperation to collaboratively work on the issues. Each element is essential for the success of the program.

References

Abe, J. A. A. (2018). Personality, well-being, and cognitive-affective styles—A cross-sectional study of adult third culture kids. *Journal of Cross-Cultural Psychology, 49*(5), 811–830.

Amir, Y. (1969). Contact hypothesis in ethnic relations. *Psychological Bulletin, 71*(5), 319–342.

Barnlund, D. C. (1976, July). Multileveled, multidimensional, multidirectional, multi-coded intercultural communication. Paper presented at the First Annual Stanford Institute for Intercultural Communication, Stanford University, Palo Alto, CA.

Barnlund, D. C. (1989). Public and private self in communicating with Japan. *Business Horizons*, 32–40.

Bonebright, D. A. (2010). Adult third culture kids: HRD challenges and opportunities. *Human Resources Development International, 13*(3), 351–359.

Clarke, C. H. (1971). Intercultural communication workshops. In D. S. Hoopes (Ed.), *Readings in intercultural communication* (Vol. 1(1), pp. 73–79). Pittsburgh, PA: The Society for Intercultural Education, Training, and Research.

Clarke, C. H. (2008). Practicing the integration of discipline and compassion. *Journal of Intercultural Communication, 11,* 1–21.

Clarke, C. H. (2016). Evolving through cultures, career, and marriages toward a transcultural identity. In C.-H. Mayer & S. Wolting (Eds.), *Purple Jacaranda—Narratives in transcultural identity development* (pp. 169–183). Waxmann: New York.

Clarke, C. H. (2017). Reflections from history: How shifting paradigms created intercultural innovations. *Journal of Intercultural Communication, 20,* 1–26.

Cohen, E. G. (1982). Expectation states and interracial interaction in school settings. *Annual Review of Sociology, 8,* 209–235.

Cohen, E. G. (1998). Making cooperative learning equitable. *Educational Leadership,* 18–21.

Cohen, E. G., & Lotan, R. A. (1995). Producing equal-status interaction in the heterogeneous classroom. *American Educational Research Journal, 32*(1), 99–120.

Festinger, L. (1957). *A theory of cognitive dissonance.* Stanford, CA: Stanford University Press.

Fiedler, F. E., Mitchell, T., & Triandis, H. C. (1971). The culture assimilator: An approach to cross-cultural training. *Journal of Applied Psychology, 55*(2), 95–102.

Flanagan, J. C. (1954). The critical incident technique. *Psychological Bulletin, 51*(4), 327–358.

Hyman, H. H. (1960). Reflections on reference groups. *Oxford Academy's Public Opinion Quarterly, 24*(3), 383–396.

Hornsey, M. J. (2016). Dissent-and-deviance-in-intergroup-context. *Current Opinion in Psychology, 11,* 1–5.

Lebra, T. S. (1983). Shame and guilt: A psychocultural view of the Japanese self. *Ethos, 11*(3), 192–209.

Lewis, J. D. (1999). *Trusted partners.* New York, NY: The Free Press.

Moran, R. T., Harris, P. R., & Moran, S. V. (2011). *Managing cultural differences* (8th ed.). Burlington, MA: Elsevier.

Nishishiba, M., & Richie L. D. (2000). The concept of trustworthiness: A cross-cultural comparison between Japanese and U.S. business people. *Journal of Applied Communication Research, 28*(4), 347–367.

Ruben, B. D. (2015). Intercultural communication competency in retrospect: Who would have guessed? *International Journal for Intercultural Relations, 48,* 22–23.

Ruben, B. D., & Kealey, D. J. (1979). Behavioral assessment of communication competency and the prediction of cross-cultural adaptation. *International Journal for Intercultural Relations, 3,* 15–47.

Sandage, S. J., & Jankowski, P. J. (2013). Spirituality, social justice, and intercultural competence: Mediator effects for differentiation of self. *International Journal for Intercultural Relations, 37,* 366–374.

Triandis, H. C., Villareal, M. J., Asai, M., & Lucca, N. (1988). Individualism and collectivism: Cross-cultural perspectives on self-ingroup relationships. *Journal of Personality and Social Psychology, 54*(2), 323–338.

Useem, R. H., & Downie, R. D. (1976). Third culture kids. *Today's Education, 65*(3), 103–105.

West, A. L., Zhang, R., Yampolsky, M., & Sasaki, J. Y. (2017). More than the sum of its parts: A transformative theory of biculturalism. *Journal of Cross-Cultural Psychology, 48*(7), 963–990.

Wiley, J., & Kowske, B. (2012). *Respect: Delivering Results by giving employees what they really want.* San Francisco, CA: Jossey Bass.

Williams, M. (2007). Building genuine trust through interpersonal emotion management: A threat regulation model of trust and collaboration across boundaries. *Academy of Management Review, 32*(2), 595–621.

Woods, P., Poropat, A., Barkera, M., Hills, R., Hibbins, R., & Borbasi, S. (2013). Building friendships through a cross-cultural mentoring program. *International Journal for Intercultural Relations, 37,* 523–535.

Yamazaki, Y. (2005). Learning styles and typologies of cultural differences: A theoretical and empirical comparison. *International Journal for Intercultural Relations, 29,* 521–548.

Clifford H. Clarke, ABD was raised in Japan by second-generation expatriate parents, whose own parents first moved to Japan in 1898 when the U.S. forced the Queen to abdicate her crown in the Kingdom of Hawaii. Since arriving in Japan at the age of 7, his favorite pastime has been exploring cultural assumptions and at the age of 10 he was asked to become a bridge-between-cultures in Kyoto.

His higher education focused on the goal of becoming an effective "bridge person" by studying world religions and philosophies (B.A.), Asian studies (PGS), counseling across cultures (M.Div.), and interdisciplinary studies in the social sciences (ABD) at Stanford University's Graduate School of Education.

His four careers have evolved through 11 years of counseling foreign students at Cornell and Stanford universities, 8 years of teaching intercultural communication at Stanford and the University of Hawaii, 30 years of intercultural business management consulting in 13 countries in Asia, Europe, and North America, and 6 years of educational program design and evaluation in the State of Hawaii.

Clarke has published 25 papers, chapters, or books in all of these areas, given 40 presentations at professional societies and universities, and been quoted by 25 newspapers and magazines in Japan, the USA, and Europe.

He also founded 3 NPOs, including the Stanford Institute for Intercultural Communication (SIIC), 2 LLCs, including the Clarke Consulting Group (CCG), and cofounded SIETAR (1971) and SIETAR Japan (1984).

Naomi Takashiro, Ph.D. in Educational Psychology, has been teaching English classes as an adjunct faculty at the Kyoto University of Foreign Studies and its junior college in Kyoto, Japan. Her academic interests are socioeconomic status and inequality in education and she has published articles in the area. She has lived in Hawaii for twenty years and has worked in multicultural organizations before coming back to Kyoto three years ago. In her spare time, she likes to read, walk, and play with birds. She has been looking for a full-time job at a university. She remains grateful to God for His guidance in writing this paper.

Chapter 19
Building a Work Culture Beyond Forgiveness—Shame as Barrier for Growth and Knowledge-Management in Working Environments

Maike Baumann and Anke Handrock

Abstract A company's success is heavily dependent on the performance of its employees. To secure a smooth workflow, structures for quality management need to be established, especially concerning the company's capital in form of the collective human expertise, in order to cover absence or leave of any working or managing staff. This requires an adequate knowledge management, including a well-structured management of failures and errors. The influence of shame and anxiety on people when expected to acknowledge their own mistakes or failures in a workplace environment is often overlooked. In this chapter, we present crucial aspects of a new approach on how to form an organizational culture where mistakes are not only perceived as forgivable, but are seen as a chance for collective growth and as a possibility to develop excellence. As a result, a successful failure management can not only enhance a company's performance, but can be used as a management tool to inspire commitment as well as a strong identification of employees with the company. The presented approach uses insights from research in Positive Psychology, Acceptance and Commitment Therapy and learning mechanisms as well as a systemic concept of leadership.

Keywords Failure management · Knowledge management · Shame · Work culture · Organizational learning

M. Baumann (✉)
Institut für Lebensgestaltung-Ethik-Religionskunde, University of Potsdam, Am Neuen Palais 10, 14469 Potsdam, Germany
e-mail: mbaumann@uni-potsdam.de

A. Handrock
Steinbeis-Transfer-Institut Positive Psychologie und Prävention at the Steinbeis Hochschule, 13467 Berlin, Germany
e-mail: info@handrock.de

19.1   Introduction

This chapter is concerned with the implementation of successful failure management in the workplace. We start the chapter with the definition of relevant terms and a general overview of failure management in the context of knowledge management. We then examine critically possible influences of the emotion of shame in the context of failures in the workplace. Next, we illustrate how the appreciation of failures as well as of successes can serve as a basis for organizational learning processes. In order to highlight the importance of the leader's behavior in the context of failure management, we introduce a set of basic principles of systemic leadership and complete the chapter with our practical approach to counterbalancing the effects of shame, feelings of rejection and feelings of inferiority on employees' fear of failure in order to ensure systematic organizational learning from one's own and the failures of others.

The frame of this chapter does not allow us to elaborate on the influence of different parent cultures on experiencing shame in the workplace environment.

19.2   Failure Management as Knowledge Management

The management of mistakes and failure is a basic aspect of organizational learning, understanding organizational learning as a "modification in organizational performance as a result of experience" (Madsen & Desai, 2010, 3). Organizational learning is crucial for stable organizational success. In the context of knowledge management, failure management is one of the most powerful and, therefore, essential aspects of the creation of new knowledge as well as of the actualization of existing knowledge within an organization.

Generally speaking, a failure may be defined as "a human act of not reaching the defined goal" (Hatamura, 2011 in Nagayoshi & Nakamura, 2017, 972). A failure in a workplace environment, where goals can be set by numerous agents, can be defined as follows: falling short of a decision maker's aspiration level that is deemed by him as only just acceptable. Success, on the other hand, reaches the decision maker's aspiration level or even surpasses it (cf. Madsen & Desai, 2010).

Recent data suggest that failing is by far a more frequent experience than success. For example, research on data collected over the period of five years in the software development industry reports that 49–56% of all projects reached partial success only and about one third of the projects were rated a complete failure (Standish Group, 2015).

Taking a systemic point of view, failures can be found at different levels, i.e. the individual level, the team level, the level of the department, the management level, the level of the organization or even at the macro level (e.g. concerning general politics or jurisdiction). Depending on the views of different decision makers at different systemic levels, one and the same outcome can be evaluated as successful, partially successful or as a failure. So in order to establish a successful failure management, a clear definition of the frame of reference is crucial. This enables the members of a system to determine the aspiration level relevant for evaluation. Once the frame is set, the members of that social system are able to judge their own performance and actions as well as other group members' performance against the agreed-upon standard of evaluation.

Humans all share some basic needs, such as the need for affiliation, and consequently also certain behavioral principles, such as applying a continuous self-evaluation in comparison to others and to their internalized rules and values. As long as a person defines himself as a member of a certain social group, e.g. a project team, the person wants to be socially accepted and integrated into that group. To reach this goal people are willing to follow the group's rules and goals and they try to fulfill set group standards. Once a person violates a valid rule of the group, e.g. by not fulfilling a given task, the person experiences shame due to moral failure and at the same time experiences a threat to his social integration into said group. As a consequence, when the aspiration level is kept unclear by the group's leader, the members of that group constantly experience a certain amount of anxiety, because they lack the possibility to judge their performance against a standard. They are thus driven to expect reprimands, to be shamed and consequently to be socially excluded at any given time.

19.2.1   Shame in the Context of Failure

For several decades shame has been proposed to be the affective core of experiences of failure. Atkinson named fear of failure as the conceptual opposite to the need for achievement and described it as "the capacity or propensity to experience shame upon failure" (Atkinson, 1957, 360).

Shame, as a secondary emotion, is subject to strong social influences during childhood. Here we present only a few exemplary findings of research on the connection between shame and fear of failure to show that the underlying binding principle between shame and fear of failure is the fear of social exclusion and, in extreme cases, of abandonment.

Developmental psychologists suggest that children experience shame when parents react with strong negative emotions to the child's failure (cf. Lewis, 1992). This is in line with Teevan's (1983) results, who demonstrated that children of mothers punishing failure in their children and reacting neutrally to their children's success have a strong fear of failure. Additionally, Elliot and Thrash (2004) showed that parents' withdrawal of love after children's mistakes leads to a fear of failure in children. This shameful reaction is typically extended as well to negative reactions of other attachment figures after failure (Downey & Feldman, 1996). The child learns from such behavior of attachment figures that failure and mistakes put people in danger of being socially rejected. The feeling of shame then indicates to the person a danger to important social bonds. People with a strong fear of failure report more relational concerns in contexts of failure than people with low fear of failure and they furthermore claim that they would be unlikely to tell their parents about an experience of failure, whereas they possibly might tell them about a success (McGregor & Elliot, 2005).

Via the internalization of third-party evaluations in childhood in achievement situations, people seem to develop a certain degree of fear of failure associated with the expectation of a threat to their social integration. In consequence this means that "for individuals high in fear of failure, … achievement events are not simply opportunities to learn, improve on one's competence, or compete against others. Instead, they are threatening, judgement-oriented experiences that put one's entire self on the line" (McGregor & Elliot, 2005, 229).

Gausel and Leach (2011) differentiate the experienced emotional qualities in the context of moral failure even further. They developed a model of reactions to moral failure that considers feelings of shame as just one possible pathway. We do understand "moral" failure directly applicable to experiences of failure in workplaces, as the term "moral" indicates transgressing a predefined social rule or convention the majority of a social group accepts and accepting the decision maker's aspiration level is part of any labour contract and holds true for the entire social group working in that social context. Gausel and Leach (2011) argue that "shame questionnaires" do not investigate only shame, but also ask for experiences of condemnation by others, of feelings of rejection and of feelings of inferiority. They remark that most people categorize all these feelings as shame even though the emotional quality and the behavioral consequences differ. Their analysis conforms very well with the developmental view presented above, in contrast to approaches that collect all the different emotional reactions possibly occurring after failure under the label of "shame". Gausel and Leach expect shame as an emotional reaction to a specific self-defect to be followed by measures of self-improvement (see Fig. 19.1). The other pathway of the model focuses on the primary experience of other-condemnation after failure, followed by feelings of rejection and inferiority. As noted above, the feelings of rejection and inferiority are often mislabeled by participants as feelings of shame.

This model illustrates that successful failure management has to counterbalance both possible appraisals (a) self-defect and (b) other-condemnation and has to take feelings of rejection, inferiority and shame into account, where only feelings of real shame motivate the person to self-improve. The two other emotional outcomes, rejection and inferiority, motivate the actor to avoid, to externalize and to hide.

19.2.2 Appreciation of Positive and Negative Outcomes in Workplace Environments

Research on the best practice of securing experiences as part of the organizational knowledge on the basis of successes and failures indicates that the performance improvement is clearest after a reflection of failed experiences (Ellis, Carette, Anseel, & Lievens, 2014). After experiences of success, on the other hand, the highest impact

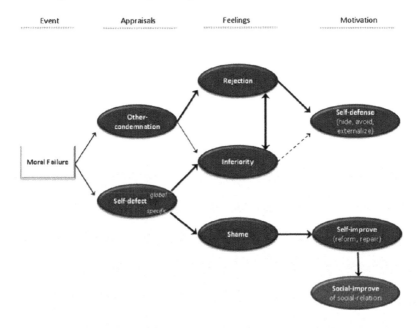

Fig. 19.1 Conceptual model of the experience of moral failure. Note that the top half of the figure shows concern for social-image, the shaded, bottom half of the figure shows concern for self-image (from Gausel & Leach, 2011, p. 470)

on performance improvement was the result of a reflection of erroneous actions only (ibid.). A further relevant finding we integrated into our practical approach discussed below showed that the combination of external performance feedback followed by additional self-explanations that were structured by reflective questions generated the most beneficial outcomes (Anseel, Lievens, & Schollaert, 2009). Reflections alone, without previous performance feedback, did not improve the performance.

Taking a person's affective state into account, the best learning results are to be expected when a person experiences emotions of a positive valence during learning (Bryan & Bryan, 1991; Bryan, Mathur, & Sullivan, 1996). In addition, positive emotions broaden people's momentary thought-action repertoires, allowing for more creativity, a wider attentional focus, enhanced cognitive flexibility and a higher variability of action. This broadening effect of positive emotions enables people to build more enduring physical, intellectual and social resources (cf. the Broaden-and-Build Theory of Positive Emotions, Fredrickson, 1998, 2002).

According to the undoing hypothesis (Fredrickson & Levenson, 1998; Fredrickson, Manusco, Branigan, & Tugade, 2000), inducing positive emotions can even "undo" the negative effect of negative emotions, as the two are assumed to be unable to coexist in parallel. Inducing a positive emotional state can be accomplished by, for instance, engaging in pleasant activities, recalling positive events of joy, fun, gratitude or happiness and by practicing relaxation (for an overview of the latter see Fredrickson, 2002).

Our practical approach integrates the above insights from emotional psychology and learning psychology. We provide a structured step-by-step process that begins with creating a strong social cohesion via a personal appreciation of all participants of the process, leads participants into a positive emotional state and later uses performance feedback and self-reflection to secure learning from failures and to generate ideas of improvement regarding already experiences of success. The structure of the process makes use of the emotional undoing effect and in this way reduces, from the beginning, negative emotions that may cause fear of failure in participants.

19.3 Contextual Descriptions—Systemic Principles and Their Influence on Work Cultures

In our practical work with teams, companies and organizations, we follow the basic systemic assumption that a person's family of origin serves as their basic model for social systems in general (for an overview of systemic thinking, see, e.g., Stanton & Welsh, 2012).

Our understanding of families as systems builds on the accounts of Varga von Kibéd (2000), Daimler, Sparrer, and Varga von Kibed (2003) and Boszormenyi-Nagy and Spark (2006). We understand families as systems that are, to a certain degree, structured hierarchically. They contain at least two subsystems, the parental subsystem and the child's subsystem. We assume that, in order to ensure the continuous existence of the entire family system, both subsystems have different tasks to fulfill, have certain rules to follow and have different ways of communication.

The application of that assumption on to work contexts leads to certain analogies between a team's hierarchy and a family system.

In the following we present some typical expectations that we often hear from clients when analyzing their personal family-related presumptions.

Assuming a functional family of origin, people tend to look at the leader for guidance, they expect fair treatment and that leaders will help in conflict resolution if they do not succeed in solving them alone. People wish for politeness, appreciation and appropriate signs of affection from their leader and the certainty that they can put their trust in the leader. In addition, they expect to receive a certain amount of information from their leader. They expect at least all the information necessary to fulfill their duty and to handle the team's social dynamics. Leaders in general are expected to protect their inferiors, to always know a solution and to have a plan. Furthermore, inferiors expect their leaders to punish wrongdoing, to enforce rules, to forgive mistakes and failures (after an adequate amount of time) as well as to allow inferiors to take appropriate risks and to prove themselves, to take some responsibility and to develop further. People also accept frustration of their wishes to a certain degree, especially if they believe that it serves the continuous existence of the overall system.

As long as leaders fulfill their role and the related expectations, people also accept that leaders have certain privileges, just as parents enjoy privileges compared to their children. So it is widely accepted that leaders receive higher payment, that they do not explain all of their actions, plans and whereabouts to inferiors and that they keep certain information secret. Different or shorter working hours are usually accepted by inferiors too as well as the use of more resources and more expensive representational objects (office, car, sports etc.) by leaders.

Under the heading of fairness, people expect leaders to respect systemic rules in promotions and in handing out privileges. Here, analogies to principles of sibling relationships can be applied: The longer a person is part of a system, the more rights that person has "earned"—analogously to different rights of older siblings compared to younger siblings. This concerns, e.g., the right to information, the right to voice an opinion in certain matters or the right to be promoted before younger team members are promoted ("younger" indicating in this case the duration of membership in the system, not age). Some additional, very basic principles that are applied in most social systems are loyalty to the system and reciprocity within the system.

Violations to systemic expectations are tolerated by the system's members only up to a certain degree. People keep a kind of internal account of costs and benefits. Systemic violations are usually booked as "costs". It is possible to get some "social credit", but only for a while. If the costs are outweighing the benefits regularly, people leave the system as soon as they can. The higher their position, the earlier they usually leave. In this respect, it is important to know that humans are subject to a certain negativity bias, letting us remember negative events and "social costs" better and for a longer time than positive events. It has been shown that it takes 3–5 positive events/memories to counterbalance one negative event/memory (Rozin & Royzman, 2001; Fredrickson & Losada, 2005; Fredrickson, 2013).

We base our practical approach to failure management partly on the use of these systemic principles. It is important to note that although we assume people to construct their schema of social systems building on their early experiences with their family of origin, we also assume that they are able to learn and to apply different systemic rules in later life. Nonetheless, given that schemata do not only account for our expectations in new situations, they also constitute our "fall-back strategy" under stress. So the assumptions drawn from early experiences in a person's family of origin are always ready to be applied in case the newly learned principles do not work properly for that person.

The principles presented may at first seem to apply only to work structures that are hierarchically managed. In our opinion it is not necessary that a social system is predefined in a hierarchic way to apply the systemic principles described above. Even in lean management systems, that e.g. try to work in just one systemic level to avoid effects of hierarchy, we observe implicit internal, short lived and self-structured micro systems that tend to establish themselves. This internal structuring occurs within any complex social system, i.e. due to project related roles, or due to different levels of expertise of team members, allowing to apply said systemic principles.

19.4   Applications

We have successfully applied the approach presented in this section to small to medium-sized companies, mostly organized in different systemic levels and mostly belonging to the health sector. To counterbalance the negative affects at the core of the fear of failure (feelings of rejection, feelings of inferiority and feelings of shame), we

- install a work culture of respect and appreciation,
- replace the widely common practice of blaming someone after failure with a set of learning- and change-oriented questions,
- normalize the naming and handling of and learning from failures, by establishing it as part of a regular weekly team meeting.

We do not want to analyze different types of errors, mistakes and failures in this chapter, there already exists a large body of practice-oriented literature in the field (cf., e.g., Reason, 2001 for an overview). Our goal here is to introduce some practical interventions in the workplace that help to counter people's fear of failure, which usually prevents them from admitting and learning from their failures.

At the center of our approach, we establish a weekly team meeting, structured and held in a special manner. When establishing this weekly meeting, it is advisable to ensure the use of a well-lit and pleasant room, big enough for the whole team to sit comfortably (shows appreciation) and containing a sufficient number of sitting options for all participants. To reduce implicit effects of hierarchy and social stress, identical chairs should be used. It is very important that all members of the team participate in this weekly meeting on a very regular basis, including the leader of the group. We recommend to make the participation mandatory, in order to accomplish a change of work culture in the entire organization. Note that this kind of team meeting is part of the organizational knowledge management and consequently should be held during regular working hours. In our experience, teams engage easily in our kind of failure management, as long as the entire team, including the leaders, participate regularly. We see our experience backed by recent research on experiences of shame in South-African workplaces. One of the results showed, that "participants felt that the organization should have procedures in place to deal with shame" (Mayer & Tonelli, 2017, p. 152).

19.4.1   Preparing the Introduction of Structured Failure Management

As shown earlier, establishing professional failure management helps to generate and secure new organizational knowledge. A crucial difficulty in introducing failure-management systems is a high degree of fear of failure in the working staff, accompanied by feelings of shame, rejection and inferiority. As discussed in connection with the developmental view on fear of failure, the degree to which people tend to fear failures seems to depend to a significant degree on early experiences with the reactions of attachment figures in achievement situations. Additionally applying our systemic view of workplace environments, we expect leaders (systemically occupying a role analogous to a parent's role in a family system) to be able to influence their inferiors work-related schemata by setting a positive example and acting as a behavioral model. When changing a person's schema concerning achievement situations and their fear of failure we see the necessity to build a firm body of continuous positive experiences with achievement situations (successes as well as failures) in order to create a stable positive basis of evaluation of achievement situations and possible failures in general. These assumptions are in line with theoretic principles of the limited reparenting interventions in schema therapy, introduced by Young (1990) and Young, Klosko, and Weishaar (2003). Such interventions are proven to successfully change dysfunctional, schema-driven behavior (Masley, Gillanders, Simpson, & Taylor, 2011).

Before handing over the responsibility for the moderation of the meetings to the team, the leader chairs a few of the meetings so as to give an example of how to do it. We advise leaders to clearly state in the beginning that the role of the moderator will be handed over to other members of the team after a few meetings. To establish a positive emotional state at the beginning of the meeting (in order to make use of the undoing-effect of negative emotions such as shame as well as to make use of the broaden-and-build effects), every member of the group is asked to share his or her "highlight of the week" (see Box 19.1). In our experience, the telling of the highlight of the week needs to be demonstrated and exercised a few times until everybody knows how to do it. In order to normalize this new process as quickly as possible the leader should demonstrate the steps in front of the team before asking other team members to follow.

Box 19.1 "The Highlight of the Week"—Instructions

Begin by saying:

> Please recall the last week and ask yourself the following question: What was my personal highlight of that week? It could be a pleasant situation you shared with a colleague, a success you achieved, maybe some difficulties you succeeded to overcome, a nice situation with a client or with a member from another department, or maybe something completely different… And sometimes it might seem difficult to identify any highlight at all. If that should be the case for you today, please think of a situation or an incident in the last week you could have been happy about, or proud of, or pleased about –even if you couldn't feel it at that time. So, what could have been your highlight of the week, if you only had had the chance to appreciate it properly at the time?

Wait for 1–2 min, then add:

> "Once you identified your highlight, please share it with the rest of the team. My personal highlight of the week is …" *or* "If I could have appreciated it at the time, my highlight would have been…"

In case the members of the group like to elaborate very long on topics you can optionally add the sentence:

When you start telling the team about your highlight, please imagine lighting a match – take as long as that match would need to burn down to tell us about your personal highlight of the week

The moderator of the meeting is the first to tell his or her highlight of the week. Then he or she asks another person to tell their highlight, and so on. When everybody has finished, the moderator thanks everybody for sharing their highlights with the group.

When a new member of the group participates in the weekly meeting for the first time, it is the responsibility of that week's moderator to practice the exercise "highlight of the week" in advance with the new participant. This ensures a positive integration of the new person right from the start and reduces the workload of the leader of the group.

The leader can also point out situations or successes of team members he witnessed or heard about during the week, that he feels worthy to be called a highlight of the week. This way he can use the exercise implicitly in a second way, to give positive feedback and to compliment (e.g., "Wow, that was great, I could imagine this might be a highlight of that week you'll tell us about in the next team meeting!"

19.4.2   The Organizational Framing

It is not necessary for the leader to be the person keeping the time and structuring the weekly team meeting. The responsibility for structuring the meetings, including the collection and preparation of an agenda, can easily be handed over to the team's members in sequence. After a first uncertainty, the members of the team typically enjoy to take the responsibility in turns once the meetings are filled with relevant input and have a clear structure they can follow. This weekly meeting is an important leadership tool and should therefore have first priority in the leader's weekly agenda. Installed correctly, it serves several purposes: It demonstrates high appreciation of the members of the team if the leader puts down all other duties once a week in order to spend time exclusively with them. To achieve that bonding effect, it is necessary to arrive in time, to respect and follow the moderation of the team member in charge, and not to attend to phone calls/emails/messengers during team meetings, not to do any paperwork unless it is part of the meetings, nor to cancel part of the meeting or leave early. Everybody's full concentration, including the leader's, is supposed to be on the team meeting. Handing over the organization and moderation of the meetings to the members of the team in sequence shows appreciation and trust to the team, while additionally enabling the team members to develop and train their organizational and moderation skills. The leader reduces his or her personal workload and can supervise and give feedback to the team's members and their performance concerning preparation and moderation of the meeting. The meetings always follow the same meta structure (see Box 19.2). This helps to ensure a straight-forward use of the time given, as it includes a pre-set overall duration of these meetings. In addition, the meta structure provides a clear framing of the task for the moderating team member.

Our process is applicable to groups and teams of up to 15 people. If the group/team/company is bigger, sub-teams need to be established for the meeting.

Box 19.2 Meta Structure of Weekly Team Meetings

(duration: 30–60 min; the single steps of the meeting are set in boldface, additional information is set in lightface)

- **Welcome by that week's moderator.**
- **Joint decision on the person taking the minutes.**
  Record-keeping should be done in turns.
- **Each person shares his or her personal "highlight of the week".**
- **Reading out of the meeting's agenda and option to add topics.**
- **Follow the agenda through.**
  The moderator is responsible for the meeting's time management.
  To keep the timeframe, the moderator can end discussions and initiate decision processes, he or she can decide to reschedule a topic if necessary or initiate further work on a topic. The moderator might sometimes need to restrict team members and even the leader in order to keep the timeframe—and he or she is entitled to do so!
- **"What could we do (even) better?" (failure management).**
  At this point everybody can share failures or difficulties that have occurred in the past week. It is essential that the person who made a mistake always has the chance to tell the incident himself. If he or she does not want to tell the incident himself, he can inform his superior beforehand and they can decide together how to name and frame the mistake/failure/accident in an anonymous way during the weekly meeting.
  The core of the appreciative failure management is the explicit orientation towards the future. During the meeting it is never (!) asked for a culprit. The question of guilt or why something was done is not at all helpful for a successful learning cycle after a failure. Whenever a failure is recalled, the moderator thanks the person for telling the team and asks what solution the person has found for himself to avoid such situations in the future. Then the team is asked for additional ideas (brainstorming is possible).
- **"What was most important to me in this week's team meeting? And what do I want to try or to implement over the course of the next week (if possible)?"**

This question is answered again in turns by everybody who is participating in the meeting.
- **The moderator thanks the team for today's meeting, he or she names the moderator of next week's meeting and bids everybody farewell.**
- **The minutes are written the same day and are handed to the leader (!), who checks them and distributes them to the team.**
- **Team members who could not participate in a team meeting (due, e.g., to sick leave) are obliged to get themselves the meeting's minutes from the team's leader within 24 h after their return and to prove it by signing the record.**

19.4.3 Additional Notes on the Implementation

In this section we provide some additional information we consider relevant to the process.

One basic principle is not to talk about people who are absent during the team meeting.

Furthermore, the leader should always respect the inferior's moderation of the meeting and understand him- or herself as "just" a member of the team for the time of the meeting. Only if the moderator is visibly distressed and overstrained by his or her task to moderate, the leader of the group should assist, and also then just as much as is necessary to have the moderator succeed with the set task.

In case the group starts breaking essential rules of the meeting and the moderator does not reinforce the given structure, the leader should see to reestablishing the basic working principles (mutual respect, inner structure of the meeting, no activities that are unrelated to the meeting etc.).

If some obvious accident or failure occurred the previous week, but no one shares this at the meeting and no one has informed their superior of it, the leader presents the raw facts known to him (never names or suspicions!) and the team engages in brainstorming in order to find a good solution. After discussing possible solutions the leader lets the entire team know that the person responsible for the mistake can still contact him during the coming week in order to see whether he or she needs anything else to finish the matter properly. If the person comes forth later, the leader thanks him or her for the courage and openness to admit to the incident and sees to it that the person really finds a good solution and secures a good learning effect from the situation.

What should never be tolerated is one team member telling on another member of the team. In such a case the leader should clarify immediately that telling is not helpful if the team wants to learn from an important experience. The leader then invites both the accuser and the accused to come to a private conflict-solving talk in his office after the team meeting. Next he or she thanks the accuser for contributing important facts to the team meeting, the leader summarizes the facts as if an anonymous failure had been named and hands over the chairing of the solution-oriented brainstorming to the moderator.

Should the leader be on holiday or not in office for another reason, then the weekly meetings should continue regardless. It is the deputy's responsibility to ensure the continuous weekly meetings of the team when the leader can not attend.

Should a mistake/accident/failure require jurisdictional consequences, the incident is always to be handled in line with the relevant jurisdiction of the country in question, ensuring the victim of the incident gains the best possible compensation.

The leader's responsibility?—Be a behavioral model to your team!

As leaders serve as behavioral models to their inferiors, we see it as condition sine qua non when installing a failure-friendly work culture that leaders also admit to failures they bear responsibility for. This does not, however, contain all types of failures and mistakes. In our experience, leaders should report failures or mistakes that concern members of the team, such as having involuntarily mistreated someone, having lost one's temper etc.

In case they do have any failures to name, leaders should always tell their failures first during the weekly meeting. They, for instance, apologize in case they mistreated someone and offer their solution/learning effect from the situation to the team. Then following the procedure, additional solution oriented ideas from other team's members are collected. This procedure includes an elegant invitation to the team for a level up feedback. We advise leaders to contribute failures and mistakes not necessarily every time, but to do so on a regular basis. A leader should never, however, make up failures just to have something to contribute to the weekly meetings.

19.5 Conclusion

In this chapter we introduced our approach to changing a team's work culture, to reframe failures as chances for joint growth and learning. Openly contributing information on a failure thus becomes reason for praise and appreciation. Due to the normalization of handling mistakes and failures openly in the team, fear of failure as well as feelings of inferiority, rejection and shame are reduced. Although the approach has not yet been evaluated statistically in its entirety, case studies and feedback from organizations and companies using the approach are very promising.

References

Anseel, F., Lievens, F., & Schollaert, E. (2009). Reflection as a strategy to enhance performance after feedback. *Organizational Behavior and Human Decision Processes, 110*, 23–35. Retrieved from https://doi.org/10.1016/j.obhdp.2009.05.003.

Atkinson, J. (1957). Motivational determinants of risk-taking behavior. *Psychological Review, 64*(6), 359–372. Retrieved from http://dx.doi.org/10.1037/h0043445.

Boszormenyi-Nagy, I., & Spark, G. (2006). *Unsichtbare Bindungen. Die Dynamik familiärer Systeme*. Stuttgart: Klett-Cotta.

Bryan, T., & Bryan, J. (1991). Positive mood and math performance. *Journal of Learning Disabilities, 24*, 490–494.

Bryan, T., Mathur, S., & Sullivan, K. (1996). The impact of positive mood on learning. *Learning Disabilities Quarterly, 19*, 153–162.

Daimler, R., Sparrer, I., & Varga von Kibed, M. (2003). *Das unsichtbare Netz. Erfolg im Beruf durch systemisches Wissen*. München: Kösel.

Downey, G., & Feldman, S. I. (1996). Implications of rejection sensitivity for intimate relationships. *Journal of Personality and Social Psychology, 70*(6), 1327–1343. Retrieved from http://dx.doi.org/10.1037/0022-3514.70.6.1327.

Elliot, A., & Thrash, T. (2004). The intergenerational transmission of fear of failure. *Personality and Social Psychology Bulletin, 30*(8), 957–971. Retrieved from https://doi.org/10.1177/0146167203262024.

Ellis, S., Carette, B., Anseel, F., & Lievens, F. (2014). Systematic reflection: Implications for learning from successes and failures. *Current Directions in Psychological Science, 23*(1), 67–72. Retrieved from https://doi.org/10.1177/0963721413504106.

Fredrickson, B. L. (1998). What good are positive emotions? *Review of General Psychology, 2*, 300–319.

Fredrickson, B. L. (2002). Positive emotions. In C. R. Snyder & S. J. Lopez (Eds.), *Handbook of positive psychology* (pp. 120–134). New York: Oxford University Press.

Fredrickson, B. L. (2013). Updated thinking on positivity ratios. *American Psychologist, 68*(9), 814–822. Retrieved from http://dx.doi.org/10.1037/a0033584.

Fredrickson, B. L., & Levenson, R. W. (1998). Positive emotions speed recovery from the cardiovascular sequelae of negative emotions. *Cognition and Emotion, 12*, 191–220.

Fredrickson, B. L., & Losada, M. F. (2005). Positive affect and the complex dynamics of human flourishing. *American Psychologist, 60*(7), 678–686.

Fredrickson, B. L., Manusco, R. A., Branigan, C., & Tugade, M. (2000). The undoing effect of positive emotions. *Motivation and Emotion, 24*, 237–258.

Gausel, N., & Leach, C. W. (2011). Concern for self-image and social image in the management of moral failure: Rethinking shame. *European Journal of Social Psychology, 41*, 468–478. https://doi.org/10.1002/ejsp.803.

Lewis, M. (1992). *Shame: The exposed self*. New York: Free Press.

Madsen, P. M., & Desai, V. (2010). Failing to learn? The effects of failure and success on organizational learning in the global orbital launch vehicle industry. *Academy of Management Journal, 53*(3), 451–476. Retrieved from https://doi.org/10.5465/amj.2010.51467631.

Masley, S. A., Gillanders, D. T., Simpson, S. G., & Taylor, M. A. (2011). A systematic review of the evidence base for schema therapy. *Cognitive Behaviour Therapy, 41*(3), 185–202. Retrieved from https://doi.org/10.1080/16506073.2011.614274.

Mayer, C.-H., & Tonelli, L. (2017). "Dream on—There is no Salvation!": Transforming shame in the South African workplace through personal and organisational strategies. In *The value of shame. Exploring a health resource in cultural contexts* (pp. 135–156). Cham: Springer.

McGregor, H. A., & Elliot, A. J. (2005). The shame of failure: Examining the link between fear of failure and shame. *Personality and Social Psychology Bulletin, 31*(2), 218–231. Retrieved from https://doi.org/10.1177/0146167204271420.

Nagayoshi, S., & Nakamura, J. (2017). Accelarate information interpretation in organizational failure learning. *Procedia Computer Science, 112,* 971–979.

Reason, J. (2001). Human error: Models and management. *British Medical Journal, 320*(7237), 768–770.

Rozin, P., & Royzman, E. B. (2001). Negativity bias, negativity dominance, and contagion. *Personality and Social Psychology Review, 5*(4), 296–320. Retrieved from https://doi.org/10.1207/S15327957PSPR0504_2.

Standish Group. (2015). *The chaos manifesto.* West Yarmouth: Standish Group.

Stanton, M., & Welsh, R. (2012). Systemic thinking in couple and family psychology. Research and practice. *Couple and Family Psychology: Research and Practice, 1*(1), 14–30. https://doi.org/10.1037/a0027461.

Teevan, R. (1983). Childhood development of fear of failure motivation: A replication. *Psychological Reports, 53*(2), 506. Retrieved from http://dx.doi.org/10.2466/pr0.1983.53.2.506.

Varga von Kibéd, M. (2000). Unterschiede und tiefere Gemeinsamkeiten der Aufstellungsarbeit mit Organisationen und der systemischen Familienaufstellung. In G. Weber (Ed.), *Praxis der Organisationsaufstellung — Grundlagen, Prinzipien, Anwendungsbereiche* (pp. 11–33). Heidelberg: Carl-Auer-Systeme Verlag.

Young, J. E. (1990). *Cognitive therapy for personality disorders: A schema-focussed approach.* Sarasato: Professional Resource Press.

Young, J. E., Klosko, J. S., & Weishaar, M. E. (2003). *Schema therapy—A practitioner's guide.* New York: Guilford.

Maike Baumann is a scientific associate at the University of Potsdam, Germany. She holds a diploma in psychology with specializations in clinical psychology/work-and organizational psychology and is currently working as a therapist, coach and trainer. Beforehand she studied linguistics and philosophy with a special focus on the philosophy of religion (University of Potsdam, Germany). Extra-occupationally she is doing a doctorate on the topic of cultural influences on social scripts at the Europa Universität Viadrina, Germany. Additionally she is internationally certified as a mediator with a special expertise in business mediation. Until now she has published various articles and monographies on Schema Therapy, Forgiveness, psychology of Self, Positive Psychology and diverse topics in the field of work and organizational psychology.

Anke Handrock (Dr. med. dent.) is a pedagogue, holds a doctorate in dentistry, is a mediator, coach and head of the Steinbeis Transfer Institute of Positive Psychology and Prevention at the Steinbeis Hochschule Berlin. She has been training medical communication for over 20 years in different Universities, such as the Humboldt University zu Berlin (Campus Charité) as well as for private organizations and clinical staff. She developed trainings in systemic leadership and is an expert in human resource development, team coaching and on corporate cultures. Besides she provides trainings in therapeutic methods and communication for a wider audience, such as counselors, psychotherapists and for institutes of several Christian dioceses in Germany. She has published several monographs and accredited journal articles on topics related to Schema Therapy, Forgiveness, Neuro Linguistic Programming, Positive Psychology and medical communication.

Part VI
Transforming Shame in Education

Chapter 20
Lecturers Through a Stay-Away Action Disowning Shame: Interventions from a System Psychodynamic Perspective

Michelle S. May

Abstract The purpose of the research was to describe the experiences of nine lecturers in a particular historically Black university (HBU), in order to analyse and interpret how through a stay way action and reflexivity about this action they could deal with shame dynamics operating in their relationship with students and management. A qualitative research method was used to explore the lecturers' experiences in a historically black university in South-Africa. The findings will illustrate how through a stay way action and their reflexivity about the stay away actions, the lecturers could move beyond hidden shame dynamics to a new story. The new story is a story of hope and creativity, which was poised to disrupt hidden shame dynamics, entrenched amongst students, lecturers and management in the HBU. By integrating the findings with systems psychodynamic literature, it will be evident how consultants and researchers through different interventions can address hidden shame dynamics in their consultancy and/or research.

20.1 Introduction

Systems psychodynamics allows for the study and interpretation of collective, interdependent unconscious and conscious individual, group and intergroup processes resulting from the interconnection between different groups and subgroups within a social system (Czander & Eisold, 2003). Systems psychodynamics provide us tools to understand and create awareness about the conscious and unconscious psychodynamics operating in an organization. Using consultancy system psychodynamic stance enables practitioners, researchers and others to work with conscious and unconscious (shame) dynamics, organizational structure and design and the interaction between the two (Amado, 1995).

M. S. May (✉)
Department of Industrial and Organisational Psychology, University of South Africa (UNISA),
AJH vd Walt Building 3-109, Preller Street, Muckleneuk Ridge, Pretoria, South Africa
e-mail: mayms@unisa.ac.za

© Springer Nature Switzerland AG 2019
C.-H. Mayer and E. Vanderheiden (eds.), *The Bright Side of Shame*,
https://doi.org/10.1007/978-3-030-13409-9_20

In the previous chapter on shame from a systems psychodynamic perspective (May, 2017) I have used the case study of the experiences of lecturers in a historically black university (HBU). In this chapter, I will use aspects of the same case study to show how that dealing with the hidden shame dynamics include working with splitting, projection and projective identification. I will show how though an unusual, yet creative action, the lecturers challenged the splitting, projection and projective identification dynamics pertaining to shame that they were stuck in. However, they could not maintain the challenge the posed to create a more functional system and I will then present an overview of how system psychodynamics can be used to address hidden shame dynamics.

20.2   Case Study

In the intergroup interaction between students, lecturers and management in a HBU in a township in South Africa in the late 1990s, hidden shame dynamics as told by the lecturers can be identified. The findings suggest that lecturers experience the manage-ment as not providing the boundary conditions required to appropriately take up their roles and do their tasks, undermining the authority of the lecturers and enhancing conflict amongst the stakeholders. An example of this is where management (after negotiation with lecturers) allowed students to have a social event at the expense of academic activities. The lecturers tried to pursue the academic activities and were attacked by some of the students without any support from management (May et al., 2012). (White) lecturers may experience shame as a signal anxiety, instigating a defence against the painful awareness of possible incompetence (not managing stu-dents and unable to manage the successful completion of a test) in the presence of the external object (the black management and students). (Black) students may expe-rience shame as a signal anxiety, instigating a defence against the painful awareness of possible incompetence or inferiority in the presence of the external object (the white lecturers). Through the envious attack the students possibly projected hidden shame as a defence against the awareness of incompetence or inferiority into the lecturers, and the lecturers may have introjected and identified with the projections and behaved as if they were shamed, linked to their apparent inability to provide an optimal learning-lecturing context for the students. This could be an instance where the lecturers experience shame resulting from narcissistic self-evaluation (through the eye of the other), which could result in social annihilation from the management of the HBU and their peers in education. In other words, the lecturers' ego-ideal (a set of standard, ideals and role expectation) (Lansky, 2005) may be under threat due to experiencing themselves a being seen as bad lecturers by students, management and peers. The lecturers probably also projected their shame into the students, the stu-dents identified with the shame, the lecturers could be free of the shame and hold onto feelings of superiority and competence. In this unconscious collusive communication through projective identification, the students can hold onto contempt for the lectur-ers who identified with the shame. In this way the students' shame remains hidden and unprocessed (May, 2017). Management not supporting lecturers and colluding with the demands of the students probably entrenched the hidden shame dynamics.

To address their experience of the (hidden shame) dynamics in the HBU, the nine lecturers went on a stay away action. The stay away action could be an attempt by the lecturers to ask for a new relationship with the students and management within a new socio-political dispensation. The new story, marked by a stay away action by the lecturers, is a story of hope and creativity, in their relationship with students, management and the wider university community, which was poised to disrupt the stable destructive dynamics, especially the hidden shame dynamics, entrenched within the HBU.

20.3 Interventions Using the Systems Psychodynamic Lens

I provide a discussion on interventions that can be used as an invitation for practitioners and researchers to use their knowledge of hidden shame dynamics to address the tensions and dynamics in their work contexts, and in so doing implement relevant changes to existing relationships and the structure of organisations. I base the discussion about interventions on the recommendations made by Powell Pruitt and Barber (2004) about how to effect change in the American school system, the use of the systems psychodynamic consultancy stance, the use the CIBART model and of role analysis. These interventions, based on the assumptions of systems psychodynamics, are made on individual, group and organisational level. It is important to guard against interventions becoming a defense against the psychodynamics that are evident within different contexts. Rather, the interventions should be used for further conversation, reflection and continuing action in different contexts (Powell Pruit & Barber, 2004).

Another important aspect when working from a systems psychodynamic lens is the system psychodynamic consultancy stance which is important with regards to the interventions proposed below. During interventions the practitioners/researchers **are not only observers** of events or the behaviour therein, but they **are actively involved** in it. They **offer interpretations and working hypothesis** about what is happening with regards to hidden shame dynamics, based upon their **own experience, observations and understanding about the matter being explored**.

20.3.1 Doing Internal Work

It is imperative that lecturers do their own internal work about their unconscious experiences of education, as well as their role as lecturers in particular. In other words, what have their educational experiences been and how do these inform their understanding of their role as lecturers, as well as the role of students and management in the university. Then of course it imperative that lecturers and other stakeholders do their own internal work about their unconscious experiences of being citizens within an apartheid and post-apartheid South Africa to make meaning of their current experiences and interactions with others across (cultural) difference (May & Cilliers, 2002; May, 2012; May & Evans, 2004). I am sure that lecturers and stakeholders to a lesser or greater degree do internal work regarding these matters, but the challenge is that they should look below the surface of their experiences and not only to that which is within the reach of their conscious understanding. Thus, it is important that practitioners and researchers, reflect on hidden shame dynamics in their contexts and how they could be complicit with them, to work continuously with these hidden shame dynamics.

20.3.2 External Holding Environments for Difficult Conversations

It is important to create external holding environments for difficult conversations to work through anxiety and concomitant destructive elements in the university—primarily between lecturers and management, among lecturers and among management. This is also an opportunity for psychologists and others to make a contribution. This does not mean that students cannot be involved in these conversations, but given that the lecturers are responsible for containing the students, and management is responsible for containing the lecturers and students (this is an overly simplistic description) (May, 2010) it seems important that the lecturers and management urgently start these difficult conversations. By doing this, these stakeholders will be working on resolving the psychodynamics, e.g. splitting, projections, introjections and projective identification, affecting their relationships and their ability to address hidden shame dynamics within the universities and in education in general. By dealing with the psychodynamics in the university, they will be more able to address difficulties pertaining to the organisational context (boundaries, authority, roles and tasks) using the SIBART model. This will afford lecturers and management the opportunity to attend more effectively to the unconscious phenomena within people, the organisational context (boundaries, authority, roles and tasks) and the complex interaction between them (May, 2010; May et al., 2012). This is also applicable to any other organisation.

20.3.2.1 SIBART (Shame, Identity, Boundaries, Authority, Role and Task) Model

The above discussion brings to the fore that system psychodynamics do not only result from interpersonal and intragroup and intergroup dynamics, but also from the socio-technical aspects of an organisation, that is, structure and design.

Therefore, to form a holistic understanding of employees' experiences, and therefore that of lecturers, one cannot only focus on unconscious processes. The focus should also be on organisational structure and design (Amado, 1995; Hayden & Molenkamp, 2004; May, 2012). Thus, the organisational structural elements that include boundaries, authority, role and task should also be explored (Hayden & Molenkamp, 2004; James & Huffington, 2004). The interaction between the unconscious processes and organisational structural elements highlights the need to work with the CIBART model. The CIBART model is a six-dimension boundary model (Conflict, Identity, Boundaries, Authority, Role and Task) which is used to study and explore conflict dynamics. The model enables practitioners and researchers to study and diagnose the dynamics of intra and interpersonal conflicts in and across groups and organisations (Cytrynbaum & Noumair, 2004; Cilliers & Koortzen, 2005). As the CIBART model is used to explore conflict dynamics, I suggest that perhaps one can consider a SIBART model (Shame, Identity, Boundaries, Authority, Role and Task) which could enable practitioners and researchers to study and diagnose the dynamics of intra and interpersonal shame in and across groups and organisations.

Shame, with specific reference to **hidden shame dynamics**, arises as a result of the splitting between the good and bad parts of a system (identity) and can manifest on different levels: intra-personally (within the individual, or between ideas, feelings and emotions), interpersonally (differences between two or more team members), intra-group (between factions, cliques, or sub-systems) and inter-group (between teams, departments or divisions in a larger system). The splitting (across boundaries, roles and tasks, as well as inappropriate autorisation) allows for projection by one part (a specific identity) onto and into the other (another identity—across boundaries, roles and tasks, as well as inappropriate autorisation), introjection (the other taking the introjection to the self) and projective identification (the other behaving as if the projection is true about the self) (May, 2017). These shame dynamics then occur because of a group's identity related to diversity characteristics, unclear or rigid boundaries, problematic authorisation, incorrect role assignment and misunderstanding about the task within and between groups. Only one or a combination of these aspects listed can entrench hidden shame dynamics:

Identity reflects the system's uniqueness in the form of its beliefs, disposition, outlook or cultural and political perspectives (Hayden & Molenkamp, 2004). Role can also be described as the personality and climate of a group or organization (Cilliers & Koortzen, 2005).

Boundaries are spaces of physical and intense psychological nature (Reciniello, 2014; Sher, 2010) across which exchanges take place in a system as well as transitional or potential space filled with unconscious (shame) dynamics which exists within and between groups, as well as the organisation's structure (Heracleous, 2004; James & Huffington, 2004). Boundaries are important in the containment of emotions (James & Huffington, 2004), such as shame.

Obholzer (2001, p. 201) stated that **"authority** is the product of organisation and structure, be it external, as in the organisation's sanction, or internal, as in the inner." This authority is used in the effective completion of the primary task or shared tasks (Eisold, 2004) and in making binding decisions for self and others (Beck & Visholm, 2014). This authority can be "given from above" from management, or "from below" from subordinates, or "from within" the group (self-authorisation) or from other groups (Eisold, 2004).

Role refers to the description of what needs to be done in order to perform with regards to responsibilities and tasks within a specific boundary (Hayden & Molenkamp, 2004; Cilliers & Koortzen, 2005). Authority is tied to positions or roles (Beck & Visholm, 2014). Three types of roles are distinguished, namely, (1) the normative (2) the existential and (3) the phenomenal role. Incongruence between these different roles creates anxiety and poor performance (Cilliers & Koortzen, 2005).

Task is the basic building block of work (Cilliers & Koortzen, 2005; Cytrynbaum & Noumair, 2004). The organisations can be a multi-task system, for example the university three primary tasks, viz. educating students, producing research publications and providing relevant community service (Rice, 1970; Rogers, 1976). According to Lawrence (1985, p. 235) the [primary] task is a tool for inquiry to understand the realities of the organisation and other social arrangements of [the workforce]. Further, the organisation can display on task, off-task and ant-task behaviour (Obholzer & Roberts, 1994).

20.3.2.2   SIBART Model: Stakeholders Toyi-Toying to the Beat of the New Story

In the case study (see Sect. 20.2) disagreements existed between lecturers and management mainly with the nature of the primary task of the HBU, role confusion experienced by the lecturers, the appropriate owning of responsibility, appropriate authorisation, the non-provision of boundary conditions and the withholding of support for lecturers by management (May, 2010; May et al., 2012). The lecturers primarily experienced the stay away action as their commitment to writing and proposing a new story for the HBU. Through the stay away action they experienced themselves as:

- Taking on new identities as lecturers in the new socio-political dispensation.
- Owning of their authority in a new socio-political dispensation within the HBU—by doing this they displayed leadership within the HBU.
- Creating of new boundaries within the HBU in order to take up their roles and do their tasks more effectively.
- Redefining their role and task more positively within the HBU, as well as the wider academic fraternity.

It is important that the lecturers asked for these new relationships with new identities, new roles, new tasks and new boundaries by taking, through the stay-away action, a clear stance about how they wanted to be treated by the students and management within the new relationships. The stay-away action was mirroring the behaviour of the students who often used stay away action to vent their dissatisfaction in the system. It seems that the lecturers were truly challenging old identities, old roles, old boundaries and old tasks and in this way working towards new relationships in a new HBU. In order to form new relationships within the HBU the lecturers through a stay-way action have taken on a denied identity because they have temporarily let go of their identity in terms of being white lecturers, in favour of another identity which usually belonged to black students, black lecturers and perhaps even black management. I propose that the lecturers may not have realised the significance of their action, on a psychodynamic level, for the HBU (May, 2010).

It seems that by authorising themselves and each other within the new sociopolitical dispensations, the lecturers have been able to create a transitional and potential space containing creativity and hope (Erlich, 2004) in which they could negotiate their relationships with the students and management. Inadvertently the lecturers were working to address the destructive dynamics, which included hidden shame dynamics, towards constructive dynamics through creative action consisting of new skills that could lead to new relational experiences (Hartling & Lindner, 2016).

It is important that the lecturers asked for these new relationships with new identities, new roles, new tasks and new boundaries by taking, through the stay-away action, a clear stance about how they wanted to be treated by the students and management within the new relationships. The stay-away action was mirroring the behaviour of the students—hoping to have their demands met as the students did through their struggle skills. It is also important that the lecturers attempted to let their voices heard through a method usually used by students and by black people. I believe, and so do the lecturers, that they were truly challenging old roles, old boundaries, old tasks and old identities and in this way working towards new relationships in a new HBU. In order to form new relationships within the HBU the lecturers through a stay-way action have taken on a denied identity because they have temporarily let go of their identity in terms of being white lecturers, in favour of another identity which usually belonged to black students, black lecturers and perhaps even black management. I propose that the lecturers may not have realised the significance of their action, on a psychodynamic level, for the HBU (May, 2010).

In the above discussion the constructs of the SIBART model was used to diagnose the psychodynamics of groups and organisations by exploring what kind of behaviour manifested, how it manifested, why it originated, what it represents and what interventions can be used (see Cilliers & Koortzen, 2005). The lecturers through their stay away action inadvertently addressed aspects which would be addressed through the model. Thus, practitioners, consultants and researchers could use the SIBART model to practically apply system psychodynamic thinking to organisations exploring organisational aspects (boundaries, authority, role and task), as well as unconscious shame dynamics (see Amado, 1995) and the complex interaction between the two (see Amado, 1995; May, 2010; May et al., 2012; Nutkevich, 1998)—see the template to work with SIBART (Fig. 20.1).

	Observed behaviour	Defence mechanism	Psychodynamic meaning of behaviour and defence mechanism	Hidden dynamics
Shame				
Identity				
Boundaries				
Authority				
Role				
Task				

Fig. 20.1 Template to work with SIBART

This table presents the complex SIBART model in a very reduced form. It can, for example, be used for self-reflection by transferring it to one's own contexts and questions, thereby contributing to the reflection of one's own psychodynamics.

20.3.2.3   Organisational Role Analysis

Role refers to the description of what needs to be done in order to perform. Taking up a specific role implies being authorised to do so and knowing the boundaries of what will be rewarded and what not. Different types of roles are distinguished, namely,

1. the normative (the objective job description and content),
2. the existential (what you believe role is you are performing), and
3. the phenomenal (what role other think you fulfil—this can be inferred by other's mostly unconscious behaviour towards you).

Incongruence between these different roles creates anxiety and poor performance and this is what the practitioners, consultant or researchers should explore. In the discussion about these three types of roles practitioners assist clients to form:

1. understanding and clarity of their roles (by using the three types of roles) versus being confused about their role comprises (often a conflict exists between the understanding on the conscious level versus what is seen and believed on the unconscious and collective levels);
2. explore the incongruence between the three types of roles ('Students think I am against them, yet I'm working so hard that I in my role as lecturer can provide them with learning opportunities!');
3. explore how willing the system is in authorising them to develop and take up new roles ('I have tried to do this correctly for very long, but no one appreciates what I do').

Through the stay away action they experienced themselves as:

- Showing personal development with regard to dealing with not always pleasing the stakeholders (reducing incongruence between normative, existential and phenomenal role).

- Showing personal development by challenging oneself personally and interpersonally to create *new alternatives to stale ideologies (reducing incongruence between normative, existential and phenomenal role)*.
- Realising that all the stakeholders, themselves included, were colluding with the old, destructive status quo—all were singing the old story and toyi-toying to the same old beat.

Through the above three aspects the lecturers were probably more aware of the labels being projected onto them and identified less with the usual projections coming their way (Powell Pruitt & Barber, 2004). Thus, the stay-away action was a crucial action in their attempts to create a new, co-constructed story (by and for all the stakeholders) though which they resisted **splitting**, **introjecting** the usual **projection** (Scott, 2011) and **preventing identification** with the **projection**.

By not accepting the "usual" projections the lecturers would make hidden shame dynamics within the lecturing-learning relationship more manageable for students. Perhaps, through the lecturers taking up the struggle, the students could become more free to attend to the task of interacting with their role and task. Through the stay-away action the lecturers may also be doing what the students have unconsciously wanted for so long, i.e. working with their own shame, rage, terror and dread and perhaps returning these experiences in a more manageable form to the students. Perhaps for a moment the students may have been "free" from the system's shame, rage, terror and dread and only needed to take responsibility for their own shame rage, terror and dread.

20.3.3 Creating Holding Environments for Lecturers and Management

It is imperative to create and support holding environments for lecturers to deal with the challenges they may face from the different stakeholders, as well as the role and task of lecturers in the current South African context. Some of these holding environments should be developed by psychologists, some by other practitioners, some by lecturers and some by other stakeholders in universities. Often in psychology thought is given to care for the practitioner. In the same way, care for the lecturers should be encouraged by creating spaces where lecturers can work, using a systems psychodynamic perspective, with their experiences and the challenges they face from different stakeholders.

Of course these lecturers may discover how they collude with the system's (hidden shame) dynamics—this could be painful and disturbing, but also liberating and filled with learning (as this research project has been for me). In this way internal holding environments (Alford, 2002; Nutkevitch, 2001) (pertaining to the intra-psychic wellness of the lecturers and to physical spaces in the university) for difficult conversations will be created. As I was writing this I became aware of the possibility of creating holding environments (pertaining to the intra-psychic wellness of management and physical spaces in the university) for management to have difficult conversation with lecturers and among themselves. These will enable management to provide appropriate (emotional) containment for students and lecturers and to manage organisational structure and design in the university as suggested by Alford (2002), Miller and Rice (1990) and Nutkevitch (2001), this highlighting the use of the SIBART model.

20.3.4   Imagining Alternatives to the (K)not of Relationships

Based on the findings, it is evident that the power struggle across many diversity characteristics creates stale ideologies which can be challenged through creating new ways of interacting with each other. Through the lecturers' stories it is evident that the lecturers are well aware of finding and creating alternatives to stale ideologies. Thus we need to imagine alternatives to create a new story (Powell Pruitt & Barber, 2004; Singer, 2006) which challenges the stale ideologies in the universities, education and South African organisations. This challenge belongs to all the stakeholders within education, especially universities. Although it seems there is a resistance to interacting in new ways with each other, I propose that as South Africans we simply do not know how to do this (see May & Cilliers, 2002; May & Evans, 2004). Therefore, by imagining and eventually actioning new alternatives of interacting with each other we will assist the stakeholders in creating a new, hopefully useful, story for education in general, universities in particular and for other South African organisations—dealing with destructive (hidden shame) dynamics constructively.

20.4   Conclusion

In conclusion I present the painting, *Eyes wide Shut* by Frier (2017), for further reflection and meaning-making about what it may mean for the lecturers and other employees to explore and work at the intersection between their hidden shame dynamics and the socio-technical aspects of organisations (Fig. 20.2).

Perhaps the individual or the individual as representation of cultural groups in making time to process, the intrapsychic and intergroup hidden shame dynamics struggle bravely to bring the hidden shame dynamics into awareness. This brave struggle is off course not without resistance and retreating from what they have to look at as they become aware of the hidden shame dynamics they may in be involved in. I propose that this struggle of looking and shying away from (Frier, 2017) hidden shame dynamics will be evident for practitioners, researchers, employees, employers and management who work with hidden shame dynamics.

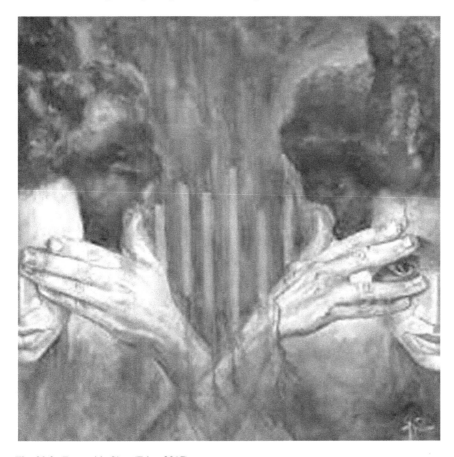

Fig. 20.2   Eyes wide Shut (Frier, 2017)

References

Alford, C. F. (2002). Is murder impossible? Levinas, Winnicott, and the ruthless use of the object. *Journal of Psycho-Social Studies, 1*(1). Retrieved from http://www.btinternet.com/~psycho_social/Vol1/JPSS1-CFA1.html.

Amado, G. (1995). Why psychoanalytical knowledge helps us understand organisations, a discussion with Elliot Jacques. *Human Relations, 48*(4), 351–358.

Beck, U. C., & Visholm, S. (2014). Authority relations in group relations conferences and in 'real life' group relations conferences. *Danish Design I* 1, *14*(2), 227–237.

Cilliers, F., & Koortzen, P. (2005). Applying the CIBART consulting model at individual, group and organisational levels. *HR Future, 113*(10), 52–53.

Cytrynbaum, S., & Noumair, A. (2004). *Group dynamics, organisational irrationality, and social complexity: Group relations reader 3*. Jupiter: A.K. Rice.

Czander, W., & Eisold, K. (2003). Psychoanalytic perspectives on organisational consulting: Transference and countertransference. *Human Relations, 56*(4), 475–490.

Eisold, K. (2004). Leadership and the creation of authority. In S. Cytrynbaum & D. A. Noumair (Eds.), *Group dynamics, organisational irrationality and social complexity: Group Relations Reader 3* (pp. 289–302). Washington DC: A.K. Rice Institute.

Erlich, H. S. (2004). Dependency, autonomy and the politics of survival. *Social and Organisational Dynamics, 4,* 285–297.

Frier, G. (2017). *Eyes wide shut.* Retrieved from https://www.saatchiart.com/art/Painting-Eyes-wide-shut/1187/2688576/view.

Hartling, L. M., & Lindner, E. G. (2016). Healing humiliation: from reaction to creative action. *Journal of Counseling & Development, 94390,* 383–390.

Hayden, C., & Molenkamp, R. J. (2004). Tavistock primer II. In S. Cytrynbaum & D. A. Noumair (Eds.), *Group dynamics, organisational irrationality and social complexity: Group relations reader 3* (pp. 135–157). Washington DC: A.K. Rice Institute.

Heracleous, L. (2004). Boundaries in the study of organisation. *Human Relations, 57*(1), 95–103.

James, K., & Huffington, C. (2004). Containment of anxiety in organisational change: A case example of changing organisation boundaries. *Social and Organisational dynamics, 4,* 212–233.

Lansky, M. R. (2005). Hidden shame. *Journal of American Psycho-analytic Association, 53*(3), 865–890.

Lawrence, W. G. (1985). Management development … some ideals, images and realities. In A. D. Colman & M. H. Geller (Eds.), *Group relations reader 2* (pp. 231–240). Washington DC: A.K. Rice Institute.

May, M. S. (2010). *The unconscious at work: The (k)not of relationship between students, lecturers and management in a historically black university.* Unpublished doctoral thesis. University of South Africa, Pretoria.

May, M. S. (2012). Diversity dynamics operating between students, lecturers and management in a historically Black university: The lecturers' perspective. *SA Journal of Industrial Psychology, 38*(2), Art. #1003, 8 pp. Retrieved from http://dx.doi.org/10.4102/sajip.v38i2.100.

May, M. S. (2017). Shame! A systems psychodynamic perspective. In E. Vanderheiden & C.-H. Mayer (Eds.), *The value of shame: Exploring a health resource in cultural contexts* (pp. 43–59). Cham: Springer.

May, M. S. & Cilliers, F. (2002). The Robben Island diversity experience 2001. Diversity dynamics a year later. In *Eight national congress of psychological society of South Africa.* Bellville: University of the Western Cape.

May, M. S., Cilliers, F., & Van Deventer, S. H. (2012). Exploring the (k)not of relationship between lecturers and management at a historically Black university: The lecturer's perspective. *SA Journal of Industrial Psychology, 38*(2), Art. #998, 10 pp. Retrieved from http://dx.doi.org/10.4102/sajip.v38i2.998.

May, M. S., & Evans, A. C. (2004). Making group relations at home in South Africa. *Journal of Psychology in Africa, 14*(1), 29–36.

Miller, E. J., & Rice, A. K. (1990). Task and sentient system and their boundary controls. In E. Trist & H. Murray (Eds.), *The social engagement of social science* (pp. 259–271). Philadelphia: The University of Pennsylvania Press.

Nutkevitch, A. (1998). *The container and its containment: A meeting space for psychoanalytic and open systems theories.* Paper presented at ISPSO. Retrieved from http://www.ispso.org/Symposia/Jerusalem/1998nutkevitch.htm.

Nutkevitch, A. (2001). Is containment relevant? *Organisational & Social Dynamics, 2,* 270–271.

Obholzer, A. (2001). The leader, the unconscious, and the management of the organisation. In L. J. Gould, L. F. Stapley, & M. Stein (Eds.), *The systems psychodynamics of organisations: Integrating the group relations approach. Psychoanalytic, and open systems perspective* (pp. 91–114). New York: Karnac.

Obholzer, A., & Roberts, V. Z. (Eds.). (1994). *The unconscious at work: Individual and organizational stress in the human services.* London: Routledge.

Powell Pruitt, L., & Barber, M. (2004). Savage inequalities indeed: Irrationality and urban school reform. In S. Cytrynbaum & D. A. Noumair (Eds.), *Group dynamics, organisational irrationality and social complexity: Group relations reader 3* (pp. 303–320). Washington DC: A.K. Rice Institute.

Reciniello, S. (2014). *The conscious leader: Nine principles and practices to create a wide-awake and productive workplace.* London: LID Publishing.

Rice, A. K. (1970). *The modern university a model organisation.* London: Tavistock Publications.

Rogers, K. (1976). Teaching and learning responsibility: A model of an educational approach for meeting the challenge of change. In E. J. Miller (Ed.), *Task and organisation* (pp. 339–359). London: Wiley.

Scott, S. (2011). Uncovering shame in groups: An exploration of unconscious shame manifest as a disturbance in communication within the early stages of an analytic group. *Group Analysis, 44*(1), 83–96. Retrieved from https://doi.org/10.1177/0533316410391168.

Singer, I. (2006). Unmasking difference, culture, and attachment in the psychoanalytic space: "Don't you make my blue eyes brown". In K. White (Ed.), *Unmasking race, culture and attachment in the psychoanalytic space* (pp. 61–74). New York: Karnac.

Sher, M. (2010). Corruption: Aberration or an inevitable part of the human condition? Insights from a Tavistock approach. *Organisational & Social Dynamics, 10*(1), 40–55.

Michelle S. May (Prof. Dr.), (D. Litt. Et. Phil., University of South Africa) is a professor at the Department of Industrial and Organizational Psychology at the University of South Africa (UNISA). She is a registered clinical psychologist. Michelle received extensive training in the field of group consultation, under which from ISLA and the Tavistock Institute (UK), and has also consulted in various programs of this nature—nationally and internationally. She has been part of the team who has designed and planned the Robben Island diversity experience (RIDE) and has been taken up the role of director, director of the training group, and associate director from 2000 until 2014. She has also been part of the Group Relations workshops at UNISA since 2000. For the last 10 years, Michelle have also contributed to the field of diversity management in South Africa as lecturer, researcher, and consultant in several organizations—her contributions have included publications in accredited journals, book chapters, as well as presentations at national and international conferences. She has chaired, consulted in, and designed many workshops in the areas of diversity management and leadership development for organizations in the public and private sectors.

Chapter 21
Shame and Anxiety with Foreign Language Learners

Paul A. Wilson and Barbara Lewandowska-Tomaszczyk

Abstract Two studies are reported that assess the moderation of shame and related emotions in Polish university students in different English L2 learning scenarios. In the first study, students on speaking and writing courses completed a questionnaire in which they rated the likelihood of their emotional responses to hypothetical situations in learning scenarios that they experienced. In both courses the main reduction in shame was shown in scenarios that provided more private as opposed to public evaluation. The corresponding decreases for fear, anxiety, anger and hopelessness were less pronounced and were dependent on the emotion and scenario. In the second study, results of regular email peer co-operation between students of English at Polish and US universities are reported. In both studies the reduction of the level of shame/embarrassment, conditioned by the presence of less formal communication scenarios, is observed, along with the development of the students' more positive linguistic self-evaluation.

Keywords Collaborative tasks · Foreign language teaching (FLT) · Foreign language learning (spoken/written) · Public/private · Shame cluster

21.1 Introduction

Strategies to reduce shame in the L2 classroom are important not only because of the direct debilitating effects it can have on learning, but also because of the influence it can have on other emotions that can also undermine progress in this context, such as fear, anxiety, anger and hopelessness. The present chapter assesses teaching methods in terms of their effectiveness in reducing shame and these other related emotions

P. A. Wilson (✉)
Institute of English Studies, University of Lodz, Pomorska 171/173 90-236, Lodz, Poland
e-mail: paul.wilson@uni.lodz.pl

B. Lewandowska-Tomaszczyk
State University of Applied Sciences in Konin, Przjazni 1, 62510 Konin, Poland
e-mail: blt@konin.edu.pl

© Springer Nature Switzerland AG 2019

C.-H. Mayer and E. Vanderheiden (eds.), *The Bright Side of Shame*,
https://doi.org/10.1007/978-3-030-13409-9_21

that were introduced indifferent L2 learning contexts involving Polish university students.

One of the main reasons for shame being central to learning contexts is that it is characterised by a negative criticism of the global self and is therefore related to evaluations of self-esteem. The central features pertaining to this global self that are particularly relevant to the classroom situation relate to the social embeddedness of shame in which a major concern is negative evaluation through the eyes of others rather than just negative assessment per se (Lewis, 1971). The powerlessness and tendency to hide, withdraw and disappear associated with shame are consistent with approaches to shame outlined by Fontaine et al. (2006). Consistent with our viewpoint on emotions, rather than considering shame as a distinct solitary emotion we underscore the conceptual arrangement of this emotion with other emotions in the shame cluster. Our decision to include in our data participant references to embarrassment in addition to shame is also based on "the blurring of their inter-categorial boundaries" in Polish and the public scrutiny that appears to be a particularly salient feature of both of these emotions in this culture (Krawczak, 2014, 457).

The importance of assessing emotions in terms of their inter-cluster in addition to intra-cluster relations is particularly pertinent to the case of shame due to its central influence on a number of other emotions. For example, McGregor and Elliot (2005) demonstrated that "shame is the core emotion of fear of failure" (227); Tangney et al. (1992) showed a close relationship between shame proneness and anxiety; and Tracy and Robins (2006) found that shame is positively associated with depression. Rather than focusing directly on depression, the present study concentrates on a similar emotion member of the same cluster, hopelessness, as it is deemed that this is potentially more relevant to learning scenarios. Finally, anger is an emotion that is relevant to the learning context as it can be a defensive response to the threat of shame (Tangney, 1995) that might arise, for example, from criticism from the teacher or other students.

21.1.1 Tend-and-Befriend

A potentially more constructive means of responding to the social threat in the L2 classroom can be achieved through the tend-and-befriend response advanced by Taylor et al. (2000). This is a stress regulatory survival mechanism, which facilitates environmental blending and hence an effective defence against many threats. Wilson (2016) argues that student collaborative writing assignments might utilise the protective elements of tend-and-befriend to reduce social threats that elicit shame and other debilitative emotions.

A specific focus of both studies centres on the function of more private rather than public, official evaluation as elements more conducive to moderating shame in foreign language teaching.

21.2 First Study

21.2.1 Aims

The overarching aim was to perform a comparative assessment of teaching strategies that were utilised in different English L2 university courses to determine which were beneficial in terms of the levels of student shame, fear, anxiety, hopelessness and anger. It is initially necessary to provide details on the specific teaching strategies or scenarios in order to highlight their different types of social threat that we predict will influence shame and the other related emotions. In the first study, two types of L2 classes were analysed: speaking course (three teaching scenarios: presentation, exam practice and an outside classroom context; writing course (two teaching scenarios: individual writing and group writing).

21.2.1.1 Speaking L2 Class

Presentation Scenario

This involved a 5–10 min English oral presentation to the other students and native English-speaking teacher in the class. Two of the students in the class and the teacher provided feedback on the quality of spoken English. A grade was also received from the teacher.

Exam Practice Scenario

This involved an exercise preparing for a forthcoming exam in which the student answered questions in English with a fellow student in a 15-min practice exam in the classroom in the presence of other students. Two other students played the role of examiners. The student examiners and the native English-speaking teacher gave the student feedback. The teacher also gave the student examinees a grade.

Outside Classroom Scenario

Two or three students were taken out of the classroom by their native English-speaking teacher to a communal area of the building. The students discussed a question orally in English for 15 min. The teacher gave feedback and a grade to each of the students.

#### 21.2.1.2	Writing L2 Class

Group Writing Scenario

Students wrote a challenging academic paragraph during the class with three other students. Afterwards they presented this as a group to the class via a projector and were given oral feedback by their native English-speaking teacher and the other students. A grade was received from the teacher.

Individual Writing Scenario

Students wrote a challenging academic paragraph on their own. They received feedback both orally (face to face) and in writing from their native English-speaking teacher. Additionally, students received feedback via email from a fellow student. A grade was also received from the teacher.

### 21.2.2	Hypotheses

On the basis of the major concern of public evaluation that characterises shame (e.g., Lewis, 1971), it is predicted that scenarios involving more private feedback will have a significantly moderating effect on the level of shame. Therefore, relatively lower levels of shame are expected for the outside classroom speaking scenario and the individual writing scenario. Evidence for the possible moderating influence of tend-and-befriend will be additionally assessed in the group writing scenario. In the group writing scenario a hypothetical email feedback condition was introduced in the questionnaire and it is predicted that this will be characterised by less social threat, and hence less shame, than face to face, class feedback. In all scenarios, ratings for shame were compared with those for fear, anxiety, hopelessness and anger.

### 21.2.3	Methodology

#### 21.2.3.1	Participants

Speaking Course

There were 9 Polish students on the speaking module of the MA English Philology course at Lodz University, Poland (mean age 23.4 years, 8 females).

Writing Course

There were 28 Polish students on the writing module of the BA English Philology course at Lodz University, Poland (mean age 20.4 years, 18 females).

21.2.3.2 Questionnaires

The speaking and writing questionnaires were adapted from the Test of Self-Conscious Affect (TOSCA) (Tangney, 1990), so that the scenarios described actual teaching procedures that the students had experienced. There were a number of questions for each of the scenarios that asked participants to imagine hypothetical events that could happen in the particular scenario and the participant had to respond on a 5-point Likert scale according to how they would feel in that situation. For each question participants had to respond to 6 Likert scales corresponding to their shame, fear, anxiety, hopelessness anger responses, with an additional filler item describing a possible positive response. The speaking questionnaire had an additional open-ended question asking participants to state which scenario had the most beneficial effect on their motions and why it had this effect.

21.2.4 Results and Discussion

A 5×3 repeated measures ANOVA was performed on the speaking class data that had two within-subjects variables (emotion: shame, anxiety, fear, anger, and hopelessness; scenario: presentation, exam practice, and outside classroom). There was a significant interaction between emotion and scenario, $F(8, 64) = 3.42$, $p < 0.01$. A 5×2 repeated measures ANOVA was also performed on the writing class data that had two within-subjects variables (emotion: shame, anxiety, fear, anger, and hopelessness; scenario: individual writing and group writing). There was a significant interaction between emotion and scenario, $F(4, 108) = 11.58$, $p < 0.01$. Additionally, a 5×2 repeated measures ANOVA was performed on the writing class data that had two within-subjects variables (emotion: shame, anxiety, fear, anger, and hopelessness; feedback: in class and via email). There was a significant interaction between emotion and scenario, $F(3.2, 86.43) = 6.19$, $p < 0.01$. The results of the simple effects analyses are shown separately for each emotion (see below).

The open-ended questionnaire results showed that 100% of the participants judged the outside classroom scenario to be the most beneficial in terms of emotions, with shame and anxiety moderation equally reported by 33% of the participants. No other emotions were mentioned in the self-reports. 67% of the participants chose the outside classroom scenario because of the lack of being observed by the rest of the class and 44% because of less judgement.

21.2.4.1 Shame

The questionnaire ratings pertaining to both the speaking and writing courses showed that the scenarios that had less public scrutiny and evaluation were characterised by relatively lower shame. The speaking course results (see Fig. 21.1) showed that the outside classroom scenario was characterised in particular by moderated shame as this emotion was rated significantly lower on this scenario than the other two scenarios and the open-ended reports referred to reductions in key elicitors of shame, namely judgement and observation, suggesting that they played a facilitating role in this reduction in shame. Although fear showed a similar pattern to shame as it was significantly lower on the outside classroom scenario than the other two scenarios ($p < 0.05$, for both), it was not referred to in the open-ended reports. Not only was anger similarly not present in the open-ended data, it was rated lower on the outside classroom scenario in comparison with only one of the other scenarios—exam practice ($p < 0.05$); however, there was no significant difference between shame and anger on the outside classroom scenario. Although an equal number of participants in the open-ended reports referred to a moderation of shame and anxiety in the outside classroom scenario (33% for both emotions), it is the references to diminished evaluation and observation that point to reduced shame compared with that of anxiety. Additionally, shame was rated significantly lower than anxiety on the outside classroom scenario ($p < 0.01$).

The higher ratings for shame in the group scenario than the individual scenario ($p < 0.05$) (see Fig. 21.2) in the writing course results suggest that it was the presentation element in the classroom context with more public feedback that was possibly responsible for this. The results showing reduced shame ratings for the relatively

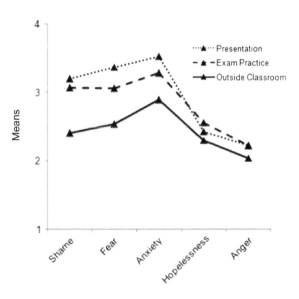

Fig. 21.1 Mean emotion ratings on presentation, exam practice and outside classroom speaking scenarios

Fig. 21.2 Mean emotion ratings on group writing and individual writing scenarios

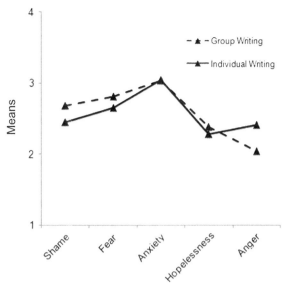

Fig. 21.3 Mean emotion ratings on class feedback and hypothetical email feedback scenarios

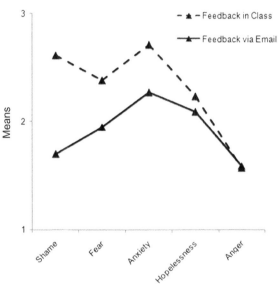

more private, hypothetical email feedback scenario compared with the class feedback scenario (p < 0.01) (see Fig. 21.3) is consistent with this. These results further suggest that there was little benefit in terms of the level of shame from collaborative writing in the group writing scenario (see Fig. 21.2), which points to a lack of influence of the potentially protective tend-and-befriend mechanism.

21.2.4.2 Fear

The lack of any significant differences between shame and fear in any of the three
speaking course scenarios results (Fig. 21.1) showed that the relatively greater similarity between shame and fear was particularly evident in the speaking course data.
Nevertheless, in comparison with clear evidence for shame reduction in the self-
reports for the outside classroom scenario, there was a lack of any corresponding
responses referring to a decrease in fear.

The dissimilarity between shame and fear in the writing course data is shown
by the relatively lower level of shame in the individual writing scenario in comparison with the results for fear, which do not demonstrate such a reduction (see
Fig. 21.2). However, fear was similar to shame in being moderated on the hypothetical email feedback scenario in comparison to the feedback in class scenario ($p < 0.05$)
(Fig. 21.3).

21.2.4.3 Anxiety

Although shame demonstrated some degree of similarity with anxiety in its pattern of
results across the scenarios, there were some notable differences. Both the questionnaire ratings data and the self-report data for the speaking course showed evidence
for both shame and anxiety reduction in the outside classroom scenario; however,
as noted above, there was relatively more shame moderation compared with that of
anxiety in this scenario.

In comparison to the difference in shame between the group and individual writing
scenarios, anxiety was similar to fear in its lack of difference between these two
scenarios. In addition, it should be noted that writing appears to be a particularly
anxiety-inducing activity as this emotion was significantly higher than all the other
emotions on both scenarios (see Fig. 21.2). However, anxiety was similar to shame
and fear in its lower ratings on the hypothetical email feedback scenario in comparison
to the feedback in the class scenario ($p < 0.05$). Nevertheless, a more pronounced
moderation effect was shown for shame in this respect as it was significantly lower
than anxiety on the hypothetical email feedback scenario ($p < 0.01$) (see Fig. 21.3).

21.2.4.4 Anger

As noted above, the moderation of anger in the outside classroom scenario appears
to be somewhat less than that for shame.

The most notable difference between shame and anger is in the writing course data
that shows that compared with the moderated shame on the individual wring scenario,
anger is significantly lower on the group writing scenario than the individual writing
scenario ($p < 0.05$) (see Fig. 21.2). Additionally, in comparison with the moderation of
shame on the hypothetical email feedback scenario there was no significant difference
in anger between this scenario and the feedback in class scenario (see Fig. 21.3).

21.2.4.5 Hopelessness

The lack of differences between the scenarios in either the speaking or the writing course hopelessness data suggests that the language competence of the students protected them from such a severe social threat that might have elicited hopelessness to a significant degree even in the more challenging scenarios.

21.3 Second Study

21.3.1 Native—Non-native Peer Collaborative Tasks

The second study focuses on the emotion profile accompanying regular online contacts between Polish MA students of English and translation at the State University of Applied Sciences in Konin and the University of Lodz, and students of technical and engineering subjects at North Dakota State University during their writing courses (Lewandowska-Tomaszczyk & Slomski, 2016) during 2015–2017 within a Trans-Atlantic Pacific Project (TAPP) (Maylath et al., 2013). The scenarios include writing tasks for the American students and writing and translation from English into Polish and from Polish into English for the Polish students and, following peer corrective feedback, production of the final versions of the relevant texts.

This part of the present analysis aims to identify the context of paired native student (NS)—non-native student (NNS) email contacts, which was shown to moderate levels of shame in the first study, and to illuminate the influence of this task type on FL learner shame/embarrassment and fear/anxiety profiles as observed in cooperation with the native language peers. A discussion of error correction and corrective feedback, including peer online interaction and accompanying emotions will follow to find out the effectiveness of a NS-NNS peer tutoring model on decreasing shame and anxiety levels with the collaborating individuals. The cooperation started in October 2015 and was conducted for five semesters (2015/16 2016/2017, 2017/2018), coordinated by an instructor from the NDSU (Heather A. Slomski) and a teacher from the Polish university (Barbara Lewandowska-Tomaszczyk). There were from 27 to 30 Polish students on average and the same number of NDSU students engaged in the project during each semester. The American classes involved different students each semester, while the classes of Polish students changed each academic year. The Polish students were all native speakers of Polish, of varied backgrounds, majoring in English studies (English philology). Their English proficiency, monitored during classes of practical English grammar, speaking and writing, evaluated according to the criteria of The Common European Framework of Reference for Languages, ranged typically between B1 and C1 levels, i.e., between the so-called independent user's threshold or intermediate proficiency or vantage or intermediate proficiency in English on the one hand and effective operational or advanced proficiency on the other. All of the NDSU students are native speakers of English, first or second generation college students, generally of middle-class background. The most common majors among them are engineering, architecture, and nursing. NSs and NNSs were paired and, in the course of a few exchanges, discussed the content and structure of the texts, provided explanation of culture-specific terms and occasionally modified their own texts in the discussion.

21.3.1.1 Peer Corrective Feedback and Emotions

As demonstrated in the introduction, a major reason for increases in shame and fear in typical everyday life contexts, even outside the classroom is the presentation of one's endeavours to public checkup and scrutiny. This is particularly frequent when it is known a priori that the individuals assessing the products, outcomes, etc. are more competent than the experiencers. Hence, corrective feedback, understood as "a more competent speaker's reaction to learners' ill-formed output" (Panova and Lyster, 2002), in the context of FLT classroom, particularly between NSs and NNSs, although considered an important facilitative strategy in second language acquisition and language development, is also a cause of the learners' shame, stress, anxiety, anger and general emotional arousal. The main objective of this part of the study is to present FLT contexts and scenarios such as paired collaborative tasks between NSs and NNSs, performed by means of email cooperation, which on the one hand will lead to shame reduction with the students and, on the other, prove more effective in developing student linguistic performance. Thus, this study complements some aspects of study one that demonstrated the ways of moderating shame feeling by creating a less formal setting for the students and providing the sense of more privacy as shown in the hypothetical email feedback scenario.

The Polish students were interviewed by the Polish teacher both before the cooperation started[1] and after the final submission of the work. Although the corrective feedback was found to bring positive results on a whole (Lewandowska-Tomaszczyk & Slomski, 2016), the Polish students reported they were worried and embarrassed before the cooperation started, which was related to the exposure of their NNS English writing to NS's judgement.

A post-task informal survey (adapted from Arnold and Ducate, 2006, 49) was administered to all Polish students at the end of each academic year. At the end of the winter term in 2017 the students were also asked 11 open-ended, descriptive opinion questions. There were 12 sentences in the first part of the survey. Out of the five possible responses—strongly agree, agree, neutral, disagree, strongly disagree—a large majority of the students (76%) reported that they fully enjoyed the electronic exchange and would enjoy participating in such a cooperation again. However, the

---

[1]The concept of *cooperation* is to be distinguished from that of *collaboration*. The former entails dividing a task into subtasks and performing them individually towards achieving the task. Collaboration also involves a common goal but implies a fully integrated work among the participants, in which there is an equal investment of efforts to achieve the purpose (see Misanchuk and Anderson 2001). In our project both forms of peer involvement were present, which is signaled by the use of relevant terms in the present paper.

students had different experiences with regard to accompanying emotions. The large majority of them (67%) marked 'strongly agree' or 'agree' with the survey statement 'The forum of the Internet exchange provided less anxiety and a more relaxed environment than classroom discussion', but some others disagreed (7%) or gave a neutral response (12%). The latter result might be interpreted in terms of the presence of prior shame and anxiety, related to exposing one's own linguistic product to direct NS scrutiny. And even though any evaluation, as mentioned above, is likely to cause negative emotional arousal, the evaluation of the language by the native language user, in the context in which NNSs forward their essays to their NS pairs, with no direct explanatory or commenting interaction, causes a degree of embarrassment and anxiety among the students. 67% of the students who highly valued the email contact mode on the other hand, positively perceived "the privacy which is provided by exchanging e-mails", which can be contrasted with more threatening face-to-face or public classroom encounters.

One of the Polish students' comments below (1) also stresses the contact with individuals of the same age, which demonstrates the reduction of negative emotions.

(1) People in a similar age often understand us better and know how to help us with problems which they also have in their education.

The results of this part of the second study support the outcomes presented in the first study, which demonstrate the effectiveness of the less public contexts in decreasing the shame level in the FLT context.

21.3.1.2 Emotions in Writing and Speaking

The Polish students experienced a certain degree of emotional tension when they contacted native speakers [see ex. (2)], but they also distinguished between degrees of anxiety and embarrassment in addressing native speakers of English in the written as opposed to spoken forms (examples 3–6), which was typically higher in the speaking context:

(2) I am not necessarily anxious, but I do feel the need to be extra careful when contacting a native speaker. I don't want to embarrass myself by making an obvious mistake, so I try to either check what I wrote before sending it over or think carefully before saying something.

(3) When I make a mistake, and I usually notice that I said something wrong right away, so I feel even more embarrassed, because I know I have the knowledge and could do better.

(4) I don't feel anxiety when I'm writing to native speakers of English, however, I feel a little bit anxious when I need to speak to them.

(5) Spoken contact is always more stressful for me, as there is more opportunity there to make some sort of an embarrassing blunder.

(6) (I may feel embarrassed) only when speaking face-to-face. It is then when I'm worried whether my English is good enough or not, etc. It may have to do with my general introversion, however.

Direct spoken contacts are judged to be a source of a higher level of embarrassment and anxiety. The sense of embarrassment when speaking English to native speakers is also experienced, when, as the students admit, their knowledge of the topic discussed is or may appear insufficient to the interactant. The feeling of embarrassment Pol. 'zakłopotanie, zażenowanie, zmieszanie' as a cluster member and manifestation of a social discomfort type of shame is generally reported to be more frequent in oral than written contexts in Polish.

The direct contacts with native peers are also perceived to reduce the students' sense of embarrassment and minimise their anxiety when they realise either that their essays were considered good and interesting by their American colleagues (as ex. in (7, 9, 10)) or else "the papers written by native speakers are not perfect" either [see also example (8)].

(7) The fact that the English of my essay was good enough to be accepted by English speakers was definitely assuring.

(8) I noticed that even native speakers make various mistakes, so I did not feel the pressure to be perfect all the time.

An important summary of the students' attitude can be given in (9):

(9) Are you more certain of your English now after this exchange?

Yes, it was nice to see that a native speaker enjoyed and appreciated my essay. Even though teachers' positive comments always make me feel better about my skills, it was especially great to hear such comments from a native speaker of English.

An observation which is worth stressing is the fact that the structure of corrective feedback seems to be governed by at least two conditioning factors. In the case of American students the cooperation involved college freshmen. At this level they are typically not yet used to carefully reading over their writing before submitting it. It is clear from some of their corrections that they were too timid to either introduce their own suggestions in their Polish partner's essays or were not assertive enough to retain their own original texts after some corrections were proposed from their NNS pairs.

21.3.1.3   The Role of *Face Work* and Politeness Strategies in Shame Moderation

Any external evaluation of one's own work is a threat to one's face (Goffman, 1967). In addition to the degree of evaluation privacy on shame moderation, another major influence is face work, which refers to all discourse and communicative strategies that deal with social prestige and personal pride, upholding one's face, face threat and face saving. Face-saving strategies are used in discourse to avoid one's own or the addressee's humiliation or embarrassment, to maintain one's dignity or preserve one's reputation. They all relate to the phenomenon of politeness.

Both the USA and Poland are characterised rather with what Brown and Levinson (1987) name 'positive politeness cultures' (contrary e.g., to the British 'negative politeness culture'), in which what counts is expressing oneself rather than not to impose one's own judgements on the interactant. However, American politeness is even more of a 'backslapping', smaller- social-distance, type than the Polish one. This is visible in the higher number of direct, friendly, strategies the American students employ in their critical comments on the Polish students' writing when juxtaposed to the Polish politeness practices in such cases. There is also another reason for a generally lower emotional arousal in the case of written email exchange, as it provides a context which is more conducive to a more descriptive, indirect metalinguistic rather than direct corrective recast strategy of corrective feedback.

As mentioned above, another possible feature that might exert an effect concerns the lower experience of the US students and their younger age. The US students are mostly freshmen, and hence they show lower assertiveness in their comments. Their corrections are typically conveyed by Indirect Speech Acts and preceded by friendly comments (ex. 10). The Polish students also try to stress some respect to their American pair's face. The Polish comments are typically of yes/no questions, which convey suggestions, by reference to authority (dictionaries/grammar books) rather than to the Polish authors' knowledge of their addressee's native language. Last but not least, the American students use a more informal, friendly style both in directly addressing their Polish pairs and in their text production, which is obviously an outcome of different routes for native as opposed to non-native (more formal in this case) language acquisition. Non-native speakers are also generally less sensitive to stylistic and register nuances in a foreign language.

The addressee-face-saving strategies on the other hand are observed both in the comments given by the Polish as well as the American students by their resorting to indirect corrections and conciliatory answers as in:

(10) NS commenting on NNS text:

> I think that this was a great beginning for you essay! Although after reading through it, I am still not 100% sure what the assignment was supposed to be on. Were you supposed to write about a specific character within a book? I think that it would help if you had an introductory paragraph that explained more what the paper was about instead of going right into the details of the character. It would help your readers understand better. Also, there are a couple paragraphs in which there should be a transition sentence so your reader isn't just jumping right into a scene. Describe what is happening before telling the reader. You have great detail within the paper which I really enjoyed reading!

(11) NNS to NS:

> NS text: Eating breakfast will make you feel more full throughout the day so you will not have to eat as much at your other meals.
>
> NNS comment: What do you think about writing 'fuller' instead of 'more full'?
>
> NS response: I'm not sure. I believe more full works well but I can also see fuller working too.

21.4 Conclusions

The significant moderation of shame in the scenario ratings in the first study pertaining to both the speaking and writing courses that provided a more private evaluation as opposed to a more public evaluation of L2 performance in the classroom context supports the hypotheses and is consistent with theories highlighting the salience of such public scrutiny in shame (e.g., Lewis, 1971). Consistent with this, the open-ended reports in the outside classroom speaking scenario specifically identified the beneficial effects of reduced observation and judgement, suggesting that they played a role in the lower shame ratings in this scenario. There was no evidence for tend-and-befriend in the group writing scenario.

The differing degrees of similarity in the first study between shame and fear, anxiety, anger and hopelessness demonstrate the complexity in the relationships between these emotions, which in this case appeared to be dependent on scenario type to some extent. Fear, anxiety and anger were all moderated in the outside classroom speaking scenario, albeit to a lesser extent than shame. In contrast, only shame was characterised as having an alleviating effect in the more private feedback associated with the individual writing scenario. It is not clear why anger had the opposite effect in this respect. However, shame, fear and anxiety were moderated to a similar degree in the hypothetical email feedback condition compared to the feedback in class condition, and this is consistent with the conclusions of the second study, thus highlighting the value of this relatively private mode of feedback in terms of minimising shame and other negative affective responses.

Additional assets demonstrated in more private, paired email contacts, involve the development of the students' higher self-assessment in language learning, the increase in their self-confidence and self-esteem, with the simultaneous respect to the interactants' pride and prestige (see also Monteiro, 2014). The rise in linguistic and communicative self-confidence can also be hypothesised to lead to lowering the level of the students' shame and fear. Collaborative communicative tasks, designed for a more private setting, can thus be considered one of the most effective strategies to reduce the emotional arousal of negative emotions in Foreign-Language-Teaching/Learning contexts.

The second study described in the present paper involved peer collaborative work between US NSs and Polish NNSs. Such pair work creates a context of privacy and encourages a more direct interaction between the students. The fact that both groups are university students, within the same age group, makes the interaction easier, in spite of a certain asymmetry between them with regard to the level of the (English) language proficiency. This context, as reported by the subjects, enhances the reduction in the students' shame and anxiety levels, originally linked to the exposure of their linguistic performance to the scrutiny of the native speakers of that language. A subsequent group discussion of these conditions and their effect on both the main learning objectives (developing higher writing/translation competences in English) and lowering the level of negative emotionality, particularly the shame and anxiety experienced by NNSs, makes the scenario a recommendable script (see 21.5.3) for the further use in classes of foreign language competence development.

21.5 Guidelines for Reducing Shame in the L2 Classroom

21.5.1 Speaking Lesson Scenario

Objectives:

1. Learning EFL objectives.

    - Presentation Scenario: Students will learn to present a 5–10 min oral presentation in good English to the other students and native English-speaking teacher in the class. Two of the students in the class and the teacher will provide feedback on the quality of spoken English. A grade will also be received from the teacher.
    - Exam Practice Scenario: Students will prepare for a forthcoming exam in which they will answer questions in good English with a fellow student in a 15-min practice exam in the class. Two other students will play the role of examiners. The student examiners and the native English-speaking teacher will give the student feedback. The teacher will also give the student examinees a grade.
    - General Speaking Scenario: Students will discuss a question orally in good English for 15 min. The teacher will give feedback and a grade to the students.

2. Emotionality component.

The aim is to reduce shame by reducing classroom exposure and scrutiny by following these guidelines:

- Presentation Scenario: Private, face-to-face feedback, or feedback via email.
- Exam Practice Scenario: Should be performed in the class without the presence of other students, or should be performed in small groups in the class simultaneously.
- General Speaking Scenario: Should be performed in small groups outside the classroom or in small groups in the class simultaneously.

Success criteria:

To meet the learning intentions students will:

- Speak English accurately, fluently, with good pronunciation, and with the use of good vocabulary.
- Decrease the sense of shame that can accompany their spoken English.

21.5.2   Writing Lesson Scenario

Objectives:

1. Learning EFL objectives.

    - Learn to write an effective, argumentative, academic piece of writing in good English.

2. Emotionality component.

The aim is to reduce shame by reducing classroom exposure and scrutiny by following these guidelines:

- Written work should not be presented and scrutinised in the public sphere of the classroom.
- Feedback should alternatively be provided in private in a face-to-face situation or via email.

Success criteria:

To meet the learning intentions students will:

- Write an academic piece of writing effectively and argumentatively in good English.
- Decrease the sense of shame that can accompany their written English.

21.5.3   Interactive NS-NNS Peer Writing Translation Scenario

Objectives:

1. Learning EFL objectives.

Learning to write compositions (argumentative essays—press-based and translations from Polish to English).

- Use of effective interactional exchanges with (native-speaker) peers.
- Familiarisation with authentic native speakers' writing and their weaknesses.
- Use of adequate writing corrective strategies in native students' (peers') essays.

2. Information Communication Technology (ICT) component.

- Complete a range of activities to become familiar with authentic English language (British National Corpus and Corpus Of Contemporary American) and corpus tools concordances, collocations, keywords.

- Students will familiarise themselves with a range of activities based on English-to-Polish and Polish-to-English parallel (translation) corpora.
- Students will use the corpus results in their own writing and in corrective exercises in their NS-NNS peer pairs.

3. Emotionality component.

- By regular peer-to-peer interaction decrease the level of negative emotionality, particularly with reference to shame and anxiety components, connected originally with presenting one's own language products to native speakers' scrutiny and judgement.

Success criteria:

To meet the learning objectives students will:

- Become regularly engaged in a cooperative exchange with NS peers from an English-speaking university.
- Complete a range of activities to achieve the learning EFL and ICT objectives.
- Familiarise themselves with the authentic language and style of the NS peers they are paired with.
- Be critical and use corrective strategies in their essays.
- Expose their own writing/translation essays to the NS peers' judgement and evaluation.
- Decrease the sense of shame and anxiety which students experience when they expose their own language production to NS's judgement.

Follow-up activities

- Students will share their thoughts and emotionality with the peers in their class and with the NS peers they are paired with.
- Students will contribute to a group discussion of their shame/anxiety/fear/helplessness/anger levels and the dynamics of these during the course of NS-NNS peer interaction.

References

Arnold, N., & Ducate, L. (2006). Future foreign language teachers' social and cognitive collaboration in an online environment. *Language Learning & Technology, 10*(1), 42–66.

Brown, P., & Levinson, S. C. (1987). *Politeness: Some universals in language usage*. Cambridge: Cambridge University Press.

Fontaine, J. R. J., Luyten, P., De Boeck, P., Corveleyn, J., Fernandez, M., Herrera, D., et al. (2006). Untying the Gordian Knot of guilt and shame: The structure of guilt and shame reactions based on situation and person variation in Belgium, Hungary, and Peru. *Journal of Cross-Cultural Psychology, 37*(3), 273–292.

Goffman, E. (1967). *Interaction ritual*. New York: Doubleday.

Krawczak, K. (2014). Shame, embarrassment and guilt: Corpus evidence for the cross-cultural structure of social emotions. *Poznań Studies in Contemporary Linguistics, 50*(4), 441–475.

Lewandowska-Tomaszczyk, B., & Slomski, H. (2016). Collaboration in language development between American and Polish university students. *Konin Language Studies, 4*(3), 305–330.

Lewis, H. B. (1971). Shame and guilt in neurosis. *Psychoanalytic Review, 58*(3), 419–438.

Maylath, B., Vandepitte, S., Minacori, P., Isohella, S., Mousten, B., & Humbley, J. (2013). Managing complexity: A technical communication translation case study in multilateral international collaboration. *Technical Communication Quarterly, 22,* 67–84.

McGregor, H. A., & Elliot, A. J. (2005). The shame of failure: Examining the Link between fear of failure and shame. *Personality and Social Psychology Bulletin, 31*(2), 218–231.

Misanchuk, M., & Anderson, T. (2001). Building community in an online learning environment: Communication, cooperation and collaboration, 22 p. In Proceedings of the Annual Mid-South Instructional Technology Conference (6th, Murfreesboro, TN, April 8–10, 2001).

Monteiro, K. (2014). Corrective feedback during video-conferencing. *Language Learning and Technology, 18*(3), 56–79.

Panova, I., & Lyster, R. (2002). Patterns of corrective feedback and uptake in an adult ESL classroom. *Tesol Quarterly, 36*(4), 572–595.

Tangney, J. P. (1990). Assessing individual differences in proneness to shame and guilt: Development of the Self-Conscious Affect and Attribution Inventory. *Journal of Personality and Social Psychology, 59*(1), 102–111.

Tangney, J. P. (1995). Shame and guilt in interpersonal relationships. In J. P. Tangney & K. W. Fischer (Eds.), *Self-conscious emotions: The psychology of shame, guilt, embarrassment, and pride* (pp. 114–139). New York: Guilford Press.

Tangney, J. P., Wagner, P., & Gramzow, R. (1992). Proneness to shame, proneness to guilt, and psychopathology. *Journal of Abnormal Psychology, 101,* 469–478.

Taylor, S. E., Klein, L. C., Lewis, B. P., Gruenewald, T. L., Gurung, R. A. R., & Updegraff, J. A. (2000). Biobehavioral responses to stress in females: Tend-and-befriend, not fight-or-flight. *Psychological Review, 107*(3), 411–429.

Tracy, J. L., & Robins, R. W. (2006). Appraisal antecedents of shame and guilt: Support for a theoretical model. *Personality and Social Psychology Bulletin, 32*(10), 1339–1351.

Wilson, P. A. (2016). Shame and collaborative learning in L2 classes. *Konin Language Studies, 4*(3), 235–252.

Paul A. Wilson (Ph.D.) holds the post of professor in the Department of English Language and Applied Linguistics at the University of Lodz, Poland. He completed his Ph.D. on the interplay between cognition and emotion at Birkbeck (University of London) in 2000. His main research interests include the conceptual representation of emotions from a cross-cultural perspective. More recently he has focused on the role of shame in educational and conflict contexts.

Barbara Lewandowska-Tomaszczyk, (Dr. habil.) Full Professor of English and Applied Linguistics at the State University of Applied Sciences in Konin, Po-land; Head of the Department of Research in Language, Literature and Translation in Konin, for many years served as head of the Department of English Language and Applied Linguistics at the University of Lodz. Author and editor of numerous books and papers in cognitive and corpus linguistics, emotion studies and translation, invited to read papers at conferences and give workshops at European, American and Asian universities.

Chapter 22
Transforming Shame in the German Educational System Using the Team Ombuds Model

Christian Martin Boness

Abstract In a majority of European countries, educational staff and systems are insufficiently prepared to deal with students from non-European cultures. The team ombuds model—inspired mostly by Scandinavian experiences—can serve as a macro-didactic concept to assist with the integration of students from different cultural orientations. Shame is often evident in learners from collectivistic cultures who easily feel shame when linked to a loss of face in the social system of the new culture. This model offers a range of facilities to help learners express themselves concerning assessments, marks, attendance during lessons, and not least, with intercultural mediation and conflict management through the ombud function. The use of this function is illustrated in the example of a migrant Chinese girl of 16 years who attends German college (Grade 11) and struggles with shame in three ways. First, in terms of language, she is shy to speak using incorrect language patterns. Second, in communication, she feels shame if required to speak directly to the teacher as representative of the educational hierarchy, and even to speak in front of her fellow learners. Third, she is inhibited in political expression because in her country of origin, political interest and expression are a matter of conformity, not of democratic discussion. By applying the team ombuds model and its implicit didactic methods, she gradually loses her shame and successfully catches up with her classmates.

Keywords Learner · Teacher · Team · Ombud · Shame · Transformation

22.1 Introduction

The majority of countries in contemporary Europe, including Germany, continue to maintain old-fashioned subject-bound curricula in their education systems. The longer a school system keeps strict subject structures and curricula in place, including the repeating of years, the more harmful it becomes to learners' chances of academic success. Furthermore, learners are likely to drop out more easily, especially if they

C. M. Boness (✉)
Göttingen, Germany
e-mail: christianboness@gmx.net

© Springer Nature Switzerland AG 2019
C.-H. Mayer and E. Vanderheiden (eds.), *The Bright Side of Shame*,
https://doi.org/10.1007/978-3-030-13409-9_22

come from disadvantaged backgrounds or ethnic minorities (Education Endowment Foundation, 2018). This situation often results in negative feelings for learners, such as anxiety (OECD, 2016), shame and fear. Generally learners do not easily cope with their shame, embarrassment and guilt feelings (Vanderheiden & Mayer, 2017, 8–23).

Educational psychologist Kurt Singer describes the situation in the school system as often humiliating and mortifying for both learners and teachers (Singer, 2000). Haas emphasises the need for teaching staff to learn about shame and its triggers (Haas, 2011). Although schools can also promote mental health if there are supportive teacher-learner relations and opportunities for self-directed learning, currently the teaching and learning activities in schools are burdened with pathological shame and embarrassment. There is a great need to move forward into a culture of mutual respect and recognition (Marks, 2005, 2013).

Recently, shame psychologists have been gradually moving from a toxic to a health-related concept of shame (Vanderheiden & Mayer, 2017, 5–8; Mayer, 2017). The protective value of shame has even been described as a guardian of dignity (Wurmser, 2010) that regulates proximity and distance by giving shelter to the self. Is there a way to transform learners' feelings of shame into positive feelings of joy and self-actualisation? Marks (2005) points out that, in comparison to the German school system, teachers in Finland are highly esteemed and valued. Finnish learners perform well in the PISA studies global rankings. According to these rankings, they score highly in *well-being* (for example in the subcategory of *life satisfaction*) while their *schoolwork-related anxiety* shows low scores (OECD, 2016).

Because Germany's educational expenditure is similar to Finland's, it appears that the aim of achieving a culture of life satisfaction, recognition and self-actualisation in German schools is not a matter of finances. *Phenomenon-based learning* was introduced mandatorily to the Finnish school system in 2016 (Finnish National Agency for Education, 2016), which demonstrates how the first country in the world experiences holistic learning. This kind of learning places the focus on an important topic, replacing pure subject-orientated learning that might disenable learners from meeting societal challenges appropriately (Brown, 2017). Inspired by Scandinavian school systems that avoid repeating years, and use *teamwork facilities* including those for learners with special needs, the *team ombuds model (tOm)* has been developed.

22.2 Theoretical Background of the Team Ombuds Model (tOm)

Since the early 1970s there has been discussion about the educational implications of modern psychological approaches. Beyond widespread psychologies, both the psychoanalytic approach by the Freudians and the cognitive behavioural-psychological approach in line with Skinner have been widely accepted in Western pedagogical settings. However, humanistic psychology seems to offer a third way of providing keys to develop self-actualisation in individuals of diverse cultures. The main assumption

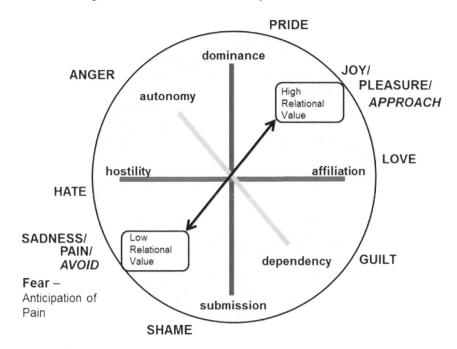

Fig. 22.1 The influence matrix. *Source* Henriques (2011)

of a positive psychology is the belief that individuals can learn to develop a stable and balanced identity if nurtured in an adequate educational environment (Vanderheiden & Mayer, 2017, 3–5).

Carl Rogers suggests that if teachers provide a "student-centered" education, it might show that teachers' "empathy, unconditional positive regard, congruence and their facilitative behaviors are associated with positive outcomes" (Rogers, Lyon, & Tausch 2013: xix). According to humanistic psychology, learning happens through cognition, feelings and (self-)experiment, in other words, in a holistic way. The good life is a process, not a state of being. It is a direction rather than a destination (Rogers, 1961).

The influence matrix, developed by Henriques (2011), plays a major role in the theoretical background of the tOm. Mainly based on Schwartz's value theory (Schwartz, 1994), Henriques constructs an influence matrix showing processes of motivational learning which can be connected to the tOm (see Fig. 22.1).

In this matrix map, motivational learning—roughly expressed—moves from low relational values to high relational values, from hostility to affiliation, from submission to dominance, from dependency to autonomy. The behaviours, feelings and beliefs of learners that are attributed to this map of motivational learning arise from observations and validations from participative work in educational environments over a longitudinal observation period of 40 years by Henriques (in press). It is evident that learners can feel shame in school contexts connected with their bodily appearance, with being blamed in front of the class, having to repeat a year, failing assessments and with exclusion from groups.

According to the matrix map, there is a *central variable* indicating *low relational value* vs. *high relational value* that is responsible for human relational processes. Migrants often are in a process of approaching low relational values because they are without their safe, familiar cultural environment. Negative personal values connected to low relational values are probably shame or even hate, sadness and feeling pain.

When living in an environment that represents significantly different cultural features from their own, learners often cannot cope easily with competitive influences of their Western host culture, and thus presumably on the dimension *submission versus dominance*, they move towards the negative pole of submission. Additionally, on the process dimension of *hostility versus affiliation*, they painfully feel the loss of cooperative influence and participation because they cannot communicate their own needs to affiliate with their fellow students. Furthermore, they cannot show appreciation and friendliness to the other learners, who usually do not warm to fellow students who cannot speak their language or reach the standards of their learners' social group. Learners can feel hate, fear or shame resulting from their social situation. Migrants are likely to feel dependent on each and every thing that is presented and offered by the host culture and its educational system. The movement towards gaining a higher degree of autonomy is usually restrained by inner and outer barriers in this third dimension of *dependency versus autonomy.* Applying the tOm might be a possible way to transform shame into something positive. The tOm offers a range of facilities, tools and methods to learners of different backgrounds to help minimise the disadvantages of the current school system in terms of traumatic shame and embarrassment, and optimise growth processes of individuals in terms of self-actualisation and success. Learners who visit schools that already have introduced the tOm can express themselves much more easily regarding assessments, attendance during lessons, participation processes and in situations of intercultural mediation and conflict management.

22.3   Working with the Team Ombuds Model (tOm) in Schools

The tOm has been in use since the 1990s in a wide range of school systems, especially in Germany. Results of PISA assessments (OECD, 2016) show that German students perform below the average in industrialised countries, especially in Mathematics, English and the sciences. Disadvantaged students with foreign backgrounds make up the bulk of students who drop out of school. Beside other models, the tOm has gained significant acknowledgement (Boness, Hoffmann, & Koch 2003; Krause & Mayer, 2010; Mayer & Vanderheiden, 2014). As a result, it can be shown that the tOm not only contributes to the development of learning competencies but also to the improvement of well-being and consequently to the motivational and volitional attitude of learners (Krause & Mayer, 2010).

The tOm begins with the mental outlook of the teachers. Only if the messages of the tOm reach the teaching staff and affect communication patterns, can curricula be altered to better comply with the challenges of contemporary education.

In terms of the daily routine in the educational system, working with the tOm means organising teaching and learning in a different way. The tOm accepts the norms and prescripts of necessary restraints, but supports autonomy and freedom of the individual and groups, following the ideas and goals of humanistic education. This model has the following characteristics:

- Stimuli are given to learners through positive reinforcement rather than through disciplinary school orders. Positive reinforcement can help to minimise disappointment in learners, and expose and clear superfluous feelings of shame.
- Communication structures are altered so that flat hierarchies can develop; the autocratic top-down teaching approach is left behind, giving way to a horizontal network of communication clusters. Learner teams are introduced to supportive peer communication on an equal base. Peers then more easily accept engagement with classmates; the danger of ostracism is thus minimised. The shame associated with language incompetency can be tackled more easily in this way than in front of the whole class.
- Lecture-style instruction becomes the exception rather than the rule; it must be carefully used. This results in more space for learning in learner teams, and more time for development of individual learner performance.
- Learning happens mainly in learner teams where students experience their own team building and team management, shaping an effective learning unit without discrimination. Personal skills, talents and responsibilities are developed to a higher degree than in class settings. Peer learner groups are likely to unlock shame feelings that hinder learners.

The five cornerstones of tOm are five different roles with different tasks and activities that contribute to unlocking learners' talents and desires to participate. The learner teams, the "ombud", the "postmaster", the teacher–facilitator and the individual learners shape and stabilise the network that keeps the tOm running.

22.3.1 Learner Teams

On average, a class of learners is made up of about 20 to 30 students. This collective learner group is divided into five or six learner teams. The tOm is based on intercultural learner teams of between three to seven students. The learner teams are created in terms of mutual attraction, so that peers with most "likes" are chosen to be in the same team. Teams have a high internal level of communication based on mutual respect and esteem. A sense of group intimacy arises, avoiding humiliation by teachers, bullying by classmates and other negative activities. Learner teams function as protective shields for shy learners. Usually the gender question is unimportant; teams are all female, all male or of both sexes. The emotional acceptance and prevailing "good vibrations" within learners' teams are the pre-condition to shaping a motivating learning environment.

If classes have a multi-ethnic structure, it is recommended that learner teams consist of members of different backgrounds. If there are outsiders, the teacher helps to connect them to a learning group that is open to "foreign" learners. The in-group and out-group issue then must be discussed in a sensitive way to avoid shame feelings. The teacher, whenever needed, supports the teams. Teams are also given a maximum of free time and space in order to work effectively. Rewards for cooperation and commitment are granted to each member of a learner team.

22.3.2   Ombuds

Ombuds are persons who are entitled to mediate between the teacher and learner teams. They play an important role in the social framework of the learner teams in balancing out opposing interests. Ombuds are supposed to bear a major responsibility for other individual learners who do not easily cope with responsibility, or who perceive it as a burden. That is the reason why ombuds are elected—not by formal procedures but by consensus of the team. Ombuds love to take responsibility for the learner team and for every single member of the team. Ombuds are highly esteemed; they are culture-sensitive and support inclusion of members with different backgrounds. They are pro-active stewards of the team in that they are the speakers of the learner team "parliament". They receive complaints, requests and petitions of the fellow learners and pass these on to the teacher. Ombuds support team members, especially those who are blocked by feelings of distress or disgrace, to implement the assignments and assessments as effectively as possible. Ombuds can—not must—report at their own discretion to the teacher.

22.3.3   Postmasters

Many learners enjoy doing official duties, especially if these duties involve digital communication and using their laptops, tablets or other devices. Postmasters are real cornerstones of the entire tOm, because they like to do their job. Postmasters are supportive to learner teams, learners and teachers in formatting and arranging the dropbox and mailbox for the entire class. These boxes collect all relevant data and documents that are produced by the learners during a term. Postmasters save and control the credit point rewards and assessments of learners and their teams. If there are differences between the teacher and teams, postmasters present the relevant documents that are collected in the mailboxes. This can lead to a solution of conflictive issues between learner and teacher.

It has been observed that learners from other backgrounds need and demand the postmasters' support more than other learners. It is also evident that postmasters who do not perform best in language can show their technical skills and be rewarded for their commitment. Postmasters experience their role in a diverse setting as being a contributor to inclusion and integration.

22.3.4   Teachers

In accordance with ideas of positive psychology, teachers redefine their traditional roles and take on new roles and duties that fall under the headings of learner-centred teaching, learner team-building, moderation, cooperation, coaching, mediation and interpersonal conflict management, didactic and professional expertise, and general responsibility.

The teachers' role is no longer characterised by chalk-and-talk teaching, but by facilitating learners' success. Learning by doing is advocated, and learning through intramural and extramural projects is supported by the tOm. The new structure of teaching and learning is far more embedded in flat hierarchies than in traditional settings of perpendicular hierarchies. Teachers gain space and time to tackle situations in which learners who need support can be approached more easily. Intimate feelings that cannot be discussed publicly in front of the class, like shame, disappointment, even hate and aggression can be addressed more easily in a private communication setting.

22.3.5   Individual Learners

In turn, individual learners are much more responsible for their own learning progress than before when they laid responsibility for all their concerns on the teachers. Now there are postmasters and ombuds who can be relied upon. As a result, they learn to be more team-orientated. Individual learners can also learn more independently because they are less dependent on the reinforcements of the teaching staff. They have more space and time to communicate with fellow students of different backgrounds. The learner teams do not feel over-controlled by the teachers and feel comfortable in a cosy team atmosphere that makes it possible to talk about emotions, even shame and fear. It seldom happens that individual learners refuse to join learner teams. In these circumstances, the choice of individual learners must be accepted, but not rewarded.

The majority of learners want to get rewards from the teacher for learning. But sometimes learners fail to pass the assessments or fail to actively take part in class. Mistakes can occur and create misunderstanding and disappointments, and in the worst case, learners have to repeat a year. Repeating a year appears to be a major source of shame for learners. The basic need for social belonging can scarcely be satisfied if repeating a year and losing friends. The credit point system is institutionalised in the tOm to avoid the sense of failure of "not passed". The **credit point system** adds chances for the silent majority of a class, for the girls who are too shy to communicate clearly, for the learners of other ethnicities who are not yet familiar with the language of instruction, and so on.

22.3.6 Credit Point System

The credit point system is based on documented efforts in **five categories** that are each rewarded by one credit point. Documents can also be written in English or in a language that is translatable by the teams and thereby understandable. Authors of written English documents are not forced to express themselves in German. They are given space and time to reduce their competence-shame at not performing like their classmates. This can also be a contribution to building awareness of other languages and cultures. The categories are detailed below.

1. In order to be rewarded with one credit point, learners are required to write **five reports** of different lessons. Individual learners can even submit drawings, designs or other creative products to explain their understanding of the content of the lessons. This particularly helps migrants to cope with the challenges of daily instruction in schools. They are given the chance to contribute something important without feeling shame or fear of the criticism of their fellow learners and educational staff.
2. To take special talents and interests of a learner into account, the learner can produce a **voluntary contribution** connected to the subject in any form. This tool of voluntary contribution often reveals unknown interests, talents and preferences of an individual learner, which can draw the appreciation of classmates when the voluntary contribution is presented. This kind of activity is rewarded with one credit point.
3. All learners are required to produce a proposal or part of a **slideshow presentation (SSP)**. The learners can do so individually or by cooperating as an entire learner team. Such a proposal shows the quality of learning progress of the team regarding their subject. Additionally it provides information about how the single learners have performed in the eyes of their own team. Every individual learner can contribute to the SSP more or less according to his or her prerogatives. Having finalised an SSP, learners who have actively taken part in the process of producing an SSP are rewarded one credit point, regardless of the standard of their contribution.
4. During the SSP, the coming out of one individual learner or a learner team standing in front of the class is a challenge, especially for shy or shameful learners. They have to overcome shame and fear while **presenting** an SSP. These activities are rewarded with one credit point, regardless of who needs less or more time presenting in front of the class. This kind of equal treatment protects learners who are in the process of learning how to present a subject properly, for example

migrants who cannot yet present an SSP because they are ashamed to show their shortcomings in the language of instruction.

5. Every individual learner needs to create a **portfolio**, a kind of diary that encompasses notes, pictures and graphs in written or visual form. Learners from different backgrounds also can make drawings that indicate issues of concern connected to the subject of that lesson. The opportunities give space to learners with culture-specific characteristics that support iconographic learning. The teacher rewards every learner's portfolio with one credit point.

The credit point system enables every learner to collect rewards of five credit points in total. Having collected them in a transparent process of assessment, learners are guaranteed not to underperform or fail in the final assessment of a term. The credit point system is an excellent tool to encourage learners who are disappointed and disgraced, or who feel humiliated by the current education system which gives poor marks and grading.

For some individual learners there is an opportunity to add one credit point reward to the five explained above, by working as ombuds or postmasters. Learners who are chosen as **ombuds** for a certain time can earn one credit point for having taken clear social responsibility on behalf of their learner teams. Learners who want to show their abilities to lead a group often strive for ombud positions. But the high requirements of the ombud position force the ombud to take care of all individual learners, whether they are weak or strong. The learners who are chosen as **postmasters** work with digital tools and earn a reward of one credit point for their technical support, and for the assistance they give to the teacher.

22.3.7 Didactic Circles for Fair Judgments

The final assessment of comprehensive performance of each individual learner is conducted in "didactic circles" that consist of a learner team including the ombuds, the postmaster and the teacher. Experiences show that this composition of assessment teams significantly lowers stress, shame and fear for the individual learner, in contrast to asymmetric relationships that obviously predominate in single teacher—multiple learner communications. Negative psychosomatic effects can be minimised, because learners from different backgrounds can be supported by their fellow learners or the ombud, or even by the postmaster.

The tOm evidently offers strong tools, positions and communication structures for supporting individual learners of different backgrounds, languages and ethnicities. The model is transparent and flexible and helps learners to cope with challenges of the school system and the host culture, effectively reducing the individual learner's feelings of shame, distress and disgrace. A summary of the tools and functions of the tOm with regard to healing shame is provided in Table 22.1.

Table. 22.1 The tOm tools and main functions. *Source* Author's own construction

tOm tool	Functions in coping with shame
Learner team	Protects and encourages shy learners
Ombud	Helps distressed learners to overcome shame
Postmaster	Supports inclusion and integration technically/digitally
Teacher	Facilitates learner-centred teaching/counselling
Credit points	Positively reinforce learners through rewards
Didactic circle	Contributes maximum of transparency for learners' assessments

The case of Li is now presented to show transformation processes from toxic shame and fear to more joy and self-esteem (Henrique, 2011) through the application of tOm tools.

22.4   The Case of Li

A 16-year-old girl named Li, who was born and grew up in China, migrates with her academic parents to a small university town in the Bundesland of Lower Saxony, Germany. She is enrolled in Grade 11 of a UNESCO secondary school at college level. She speaks some English, but not German—the language of instruction. At school, Li is silent. At the end of a lesson on the subject of Politics and Economy, the class teacher asks about her comprehension and well-being in the class. She responds in English, whispering in a low voice that she has no clue at all. Li does not yet know where she belongs. She behaves in a very shy manner and seems to feel shame. Li never participates actively during periods as other learners do.

The teacher then suggests that Li joins a learner team of her choice. But she is hesitant, and asks the teacher to decide for her. During the working periods, the ombud of the team calls the teacher to help with the integration of Li into the complex situation of group-learning. They agree that Li should be given time and space to adjust. They observe that Li enjoys drawing or copying whatever she thinks is of interest.

At the end of each Politics and Economy lesson, the teacher exchanges ideas with Li about her learning process, good feelings and well-being. After one month, Li presents a calligraphic opus to the teacher—her personal portfolio—containing drawings of Chinese icons, and information about Chinese celebrations. This is all written in English; not one word is in German.

The teacher and learners within her learner team discuss the very special circumstances of Li's attendance at school. There are many lively questions about Li's background, her stay in town and what she aims to do. The whole learner team is able to speak English, apart from one learner who remarks that this is a German school, not an English school. But this remark is not echoed by anyone else in the team, and they continue with their work on the subject of the lesson. After six weeks Li offers to contribute a topic on Chinese public holidays and the meaning of these in China.

Li fails the first class test but passes the subsequent one, using the correct terms. She demonstrates her cognitive intelligence with some understanding, although with many gaps. When the teacher asks her how she managed to pass the second test, Li responds that in the night hours she would read the handouts of the learning teams and learn all phrases by heart, admitting that she does not understand the meaning of many of the terms yet.

Li seems to feel comfortable in her learner team. She produces five reports about selected subjects as expected, using drawings, English comments, and later on some German terms. She also works through and understands the notes on the blackboard. While her fellow learners present an SSP on their topic of "civil participation in political decision processes", she stands smiling but silent, with her team in front of the class. Li then delivers a special contribution about Chinese holidays. Obviously her shame feelings have diminished and she feels at ease. She feels proud to have gained five credit points, as have many other individual learners in class.

The end of the six-month term approaches and the didactic circle meets. Li's learner team conclude that Li has passed and achieved the main goals of the subject Politics and Economy. Her scoring shows first, an individual development in learning from level zero to a medium level of understanding and language performance. Second, it indicates that Li has enriched her learner team with a great deal of information about her background in China, and additionally has helped her team in taking on some tasks to produce the SSP, although she did not say a word during the presentation itself.

Teacher, postmaster and ombud all confirm Li's final performance assessments, full of confidence, surprise and acknowledgement. Clearly, Li's feelings of shame that were predominant in the beginning of her attendance at school, have gradually given way to joy and a little pride.

As soon as the information about Li's performance is released, there is much discussions in class. Some learners complain that she never gives any oral contribution and so cannot get a "passed" score. Furthermore, everybody knows that she failed her first class test. A majority of learners do not understand how Li manages to get along and continue in class. Members of Li's learner team respond by explaining patiently what they have gained from Li's presence in their team: discovering that a Chinese learner, according to culture, is supposed to be silent in class until asked by the teacher; that what constitutes a "good performance" in China is to recite prescribed passages rather than to criticise an issue; that performance is built more on collective congruence and less on individual performance. The postmaster and the ombud then inform the class that Li has been rewarded with a total of five credit points, and therefore has passed.

This outcome of her first term in a German school triggers joy and happiness in Li. She is proud to have caught up a great deal. Belonging to her learner team and the commitment of having given a valuable contribution to the fellow learners in her Grade 11 class makes her self-confident and happy.

22.5 Conclusions

It is assumed that Li has been brought up in a Chinese cultural context with a distinct social distance maintained from teachers or other authorities. She has been socialised in a culture of collective activities with less emphasis on individualism. Li loves celebrations, but her emotions of joy or hate are carefully controlled. Her basic need of belonging to a certain social group is finally met when she is welcomed in the learner team.

In the German school, Li is confronted with three aspects of shame, discussed below.

1. Li struggles with language: she is a shy girl and fears to speak using incorrect language patterns. She anticipates painful feelings being negatively reinforced by teachers and German learners. As a result she is distressed and keeps quiet. But under the protection of her learner team, she begins to unfold her talents in drawing and design. She is given space and time to show her mastery of shape, colour and structure through her creative products. Additionally she receives intensive language support from the team. A transformation process in Li's motivational behaviour could be observed on the move towards a higher relational value (Henrique, 2011).
2. Li struggles with culture differences: she feels ashamed to speak directly to the teacher as representative of the educational hierarchy, or even to speak in front of her fellow students. Li has to cope with and transform this difference by learning in a team with her "egalitarian" peers. She experiences her peers as more relaxed and open, and adjusts her role from a silent learner towards becoming a cooperating learner. Moreover, she moves towards affiliation and social esteem. She can feel proud of herself for delivering helpful assistance to her learner group.
3. Li grapples with the subject of political science: in her country of origin, China, politics is a matter of conformity, not of democratic discussion. Although in Germany a critical attitude towards society and political parties is highly valued, Li stays with her Chinese background which requires a traditional and conforming attitude regarding society and a one-party system. However, she receives a reward for copying and learning about the political system in Germany successfully.

It can be observed how Li's original shame and fear complex transforms from a negatively experienced emotion into positive mental health. At the end of the term, Li seems to have won peers as reliable partners or even friends. In comparison to the original situation at the start of the process, her need for belonging is being met, as is her need to be esteemed by her fellow learners and teachers. Learning in a team that protects and supports her, fulfils her need for safety.

Li's personality settles into more relaxed and happy patterns, showing the progress she has made from self-relatedness to other-relatedness. And this phenomenon can be considered as one more step to her self-actualisation. Her growth potential has been unlocked through application of the tOm in terms of her team members, the ombud, postmaster and last but not least, the teacher. Additionally the credit point system and the didactic circle have given her a feeling of success, acceptance and pride.

Li is likely to continue positively with her cognitive and emotional development and in activating mental health resources, provided that her learning conditions and personal environment offer support in future years at her secondary school in Germany.

References

Boness, C., Hoffmann, A., & Koch, K. (2003). Das Team-Ombuds-Modell. Eine Antwort auf fehlende Standards und divergente Erwartungen bei schulpraktischen Studien. *Die Deutsche Schule, 2,* 220–231.

Brown, K. (2017). *Finland to become the first country in the world to get rid of all school subjects.* Retrieved February 10, 2018, from http://www.collective-evolution.com/2017/04/04/finland-to-become-the-first-country-in-the-world-to-get-rid-of-all-school-subjects/.

Education Endowment Foundation. (2018). *Repeating a year,* Department for Education, London. Retrieved February 27, 2018, from https://educationendowmentfoundation.org.uk/evidence-summaries/teaching-learning-toolkit/repeating-a-year.

Finnish National Agency for Education. (2016). *Curriculum reform 2016.* Retrieved February 28, 2018, from http://www.oph.fi/english/education_development/current_reforms/curriculum_reform_2016.

Haas, D. (2011). Roter Kopf – gesenkter Blick. Was Lehrkräfte über Scham wissen sollten. *Zeitschrift für Religionspädagogik, 10*(H.2), 109–115.

Henriques, G. (2011). A new unified theory of psychology. *The influence matrix* (pp. 81–95). New York: Springer. ISBN 978-1-4614-0057-8.

Krause, C., & Mayer, C.-H. (2010). *Salutogenese und interkulturelle Gesundheitspädagogik.* Universität Göttingen, unpubliziertes Dokument.

Marks, S. (2005). Von der Beschämung zur Anerkennung. *Bildung und Wissenschaft, 10,* 6.

Marks, S. (2013). Scham im Kontext von Schule. *Soziale Passagen, 5*(1), 37–49.

Mayer, C.-H. (2017). Shame—"a soul feeding emotion": Archetypal work and the transformation of the shadow of shame in a group development process. In E. Vanderheiden & C.-H. Mayer (Eds.) (2016). *The value of shame—exploring a health resource in cultural contexts* (pp. 277–302). Cham, Switzerland: Springer.

Mayer, C.-H., & Vanderheiden, E. (2014). *Handbuch interkulturelle Öffnung.* Göttingen: Vandenhoeck & Rupprecht.

OECD (2016). PISA ranking. Retrieved February 25, 2018, from http://www.oecd.org/pisa/pisa-2015-finland.htm.

Rogers, C. (1961). *On becoming a person: A therapist's view of psychotherapy.* Excerpts. London: Constable.

Rogers, C. R., Lyon, H. C., & Tausch, R. (2013). *On becoming an effective teacher—person-centered teaching, psychology, philosophy, and dialogues with Carl R. Rogers and Harold Lyon.* London: Routledge.

Singer, K. (2000). *Wenn Schule krank macht.* Weinheim: Beltz Taschenbuch.

Schwartz, S. H. (1994). Are there universal aspects in the content and structure of values? *Journal of Social Issues, 50*, 19–45. Retrieved from http://dx.doi.org/10.1111/j.1540-4560.1994.tb01196.x.
Vanderheiden, E., & Mayer, C. (Eds.). (2017). *The value of shame. exploring a health resource in cultural contexts*. York: Springer. ISBN 978-3-319-53100-7.
Wurmser, L. (2010). *Die Maske der Scham*. Eschborn/Frankfurt, M: Klotz.

Christian Martin Boness (Dr. disc. pol.) Dipl. Theology, M.A. Education, Dr. disc.pol. with focus in intercultural didactics (Georg-August-University, Göttingen, Germany). He has been working as a teacher in high schools in Germany for about 30 years and has spent several years in Tanzania, working as a missionary and students pastor. Since two decades he works in international management consultancy. He has conducted various international research projects on transcultural conflicts and mediation in East Africa and is author of several books and articles on intercultural research in African contexts.

Part VII
Transforming Shame in Medical Contexts

Chapter 23
Dealing with Shame in a Medical Context

Iris Veit and Kay Spiekermann

Abstract Shame is an exceedingly important social feeling that has not adequately been incorporated in the pre-and post-qualification training of doctors. Shame in health-care settings is something experienced by patients and doctors alike. In medical institutions personal privacy of patients is restricted. The questions the doctor asks about the patient's private life while taking the medical history can be humiliating for the patient as indeed can the feelings of helplessness and inadequacy which often accompany the state of being ill. Getting undressed and being examined can make the patient feel ashamed, particularly in the case of invasive internal examinations. Diseases and their treatment may cause shame especially when they mar the patient's physical appearance and/or carry a social stigma. Doctors too may undergo shame, notably when they make mistakes or near misses. Feelings of humiliation can also arise when boundaries are violated by patients behaving over-familiarly or coquettishly. And it is also demeaning when one's professional competence is questioned by patients and colleagues. A sensitive and cooperative demeanour, particularly during the physiological examination, is an important skill for medical practitioners. In essence, doctors should always treat their patients respectfully, mindful of their feelings and trying to avoid subjecting them to embarrassment. Doctors have to find a way of being honest with their patients without their losing face. The verbal interventions which are helpful when dealing with feelings of shame are listed. Special emphasis should be placed on pre-empting shame by specifically addressing it beforehand, as well as on counselling techniques which involve creating a degree of detachment by putting unwelcome words into a third person's mouth. To ensure empathetic interaction in the patient-doctor relationship the latter should include the sense of shame in their self-reflection and introspection.

Keywords Shame · Patient · Medical practioner · Personal privacy and dignity · Physical examination · Dealing with errors

I. Veit (✉)
Bahnhofstr. 204, 44629 Herne, Germany
e-mail: info@irisveit.de

K. Spiekermann
Schürmesweg 16, 47802 Krefeld, Germany
e-mail: kaysp@web.de

© Springer Nature Switzerland AG 2019   349
C.-H. Mayer and E. Vanderheiden (eds.), *The Bright Side of Shame*,
https://doi.org/10.1007/978-3-030-13409-9_23

23.1   Shame in the Context of Medical Practice—Theoretical, Psychodynamic Reflections

Shame is a social emotion. The word social in this connection means that it impacts on people's relationships to one another. Shame has this capacity because it is intrinsic to the process of individuation. It arises, when a person's self-image is threatened, when one's personal space is invaded or when one's very essence meets with public rejection. A sense of shame helps to ensure that social values and norms are followed. Humiliation incurs such a disagreeable physical response that abiding by social rules is preferable to dealing with the ramifications of not doing so. An example of this is given by the philosopher Spinoza, who cites that the vogue of that time for young girls to commit suicide came to an end when it was announced that the bodies of such girls would be put on public display (Spinoza, 1986).

The gestures and facial expressions which are associated with feelings of shame such as averting one's eyes, making oneself smaller as well as blushing seem to be familiar to every culture (Ekmann, 2006). This is an indication that these physiological reactions follow a phylogenetic pattern. Gestures and facial expressions of this kind are also seen in the work of Michelangelo, the Expulsion from Paradise. This is a masterpiece which makes the connection between shame and individuation. The story of the expulsion from paradise is an important metaphor which helps us to understand that the knowledge of good and evil, in other words understanding the norms of social interaction, and **the development of the self and self-identity are all connected with shame**. The message of this metaphor is backed up by findings made by developmental psychology and by psychoanalysis. The development of self requires the presence and participation of others—especially from the perspective and in the mirror image of his or her former attachment figures—from a bodily based core self onto a subjective self and then further on to a self capable of verbal expression (Stern, 2016). This view is supported by Grossmann's Infant Observation as well as by Thorton's Still Face Experiment (Grossmann & Grossmann, 2007, 2009). The more sensitively the attachment figure reacts to the baby's signals and mirrors them, and the stronger the flow of this exchange of signals is, and the more harmonious this "communicative dance" (Buch, in this book) between the two develops, the more inherently confident, self-assured and inquisitive the child will become. Ideally the child will come to the conviction, "I am acknowledged, I am worthy, other people value me too." Subject to the strength of this confidence the individual's roles in the family will eventually shift and self-perceptions of identity will form, including those which are related to gender.

The formation of stable self-esteem can be disrupted and feelings of shame arise. This can happen when, for example, a parent suffers from some kind of addiction or another serious psychiatric illness or was himself traumatised in childhood. Such parents are then not able to react adequately to the needs of the child, their demeanour changing from friendly to impersonal at random. One minute they overwhelm the child with teary affection, only to lash out again at the next. The attachment figure's behaviour finally becomes unpredictable for the child. Sometimes there is only a single parent who may then misuse the child as an emotional crutch. Sometimes attachment figures are perpetrators who traumatise the child physically and sexually. Then the consequences are more profound and affect the child's physical core self as well (Egloff, Bischoff, Kipfer, Studer, & Holtforth, 2016).

The spectrum of feelings of shame range from shame for not being seen or acknowledged adequately to the shame of even being someone who has no identity at all.

Shame takes place in the eye of the beholder (Sartre, 1943). The earlier adequate mirroring communication is hampered, the more far-reaching the consequences for the development of the self will be, the later in life relationships with other people will also suffer. In what ways can the person concerned react to the described disturbance in the self-development? One possibility is to make oneself grander than one actually feels and develop an idealized self-image, in other words to put on the **mask of grandiosity** (Kernberg, 1988; Wurmser, 2007). Such an individual will in later life remain especially sensitive to being slighted and will feel more shame than others when their idealized self-image is damaged. Changes in one's physical looks due to illness or age can cause shame as indeed can simply being ill. Recommendations on changes in lifestyle may be interpreted as reproaches. Feelings of unworthiness are brought on by lack of recognition and appreciation at work or by a separation from a significant attachment figure. Situations like these can bring on a life crisis marked by feelings of shame and even precipitate suicide.

23.1.1 The Context of This Chapter

Thus doctors will encounter patients who have a damaged self to a lesser or to a greater extent and so some patients will become more embarrassed or feel humiliated sooner than others. This is the author´s experience after 30 years working as a general practitioner in Germany, as a leader of Balint-groups for more than 20 years, as a teacher of nurses and medical students and a teacher for basic psychosomatic skills called Psychosomatische Grundversorgung in Germany (Veit, 2018). All the later described cases are real patients she met in her own office. The verbal interventions results from videotaped interaction with patients and their discussion with other medical practitioners. There is a lack of research concerning the emotion of shame in a medical context. This statement is combined with the hope, that this book might lead to further research.

23.2   Shame of the Patient

23.2.1   Sparing the Patient Shame

The sense of shame is something which is not paid much attention to in medical practice, although it is exactly in this setting where feelings of shame can be triggered because medical examinations and treatment are more often than not invasive and violate personal boundaries with little regard to the privacy of the patient. Because the purpose of shame is to protect the individual, the situations incuring shame are many and varied.

- Privacy and dignity can not always be maintained in medical institutions (shared rooms, the monitoring of excretory functions).
- A sick person in nursing care may feel as if he or she were a small child again that has to be fed and washed. Undergoing this kind of dependency can make the patient feel anything from somewhat embarrassed to deeply ashamed.
- Getting undressed and being naked can be humiliating, and this can be even more the case with invasive internal examinations, which include endoscopic interventions and urinary catheterisation which involve exposing and inspecting the most intimate areas of the body.
- When the medical history is taken patients are confronted with questions about intimate details of their private life including substance misuse, sexual practices and/or dysfunctional relationships for example, which could all be considered to be stigmatising. They are ashamed when they deviate from social norms in that for instance, they are overweight, illiterate, belong to a sexual minority or simply because they are unfamiliar with the prevalent cultural conventions. They feel ashamed about situations where they have lost their dignity. It is especially awkward for patients to talk about embarrassing physical symptoms, such as fecal or urinary incontinence. Uncertainty about which words to use can often lead to the patient preferring to keep quiet about their affliction. This problem is heightened when the doctor-patient dialogue can be overheard by others, as is the case if the patient is in a ward together with others.

An important ethical task for doctors and nurses with regard to these feelings of shame remains to be addressed by both doctors and nurses:

Spare the patient the misery of shame!

Whenever possible the patient's privacy should be respected and any interaction should remain discreet. It can be helpful to start off by reassessing institutional procedures in terms of to what extent they might violate the patients' dignity. This could result in medical histories only being taken in private from there onwards. Physical examinations, particularly invasive ones, should not be interrupted by third parties. And the intimacy of the doctor-patient consultation should not be disturbed by telephone calls or other conversations that have nothing to do with the patient. These are just some examples.

Doctors on their part can experience shame too, feeling uncomfortable talking about awkward issues with the result that the medical problem may be left unaddressed. However it should be mentioned that (research shows that) female patients who are the victims of domestic violence would wish for their physicians to bring up the subject (European Agency for Fundamental Rights, 2014). The broad consensus in Germany with regard to the doctor-patient relationship i.e. medical confidentiality and the subsequent belief that findings will not be made public, seem to provide the necessary secure setting for confiding intimate problems, so doctors should feel free to broach potentially awkward issues. They will find this easier if they adopt a non-judgemental approach.

When addressing taboo topics it may help if the doctor leads the way with the choice of words or level of language for both to use (nursery language, slang, medical terminology), "What do your stools look like, runny, soft or formed?, "Does your penis become stiff enough, or does it go limp again too quickly?"

23.2.2 Feelings of Shame During the Physical Examination

Getting undressed and being touched can be very embarrassing for any patient. However, the physical examination is indispensable for doctors who carry out most of their examinations manually. Quite apart from the direct result of the examination, other information may be gathered that perhaps did not become clear during the medical history taking. The doctor can immediately tell how the patient feels about his or her body, how he treats it and how he presents his body when others are present. Does he put away his clothes neatly? Does he hesitate before he gets undressed or does he flaunt his body? Considering that the patient's body has been there from the very beginning of his life and been involved interactively in everything he has ever done, it represents a kind of mirror of his biography into which the examining physician can take a direct look.

No words are needed, instead it is enough to observe the patient to know whether he perceives his body as being alien or shameful, or whether he neglects himself or not. Thus there is much more to learn than might be revealed by the straightforward results of the examination. What is more, physical contact can have a soothing effect, and the thoroughness of the procedure shows the patient that he and his afflictions are being taken seriously.

How can the doctor keep the embarrassment of the intimacy of the physical examination to a minimum?

If the case history was already taken in a tactful and respectful way, this demeanour will later help to make the actual physical examination easier. As has already been mentioned, the physical dignity of the patient is to be respected. Their individual boundaries to physical examination might be different depending on culture and combined gender roles, on learned family tradition or individual traumatic experiences. It should be pointed out that some rules of hygiene (wearing gloves for the examination of the genital area are less about hygiene but more about maintaining physical boundaries. The same goes for clinical apparel. The patient may also feel reassured that his physical privacy is being treated with respect when **transparency** about the entire examination procedure is provided. This is achieved by the doctor saying what he is going to do beforehand and using wording like, "I am now going to…" during the examination. Furthermore the patient should be assured that he retains **control** over the procedure, "If you want something to be done differently, we can stop whenever you want. You can say "No" at any time." Potential embarrassment may be forestalled by saying, "You might find this difficult…"

Excessive embarrassment about exposing the body can be a diagnostic indicator that the patient's physical boundaries were breached at some time in the past. The possibility of abuse or molestation should not be ruled out.

23.2.3   Diseases Themselves Can Be Humiliating

Diseases which cause the patient emotional distress include:

- disorders, which damage one's appearance such as skin diseases, or affect the patient's sexual identity. Therapies too, can have an adverse effect (hair loss, skin changes, amputations such as mastectomies) and cause more disfigurement and upset to one's self-image. This can be true for every patient, but particularly so for those who use their looks to mask their damaged self.
- medical conditions, which are associated with loss of control of bodily functions leading to urinary and fecal incontinence, for example. Patients suffering from chronic inflammatory bowel diseases with increased uncontrollable diarrhoea are especially likely to report being so afraid of the humiliation of being caught out or giving off a noticeable offensive smell that they adjust their lives accordingly, perhaps not even leaving the house any more.
- illnesses such as Hepatitis C, HIV infections and alcoholism which carry a special social stigma.
- ill health connected with life-style choices made by the patients which make them feel ashamed of their own failings, and of being helpless and incapable. Shame and a guilty conscience often appear together and are difficult to separate. Patients are ashamed of being overweight or of not doing any sport. In the expectation of being berated by the doctor, they may react with futile attempts to excuse or justify their behaviour or just avoid the doctor's office altogether. Physicians may well become annoyed when they are faced with such apparently unreasonable patients.

Mrs Schulz, who is 63 years old, is overweight and suffers from Diabetes mellitus. She was not able to carry on working in her job as a carer for the elderly and has been a pensioner for two years. As a single mother of two daughters she has had to work hard. She separated from her alcohol dependent husband decades ago. After her retirement she fell into a deep hole. She lost many of her social contacts. For the last two years she has been neglecting herself, has put on weight and has ignored all the rules about living with diabetes. She has however now decided she wants things to change and has finally come to see the doctor again. At the doctor's office she is pleased that she does not have to get on the scales before she has even seen the doctor. As she expected the laboratory results the doctor has in front of him are not good at all. He might now well start to reproach her saying, "You are too fat. You have to lose weight and be more active!". She will feel disappointed and humiliated. She has already given herself this advice—without avail. She will probably defend herself by saying, "But I don't eat much." Better results could be achieved if the doctor started by praising the patient for finding the courage to come and see him, and acknowledge this as a first step in the right direction.

Some patients see their illness as shameful and the enhanced image they may have of themselves becomes impaired. Being sick forces the patient to confront ageing and death. The damage caused by the disease and the associated shame are met with denial. This denial may be of help to get through the first phase of coming to terms with the illness, but later on when the disease progresses, denial exacerbates the situation. The patient does not turn up for necessary check-ups, for instance. The patient thinks, "That doesn't apply to me. I'm different!" Such patients behave as if he were indestructible and in no need of therapy.

Mr Meier, a 50 year old patient, who is always conservatively well-dressed, always engaging and self-assured, had a myocardial infraction when he was a young man. He works in the middle management of a bank and has been married for a long time. He downplays the great pressure he is under at work and even does voluntary work for various charitable organisations. "Always be the best" is his motto. With regard to how and when to take his medication, his lifestyle and medical monitoring he does as he pleases. He tells the doctor quite clearly but also charmingly that he knows best.

He grew up without a father. His mother is a very assertive woman with a theatrical manner, who never remarried after her husband died. She admires her son and ensures his dependence on her by being seductive and controlling, meddling in his affairs well into his adult life.

The patient acquiesces to his mother's interfering behaviour without demur and has always remained living near her. The roles that he tries to fulfil are not appropriate to his stage of development. In his self-experience he is torn back and forth between the feeling of worthlessness and the feeling of omnipotence, between self-doubt, fear of criticism on the one hand and his own maxim, "Be the best" on the other. The severity of his illness does not fit into the self-image as that of a successful doer. So illnesses and their consequences are met with denial. The patient would rather have the doctor's admiration and approval. This jeopardises the course of the disease and also puts the doctor into an emotionally trying position.

Some health problems actually derive from a patient's exaggerated feeling of shame. The following example could explain bodily distress symptomes compounded with a narcissistic conflict.

A female executive secretary to a large company, feels unable to return to work. She complains of ringing in her ears and symptoms of exhaustion. She puts the blame for this on her boss's obnoxious behaviour. For years he had used her to stabilise his erratic mood swings, paid her compliments, and inappropriately involved her in the organisation of his personal life. For many years she had been flattered by this. She comes from humble beginning, her mother was a market worker, father unknown. She has always been ashamed of her background and especially of her mother. A while ago the patient, who is not quite so young any more, approached her boss about a small disagreement. He was offended by this and reacted by telling her that she no longer looks like a model and she, too, is indeed replaceable. These upsetting remarks, which were sparked by a narcissistic collision, are the root of her "burn-out" symptoms. The doctor could help the patient if he succeeded in placing her feelings of hurt in a biographical context and then modifying her further treatment to include psychotherapy.

Some patients with inflated self-esteem can react to being slighted with a major depressive episode. Seemingly small offences at work, such as a promised promotion not materialising, can trigger a profound crisis and complete social withdrawal sometimes even culminating in suicide. These are the usually successful and very violent suicide attempts such as by jumping in front of a moving train or from a great height like a bridge.

23.3 Shame on the Part of the Medical Practitioner

23.3.1 Shame Is Contagious

Like any other feeling, shame is contagious. That goes for doctors, too. Because they sense shame on the part of their patients, perhaps subconsciously, they can avoid addressing embarrassing or taboo subjects in the consultation. This may be particularly true for doctors, who are able to easily empathise with the patient. Acknowledging one's own inhibitions and interpreting them as those projected by the patient is helpful for these doctors. Some useful verbal interventions were given earlier.

23.3.2 Dealing with Errors and Near Misses

Doctors too have a personal history and have been through their own specific socialisation process, factors which impact on their own feelings of self-worth and can be linked with a sense of shame. Nothing seems to be so ignominious for doctors as medical errors, or near misses, that have harmed or might have harmed patients. A study carried out in New Zealand looked at the long-term effects on doctors who have had a patient filing an official complaint against them or have been criminally charged because of faulty treatment. Two thirds of these doctors felt angry and depressed for weeks after being notified of the complaint. A third felt guilty and ashamed. A third lost all joy in their profession. The feelings of humiliation went on for years (Cunningham & Dovey, 2000). A medical error, or near miss error, seems to have the same effect as a trauma. Self-image is shaken to the core. The accompanying shame brings with it a strong urge to hide. Doctors who are experiencing this describe their feelings by saying, "I wish I could just disappear." This state of mind is not ameliorated by superiors and colleagues who do not openly discuss making errors or offer their support (Ofri, 2013). Hospitals are increasingly providing complaint management to patients. This is certainly to be welcomed, however they omit to support doctors with opportunities for open discussion about medical blunders. That doctors affected by such incidents miss social support is corroborated by Balint groups.

Shame affects one's self-image. The question arises as to why the medical profession is particularly susceptible to feelings of shame when errors are made. There seem to be unrealistic expectations of perfection which are generated by our western culture. "Grey's Anatomy", an American medical drama series, may serve to illustrate this point. One of the principal characters says before the start of a difficult operation with appropriately theatrical music playing in the background, "It's a beautiful night to save lives!" This example may go to show how the narcissism of the medical profession is nurtured by various cultural sources. Of course the notion of a doctor as being a kind of magic healer contributes to the way the profession is presented in soap operas, an image, which can be utilised in the healing process. A more rational way of looking at doctors as being "good enough" could be detrimental to this magic effect. Or to put it slightly differently, trust is an important foundation for healing. This perspective may seem to justify doctors overrating their capabilities, however this mindset makes them more vulnerable to criticism. Moreover it is an established fact that honesty towards the patient about mistakes that were made or nearly made contributes to a relationship of trust and reduces negative feelings on the doctor's part.

Although it is widely known that apologising to patients in such cases results in fewer lawsuits being filed, and that doctors who do apologise to their patients suffer less psychological stress, saying sorry is not something that is sufficiently encouraged in the pre- and post-qualification training and development of doctors. Instead, medical self-overestimation is reinforced by evading the issue of medical errors altogether, and shame is something that is just not spoken about. Indeed such discussions are already very constrained by indemnity clauses.

A culture of being open about medical fallibility will only then become the norm when and if the issue of shame is specifically addressed. Systems to reduce errors as well as quality assurance are important but they do not suffice. The experience of feeling shame should be on the agenda of every pre and post qualification training course to be discussed and shared by all.

23.3.3   Patients Who Cross Boundaries

Medical practitioners or carers can also be made to feel ashamed when patients cross boundaries in their dealings together. This is something which nursing staff in particular can confirm. They are embarrassed by the exhibitionistic behaviour on the part of some patients during a bed bath for example. Similarly doctors report feelings of awkwardness when patients conduct themselves in a seductive manner. However it is not only sexualised behaviour, which causes feelings of unease. A doctor may be discomfited by patients encroaching on his personal space by suddenly giving him a hug, or by their trying to establish intimacy by giving exorbitant gifts, or by revealing too much of their own private affairs.

How can an appropriate distance be maintained? When a health worker starts to feel awkward or embarrassed, it is important to interpret this is as a signal that boundaries need to be put more clearly in place. A doctor receives an overgenerous gift for instance. He might then say, "I feel honoured, that you are showing your appreciation to my team and myself in this way. But I am surprised that you think that only by doing this can you really be sure of our good care."

In any event it is important to be aware of the uneasy feelings that arise when professional boundaries are crossed and to kindly but firmly draw a line.

23.4 Interventions for Handling Shame

Because feelings of shame are of such general significance in the day-to-day routine of medical institutions, *tact and respect* are indispensable and of utmost importance. Respect is an attitude that is conveyed right at the start of the interaction by the way in which the patient is greeted. Does, for instance, the doctor know the patient's name and does he when introducing himself give his own name and job title? Does he in so doing make the patient from the outset feel that he *actually sees* him? Respect is conveyed in every doctor-patient interaction in medical institutions by *listening to—and enquiring about—the patient's perspective.* The patient should have enough time to describe his health problems and not be interrupted by the doctor's train of thoughts. The doctor should be proactive in trying to find out what the patient makes of his symptoms. Proceeding in this way creates an atmosphere of trust which is essential for potential confrontations with unpleasant facts as well as for making the physical examination easier.

How can doctors and other carers face patients with unwelcome facts such as the consequences of their chosen lifestyle—suspected alcohol abuse perhaps—without making them feel overly ashamed? Being confronted with "reality" is a challenge in every interpersonal interaction. Since shame is a universally unpleasant feeling some doctors and other practitioners find it easier if they make light of the check-up results, playing them down.

A young woman appears in the emergency department with injuries, haematoma on her forearms and face. She says she fell down stairs the previous evening. She is now in need of a sick certificate because she is in no condition to do her job as a sales assistant. The person treating her sees her injuries as unequivocal evidence of domestic violence. Instead of keeping quiet about this suspicion, he could choose to put the difficult words into someone else's mouth, so to speak. For instance, he might let science do the talking, "According to scientific experience those kinds of injury are signs of physical violence." Or he could quote someone with authority, "My former consultant would have said…" He might even tell a little story, "I once had a patient who…" This kind of technique has the effect of taking the patient to his side, and then looking at the situation from a certain distance together.

The subjunctive mood also has its uses, "I would love nothing more than to be able to say to you…"

Surprise and worry are also possible tools. One could say, "When I look at your injuries, then I worry that…"

In addition to the aforementioned counselling techniques for creating the necessary distance between the doctor and patient it can be helpful to pre-empt the patient's feelings of shame by naming the problem, "It might make you feel awkward, if I have to tell you that…"

When talking about difficult subjects the doctor should avoid making value judgements. If the patient with injuries associated with domestic violence were confronted with the question, "Why don't you just finally get around to leaving him?", the patient might only fall silent, and the next time he is physically abused choose not to see this doctor again.

The doctor should altogether *avoid reproaching* the patient, and instead of directly imposing his own set of values, ask questions that tap into the patient's potential ambivalence, "What would it be like if you left this marriage?"

In the case of the diabetes patient Mrs Schulz it is essential for the doctor to adopt an approach which focuses on the patient's strengths and achievements. This kind of encouragement makes it easier for patients to cope with negative emotions, especially those who are stricken with shame and guilt. A *resource-oriented* physician will find it easier to help the patient find a solution.

People who have an ashamed self and a pathological sense of shame tend to have a derogatory attitude towards other people. On account of their self-doubt on the one hand and their need to be the best on the other their manner can be arrogant and presumptuous and they react to the smallest affront with belligerence. Indignant rage can be ignited by the slightest feeling of being disregarded. A long wait at the doctor's surgery may already make such a patient feel he has not been treated with enough respect and end up in him shouting abuse.

When Mr Meier, the afore-mentioned heart attack patient, is turned away from the surgery where he has an appointment with the junior doctor without being told that the chief physician is not available to him, he berates her by saying, "Have you even learnt enough to be able to treat me?" as well as, "Next time I want to see the senior doctor again!" Naturally the junior doctor is annoyed that her competence is being questioned. She could now react by being offended and either justify herself or throw the patient out of the surgery or demand that her superior gives him a good telling off. It would be far better if she were able to keep calm and sidestep the patient's fury in the same away a toreador dodges the attacking bull by apologising to the patient for him being kept waiting, "I'm very sorry for any inconvenience". Trying to see and to name the problem from the patient's perspective usually helps to dissipate any anger.

Being able to apologise is quite generally an important capacity for people working in medical institutions. This is especially true in the case of errors and near miss errors. Saying sorry takes the pressure off the medical practitioner and also reduces the number of court cases (see Sect. 23.3.2). This is also true for alleged errors which the patient regards as being genuine ones. This is not about the doctor accepting the blame but about mirroring the patient's viewpoint and conveying to the patient that his viewpoint has been understood.

23.5 Summary

Shame is an emotion which is not paid much attention to, but one which is a common issue in the everyday life of medical institutions. Introspection can help practitioners to be aware of their own shame and that of the patients (Veit, 2018).

This is something to be practised in undergraduate and postgraduate training. Following interventions have been proven in the daily work of general practitioners, in the training for psychosomatic primary medical care in Germany (Psychosomatische Grundversorgung) and in communication skills courses at the Ruhr-University in Bochum (Table 23.1).

Table 23.1 Summary of recommended approach and interventions for dealing with shame in medical institutions (Veit, 2018)

Spare the patient shame whenever possible	
Ensure transparency and extend the patient's control over the procedure particularly during the physical examination	"I am now going to…" "If you want something to be done differently, we can stop whenever you want. You can say "No" at any time."
Treat the patient with respect from taking the medical history onwards by listening to the patient's perspective and taking it into consideration, and also by giving the patient authentic praise where possible	"What is your opinion about the origin of your complaints?" "I can understand, it must be a difficult situation." "It might be difficult to talk about this theme."
Take heed of personal feelings of shame	
Managing the confrontation with unwelcome facts	"It might make you feel awkward, if I have to tell you that…" "My former consultant would have said…" "According to scientific experience those kinds of injury are signs of physical violence." "I would love nothing more than to be able to say to you…" Ask questions that tap into the patient's potential ambivalence
Be resource-oriented	
Set boundaries with regards to patients' encroaching and presumptuous behaviour	"I feel honoured, that you are showing your appreciation to my team and myself in this way. But I am surprised that you think that only by doing this can you really be sure of our good care."
Apologise for real as well as near miss errors Circumvent vilification with aplomb	"I'm very sorry for any inconvenience."

References

Cunningham, W., & Dovey, S. (2000). The effect on medical practice of disciplinary complaints: Potentially negative for patient care. *New Zealand Medical Journal, 113,* 464–467.

Egloff, N., Bischoff, N., Kipfer, S., Studer, M., & Holtforth, M. (2016). *Stressinduzierte Hyperalgesie. Ärztliche Psychotherapie, 11,* 130–137.

Ekman, P. (2006). *micro expression training tool*. MOZGOmedia.

European Agency for Fundamental Rights (2014). Retrieved from http://fra.europa.eu/en/publication/2014/violence-against-women-eu-wide-survey-results-glance.

Grossmann, K. E., & Grossmann, K. (2009). Bindung und menschliche Entwicklung. *John Bowlby, Mary Ainsworth und die Grundlagen der Bindungstheorie*. 2. Aufl. Stuttgart: Klett-Cotta.

Grossmann, K. E., & Grossmann, K. (2007). Die Entwicklung psychischer Sicherheit in Bindungen. Ergebnisse und Folgerungen für die Therapie. *Z Psychosom Med Psychother, 53,* 9–28.

Kernberg, O. F. (1988). *Innere Welt und äußere Realität*. Anwendung der Objektbeziehungstheorie: Stuttgart, Verlag Internationale Psychoanalyse.

Ofri, D. (2013). *What doctors feel*. Boston: Beacon Press.

Sartre, J. P. (1943). *Das Sein und das Nichts*. Reinbek: Rowohlt.

Spinoza, B. (1986). *Die Ethik*. Ditzingen: Reclam.

Stern, D. N. (2016). *Die Lebenserfahrung des Säuglings*. Stuttgart: Klett-Cotta.

Veit, I. (2018). *Praxis der Psychosomatischen Grundversorgung. Die Beziehung zwischen Arzt und Patient*. Stuttgart: Kohlhammer Verlag.

Wurmser, L. (2007). *Die Maske der Scham Die Psychoanalyse von Schameffekten und Schamkonflikten*. Magdeburg: Verlag Dietmar Klotz.

Iris Veit (Dr. med.) has been working as a general practitioner in her own medical office together with other GPs for the last 30 years. Her academic work is in collaboration with the Ruhr Universität Bochum where she mainly teaches communication skills in patient-doctor interactions.

She is a supervisor and leader of Balint groups. She is committed to establishing local medical networks specifically for women. She is an active member of the German society for General Practitioners and Family Medicine DEGAM. Dr. Veit is especially involved in the postgraduate training for psychosomatic medicine in primary care and this is also the subject of her book Psychosomatische Grundversorgung—Die Beziehung zwischen Arzt und Patient, Stuttgart: Kohlhammer which was published in 2018. Besides this she has written articles for various accredited medicals journals.

Kay Spiekermann The text of Iris Veit was translated by Kay Spiekermann, who is a native speaker of British English. She trained to be a teacher and then studied education in Germany. Amongst other things she has taught parenting classes and for many years also worked on a voluntary basis as a telephone counsellor on a German helpline for young people. With this background she is regularly asked to translate papers of a psychological or psychoanalytical nature from German into English.

Chapter 24
From Shame to Pride—Initiation of De-stigmatisation Processes in Review Dialogues

Ottomar Bahrs and Karl-Heinz Henze

Abstract People with chronic conditions often experience marginalisation, discrediting and lack of social support. Their primary contact person is usually the family doctor, who not only serves to guide the patient to appropriate support systems, but can also help with the important task of verbalising emotions and taboo topics. This chapter discusses in which ways the review dialogue, as a specific type of conversation in the context of long-term care, may explore and reflect on the process of labelling and stigmatising. Our focus is specifically on the general practitioner's (GP's) setting, although review dialogues are also useful in other contexts. Within the framework of the BALANCE study (DRKS00004442, 2016), a total of 125 encounters from 14 voluntarily participating GPs were videotaped and analysed using mixed methods. The case of an almost 40-year-old female patient, born in Turkey, but having grown up in Germany, was selected for our exemplary analysis. She had been treated for chronic diseases (including hypertension and depression) by her present family doctor for 10 years. The review dialogue illuminates not only the significance of her symptoms in everyday life but also the biopsychosocial multidimensionality of the situation, illustrating the psychodynamics of the family of origin and the present family. The process of review dialogue brought shame-based, suppressed and thus hidden conflicts to light, which the patient was not allowed to carry to the outside world. A key challenge of the bicultural doctor–patient interaction is to re-establish a new personal identity. Just this realisation can already contribute to the empowerment of the patient. This long-term-care case study illustrates that the review dialogue can deepen the understanding of previously collected information, possibly even leading to corrected expectations as well as interpretations by both the patient and the GP. In this way, review dialogues can contribute to an increased bridging effect between the medical world and life world, while supporting the patient's

O. Bahrs (✉)
Institut für Allgemeinmedizin, Freier Mitarbeiter an der Heinrich-Heine-Universität Düsseldorf, Immanuel-Kant-Str. 12, 37083 Göttingen, Germany
e-mail: obahrs@gwdg.de

K.-H. Henze
Freier Mitarbeiter am Lou Andreas-Salomé Institut für Psychoanalyse und Psychotherapie, Göttingen, Germany
e-mail: khenze@gwdg.de

empowerment. The chapter describes which strategies, conversational techniques and attitudes have proven to be helpful and how the patient is able to increasingly use the offered possibilities by the review dialogue. Here, a protective setting of the doctor–patient relationship that has been experienced as safe by the patient, is crucial for the outcome.

Keywords Doctor–patient interaction · Shame · Salutogenic orientation · Long-term conditions · Patients with migration background · Stigma

24.1   Introduction

The living situation and healthcare of people with chronic conditions pose special challenges—for those affected, for their relatives, as well as for professional helpers. People with chronic conditions often experience marginalisation, discrediting and lack of social support, leading to feelings of shame. Common behavioural responses are avoidance and withdrawal.

The primary contact person is commonly the family doctor, who not only serves to guide the patient to appropriate support systems, but can also help with the important task to verbalise emotions and taboo topics.

Although surveys show that patients are largely satisfied with their family doctor (Grol et al., 2000; Böcken, Braun, & Landmann, 2009), a closer analysis of conversations and interaction processes reveals that the potential "hidden agenda" of patients is rarely addressed in daily practice (Barry, Bradley, Britten, Stevenson, & Barber, 2000; Peltenburg, Fischer, Bahrs, van Dulmen, & van den Brink, 2004). Existing diagnoses often provide the framework for what can become an issue, and the knowledge acquired in many encounters gives the impression of a familiarity that requires no further questions. This ritualising of interactions and treatments involves the risk of underestimating the effects of "chronification" on one hand and health resources on the other (Balint, Hunt, Joyce, Marinker, & Woodcock, 1975; Malterud & Hollnagel, 1998). Apparently it requires a targeted interruption and re-framing of normal daily patient–doctor interaction routines, to allow a conversation from an extended perspective. For this target, the concept of a review dialogue as a result of practice-based research, was developed in cooperation with practising physicians, other health service providers, self-help representatives and accompanying social science researchers (Bahrs & Matthiessen, 2007). During a review dialogue of about 20–30 min, the doctor invites a chronically ill patient to specific conversation, gaining an overview of the patient's overall situation, the patient's priority health goals and discussing implementable and expedient ways of achieving them for both parties involved (Bahrs, 2011). The follow-up BALANCE study (Bahrs, Heim, Löwenstein, & Henze, 2017) was used for the evaluation. One of our basic assumptions was that, in particular, people who have experienced discrimination can benefit from this setting. We would like to illustrate this by tracing the course of treatment of a Turkish-born patient.

In this chapter, we briefly present the theoretical background concerning concepts of shame, as well as the guiding principles and procedure for the review dialogue. We illustrate the interaction and transformational processes of this case study and draw conclusions regarding helpful techniques and possible applications of the review dialogue.

24.2   Shame—Theoretical Aspects

Shame can be viewed from a variety of theoretical viewpoints. Here, we focus on views that are of particular relevance for understanding the illustrated case study. We understand shame as a complex, self-reflective affect (Seidler, 1997; Tiedemann, 2007) which influences physical, mental, social, and existential dimensions. Shame is mostly interwoven with feelings of fear and guilt.

24.2.1   Shame: Cross-Cultural and Culture-Specific

From an anthropological perspective, shame is understood across cultures as a basic human feeling. People are the only living beings who are able to simultaneously reflect themselves (subject) as well as their environment (Plessner 1982, cited in Lietzmann, 2003, 9). However, different situations and forms of shame-expression, the meaning of shame, and how to deal with it, are socially and culturally specific (Landweer, 1999; Vanderheiden & Mayer, 2017). They depend on culturally conveyed values and the specific biography of the affected person—especially in terms of the internalised history of shame (Landweer, 1999; Vanderheiden & Mayer, 2017). A potential shame-inducing behaviour can indeed be perceived as shameful.

24.2.2   Shame: Intersubjective and Intrapsychic

In Sartre's existential-ontological view (Sartre 1977–79; 1980), the gaze and the judgment of the other is fundamental to the structure of shame: "I am ashamed of myself in front of others." (Sartre, 1993, cited in Lietzmann, 2003, p. 26, translation by the authors). It's not only about a specific behaviour and the experience of being a discredited object, but also about "just being an object. Meaning to recognise oneself in this diminished, dependent, and frozen object that I am for the other" (Lietzmann, 2003, 27, translation by the authors).

In general, shame has an "intersubjective texture"; there is a confrontation of an observing object with external reality or of an (imaginary) object with inner reality (Altmeyer, 2008, 303; Altmeyer, 2003 in Tiedemann, 2007, 380, translation by the authors). According to Moser and Zeppelin, on one hand, the opponent of the subject of shame is perceived as threatening and superior, while on the other hand, it is an existentially needed subject of relationship development. The latter already unfolds during the early stages of childhood. "Shame signals a self-change according to the assumed intention" of the significant other (Moser & Zeppelin, 1996, cited in Tiedemann, 2007, p. 374, translation by the authors). Thus an unacceptable action within the relationship is signalled by the other and triggers the feeling to be ashamed and shame. This results in both seclusion and withdrawal, as well as the wish to restore the relationship with the significant other, by interacting to once again build a level of understanding.

Wurmser focuses on the psychodynamics of inner shame, which initially appears as a fear of shame. Shame is both the cause of conflict and the product of internal conflict situations (Wurmser, 1993, XVI), and threatens the self (the ego identity). Why one is ashamed, is particularly affiliated with a no longer integrable distance between the (self-)observing ego functions ("so I am") and the ego ideal as element of the super-ego ("so I want to be"). Shame can also be understood as failure with regard to one's own expectations, mostly based on a negative self-evaluation as well as a real (or feared) negative evaluation by significant others (Lietzmann, 2003; Landweer, 1999). According to Wurmser (1993, 79), shame results from not fulfilling an expectation, as a wanted "global ideal" of oneself perceived by significant others and their corresponding group of expectations.

In order to protect the self, and to reduce hard-to-endure experiences, unconscious defence mechanisms appear. Examples are "externalisation", where the inner fear of being exposed to discreditation is overlaid through activities (for example, provoking contempt) (Wurmser, 1993, 16) as well as "reversal into the opposite", where shame is transformed into embarrassment of another subject (Wurmser, 1993).

24.2.3 Shame and Power

Shame refers to an inadvertent breach of norms, which are at least partially shared with the person involved. Thus, it can be understood as a gesture of submission to the prevailing norms of the respective reference group, as well as a statement that henceforth, norms will be complied with (Vanderheiden & Mayer, 2017; Neckel, 1991). Shame acts as a medium of social control in the form of self-assessment and self-control (see Landweer, 1999; von Scheve, 2013; Neckel, 1991). The subjects in the triangle of subject–object–significant other, "see themselves with the eyes of those who signal a normative condemnation" (Neckel, 1991, 199 ff., translation by the authors). Social inequality is also consolidated by the different appreciation of social milieus, solidified, for instance, in the form of specific habitus formations (Neckel, 1991).

The risk of feeling ashamed through a perceived complete deviation of values and norms, is much higher if one's own normative standards have not been established as valid social norms (Neckel, 1991, 197). In addition, the milieu, subculture or specific reference group determines divergent role expectations. A self-presentation which is accepted in one (familiar) environment can be normatively unacceptable in another environment, potentially leading to discreditation or stigmatisation (Goffman, 1994, cited in Schorn, 1996, 110).

Repeated experiences of embarrassment are stored in the body and may no longer be consciously perceived as inappropriate. Therefore it requires special situations/reflections, in order to distance oneself from the internally stored shame, so as to be able to re-evaluate (Neckel, 1991). Obviously, members of the social underclass and of minorities (such as people with migration experience) are more frequently affected than others (Neckel, 1991; Peacock, Bissell, & Owen, 2013; Wettergren, 2015).

24.2.4   Editing and Repealing of Shame as Well as Other Perspectives of Shame

One significant factor of the shame experience is its extent. If shame occurs in a manageable or bearable form, it may contribute to the further development of ego identity (Erikson, 1973), such as the subject is able to face up to this experience, to question the self and to learn. In other cases, as for example, if a change of perspective (Vanderheiden & Mayer, 2017) happens, this development is rather unlikely within the so-called *Schamsubjekt*. Here, the potential initiation of a re-evaluation process, would require a change of circumstances or suggestions from outside. In terms of the doctor–patient discussion, one crucial requirement for this process is the relationship experience and the design of the interaction. In the conversation, feelings of being ashamed and shame can become virulent again, both in the context of sharing past experiences as well within the current relationship. Therefore, it is required that the dialogue with the doctor can contribute not only to the solidification of the situation, but also to the potential of creating a new perspective of existing relationship experiences. Thus, the reflection on shame questions regarding the patient's own reference values can be facilitated. As a consequence, "pride" (Wurmser, 1993) or outrage may take the place of shame. The shame which is now no longer considered appropriate, can become the motor of change and empowerment (Vanderheiden & Mayer, 2017; Landweer, 1999; Peacock et al. 2013).

For a feeling of shame to arise, it can be sufficient that one's own actions do not correspond to one's inherent values, even if there are no others who live up to these expectations. Typically, this is interpreted as an indication of "unrealistic" claims, but in individual cases, it may be also understood as orientation towards concrete utopias, which can be counterfactually maintained. Then, shame could be seen as a resource (Vanderheiden & Mayer, 2017).

24.3   The Review Dialogue

Usually, the conversation between the patient and the GP is patient-initiated on an ad hoc-basis, or it is disease-related and initiated by the physician. However, a different framework is chosen for the review dialogue. Here, the family doctor invites the (chronically ill) patient for a 20–30 min conversation outside the consultation hours, so that together, they reflect on the overall situation as well as the previous course of treatment. The aim is to identify the patient's guiding life and health goals, to mutually to agree on a potentially new formulated treatment plan and to define respective responsibilities.

The concept of the review dialogue was developed in an applied study involving physicians, other healthcare providers, patient representatives and social scientists (Bahrs & Matthiessen, 2007). It was redesigned and evaluated in the recently completed BALANCE study (Bahrs et al., 2017). The concept incorporates elements of relational medicine (Balint et al., 1975), narrative based medicine (Greenhalgh & Hurwitz, 2005), salutogenesis (Antonovsky, 1997; Malterud & Hollnagel, 1998), systemic family therapy (Welter-Enderlin & Hildenbrand, 2004) and shared decision-making (Härter, Loh, & Spiels, 2005).

24.3.1   Conceptual Assumptions

The review dialogue is understood as a meeting of experts. The patient is considered as the expert on the patient's own health and illness, while the GP offers expertise in medical knowledge and relationship-building capacities. The physician has the task of organising the medical interview as a combination of personal meeting and medical talk, as a "case understanding in the encounter" (Welter-Enderlin & Hildenbrand, 2004, translation by the authors). In order to be able to tailor the treatment to the patient's needs, desires and possibilities, doctor and patient need to agree on what the particular health and illness implies for the patient, and what it is worth to the patient to be healthy. Personal health goals usually open in the light of often unspoken life goals. Implementation options and the need for help depend on the patient's life situation. Within the context of the longer history of customary treatment, patient and doctor usually have an implicit knowledge of what is important to the patient. However, they can only share it, if it becomes explicit. Therefore, the review dialogue needs to create an overall picture of risks and resources (Malterud & Hollnagel, 1998) and to simultaneously take into account the framework-specific constellation of the doctor–patient relationship (Welter-Enderlin & Hildenbrand, 2004) (see Fig. 24.1).

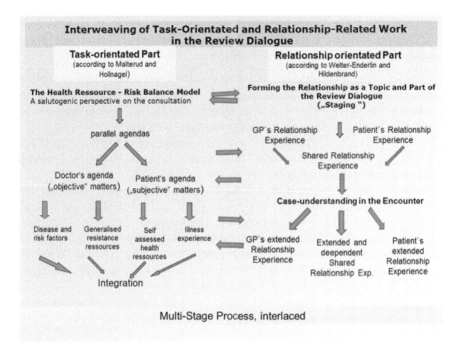

Fig. 24.1 Content and relationship-related work in the review dialogue (Authors' own construction based on Malterud & Hollnagel, 1998; Welter-Enderlin & Hildenbrand, 2004)

24.3.2   Attitudes and Techniques

In the review dialogue, the GP becomes listener and companion, an initially unusual role for the patient, which requires justification. In order to enable the patient to make use of the open conversation space, an introductory instruction (framing) is required. Here, the relevance of this approach becomes just as comprehensible as the interest of the physician and the specific tasks of both actors. The doctor thus enables the patient's narratives, supports with interest and deepening questions, verbalisations, occasional summaries, or hints about alternative thinking. In particular, the doctor asks for success and coping experiences, unless the patient addresses them on his/her own, and highlights resources that the patient has already successfully used or could use in the future.

24.3.3   Procedure of the Review Dialogue

The course of review dialogues differs from conventional doctor–patient conversations. Although it is possible to describe the logical structure as a flowchart

(Bahrs et al., 2015), the review dialogue should be designed jointly and, consequently, should be implemented on a case-by-case basis. Below, we introduce essential segments and give examples of possible applications.

- **Opening**: "Nice that you have come. Thank you! The purpose of the conversation today is to find out what is important to you, in terms of health and what you want to achieve next year. I also want to get to know you better and work with you, to find ways to achieve those goals. Would you agree with that?"
- **Narrative stimulus (reviewing)**: "How did you feel during the last year?" For detailing: "What was good for you?" "Was there anything that you would say you do not want to experience again?"
- **Evaluation and (re-)formulation of the treatment assignment**: "What did you expect from this, or expect me to do during this time?" "What would have to happen to get you out of here and say, 'I feel really good!'?"
- **Future orientation**: "What is it worth for you to be healthy?"
- **Prioritisation of (initially 1–2) health goals**: "What would you say: Where is your most important weak point?" "If you now imagine that we will meet again in a year, what would you like to have achieved by then?"
- **Negotiating ways to achieve health goals**: "Now there are various ways in which you can approach this goal (such as weight loss). What do *you* think, how will you handle this?"
- **Agreeing on patient's and physician's responsibilities**.
- **Evaluation of the interview itself**: "How did this conversation feel for you today?" "Do you have anything else on your mind?"
- **Closing**: Appointment, thanks, farewell.

24.4 Case Study

The information for the following case study had been collected within the context of the BALANCE study, that was conducted between 2011 and 2015 and used a mixed methods design. The purpose of the study was to find out wether the use of review dialogue encourages patients and physicians to agree on shared health goals and to better achieve them. A total of 52 general practitioners and 438 chronically ill patients participated in BALANCE. Within one year, physicians performed between two and four goal setting interviews with volunteering patients. The agreed health goals, as well as ways to achieve them, were documented for all review dialogues. Patients and physicians were asked to individually assess the extent of goal achievement. The data from a total of 286 patients and 36 doctors has been evaluated. For the qualitative sub-study involving 14 GPs and 50 patients, a number of review dialogues were recorded on video (Bahrs et al., 2017). The case study now described, was selected for its relevance in dealing with the topic of shame.

24.4.1 Starting Situation

Dr. Angela Mead is a GP, 50 years old and established her practice 12 years ago. Her patient, Mrs Bulut, 37 years old, is of Turkish origin. She migrated to Germany at the age of two, where she was raised. She is married, has two children (9 and 14 years old) and works as an administrative clerk.

Dr. Mead has been taking care of her patient for 12 years. She believes she knows her patient "pretty good" (score 4, range: $1 = $ "not at all" to $5 = $ "very good") and considers her patient's salutogenic resources to be low (2 out of 5). Last year, 10 visits of Mrs Bulut were registered. The doctor selected this patient for the project, because of recurring problems regarding hypertension and depressive episodes); other diagnoses include grade II obesity and autoimmune thyroiditis.

24.4.2 History of Review Dialogues

Within a year, a total of four review dialogues were performed, of which three were recorded on video. Because the **review dialogue II** was not recorded, apart from brief written information, it was not considered for our analysis.

Review Dialogue I: Problem Dimensioning—Lack of Recognition and Lack of Energy in the Cycle of Excessive Demands

The GP opens the conversation with questions regarding how the patient copes with the present situation, exploring the biographical background, how stress and demands are rebalanced, assuring understanding and leading back to the present situation. In view of the problem constellation, the two most important health goals for the coming year are being developed and both actors agree on the measures they must take in order to achieve the goals. The consultation lasts 42 min and ends with an evaluation of the review dialogue itself.

At this point, the diagnosis "depression" is re-established and both participants agree on the health objective "strengthening self-esteem". The encounter results in referrals to a neurologist/psychiatrist and a dietician—which are apparently not accepted by the patient.

Once again, the patient, Mrs Bulut, complains of the already familiar symptoms: tiredness, fatigue, exhaustion, headache, high blood pressure, irritation and sleep disturbances. Her everyday life is characterised by a heavy workload, and she feels that her efforts are not recognised. She also has to cope with the "double burden" of paid work and housework. Her husband hardly supports her; his shift work also leaves little room for it, and the spouses hardly see each other. Mrs Bulut criticises herself for not being able to set boundaries, being a perfectionist and occasionally losing control. She then yells at her children, sometimes even throws objects and has "bad feelings". That feels very bad for her, because she wants to be a "good mother". The GP asks in depth:

A20: What's wrong with having such feelings? So, who told you that or how did you get that?

P20: Yeah, my dad used to be that way, he was always gone, and [*P starts crying, sobbing*] I do not know, I did not really want to be like Dad.

A21: Okay, okay. Uh-huh. So, he is a negative role model for you? Uh-huh. Did he have other sides?

P21: Yeah, good sides, too, but he was always working and [*pause, crying*] Papa was a bit older/A21a: Yeah./I do not know why I have to cry like that. [*Crying*]

A22: Because that reminds you. And then you also understand what load weighs on you, that you try to be by no means in this way. But do you think you are like that?

P22: Sometimes already.

For a lengthy period, the patient now recalls memories of her father, who had come to Germany as a Turkish immigrant, a simple, hardworking man committed to his traditions, who wanted to rigorously protect his children from Western influences and occasionally slipped his hand. She responded with provocative behaviour, both helpless and speechless, both retreating. Mrs Bulut is overwhelmed by the feeling of sadness of the recalled situation, especially as she was unable to communicate with her father, who died 15 years ago. Now she tries to discuss conflicts with her own children, but Dr. Mead's dig deeper makes it clear that this usually means she tries to explain her behaviour and apologises.[1] At this point, the diagnosis "depression" is restored and both actors agree with the health goal of "strengthening self-esteem". In considering the practical consequences, the patient and doctor fall short of what had already been discussed: the life-world aspects recede into the background. The encounter ends with referrals to a neurologist or psychiatrist and a nutritionist. Both proposals are reluctantly accepted by the patient. When asked for feedback on the review dialogue, Mrs Bulut emphasises that it was beneficial to have time and to not confine herself to one problem.

In this conversation, the patient's shame becomes clear in her failure to set her own standards. Furthermore the biographical anchoring of the shame clearly emerges. In addition, the power of shaming experiences as well as Mrs Bulut's burden become apparent and recognisable. Dr. Mead succeeds in creating an open atmosphere of conversation, in which Mrs Bulut is able to express herself without fear, and apparently she experiences this as liberating. Dr. Mead uses the following techniques:

- *Focusing on resources*: How did you manage to cope with your well-known problems?
- *Reinterpretation*: Disengaging is a warning signal, indicating that something becomes "too much".
- *Stimulation to self-reflection*: Why do you think that "evil feelings" are bad?
- *Stimulation to self-reflection*: Do you believe that you are like your father?

[1]The self-stigmatisation of Mrs Bulut as a "bad mother" has her biographical forerunner in the behaviour of the "bad child". As a child she had no opportunity to justify herself to one-sided blame, even though, in her eyes, both father and child were responsible. She wants to spare her children this experience and takes the blame again.

- *Reinterpretation and appreciation*: You think that you don't do enough, because you are tired and powerless. On the contrary, you are doing too much, and that's why you lack energy.

Review Dialogue III: Problem-Solving—Stigma, Outburst Fantasies and the Need for Talking

In Review Dialogue III, a change of direction takes place. First, the patient takes the initiative and insists on the physical aspect of her complaints and does not want to be seen as "only psychogenic". The GP asks, what "psychogenic" means for her and her surroundings; is this seen as shameful? As a result, Mrs Bulut is able to explain that neither her problems, nor her views are accepted by her environment:

> P8: Friends say you have to slap me once, and then everything would be all right again. They don't think. They say: "You're fine. You have got it all, you have a good job." And I guess they accept the situation; they say I'm lazy.

Having been reminded of stressful experiences in work and family relations (which are known to the GP from former consultations), the patient complains that her husband had two affairs and that she felt deeply hurt. She has accepted his mistakes and taken him back, but cannot forgive him.

> P10: Somehow I have no satisfaction. That's my problem!

However, everybody sees the situation as "normal" again. Asked for the perspective of her husband, Mrs Bulut states that he does not see any problems, nor does he accept a separation. Therefore, Mrs Bulut is forced to conceal her separation fantasies, which can be seen as the social genesis of her grumbling. Obviously her ambivalence becomes a weighty decision-making problem, paralysing her in everyday life. Mrs Bulut suggests that perhaps a partner counselling is necessary—but Turks do not go to psychotherapy.

> P12: In the beginning I was always thinking: "Okay, I am the patient now." My husband has always said: "Oh, you have screw loose!" And that my nerves are just blank. /Mhm. /Then I thought, "Okay, I'm the sick now, so I'm always so aggressive, or unbalanced." Then I took the pills, did the therapy, was in the cure, and he always kept out, right? (…) My husband has never dealt with it, such as psychologists or therapies or partner talks. He never made any suggestions. He always says: 'Oh, you're not feeling well? Then go to the doctor! [Laughs] But that's not a solution.

Since neither talking nor soothing helps, the GP suggests family counselling—with, or without her husband. It is important for Mrs Bulut to think about her priorities—this is what her family doctor gives her as a *"homework assignment"*.

In this conversation, similar to Review Dialogue I, Mrs Bulut's suffering owing to a long-standing unsolved family problem emerges, which is a matter of overcoming everything else and cannot be talked about. While Review Dialogue I deals with her paternal conflicts, Review Dialogue III refers to problems with her husband. Therefore, in both cases, disputes with the male family leader are addressed. Apparently, cultural features play a significant role, and instead of support, Mrs Bulut is more likely to be confronted with derogatory and discrediting statements in her milieu. Dr. Mead encourages her and supports her aspirations for autonomy.

Mrs Bulut describes her experiences of powerlessness and embarrassment which happen in her social environment. Paradoxically, the assumption of her imposed role of "the sick one in the family" gives her the chance to break the silence-taboo and speak openly to Dr. Mead. The GP accompanies the self-discovery process of her patient and uses the following helpful techniques:

- *Deputy addressing of taboo topics*: There are circles, where it says: 'Well, if you would really pull together, then it would work out!'
- *Reinterpretation*: I do not even know if it's a question of energy. Maybe you also carry the infidelity of your husband around with you?
- *Circular questions*: Did you ever talk to your husband about what he imagines? What do you think about what's going on in his head?
- *Future orientation*: What is your vision for yourself? How would you like to have it for yourself sometime? What projects do you have in mind?
- *Confrontational interpretation*: You didn't make a decision for a long time and did not actually say 'yes' to continue living with your husband.
- *Focusing on the patient's wishes*: For a moment, forget the question of whether or not this will work. Listen to yourself: What about your own wish?
- *Homework*: I want you to think this through and make a conscious decision as to whether or not to do a couple counselling. Can you take this as a homework assignment?

Review Dialogue IV: First Achievements and Future Planning—Being Recognised, Resources, Ownership

The fourth 40-min review dialogue completes the project one year after the first review dialogue. As in the other dialogues, the goal is to clarify the upcoming joint tasks. The focus is also on evaluating the achievements and setting up further treatment, which should not fall back into the previous routine, but still to accomplish it with a smaller time quota, as long as review dialogue is not yet implemented as a fixed supply module.

When asked about her well-being, Mrs Bulut initially describes symptoms similar to those in Review Dialogue I, but restricts, that she feels better now and that she can help herself. She is aware of her weak points and knows how to defend herself: "I give back words now". She has not taken the prescribed medication (it is in the refrigerator), but she confirms that everything else has been done as agreed. She has talked to her husband and has decided to continue living with him. He grew up in Turkey and does not see some things as relaxed as she does, but she is now able to communicate with him and has "brought him up a bit". Now, he participates with housework, and she has managed to go to a vocational training. Her husband made a scene in front of her, but she did not change her mind. It was good for her to talk to like-minded and educated people. She usually did not have this kind of exchange in everyday life: "It was beautiful". She had felt that she was being taken seriously and thought:

P27: "Oh God, there are also people who are respecting you".

When asked by the doctor how it was after her return, Mrs Bulut states that she felt that she had changed. Only then, she noticed how much energy her daily life required and how little was left for other things. She will now treat herself to more "time out"s.

Table 24.1 summarises the relevant dimensions and developments of the review dialogues.

24.5 Summary

In the course of the described case, the review dialogue acts as support and assistance for a re-evaluation and transformation process of the patient. An important requirement for this is the shaping of the relationship and interaction, so that past and current (shameful) experiences can be reactivated and be processed. In this reflection process, one's personal shame reference values may be questioned. In this case study, examples of stigmatising and discrediting experiences through family members, based on milieu-specific norms are described. The protagonist is potentially marginalised and ashamed, because she could be shameful for the family. In the review dialogue, the subsequent experience of being able to emotionally face oneself and to endure shame and embarrassment, as well as to be able to initiate some change, leads to an extension of the evaluation. Furthermore, the potential of a change in self-representation, contribution to empowerment, seems possible. Mrs Bulut now experiences pride as the antipode of shame (Wurmser, 1993). She has made new experiences in dealing with shame and embarrassment and made herself aware of her own resources. The physician's specifying, clarifying and promoting remarks, as well as her referral to further resources and encouragement towards the patient's abilities, have contributed to this outcome.

The described transformation process has neither started with Review Dialogue I nor ended with Review Dialogue IV. Generally, it should be noted that the review dialogue is a flexible instrument, potentially promoting long-term relationship-building, mutual appreciation and understanding. It has a developing character.

The described relationship-shaping tools used within the review dialogue allowed shame to become visible, either entirely without embarrassment, or in the form of manageable embarrassment. The questioning of internalised views, the offered shared decision-making, based on the introduction of one's own expertise, as well as the promotion of approaching situations of shame with different actions, all contribute to the successful examination and transformation of shame itself.

The review dialogue has been developed in a GP setting, but can be used in other settings, wherever long-term support is required, as for example in specialised care, for patients with rare diseases or with other serious chronic diseases. It is applicable to other health and social professions such as physiotherapy, respiratory therapy or work counselling, in modified forms, if necessary.

Table 24.1 Changes in the course of the review dialogues

Dimension	Review dialogue			Development
	Review dialogue I	Review dialogue III	Review dialogue IV	
Emotion	Powerlessness/helplessness; Shame and description of shaming experiences	Anger, ambivalence; stigmatisation; Internal conflicts	Experience of being appreciated, self-esteem, pride	From passivity to activity
Time perspective	Primarily past-related; Problem with father is really no longer solvable; So far, aspired ideals have not been achieved	Primarily present-related; problem with husband; Although offense cannot be undone, relationship issues must be tackled; the patient is considered a shameful significant other by her family members and feels ashamed	Present-related and future-orientated; Overcoming current problems through future orientation and trialling (Probehandeln)	From the latent orientation of the past to the latent future orientation
Main topics	Recognition problem in everyday life and treatment	Female doctor strengthens the autonomy-conscious part of the patient	Patient has received recognition apart from family and therapy and is experiencing this again in the encounter; Tendency to turn from shame to pride in achievement	From the repetition of the problem in the treatment relationship through the scenic enactment in the treatment relationship to the (re) production of solutions also in the treatment relationship
Diagnosis	Depression	The sick one of the family	Everybody is vulnerable	From life as a problem to a problem to living with problems
Central intervention	Engaging in narration; Specification, concretisation, stimulation for self-reflection; Reinterpretation	Resolution of the diagnosis in the history of stigmatisation; Instruction on the activity and first perspectival orientation forward; "Auxiliary ego"	Verbalisation regarding changed identity and self-acceptance; Mutual recognition	From interpretation to inviting and accompanying narrations to mirroring
Relationship and roles	GP as guide—patient is partly relieved of self-responsibility	GP as a coach—patient seeks responsibility	GP as professional and personal counterpart—both actors take responsibility	From the expert–patient relationship through advocacy to mutual expertise

Working with review dialogues initiates a change of roles within the patient–doctor relationship, and requires time for adjustment of both actors. Therefore, we suggest accompanying the implementation with supporting development processes, such as quality circles and participatory research (Wright, 2010).

References

Altmeyer, M. (2008). Von außen nach innen. Zu Jens Tiedemanns Beitrag „Die intersubjektive Natur der Scham". *Forum der Psychoanalyse, 24*(3), 300–304.

Antonovsky, A. (1997). *Salutogenese*. Tübingen: Dgvt-Verl.

Bahrs, O. (2011). Der Bilanzierungsdialog—Eine Chance zur Förderung von Ressourcenorientierung in der Langzeitversorgung von Patienten mit chronischen Krankheiten. *Gesundheit und Gesellschaft, Wissenschaft, 11*(4), 7–15.

Bahrs, O., & Matthiessen, P. F. (Eds.). (2007). *Gesundheitsfördernde Praxen—Die Chancen einer salutogenetischen Orientierung in der hausärztlichen Praxis*. Bern: Hans Huber.

Bahrs, O., Henze, K. H., Löwenstein, F., Abholz, H. H., Ilse, K., Wilm, S., et al. (2015). Review dialogues as an opportunity to develop a person-related overall diagnosis. *International Journal of Person Centered Medicine, 5*(3), 112–119.

Bahrs, O., Heim, S., Löwenstein, F., & Henze, K. H. (2017). Review dialogues as an opportunity to develop life course specific health goals. *The International Journal of Person Centered Medicine, 7*(2), 98–106.

Balint, M., Hunt, J., Joyce, D., Marinker, M., & Woodcock, J. (1975). *Das Wiederholungsrezept – Behandlung oder Diagnose?*. Stuttgart: Ernst Klett.

Barry, C. A., Bradley, C. P., Britten, N., Stevenson, F. S., & Barber, N. (2000). Patients' unvoiced agendas in general practice consultations: Qualitative study. *BMJ, 2000*(320), 1246–1250.

Böcken, J., Braun, B., & Landmann, J. (Eds.). (2009). *Gesundheitsmonitor 2009—Gesundheitsversorgung und Gestaltungsoptionen aus der Perspektive der Bevölkerung*. Gütersloh: Verlag BertelsmannStiftung.

DRKS00004442. (2016). *Bilanzierungsdialoge als Mittel zur Förderung von Patientenorientierung und zur Verbesserung hausärztlicher Behandlungsqualität bei Menschen mit chronischer Krankheit (BILANZ)*. Retrieved from http://www.drks.de/drks_web/navigate.do?navigationId= trial.HTML&TRIAL_ID=DRKS00004442.

Erikson, E. H. (1973). *Identität und Lebenszyklus*. Frankfurt a.M.: Suhrkamp.

Greenhalgh, T., & Hurwitz, B. (Eds.). (2005). *Narrative-based medicine*. Bern: Hans Huber.

Grol, R., Wensing, M., Mainz, J., Jung, H.P., Ferreira, P., Hearnshaw, H., Hjortdahl, P., et al. (2000). Patients in Europe evaluate general practice care: an international comparison. *British Journal of General Practice, 50*(460): 882–887.

Härter, M., Loh, A., & Spiels, C. (2005). *Gemeinsam entscheiden—erfolgreich behandeln: Neue Wege für Ärzte und Patienten im Gesundheitswesen*. Köln: Deutscher Ärzte-Verlag.

Landweer, H. (1999). *Scham und Macht—Phänomenologische Untersuchungen zur Sozialität eines Gefühls*. Tübingen: Mohr Siebeck.

Lietzmann, A. (2003). *Theorie der Scham. Eine anthropologische Perspektive auf ein menschliches Charakteristikum*. Tübingen: Dissertation zur Erlangung des akademischen Grades Doktor der Sozialwissenschaften in der Fakultät für Sozial- und Verhaltenswissenschaften der Eberhard-Karls-Universität. Retrieved from http://nbn-resolving.de/urn:nbn:de:bsz:21-opus-9350.

Malterud, K., & Hollnagel, H. (1998). Talking with women about personal health resources in general practice—Key questions about salutogenesis. *Scandinavian Journal of Primary Health Care, 16*, 66–71.

Neckel, S. (1991). *Status und Scham. Zur symbolischen Reproduktion sozialer Ungleichheit*. Frankfurt am Main: Campus.

Peacock, M., Bissell, P., & Owen, J. (2013). Shaming encounters: reflections on contemporary under-standings of social inequality and health. *Sociology*. Published online July 18, 2013; Retrieved February 7, 2018 from http://journals.sagepub.com/doi/abs/10.1177/0038038513490353.

Peltenburg, M., Fischer, J. E., Bahrs, O., van Dulmen, S., & van den Brink, A. (2004). The unexpected in primary care—A multicenter study on the emergence of unvoiced patient agenda. *Annals of Family Medicine, 2*(6), 534–540.

Sartre, J. P. (1977–79). *Der Idiot der Familie* (Vol. 5). Reinbek bei Hamburg: Rowohlt.

Sartre, J. P. (1980). *Das Sein und das Nichts*. Reinbek bei Hamburg: Rowohlt, unchanged ed.

Scheve, C. V. (2013). Sighard Neckel: Status und Scham. Zur symbolischen Reproduktion sozialer Ungleichheit. In K. Senge & R. Schützeichel (Eds.), *Hauptwerke der Emotionssoziologie* (pp. 235–242). Wiesbaden: VS-Verlag.

Schorn, A. (1996). *Scham und Öffentlichkeit. Genese und Dynamik von Scham- und Identitätskon-flikten in der Kulturarbeit*. Regensburg: Roderer Verlag.

Seidler, G. H. (1997). Scham als Mittlerin von Innen und außen: Von der Objektsbeziehungsthe-orie zur Alteritätstheorie. In R. Kühn, M. Raub & M. Titze (Eds.). Scham—ein menschliches Gefühl. *Kulturelle, psychologische und philosophische Perspektiven* (pp. 107–123). Opladen: Westdeutscher Verlag.

Tiedemann, J. L. (2007). *Die intersubjektive Natur der Scham*. Dissertation. FU Berlin, FB Erziehungswissenschaft und Psychologie. Retrieved from http://www.diss.fu-berlin.de/2007/659/.

Vanderheiden, E. & Mayer, C.-H. (2017). An introduction to the value of shame—exploring a health resource in cultural contexts. In E. Vanderheiden & C.-H. Mayer (Eds.), *The value of shame. Exploring a health resource in cultural contexts* (pp. 1–39). Cham: Springer International Publishing.

Welter-Enderlin, R. & Hildenbrand, B. (2004). *Systematische Therapie als Begegnung*. Stuttgart: Klett-Cotta, 4, completely revised and expanded version.

Wettergren, A. (2015). Protecting the self against shame and humiliation: unwanted migrants' emotional careers. In J. Kleres & Y. Albrecht (Eds.), *Die Ambivalenz der Gefühle* (pp. 221–245). Wiesbaden: Springer Fachmedien. Retrieved from https://doi.org/10.1007/978-3-658-01654-8_12.

Wright, M. T. (Ed.). (2010). *Partizipative Qualitätsentwicklung in der Gesundheitsförderung und Prävention*. Bern: Huber.

Wurmser, L. (1993). *Die Maske der Scham. Die Psychoanalyse von Schamaffekten und Schamkon-flikten*. Berlin, Heidelberg, New York: Springer Verlag.

Ottomar Bahrs (Dr.) is a medical sociologist, supervisor and facilitator of quality circles in medicine and social work. He is a freelance researcher at the University of Düsseldorf, lecturer at the university of Göttingen and speaker of the umbrella organization on salutogenesis. He has published several monographs, text collections and journal articles on coping with chronic ill-being, doctor-patient-interaction, hermeneutics, interprofessional cooperation, quality improvement, health promotion and salutogenesis.

Karl-Heinz Henze (Dr.) is a psychologist and psychotherapist. Until recently resarcher and lec-turer at the Georg-August University of Göttingen, since then active in his own psychotherapeutic practice. Fields of work: psychosocial aspects of chronic illness, death and dying, doctor-patient-interaction.

Part VIII
Transforming Shame in Therapy, Counseling and Self-development

Chapter 25
Working with Shame in Psychotherapy: An Eclectic Approach

Aakriti Malik

Abstract Shame as an emotion is a deep rooted one. Being a widely felt emotion, its presence in the context of psychopathology and psychotherapy with clients is of special importance. Shame as experienced by clients, often hides under the façade of secondary emotions of pain, embarrassment, grief or anger. Uncovering shame therefore requires great skill, patience and knowledge on the part of the therapist. At times, it is through the client's repetitive experiences and narratives that inklings of shame may be revealed. The repertoire of other emotions makes shame so distant for the client that it can take a long time accepting it as one's own. Working with shame in psychotherapy effectively has found to alleviate symptoms, decrease distress thus creating opportunities for accepting the self as it is. The current chapter aims at understanding shame from different theoretical perspectives, it's link with psychopathology and how it showcases in therapeutic settings. Selected cases of shame and working with it have been presented in the Indian context. Conclusions on effective possibilities for healing shame in psychotherapy in addition to suggestions for future research have been discussed.

Keywords Shame · Psychotherapy · Culture · India · Client

25.1 Introduction

The Oxford dictionary on-line defines shame as "a painful feeling of humiliation or distress caused by the consciousness of wrong or foolish behaviour". Researchers (Karlsson & Sjoberg, 2009) have found the root of the word "shame" to be traced to Indo-European word kam/kem meaning to "hide", "conceal" and "cover up". Amidst the realm of the positive and negative emotions, shame confines itself in the zone of self-conscious emotions which includes guilt, embarrassment and pride. These feelings consist of an inherent capacity of the self to evaluate itself thus making them

A. Malik (✉)
D-31-7, PJ8 Service Suite, Block D, Jalan Barat, PJ Seksyen 8, 46200 Petaling Jaya, Selangor, Malaysia
e-mail: aakritimalik26@gmail.com

© Springer Nature Switzerland AG 2019
C.-H. Mayer and E. Vanderheiden (eds.), *The Bright Side of Shame*,
https://doi.org/10.1007/978-3-030-13409-9_25

'self-conscious' (Tracy & Robins, 2006). Even as guilt and shame continue to be used synonymously for the longest time, researchers have outlined clear distinctions between the two (Tangney, Stuewig, & Mashek, 2007). As theorized by Tomkins (1963) the response of hanging the head or lowering the eyes when one feels ashamed leads to an instant reduction of facial visibility. This is the reason why shame is often equated to 'loss of face' or to lose one's honour.

Shame has been primarily found to consist of two major components. The first is referred as an *external shame* which consists of thoughts and feelings on how one exists in the mind of others (Gilbert, 1997, 1998 Gilbert, in this book). It constitutes feelings of anger, contempt, rejection which others might have of one's self. The second component, *internal shame*, is experienced when one looks at one's self and criticizes and devalues it (Gilbert & Procter, 2006).

Additionally, shame has also been attributed to a person's current state or personality trait. When expressed as an emotion in specific situations, shame, becomes a state of the individual. However, when a person finds themselves ashamed more than often it is said to be rooted as their personality's trait. Repetitive childhood experiences of hearing oneself as "I'm bad and unattractive" or "Something is wrong with me" usually falls in this category (Claesson, Birgegard, & Sohlberg, 2007). This has also been described as "core shame" and shame proneness wherein a person experiences frequent episodes of shame states (Tangney et al. 2007; Cozolino & Santos, 2014).

As an emotion, researchers have often questioned the delay of the scientific field to be intrigued by the psychology of shame and a willingness to comprehend it (Kaufman, 1996; Zaslav, 1998).

25.2 Conceptual Framework: Understanding Shame Through Theories

Of the different theorists who've discussed about shame, some of the prominent theoretical perspectives have been offered by the evolutionary or functionalist, psychodynamic perspectives (Eriksonian, Attachment theorists, object-relationists), cognition and attributional approaches.

With respect to the evolutionary approach (Gilbert and Elison, in this book), humans have been found to be social beings carrying a social threat warning system. The behaviors associated with shame (such as averted gaze, slumped posture, lowered head) are submissive and strategies to disengage from a conflict (Dickerson, Gruenewald, & Kemeny, 2009). Theorists are of the view that shame, from an evolutionary perspective, can be both adaptive and maladaptive, facilitating relationships at one end and leading to defensive behaviors on the other, especially if frequently shamed as a child (Dickerson et al., 2009; Leeming & Boyle, 2013).

In the psychoanalytical tradition, Piers and Singer (1953) described shame as arising from the conflict between the ego and ego ideal in contrast to guilt emanating from the tension between ego and superego. Erikson (1950) in his theory of lifespan development considers shame as a consequence of the child being unable to claim his autonomy as s/he learns toilet training in the second stage. Pioneers in the field of object relations emphasized on the internal mental representation the child has of his caregiver. As the child alternated between the experiences of union and autonomy with the other, it was in such moments that shame found its presence (Stadter, 2011). Attachment theorists (Bowlby, 1973, as cited in Mills, 2005) posited shame to be felt whenever the mother-infant bond faced disruption. According to Bowlby a child who feels unwanted by his/her parents also comes to believe that s/he is "essentially unwantable, namely unwanted by anyone."

Cognitive psychologists (Tangney & Fischer, 1995) have viewed shame as related to a global and 'pervasive sense of self as bad, defective or deficient'. This ability to self-evaluate oneself is believed to develop in children between the ages of two to three years. In contrast, theorists (Tomkins, 1962, 1963 as cited in Zaslav, 1998) of affect theory consider shame to be a negative emotion which impedes the occurrence of positive emotions such as interest-excitement or enjoyment-joy. According to Tomkins, this emotion allows individuals to both master and overcome obstacles that may prevent positive effects from occurring.

Thus, while different theorists have posited their understanding of shame and its expression, the common thread that is seen through all the perspectives is an understanding of shame as a social emotion capable of alerting an individual of their societal boundaries. Additionally, it is through an individual's internalisation of a behaviour that shame comes to be either adaptive or maladaptive.

25.3   Shame and Psychopathology

Research suggests that shame and shame proneness have been linked with psychological difficulties and mental illnesses. Shame has been found to be associated with depression, eating disorders, bipolar disorders, anxiety disorders, personality disorders (borderline and narcissistic and mood disorders) (Tangney et al. 2007; Candea & Szentagotai, 2013; Scheel et al., 2014). People suffering from borderline personality disorder have been found to report significantly higher levels of shame compared to those diagnosed with mood disorders. (Rüsch et al., 2007; Scheel et al., 2014). Shame has also been reported in people suffering from Post-Traumatic Stress Disorder, both, as a primary emotion seen at the time of trauma and a secondary emotion seen after the appraisal of the event. (Grey, Holmes, & Brewin, 2001; Ehlers & Clark, 2000). The role of shame has also been found in constant worrying present in Generalised Anxiety Disorder (Gosselin et al., 2003) and potential consequences of Panic Attacks which lead to catastrophic misinterpretations of body sensations in Panic Disorder (Austin & Richards, 2001).

Thus, shame as an emotion finds its place in a wide variety of mental illnesses which may or may not have been studied yet, leading to the need to understand its effect on both the client and the symptoms of the illness they are diagnosed with.

25.4 Shame and Culture

Emotions have been found to play a central role in social relationships (Oatley, Keltner, & Jenkins, 2006; Mesquita, 2010). Expression of an emotion allows one to express one's concerns, reveal strategies, goals, intentions to act, thereby allowing an individual to take a stance in the social world. (Solomon, 2004; Griffiths & Scarantino, 2009). Universally, emotion regulation seems to be motivated by a person's need to establish and maintain proper and good relationships (Thompson, 1991; Gross, Richards, & John, 2006). Different cultures have different standards, and great variation on what will illicit shame. Studies in the area of culture and emotions have found East Asian cultures (Bhawuk, Wang, & Sang, Sueda and Clarke & Takashiro, in this book) to be interconnected, interdependent and adjust to each other's expectations (Kim & Markus, 1999; Oishi & Diener, 2003).

Interestingly, while Western literature clearly contrasts shame and guilt as having an "external" (being oriented to others) versus an "internal" orientation (being oriented towards self), studies on collectivistic cultures give mixed findings on the differences and similarities between shame and guilt (Breugelmans and Poortinga, 2006; Wong & Tsai, 2007). It is purported that since collectivistic cultures do not view themselves as separate from their relationships with others, their contexts or actions, shame and guilt acquire less differentiations from each other. These two emotions are considered conducive, in building strong relationships as they highlight flaws and shortcomings, thus encouraging alignment with social rules and relational embeddedness (Leersnyder, Boiger, & Mesquita, 2013). The ability to focus on one's flaws allows one to experience self-criticism which pushes individuals to live up to other's expectations, especially observed in countries such as Japan (Lewis, 1995; Nisbett, 2003). Thus, less focus is put on "internal" orientation in collectivistic cultures as compared to western cultures (Morling, Kitayama, & Miyamoto, 2002).

Additionally, both Western and Collectivistic cultures differ in the value they attach to shame itself. It has primarily been found that cultures such as Indian, Chinese, Japanese view shame as one of the positive emotions as compared to Americans, who see it as a negative emotion. For instance, Rozin (2003) in a research found that Americans viewed shame and anger as similar as they are both negatively valenced in contrast to Hindu Indians who considered happiness and shame as similar as they are both socially constructive. It is owing to this reason, that shame in collectivistic contexts plays a salient role in everyday life. (Crystal, Parott, Okazaki, & Watanabe, 2001).

Since the emotion of shame is intricately woven in the fabric of Asian cultures, it's no wonder that both the client and the therapist may find it difficult to exterminate it from the narrative. In extreme cases, hypothetically speaking, a therapist may even talk of emotion regulation with complete negation of the emotion "shame". Thus, it may take a personal experience on the part of the therapist themselves to be capable of recognising shame and seeing its effects on the client's psyche, personality and their lived life.

25.5 Shame in Psychotherapy

Lewis (1971), a pioneer in recognising the importance of shame in psychotherapy, posits that shame represents a family of emotions such as humiliation, belittlement, feelings of low self-esteem and stigmatization. Additionally, it can represent itself as a core ingredient in experiences of feeling hurt, inadequate, rejected, exposed, defeated, intimidated, peculiar, powerless and helpless.

In other words, the emotion of shame can often mask itself in a variety of other feelings. It is because of this reason that it can elude both the client and the therapist for a long time, that even when identified, its' presence may bring a kind of a denial or confusion in the client as if the word "shame" had suddenly become foreign. Nonetheless as therapists, one needs a keen eye to detect the presence of shame, a skill which requires great clinical acumen, knowledge and experience.

25.5.1 Who Am I?

A client named Neetu, shared in our seventh session, her uncertainty on feeling ashamed about her personality during her teens. Neetu was a thirty-three years old married woman, who stayed with her husband and child, from a middle-income family, with a Masters degree in Education. Her spontaneous reaction to feeling ashamed was that of confusion. Neetu had brought concerns about her workplace into psychotherapy which would often manifest in forms of constant chatter and ruminations in her mind. She would spend hours worrying over her thoughts, perceiving them to be real at the pretext of household chores being left unattended to.

Thoughts such as "*What will they think of me*" or "*They will seclude me*" would disturb her to the extent of making her feel inferior, inadequate, worthless, small and useless. She was diagnosed to have Obsessive Compulsive Disorder and was seeking both pharmacological help as well as psychotherapy for the same. Neetu had given her colleagues at work all the power to decide her worth. In other words, a supervisor's praise would make her feel elated while a critical comment was taken at heart, making her lose her worth and confidence. With respect to social situations she found herself repeatedly getting "*hurt and betrayed*" as she would realise the motive of the colleague much later than the occurrence of an event. Over the course of initial sessions, it was found that Neetu was discouraged to make friends in her teen years, which took away the core knowledge and skills required to befriend people, recognise their intentions and protect oneself in accordance to different situations.

One particular session vividly brought to the front the aspect of shame. As she recalled her colleagues mocking at her in a meeting where she was presenting, tears filled her eyes and began streaming down her cheeks. In a few seconds a pain so deep unleashed itself through a generous cry wherein she averted her gaze, bit her lips and looked down and away. After a few moments of silence, I gently asked her "*What do you feel right now?*". She replied "*Inferior*" through her sobs. Tugging along through her tears she said "*I felt like a demon in the story which I was talking about*". I calmly enquired "*What does being a demon means to you?*". She replied "*Not being sincere in my work*". I asked if she felt she was being insincere. To this she replied "*I feel like I'm not a correct person*". It is important to note here that this was not the first time Neetu felt like this. On other occasions in the past she had taken her superior's criticism at heart, personalising it to herself rather than the task which required re-working. Having read about shame and its' mechanisms in therapy I was particularly interested in exploring the emotion with Neetu. I recognised the *shame behind her repeated narrations of feeling "inadequate, small, inferior*" as put by her in prior sessions. Some enquiry about her childhood led her to share how her grandmother and aunt would constantly compare her with her sister. "*I wanted to be a correct person*" she uttered with emphasis on the word "correct". I asked what she meant by it. "*A person who is not very serious, jovial*". Further enquiry led her to share her elder's focus on wanting her to be "*studious, docile, quiet and polite*". Some of the principles offered by them to her included "*Find happiness in others' happiness*" and "*Don't allow others to point fingers at you*". It is here that the shame Neetu experienced in being herself became all the more evident.

The session saw great ambivalence from Neetu's end about her personality. While she had idealised the "*docile, polite*" person and aimed to be like that, she often felt ashamed about putting forth her perspectives to others or speaking her mind assertively. This also led her to feel '*inadequate and lacking*' every time she saw someone be confident and assertive in her approach. Lerner in her book (2004) The Dance of Fear, writes "Whatever is shamed, stigmatized or misunderstood in the larger culture gets absorbed as someone's personal shame". This is precisely how Neetu had internalised herself as an "*incorrect person*". In a culture like India, parents are often seen comparing their child either to their siblings, cousins or neighbours' children. While their intention is to encourage the child to hone their skills and capacities to be able to compete with the world at large, children sensitive to criticism often get emotionally affected by their elder's comments than motivated.

Some of the factors which were taken into account while formulating the role of shame in Neetu's narrative included the object relationistic perspective, wherein her urge to be the "only good person" in the eyes of a Supervisor or an elder was highlighted; the cognitive perspective, which accounted for her global attributions towards herself as "*bad, deficient and defective*" and the role of the Indian culture in shaming her for not possessing the necessary and favourable feminine qualities (of being "*quiet, docile and polite*") desired in an Indian girl.

Thus, the psyche quite literally internalizes words such as "*incompetent*", "*incorrect*" and "*lacking*" thinking them to be an inherent flaw in one's self. It was not long after the repetitive experiences of 'feeling inferior' that were brought in the sessions that I recalled something interesting. The therapist who had referred Neetu to me had emphasised her unending need for 'striving to be perfect' which further highlighted how flawed or incomplete she saw herself.

25.5.2 The Multiple Facets of Shame

What is essential to understand is that every time a client brings a particular emotion to therapy, that emotion itself has had its' share of trajectory-hiding, flowing, falling, rising, plundering, wrecking through the clients' many lived experiences. Like a river, shame brings along the many particles, debris, boulders of other emotions which have eventually submerged themselves so well in shame that shame loses its identity as an individual feeling. It took me seven sessions to comprehend the dynamics present in Neetu's case. Once shame came into the view, what was earlier seen as mere lack of confidence owing to depressogenic thoughts, that disturb client with OCD, changed.

25.5.3 Bringing Shame on the Table

The therapeutic approach I had envisioned for Neetu involved understanding her obsessions, compulsions and their content and psychoeducating her utilising the Cognitive Behavioral techniques. To address her feelings of inferiority and difficulty in handling anxiety a compassion focused and mindfulness approach was planned in addition to the primary humanistic stance I would adopt in therapy.

In the session described above when Neetu expressed her ambivalence on the parts of herself as being 'rebellious' versus wanting herself to be 'docile and soft spoken' I reflected back to her the continuous tug-of-war she felt within herself. I said *"It seems that a major part of you has been so driven to be docile and soft spoken that whenever the rebellious part of you comes forth there is shame associated with it. How do you connect with this?"* While Neetu understood about her conflicting parts of herself, she expressed surprise and confusion on my usage of the word "shame".

As I wrote my reflection post the session, going through previous session's notes I found something extremely captivating. Neetu in one of the earlier sessions had remarked *"I need to 'full' myself. Others are full vases, I have a lack, I'm empty, constantly running and not enjoying time with my family"*. Her inability to process shame brought to mind Lerner's words and I quote *"Shame drives the fear of not being good enough. You may carry the shame around with you all the time but be aware of it for only brief moments"* (p. 118).

25.5.4 Unpeeling of Shame and Its Experience

At times the progress of therapy itself may become a problem wherein the therapist looks for quick-fixes or tools to work on the machine (a client) so as to be able to bring it back to its original working state. That said, psychotherapy is a process in itself, a space which allows the client to paint their life on a blank canvas which the therapist offers. Some of the essential aspects which I focused on working with Neetu involved reflecting, mirroring, psychoeducating about her obsessive and compulsive phenomena and allowing a vast space for her to simply "be" sans any judgments, opinions, criticism or rebuke. Amidst these and other CBT techniques or tools of therapy, one of the most essential intervention used was borrowed from the therapist's basic humanistic stance and an eye on the therapeutic relationship (borrowed from Yalom's Gift of Therapy). My belief in Neetu's capacity to learn from her experiences, too see a world outside her "obsessional fantasy", to bring her back to the session than getting "lost" in her "obsessional narrative" played a key role in helping her understand the dynamics of her life viz a viz the OCD.

More details on the effectiveness of the interventions used were shared when Neetu was enquired for her feedback on her progress in the psychotherapy. She shared an increased capacity to filter her thoughts, to understand the difference between "real world versus an ideal world" and emphasised on the therapist's capacity to quickly catch her emotion and feeling state. Additionally, the homework tasks assigned and her writing brought immense clarity and perspective, for her, in work situations. Something which the therapist found very interesting, was revealed. Neetu also shared some of the metaphors which the therapist had used in various sessions to help her understand her state.

The cumulative effect of these interventions was seen in the tenth session wherein Neetu brought her confident, creative, ambitious, self-aware, socially-aware side of her, with traces of shame gradually processed. She shared her capacity to become indifferent towards her colleagues' comments and opinions, an ability to assert herself in dialogues wherein she earlier found herself speechless and a resolve to focus on her inner capacity and strengths.

Thus, in summary, the therapy process offers an amalgamation of skills, interventions and techniques used. With it is included the therapist's innate capacity to judge and customize techniques according to the needs of the client. In Neetu's case, the therapist-client fit felt just right.

25.5.5   Of Boundaries and Borders

Another client named Aastha, twenty-seven years old, single, with an educational background of Masters in Literature, came to psychotherapy with complaints of *"feeling disoriented, inefficient at work, difficulty in handling emotions and carrying an intense ball of pain inside her"*. At the time of seeking therapy, she was working from home, accompanied by her parents, with her office based in another city. Initial sessions revealed history of a broken engagement wherein she found herself being cheated by her fiancé for another woman which left her feeling inadequate and perplexed about issues concerning loyalty. Aastha came from a family which was dysfunctional and had severely hampered her sense of 'self' in the early years. Sexually abused by a stranger at the age of eight (which was kept as a secret) and losing her grandmother, the only person who understood her, were losses too potent for her. It was no surprise then why Aastha would find herself repeatedly getting caught in relationships which pulled her for love and affection even as a part of her would want to withdraw from the very person she admitted to being in love with. Despite her high intellect, florid vocabulary and deep potential to express herself she lacked on social skills and described herself as *"lacking a judgment over people's intentions"*.

Very early in the sessions it was understood that Aastha had borderline personality traits. In sync with her diagnosis and goals for learning social skills and controlling her emotions, Linehan's (1993) Dialectical Behavior Therapy plan was followed.

25.5.6 *"I'm Always Apologetic"*

In one of the sessions Aastha shared how she found herself profusely apologising to people even as they were responsible for something wrong. As she expressed herself, I sensed a confusion within her which seemed to emanate from a place of ambivalence; a space where she believed herself to be inherently "wrong" (*"I must have done something wrong, even though I do not remember, because I'm wrong"*) versus a space wherein she apologized to save the relationship (*"I have not done anything wrong but anything to save this relationship from going bad"*). With reference to this, Aastha shared an incident when she had to, literally, hold her heart as she apologized to her parents for something she did not agree with.

25.5.7 *The Eternal Conflict*

Time and again, in the sessions, Aastha would make references to a part of her which wanted to do something versus a part of her which was against it. Lost amidst the two voices she would either engage in actions that were impulsive, later to regret them, or completely shut herself and withdraw so as to avoid making any decision. On one such occasion she talked about the heated atmosphere at home in the midst of a fight. She exclaimed how fearful she was of fights and how nervous she felt about them. Further in the session she said *"I feel like a child at times, stubborn as a rock which says no to this and do something else instead. At the same time there is an adult which asks me to handle my situation well"*.

On a later occasion, it was found that the contrary voices which would often entangle Aastha belonged to her father and mother. This expression of hers was utilised in therapy. Through reflection and psychoeducation, the Transactional Analysis model of the Adult, Parent and Child figures was explained; and the conflicting voices were attributed to her internalised scripts of her parents. Amidst the many aspects of an invalidating environment, as a child, she was often left confused about which parent to follow and to ignore. At this she remarked *"As kids we had the ability to forget, now we can't"*.

Thus, shame at times becomes so imbued in one's behaviour that one forgets which part of the self it refers to. In Aastha's case shame got associated with not knowing which voice to hear. Even as she would choose a voice to which she believed in, it brought with it a shame so unbearable that was difficult to bear, a splitting which felt like a trap with no "grey's" in between. At this Brené Brown, in her book Daring Greatly (2012), writes "Sometimes shame is the result of us playing the old recordings that were programmed when we were children or simply absorbed from the culture".

25.5.8 Shame for What One Is not Guilty About

On one occasion Aastha forgot about the scheduled session. This led her to profusely apologise in the next session which was accepted by me non-judgmentally. The discussion about guilt led us towards understanding the role of shame in her life. Recognising the many traumatic experiences, she had faced as a child, leading to discordant voices within her, an effort was made to experience the child and the adult within her. Borrowing from the Gestalt therapy's empty chair technique, she was asked to imagine herself as a five-year-old Aastha and an Aastha of today. Through a guided visual imagery, she was asked to view the five-year-old as having done a mistake, hold her hand and say *"I'm there with you. I'll always be there with you"*. Aastha began sobbing as she imagined her own compassionate self. Of all the situations she blamed herself for in the past, one of the biggest mistake she was reminded of by her family was of losing her virginity before marriage. Indian culture has for decades associated virginity and feminine integrity as being equivalent, wherein losing virginity is considered shameful for the entire family, for it brings bad name to the girl and her parents. On the other, nothing is asked of the man who may have had multiple sexual partners before he decides to marry.

As she composed herself after the imagery, Aastha shared the experience as feeling the warmth of an accepting hug, *"for the first time I felt completely accepted...it was amazing to be loved like that"*. She continued *"That little girl was so scared, she felt bad that she was supposed to feel guilty."* She shared how she did not feel guilty about losing her virginity, which she considered an act of love, even as she was "made to feel ashamed" about it.

Of essential importance here is to highlight the usage of words "guilty" versus "ashamed". While many clients may use these words synonymously, Aastha clearly understood the difference between the two and was one of the high cognitive functioning clients in psychotherapy.

Her experience very delicately differentiated the boundaries between 'the self' and 'the other' juxtaposing itself to the definition of shame versus guilt. Her experience of connecting with her childhood self was one of the highlights of the therapy. It marked an ego integration which every therapist dreams for their client with borderline traits. The therapist in me was amazed at the wisdom that flowed from her. Her affirmative words brought a deep knowledge of how cultures alone can 'make' a woman feel ashamed even as she isn't. The experience is akin to the image of a shame that is literally and metaphorically injected by others making one feel wronged even as one doesn't.

Aastha's case was primarily formulated from a psychoanalytical perspective wherein the role of shame found itself switching between the ego and the ego ideal on one hand and at other, displayed itself in the form of an inherently insecure attachment style. Her relationship with her primary caregivers left her feeling "essentially unwantable, namely unwanted by anyone", thus leading to high unacceptance of herself for the person she was. Keeping this in mind, a Gestalt approach along with the Dialectical Behavioral Therapy was envisioned for her to strengthen her ego functioning, be mindful of her emotional disturbances and coalesce her conflicting parts of the self.

25.5.9 The Space of Therapy

Shame as an emotion is not to be looked down upon. It will be a huge irony if we pity, belittle "shame" for existing in the first place. It's an emotion that needs to be pulled out of the closet of human heart and mind and be given a space worthy of compassion, care, love and vulnerability. It needs an atmosphere inherently warming and comforting that even as one feels like breaking into a thousand pieces, one knows that they'll join to make something beautiful out of them. A therapeutic environment, described by Winnicott as "holding" comes the closest to this. It is this compassion weaved with vulnerability, courage and a capacity to deconstruct shame that Brown (2006) emphatically focuses in her Shame Resilience Theory and Gilbert and Procter (2006) describes in Compassionate Mind Training (Gilbert, Oousthuizen, Merkin und Vanderheiden, in this book) approach.

25.5.10 Measuring One's Words

It is essential to note that certain processes demand a client to live them wholly, the same holds true for shame. While Neetu expressed her confusion at the word 'shame', Aastha came to process it at a much inherent level, differentiating it from being owned by self or being 'made to' felt. A greater learning from the beautiful individual differences of these two cases is the need to measure one's words as a therapist. In other words, as therapists we cannot impose our learning onto a client to make it 'their insight'. Every client carries within them a treasure trove of strengths, capacities and wisdom that nudges them to grow forward in life. Like a caterpillar waiting for the cocoon to break, this too is a process which needs immense patience, struggle and cracking open on a client's part, something, we as therapists can and in no way should take away from them. That said, it's essential to reflect, psychoeducate clients about shame, it's healthy and unhealthy components.

25.6   Conclusion

By sharing the two case vignettes an attempt was made to understand how shame often creeps in psychotherapy, plays hide and seek some times and masks beneath various other emotions on other occasions. From the view of psychotherapy, an effort was made to utilise shame sensitively with the material the client brings in the therapy, thus highlighting the existence of symptoms as well as the deep roots for their cause.

While research in the realm of shame is still nascent, it continues to be a domain of huge interest to both people and mental health professionals at large. It is essential for psychotherapists to correctly identify it and work through it with the client; for shame can be as powerful as a quicksand, sucking in people, their worth, their integrity; sometimes alone, other times with families and cultural baggage tangled with it.

References

Austin, D. W. & Richards, J. C. (2001). The catastrophic misinterpretation model of panic disorder. *Behavior Research and Therapy, 39*, 11. Retrieved from https://doi.org/10.1016/S0005-7967(00)00095-4.

Breugelmans, S. M., & Poortinga, Y. H. (2006). Emotion without a word: Shame and guilt among Raramuri Indians and rural Javanese. *Journal of Personality and Social Psychology, 91*, 1111–1122.

Brown, B. (2006). Shame resilience theory: A grounded theory study on women and shame. *Families in Society: The Journal of Contemporary Social Services., 87*(1), 43–52.

Brown. B. (2012). *Daring greatly how the courage to be vulnerable transforms the way we live, love, parent and Lead.* Penguin Group.

Candea, D., & Szentagotai, A. (2013). Shame and psychopathology: From research to clinical practice. *Journal of Cognitive and Behavioral Psychotherapies, 13*(1), 101.

Claesson, K., Birgegard, A., & Sohlberg, S. (2007). Shame: Mechanisms of activation and consequences for social perception, self-image and general negative emotion. *Journal of Personality, 75*(3), 595–627. Retrieved from https://doi.org/10.1111/j.1467-6494.2007.00450.x.

Cozolino, L. J., & Santos, E. N. (2014). Why we need therapy—and why it works: A neuroscience perspective. *Smith College Studies in Social Work, 84*(2–3), 157–177. Retrieved from https://doi.org/10.1080/00377317.2014.923630.

Crystal, D. S., Parott, W. G., Okazaki, Y., & Watanabe, H. (2001). Examining relations among shame and personality among university students in United States and Japan: A developmental perspective. *International Journal of Behavioral Development, 25*, 113–123.

Dickerson, S. S., Gruenewald, T. L., & Kemeny M. E. (2009). Psychobiological responses to social self threat: Functional or detrimental? *Self and identity*, 8, 270–285. Retrieved from https://doi.org/10.1080/15298860802505186.

Ehlers, A., & Clark, D. M. (2000). A cognitive model of posttraumatic stress disorder. *Behaviour Research and Therapy, 38*, 319–345.

Erikson, E. H. (1950). *Childhood and society*. New York: Norton.

Gilbert, P. (1997). The evolution of social attractiveness and its role in shame, humiliation, guilt and therapy. *British Journal of Medical Psychology, 70*, 113–147.

Gilbert, P. (1998). What is shame? Some core issues and controversies. In P. Gilbert & B. Andrews (Eds.), *Shame: Interpersonal behavior, psychopathology and culture* (pp. 3–36). New York: Oxford University Press.

Gilbert, P., & Procter, S. (2006). Compassionate mind training for people with high shame and self-criticism: Overview and pilot study of a group therapy approach. *Clinical Psychology and Psychotherapy. 13*, 353–379. Retrieved from https://doi.org/10.1002/cpp.507.

Gosselin, P., Ladouceur, R., Langlois, F., Freeston, M. H., Dugas, M. J., & Bertrand, J. (2003). Développement et validation d'un nouvel instrument évaluant les croyances erronéesà l'égard des inquiétudes [Development and validation of a new instrument to evaluate erroneous beliefs about worries]. *European Review of Applied Psychology/Revue Européenne de Psychologie Appliquée, 53*(3–4), 199–221.

Grey, N., Holmes, E., & Brewin, C. R. (2001). Peritraumatic emotional "hot spots" in memory. *Behavioural and cognitive psychotherapy, 29*, 367–372.

Griffiths, P. E., & Scarantino, A. (2009). Emotions in the wild: The situated perspective on emotion. In P. Robbins & M. Aydede (Eds.), *Cambridge handbook of situated cognition* (pp. 437–453). Cambridge: Cambridge University Press.

Gross, J. J., Richards, J. M., & John, A. P. (2006). Emotion regulation in everyday life. In D. K. Snyder, J. A. Simpson, & J. N. Hugh (Eds.), *Emotion regulation in families: Pathways to dysfunction and health*. Washington, DC: American Psychological Association.

Karlsson G. & Sjoberg L. G. (2009). The experience of guilt and shame: A phenomenological-psychological study. *Humanistic Studies, 32*, 335–355. Retrieved from https://doi.org/10.1007/s10746-009-9123-3.

Kaufman, G. (1996). *The psychology of shame: Theory and treatment of shame based syndromes* (2nd ed.). New York: Springer Publishing Company.

Kim, H., & Markus, H. R. (1999). Deviance or uniqueness, harmony or conformity? A cultural analysis. *Journal of Personality Social Psychology, 77*, 285–800.

Leeming D., & Boyle M. (2013). Managing shame: An interpersonal perspective. *British Journal of Social Psychology. 52*, 140–160. Retrieved from https://doi.org/10.1111/j.2044-8309.2011.02061.x.

Leersnyder, J. D., Boiger, M., & Mesquita, B. (2013). *Cultural regulation of emotion: Individual, relational and structural sources. Frontiers in Psychology, 4*, 55. Retrieved from https://doi.org/10.3389/fpsyg.2013.00055.

Lerner, H. (2004). *The dance of fear rising above anxiety, Fear and Shame to Be Your Best and Bravest Self*. Harper-Collins: New York.

Lewis, H. B. (1971). *Shame and guilt in neurosis*. New York: International University Press.

Lewis, C. C. (1995). *Educating hearts and minds*. New York: Cambridge Press.

Linehan, M. M. (1993). *Skills training manual for treating borderline personality disorder*. The Guilford Press.

Mesquita, B. (2010). Emoting: A contextualized process. In B. Mesquita, L. F. Barrett, & E. R. Smith (Eds.), *The mind in context* (pp. 83–104). New York: Guilford Press.

Mills, R. S. L. (2005). Taking stock of the developmental literature on shame. *Developmental review, 25*, 26–63. Retrieved from https://doi.org/10.1016/j.dr.2004.08.001.

Morling, B., Kitayama, S., & Miyamoto, Y. (2002). Cultural practices emphasize influence in the United States and adjustment in Japan. *Personality Social Psychology Bulletin, 28*, 311–323.

Nisbett, R. E. (2003). *The geography of thought. How Asians and Westerners think differently… and why*. New York, NY: Free Press.

Oatley, K., Keltner, D., & Jenkins, J. M. (2006). *Understanding emotions* (2nd ed.). Malden, MD: Blackwell Publishing.

Oishi, S., & Diener, E. (2003). Goals, culture and subjective well-being. *Personality Social Psychology Bulletin, 29*, 939–949.

Piers, G., & Singer, M. B. (1953). *Shame and guilt: A psychoanalytic and a cultural study*. Springfield, IL: Charles C Thomas; reprint ed. (1971). New York: Norton.

Rozin, P. (2003). Five potential principles in understanding cultural differences in relation to individual differences. *Journal of Research in Psychology, 37*, 273–283.

Rüsch, N., Lieb, K., Göttler, I., Hermann, C., Schramm, E., Richter, H., et al. (2007). Shame and implicit self-concept in women with borderline personality disorder. *The American Journal of Psychiatry, 164*(3), 500–508. https://doi.org/10.1176/appi.ajp.164.3.500. [PubMed: 17329476].

Scheel, C. N., Bender, C., Tuschen-Caffier, B., Brodführer, A., Matthies, S., Hermann C., et al. (2014). Do patients with different mental disorders show specific aspects of shame? *Psychiatry Research, 220*(1–2), 490–495. Retrieved from http://doi.org/10.1016/j.psychres.2014.07.062.

Solomon, R. L. (2004). Back to basics: On the very idea of basic emotions. In R. L. Solomon (Ed.), *Not passion's slave* (pp. 115–142). Oxford: Oxford University Press.

Stadter, M. (2011). The inner world of shaming and ashamed: An object relations perspective and therapeutic approach. In R. L. Dearing & J. P. Tangney (Eds.), *Shame in the therapy hour* (pp. 45–68). Washington: American Psychological Association.

Tangney, J. P., & Fischer, K. W. (1995). Self-conscious emotions and the affect revolution: Framework and overview. In J. P. Tangney & K. W. Fischer (Eds.), *Self-conscious emotions: the psychology of shame, guilt, embarrassment and pride* (pp. 3–22). New York: Guilford.

Tangney J. P., Stuewig J., & Mashek D. J. (2007). Moral emotions and moral behavior. *Annual Review of Psychology, 58*, 345–372. Retrieved from https://doi.org/10.1146/annurev.psych.56.091103.070145.

Thompson, R. A. (1991). Emotional regulation and emotional development. *Educational Psychology Review, 3*, 269–307.

Tomkins, S. S. (1962). Affect, imagery, consciousness, volume 1: The positive affects. New York: Springer.

Tomkins, S. S. (1963). Affect, imagery, consciousness, vol 2: *The negative affects*. New York: Springer.

Tracy, J. L., & Robins, R. W. (2006). Appraisal antecedents of shame and guilt: Support for a theoretical model. *Personality and Social Psychology Bulletin, 32*, 1339–1351. https://doi.org/10.1177/0146167206290212.

Wong, Y., & Tsai, J. (2007). Cultural models of shame and guilt. In J. L. Tracy, R. W. Robins, & J. P. Tangney (Eds.), *The self-conscious emotions: Theory and research* (pp. 209–223). New York: Guilford Press.

Zaslav, M. R. (1998). Shame related states if mind in psychotherapy. *The Journal of Psychotherapy Practice and Research, 7*, 154–156.

Aakriti Malik is a lecturer at the Department of Counselling and Guidance, School of Education and Social Sciences at Management and Science University, Shah Alam, Malaysia. A licensed Clinical Psychologist from India, she completed her Masters in Psychology from Ambekar University, Delhi and MPhil in Clinical Psychology from NIMHANS, Bangalore, an institute of national importance for its' contribution to mental health treatment, training and research. Having seen children, adolescents and adults from diverse backgrounds in psychotherapy for the past six years, she considers her profession a privilege. It allows her to connect to the deeper realities of people and encourage them to reach their true potential. Her research interests have been diverse, ranging from bullying in schools, history of hysteria to client expectations from mental health professionals. She has taught undergraduates of psychology, counselling, nursing, occupational therapy, physiotherapy and education in various Government colleges in India and abroad. Her publications include articles and books chapters on bullying, psychotherapy with cancer afflicted patients, mental health in nursing and expectations from Mental Health Professionals. Additionally, she has to her credit multiple workshops and seminars conducted for school students, undergraduates, postgraduates, school counsellors, teachers, principals, nurses and doctors. She has also been an expert columnist in renowned newsletters such as the New Indian Express and Times of India. In her recent move to Malaysia, she aims to enrich her understanding about the Malaysian culture thereby increasing awareness of mental health among the people and mental health community.

Chapter 26
Interpreting Instances of Shame from an Evolutionary Perspective: The Pain Analogy

Jeff Elison

Abstract From a basic emotions perspective, shame can be viewed as a family of emotions (e.g., embarrassment, humiliation, guilt), which share a common antecedent—devaluation. As an evolutionary adaptation, shame can be either adaptive or maladaptive, depending on context and one's response. Findings on the affective neuroscience of social pain suggest the physical pain system was co-opted for adaptive social functions. Thus, physical pain is an appropriate analogy for understanding shame, the two sharing many features. Both are elicited by injury; with shame the injury is to a relationship or status. Both direct attention to the injury and make us care. Both motivate immediate and future behavior. We may lash out or cease what we are doing to end the pain, make attempts to repair reputational damage, or hide the source of shame. Both motivate attempts to avoid reoccurrence of the pain in the future. One may improve to avoid performance-based shame, or learn to avoid behaviors that elicit shame, just as one avoids cuts. Finally, both are communicated via physical expressions that often elicit empathy or forgiveness. Clients understand the functions of physical pain and how it protects us. Using the shame-pain analogy helps clients view shame in an adaptive light and helps them distinguish adaptive from maladaptive responses.

Keywords Shame · Pain · Evolution · Coping · Emotion regulation · Shame-pain analogy

26.1 Shame: An Evolutionary Perspective

An evolutionary perspective means looking first for function. Evolutionary perspectives on shame, bolstered by findings from affective neuroscience, illuminate shame's functional value and guide therapeutic approaches. In brief, shame is a basic emotion, an evolutionary adaptation piggy-backed on the physical pain mechanism (i.e., an

J. Elison (✉)
Psychology Department, Adams State University, 208 Edgemont Blvd,
Alamosa CO 81101, CO, USA
e-mail: jeffelison@adams.edu

© Springer Nature Switzerland AG 2019
C.-H. Mayer and E. Vanderheiden (eds.), *The Bright Side of Shame*,
https://doi.org/10.1007/978-3-030-13409-9_26

exaptation; Elison, 2005). Therefore, a very tight analogy exists between pain and shame in terms of antecedents, attentional effects, motivation, and coping. Like pain, shame serves valuable survival functions. Nevertheless, just as pain and efforts to cope with pain may be maladaptive, the same is true of shame.

An example comparing occurrences of pain and shame serves as an overview. Imagine two events: stubbing your toe and damaging a relationship. The first elicits physical pain, the second elicits social pain (shame). The antecedents in both cases are injuries: physical versus social/relational. Both activate a common brain structure (dACC; Eisenberger, 2011). Both direct our attention to the injury. Both motivate actions to address the injuries, such as repair. Finally, both motivate future avoidance: watch where you are walking; watch what you say.

Life without a functioning pain system is difficult and dangerous; so is life without the capacity to feel shame. Nevertheless, there are problems and pathologies associated with pain and shame.

26.2 Shame as an Evolutionary Adaptation

Shame is universal, an evolutionary adaptation (Elison, 2005; Tomkins, 1963). Emotions, as adaptations, are characterized by certain universal attributes: antecedents, expressions, feelings, attentional effects, action tendencies (motivational effects), and coping. Although a specific instance of any emotion may be maladaptive, emotions are thought to be adaptive overall.

26.2.1 Scope of Shame

As an emotion family, shame is viewed broadly to include embarrassment, humiliation, guilt, rejection, and "hurt feelings," even when so mild as to be unconscious (Cooley, 1922; Elison, 2005; Scheff, 1988; Tomkins, 1963).

26.2.2 Shame's Antecedents

Cooley (1922) cogently described shame's antecedents with the analogy of the Looking Glass Self. We see ourselves mirrored in the eyes of others and those mirrors convey judgements. Negative judgements elicit shame. Thus, the shame family represents social pain elicited by *devaluation*.

Basic emotions, just like physical pain, evolved in response to recurring challenges (e.g., injuries) to motivate adaptive responses (e.g., repair). Devaluation is a challenge because it threatens loss of status. Access to resources and mates depends on the quality of one's relationships and social status. Social exclusion, especially in our ancestral past, is life threatening. Shame, as a response to devaluation, is an alarm system (like pain) to warn us and motivate us when our rank or relationships are threatened.

Findings from affective neuroscience suggest shame is an exaptation that co-opted one of the brain regions associated with physical pain (dACC; Eisenberger, 2011). The dACC is responsible for pain's affective component, making us care. Evidence for the parallel roles of the dACC comes from fMRI studies showing activation during physical and social pain (i.e., social exclusion).

Cooley (1922) and Scheff (1988) maintain that the Looking Glass Self is always operational, even when alone. We automatically and unconsciously monitor our social environments.

26.2.3   Shame's Functions

The parallels between shame and physical pain make pain a useful analogy for understanding shame. Pain and shame are alarm systems to make us aware of "injuries," make us care about them, and motivate us to take reparative or preventative actions. Shame inhibits current behavior and makes us defer to the judgments of others. Thus, Scheff refers to shame as the "deference-emotion system" (1988).

26.2.3.1   Shame's Attentional Effects

Like any emotion, shame provides information. It directs attention to the relational problem ("someone thinks less of me") and self-consciousness ("what have I done?").

26.2.3.2   Shame's Feeling

The painful feeling of being small, weak, shrinking is inhibitory. We lose agency and stop what we are doing. Over longer periods, shame's pain motivates coping, described below. Shame keeps us aware of our social status and motivates its care. Just as a patient is more likely to remember to take medications when in pain and lapse when the pain is gone, we are more likely to follow norms when others are watching than when alone.

26.2.3.3   Shame's Behavioral Effects

Responses to shame are like those for any alarm. The immediate effect of shame is behavioral and cognitive inhibition. We are stopped mid-sentence when we see we have offended our listener. The cessation of immediate behavior is a form of deference. Attention turns self-conscious. A series of evaluations follows. Why the alarm; why am I feeling shame? Who is judging me, for what? Is this a false alarm; do I care? Should I respond to the alarm: do I repair, cover up, or rationalize? Or do I ignore it, like pretending not to smell smoke?

Sometimes this series of evaluations is explicit and conscious. At other times, it is short-circuited by automatic, scripted behavior. These can be adaptive or maladaptive, ranging from reparation and personal improvement to hiding or violence.

Ultimately, shame motivates us to maintain our relationships and status, to avoid exclusion. Maintenance is achieved via change, conformity, reciprocity, and socialization. These mechanisms work both directions—others change and conform to our expectations, and reciprocate our favors.

The analogy with physical pain is clear, as both can be used to force others to conform or reciprocate. Socialization is often achieved through physical or social pain, but the desire to maintain positive relationships may be the best motivator for adopting others' norms.

26.2.3.4 Shame's Expression

The universal expression of shame (head-down, gaze-averted, shoulders slumped) provides potent non-verbal communication. It communicates deference: "I have perceived your negative evaluation," "I value your judgment, our relationship," "I feel bad." When appropriate, a clear display of shame is functional; others are more likely to forgive us or even feel empathetic. Empathy makes sense considering the pain analogy; shame and embarrassment are recognized as painful.

26.3 Shame in the Evolutionary Context

Shame is an adaptation, yet shame-coping responses complicate whether shame is adaptive or maladaptive in any given case. Nonetheless, the evolutionary perspective and the pain analogy have strong implications for working with shame in any context: intimate relationships, parenting, sports, work, legal, and therapy.

26.4 Applied Approaches to Dealing with Shame

The focus of this section is identifying shame (feelings, thoughts, and behaviors) and identifying common adaptive versus maladaptive responses. Most of an individual's responses to emotions are scripted to some degree, meaning automatic and largely unconscious. They are emotion habits involving perception, feeling, behavior, and coping. Changing problematic shame involves identifying these scripts so they may be raised to awareness, finding a more adaptive substitute reaction, and then practicing the new reaction until it becomes scripted.

Given the claims that shame is an alarm and emotions are information, it is adaptive to switch attention to the problem and evaluate one's immediate situation. The immediate situation is relational, the shamed reacting to one or more looking glasses. Elements to evaluate include: accuracy of perceptions, history between the shamed and the other, the "offending" behavior, and options for responding. Understanding these elements opens doors to alleviating maladaptive shame.

26.4.1   Shame Is Useful

A place to start is with the big-picture perspective that life would be impossible without the capacity to feel shame. In this respect, shame is just like pain. Congenital analgesia (pain insensitivity) is dangerous. Those afflicted may fail to recognize illness or injury, reducing life expectancy. Similarly, those who feel no shame suffer socially and society suffers. They may fail to recognize their effects on others, at a cost to relationships or status. They may fail to conform or be socialized to the norms that make societies possible (e.g., psychopathy). Few of us are thankful for pain, but we should be thankful for the valuable alarm functions provided by physical and social pain. Being called shameless is not a compliment.

On the other hand, some people experience shame too intensely or too frequently, most likely due to being shame-prone or being in a shaming environment. Shame-prone refers to the tendency to experience maladaptive shame or inordinately intense shame (Tangney & Dearing, 2002), like experiencing pain in the absence of painful stimuli. People who are shame-prone or living in shaming environments often exhibit psychological symptoms and maladaptive behaviors.

26.4.2   Before the Looking Glass: Desired Images

Understanding Cooley's looking glass analogy and the dynamics of devaluation point to several elements of shame that may be problematic, providing targets for intervention. Devaluation occurs when the impression of one's self that one desires to see in the eyes of others falls short of the impression one perceives in the eyes of others (Elison, 2005). This definition involves three components—desired image, others' images of one's self, and the act of perception—discussed in the following sections.

An effective place to start self-change or therapeutic intervention is with desired images of self. Much has been written about a similar concept, the ideal self, and targeting its content. For example, perfectionism can result from an unattainable ideal self. All of that is relevant here—individuals can identify and re-evaluate the goals and standards that make up the ideal self. Are they realistic? Do they truly match their own desires, or have they internalized poorly fitting parental or societal standards?

Embracing the evolutionary perspective (Gilbert and Malik, in this book), a superordinate desired image of self arises: acceptance/inclusion. Death (or inability to reproduce) due to social exclusion is the extreme form of the selection pressure that led to the social pain adaptation. Humans fear exclusion and desire acceptance. Consistent with Cooley (1922) and Scheff (1988), evolutionary accounts include constant, automatic vigilance for social threats. Thus, the mere perception of disapproval triggers the alarm. Cognitive evaluations and coping follow. The classic analogy in evolution is the snake-stick scenario. Which is more costly: not reacting when you step on a snake or needlessly reacting when you step on a stick? Certain classes of false positives (jumping off the stick) are much less costly than their concomitant false negatives (failing to jump from the snake).

The study that revealed the neurobiological support for shared physical-social pain mechanisms illustrates our acute sensitivity to exclusion (Eisenberger, 2011). Participants where monitored by fMRI while playing ball-toss on a computer, believing they were playing with real people, when in fact the game was rigged to exclude them. Participants were distressed by exclusion in a kids' game, played on a computer, with "strangers," while lying in the noisy cramped scanner! The implications for human nature are striking: humans are exquisitely sensitive to exclusion. Sensitivity is hardwired, normal.

The simple message that sensitivity to exclusion is normal can be comforting, especially for those living in individualistic cultures where "needing others," "caring what others think," and conformity are often viewed as weaknesses.

26.4.3   What's in the Looking Glass? Accuracy of Perception

To perceive devaluation, one must first perceive or imagine a negative judgment. The act of perception is fallible, misreading what others think. Imagination opens the doors for misreading farther. If the appraisals involved in the looking glass self are unconscious and automatic (scripted), they can be difficult to change, but not impossible. By identifying maladaptive tendencies and raising them to consciousness, we can slow down the process and question the accuracy of impressions.

26.4.4   The Fun-House Looking Glass

The third component of devaluation is others' images of one's self. It is helpful to consider the identity of the other (stranger vs. parent) and the others' standards. Because we respond rapidly and automatically to others' facial expressions or words, it is impossible to simply "turn off" shame. Rather, we must respond to the feeling in the moments or hours that follow. Conscious assessment and reframing of shame may reduce its intensity or eliminate the feeling. A place to start the conscious process is to ask whether this is a person about whose evaluations you care.

It may be more important to consider why we are being judged. Because people hold opposing standards (eating meat is immoral vs. natural), we can never be free of negative judgments. If I care about doing a good job at work *and* want to keep my job *and* my boss thinks my work has fallen short, then it makes sense to answer shame's alarm. However, I just don't care what strangers think about my old car. Perhaps a facile example, but there will always be someone with a different view of religion, politics, diet, sex, etc.

"Fun-house" mirrors distort images to make people look squat, wavy, or otherwise unreal. People often do the same, distorting images of others. Rock climbers use "climber fat" as slang, capturing the experience of being thin and fit by normal standards, but feeling overweight in comparison to climbers. Ballet dancers, gymnasts, and endurance athletes experience something similar. Children, partners, and employees of perfectionists may as well. The "fun-house" mirror analogy is valuable as it makes light of others' distorted standards and illustrates Cooley's looking glass.

26.4.5 What Consequences?

Evolution operates according to relative probabilities and consequences. An example is the snake-stick dilemma. The probability that the thin, vibrating object underfoot is a snake is small, the probability that it is dangerous is smaller. Yet, we react with fear and jump. Here, human nature is usually wrong; we needlessly feel fear, shift attention, and waste energy. The key to understanding this paradox is the relative consequences of false positives versus false negatives. The false positive (stick for snake) resulting in a little bit of fear and wasted energy presents a small cost in comparison to the risk from the false negative (snake for stick). Thus, human nature is to jump.

Similar calculations apply to devaluation. The existence of shame as an adaptation points to the importance of true positives—devaluation can be as threatening as the poisonous snake. Nevertheless, we often experience false positives due to misperception. Perhaps more commonly, we correctly perceive the devaluation, but like the non-poisonous snake, the consequences are negligible. Negative judgments of strangers generally fall in this category. Counter-intuitively, our mistakes and shortcomings may not have serious consequences among friends and loved ones. True loved ones accept us. In these cases, shame should be "let go" to the extent possible.

Understanding the biological/organic nature of shame and the frequency of false positives suggests that we should not dwell on shame's pain without evaluation. Focusing on the feeling makes us weak and powerless, activating memories of past shame. Far from denial, reframing shame as a mistaken alarm (like a smoke detector with low batteries) *can be* the adaptive response.

26.4.6   Shame Is Adaptive: Do the Right Thing(s)

26.4.6.1   Reducing Devaluation

An adaptive response is to pay attention to shame, rather than to ignore the alarm. If, after evaluating the factors above, the devaluation is real and important, then it makes sense to consider what can be done to reduce the devaluation and improve others' images of us. If the reasons for devaluation are unclear, asking for clarification may be appropriate. If the reasons are clear, can they be addressed to reduce the devaluation and repair one's injured status?

Apologies may be in order and may alleviate the devaluation. An explanation may help, if an action or statement has been misunderstood, as when a joke is taken seriously. A discussion may help, if our norms or values conflict with those of the other. Taking responsibility and actions to address shame are often respected, especially in contrast to the resentment and further devaluation that follow when the issue is ignored, denied, or hidden.

26.4.6.2   The Value of Showing Shame

Part of the nonverbal shame display is to break eye contact. The display also communicates awareness of the shame issue, deference to the other, and pain. Shame's nonverbal display most likely evolved from the submissive behaviors associated with threats of aggression. The displays show similarities: physical, contextual, and functional. The context is threatened status or rank—via aggression versus opinion. The function is appeasement—to reduce or stop the aggression versus devaluation. The displays are adaptive.

The submissive display of shame affects others. Just as the display of a submissive dog controls the dominant dog, making attack less likely, the shame display reduces devaluation. Others are more likely to accept apologies or explanations that are accompanied by a shame display because they interpret them as sincere. Because the shame display conveys pain, the other may even feel empathy.

When ashamed, we are tempted to hide from others, so we are also tempted to hide our displays of shame. They seem to broadcast our flaws. Understanding the adaptive value of shame and its display implies that we should not be afraid to let our shame show.

26.4.6.3   Avoidance: A Lesson to Be Learned?

The best response to shame is often future avoidance. Pain dramatically shapes our behavior, narrowing or expanding it to avoid more pain. We quickly narrow behavior and avoid pain when we learn not to touch hot stoves. We expand behavior and avoid pain when we learn to store knives safely. The shame-pain analogy holds with respect to avoidance.

An adaptive response to valid shame is to look for the lesson to be learned, which is often avoidance. We learn to avoid mistakes, certain topics of conversation, and specific people. We learn to take the precautions necessary to avoid a shame-inducing scene. We act to avoid shame before even leaving the house: shower, shampoo, apply deodorant, brush teeth, dress. Many of these behaviors benefit us directly, but they all reduce devaluation.

26.4.7 Maladaptive Responses: The Compass of Shame

Having discussed adaptive responses, examining maladaptive responses illuminates the contrast between the two and aids in identifying problematic scripts. Because shame is an alarm, ignoring it can be dangerous, like ignoring the fire alarm. Similarly, morphing shame into a more palatable emotion, like anger, can be counterproductive. We also pay a price when we make too much of shame. Perseverating on a minor embarrassment is like deploying the fire extinguisher when the alarm clock rings. One model that encompasses a broad range of these potentially maladaptive responses is Nathanson's (1992) Compass of Shame (Wang & Sang and Larsson, in this book). Nathanson grouped shame-coping into four categories (Withdrawal, Attack Self, Attack Other, Avoidance) and located them at the points of the compass (Fig. 26.1). Webb suggested modifying Nathanson's diagram by adding the emotions used to mask shame in the four quadrants and the clarifying labels *Hide from Self/Other* (T. Webb, personal communication, December 16, 2017). Shame, broadly defined, lies at the center.

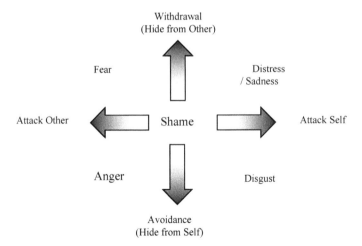

Fig. 26.1 The compass of shame. Adapted from Nathanson, 1992; modifications by Webb

The four shame-coping styles encompass families of scripts; each style manifests in many ways. The styles are viewed as relatively stable personality traits, and thus there are individual differences in their use. Nathanson (1992) devotes chapters to each of these categories, described briefly here. Nathanson's model provides a useful visual, and readily recognizable categories, that can anchor therapeutic discussions.

26.4.7.1 Withdrawal: Hiding from Others

As an adaptation, shame produces a display and behaviors associated with inhibition and submission. Withdrawal may be the primary behavioral response—escape painful gaze and devaluation. People describe wanting to disappear or wishing they were invisible. Withdrawal as a conscious behavior varies from cessation of conversation or actions to fleeing from important environments (e.g., quitting school).

Withdrawal can be adaptive: from toxic environments; when it appeases others; when others might aggress. Nevertheless, withdrawal can be maladaptive when an opportunity to reduce devaluation (e.g., apology) would have been effective. As much as we might want to disappear, leaving school or a job is almost always an overreaction, with serious costs.

Research demonstrates that Withdrawal has serious consequences for psychological health, being correlated with: depression, low-self-esteem, anxiety, and interpersonal sensitivity (Elison, Lennon, & Pulos, 2006). Among the four styles, it shows the highest correlations with social anxiety/phobia, which makes sense given the self-chosen isolation. Among the four styles, Withdrawal and Attack Self are the most highly correlated pair. Both are internalizing responses. When the two are paired, they result in social isolation and rumination, a damaging combination.

Addressing Withdrawal, or any of Nathanson's shame-coping styles, involves recognizing them and replacing them with more adaptive responses. Flexibility is a sign of psychological health. Over-deployment of any shame response is likely to be problematic. Clients should be encouraged to fight the urge to run, and to instead evaluate the validity and consequences of the shaming event, only withdrawing when deemed effective. The motivation to change can be encouraged by discussing Withdrawal's costs to psychological health, happiness, and relationships.

26.4.7.2 Attack Self: Inward-Directed Anger

Just as we may be angry with ourselves when we cause our pain (e.g., stubbed toe), it is natural to be angry with ourselves when we cause ourselves shame. Attack Self involves inward-directed anger, self-blame, self-loathing, and rumination. Tomkins (1963) wrote of scripts that magnify emotions; in everyday language we refer to "blowing things out of proportion," apt descriptions of Attack Self. People who favor Attack Self, tend to do the opposite of adaptive evaluations; they misinterpret neutral reactions as devaluation, they overestimate the seriousness of their mistakes or inadequacies, and they place too much blame on themselves. They may say they hate themselves, they are worthless, or they will never be successful. Attack Self is part of maladaptive perfectionism.

Deployed strategically it is effective in reducing devaluation. Being the first to call attention to our mistake may impress others, diminish their power to shame us, allow us to joke about it, and even garner empathy. Self-deprecating humor can be endearing.

Due to the internalization, rumination, and magnification that make up Attack Self, it shows the highest correlations with a wide range of psychological symptoms: depression, low self-esteem, anxiety, perfectionism, and fear of failure (Elison et al., 2006).

Addressing Attack Self involves reality testing, revealing the clients' tendencies to misread others and to respond introapunitively. Although habitual and therefore difficult to change, most clients are likely to be motivated to try, due to the high costs.

26.4.7.3 Attack Other: Outward-Directed Anger

Just as we may be angry with others when we blame them for pain (e.g., stepping on our toes), it is natural to be angry with others when we feel shame. Attack Other involves outward-directed anger and blaming others. Another ploy is to find someone to bolster our status via comparison: "I may have gotten a D, but he got an F." Responding with anger-aggression appears paradoxical—if a person is concerned with (de)valuation by others, why would they risk further damage by responding with hostility? The pain analogy provides an explanation. If social pain is an exaptation of physical pain, then the threat-defense responses (i.e., fight or flight) that evolved in response to physical pain are likely to be deployed in response to social pain (Elison, Garofalo, & Velotti, 2014; MacDonald & Leary, 2005). There is a biological basis for the fact that anger and aggression are common responses to shame.

An evolutionary connection does not necessarily imply that anger is an adaptive response. The benefits of the physical pain exaptation (i.e., the alarm and motivational components) could have outweighed the costs of the linked threat-defense responses (i.e., attention and flight may generally be adaptive, while fight may be generally maladaptive). Thus, anger-aggression may be adaptive or maladaptive, depending on context. They will often make the situation worse, in that others may think less of us. In other cases, such as being humiliated by a bully, standing one's ground could be adaptive.

Attack Other correlates with depression, hostility, distancing, and psychopathy (Campbell & Elison, 2005; Elison et al., 2006).

Addressing Attack Other involves reducing the clients' tendencies to externalize and discussing its counterproductive nature. Clients may appreciate learning that anger "came along for the ride" in our evolutionary history, yet it may be less adaptive in response to social pain. Aggression comes with a high cost, socially and legally. The externalization component makes Attack Other difficult to address.

26.4.7.4 Avoidance: Hide from Self

Avoidance involves denial, disavowal, and emotional distancing. The goal is to minimize conscious recognition of shortcomings and shame. We can deny caring: "She dumped me, but she's not that great." We can use disavowal when we adjust priorities to protect self-image: "Chemistry is silly; I'll switch to psychology." We can distance ourselves by joking about a failure or via addictions.

As always, context matters when evaluating whether avoidance is adaptive in a given instance. Avoidance via reframing, when a situation cannot be changed, could be adaptive. Dropping important goals or ignoring situations that could be improved are maladaptive. An interesting finding indicates that others can interpret our Avoidance as being passive-aggressive. Specifically, when someone offers constructive criticism and we dismiss it, they may feel ignored or worse.

Avoidance correlates with emotional minimization and psychopathy (Campbell & Elison, 2005; Elison et al., 2006).

Addressing Avoidance involves raising the clients' awareness of their defensiveness and increasing their tolerance for negative emotions and realistic self-assessment. The denial and distancing components make Avoidance difficult to address. Clients may not want to face the negative emotions or realistic self-images and derail the conversation or quit therapy.

26.4.7.5 Coping by Degrees

Another useful visual is to think of the Compass of Shame as a bullseye, as in darts. The bullseye represents adaptive coping—we acknowledge shame, evaluate the situation as outlined above, and address it if possible and appropriate. The four arrows of the compass represent our tendencies to respond defensively. The range of behaviors along each arrow can be arranged with distance representing intensity or severity. For example, brief thoughts of "I'm stupid" before addressing a minor mistake represents mild Attack Self. Extended rumination over inadequacies or suicidal ideation represent extreme Attack Self. Application with clients is discussed in Sect. 26.5.

26.5 Applied Methods and Applications

26.5.1 The Compass of Shame

The goal in using the Compass of Shame model in therapy or self-reflection is to identify problematic responses to shame (i.e., habitual scripts) and replace them with adaptive responses. The change process is enhanced when clients are partners in identifying how the compass model manifests in their own experiences. Descriptions of the four styles that include typical feelings, thoughts, and behaviors appear above and elsewhere (Elison et al., 2006; Nathanson, 1992). But the possible manifestations are endless, so personalizing these experiences is necessary.

26.5.1.1   Assessment: The Compass of Shame Scale

The Compass of Shame Scale (CoSS; Elison et al., 2006) was developed to quantify use of Nathanson's four families of shame responses (Fig. 26.1). The CoSS is a self-report instrument comprised of 12 shame-inducing scenarios (stems), to which respondents rate their frequency of use of the four styles. A sample item is:

> When an activity makes me feel like my strength or skill is inferior: (stem)
> 1. I don't let it bother me. (Avoidance)
> 2. I get mad at myself for not being good enough. (Attack Self)
> 3. I withdraw from the activity. (Withdrawal)
> 4. I get irritated with other people. (Attack Other)
> * Labels in parentheses are only provided here for clarity.

Respondents rate all four options for each scenario on a frequency scale: *Never* to *Almost Always*. Scores are calculated by adding all 12 responses for each family.

Data on many of the correlates described above come from studies employing the CoSS. However, the CoSS has also been used in therapy. Interpretation of scores is aided by norms (available from the author), but these are not necessary. Therapists and clients can use the scores, or even just clients' responses to individual scenarios, as a guide for discussions:

> • Which of the 12 stems are most painful for you? (inferiority, rejection, guilt)
> • Are there other situations that are especially painful?
> • Which types of response do you use the most?
> • How have these types of responses caused problems for you? (work, relationships, legal)
> • How could you respond to a given situation in a better way?
> • Does your response to a situation change over time? (discussed below)

Version 3 of the CoSS was published in Elison et al. (2006); however, Version 5 incorporates several improvements (contact: jeff_elison@msn.com) and has been translated to 13 languages.

26.5.1.2 Dynamic Shame-Regulation

Shame can last for minutes, hours, or days. Thus, shame-regulation strategies play out over time. Just as one's preference for Attack Self shows stability over time, so do sequences of shame-coping responses. For example, imagine snapping at a loved one when he offers constructive criticism, Attack Other. As the shame over the criticism subsides, it may be overshadowed by shame over the Attack Other response: "He didn't deserve that." Self-blame commonly follows: "I'm a bad person," Attack Self continuing the maladaptive trajectory. An adaptive response would be a heart-felt apology. Discussing and identifying these typical sequences add another level to therapeutic interventions.

Because other-directed anger and self-directed anger are correlated, they often appear in sequence (previous paragraph); however, the order can reverse. Those who automatically internalize will start with Attack Self, but given time, they may reframe the situation, realistically or not, and switch to Attack Other ("who are they to judge?").

Attack Self and Withdrawal are the most highly correlated of the CoSS responses. The evolutionary response to run away or hide comes immediately. Then, once safely away from judging eyes, one switches to Attack Self and rumination. Attack Other is correlated with Withdrawal, to a lesser degree, and may also follow, possibly appearing passive-aggressive.

Reframing is an often conscious cognitive process that takes time, and so, Avoidance or Adaptive responses may follow the others.

Beyond the obvious discussion points of why these sequences may be maladaptive, their presence begs the question: why not take a shortcut to an adaptive response. Indeed, instantly banishing maladaptive responses is an unrealistic goal. Lest clients Attack Self over their lapses toward an unrealistic goal (as with dieting), it is better to strive for progress, defined as using them less often or spending less time getting to an adaptive response. This point is especially important for those prone to internalization or perfectionism.

26.5.1.3 The Bullseye

The Compass of Shame model is useful even without CoSS scores. An exercise employing a CoSS-bullseye diagram is to identify a response to a specific shame experience and then classify it in terms of which family it belongs to and how far out on the arrow it falls. Doing this repeatedly can reveal characteristic and problematic responses, as well as progress. The visual aid makes the categories easier to understand and remember, as well as providing a reminder that the goal is a bullseye of adaptive responding.

26.5.1.4 Walking the Compass

Clients can more fully explore their shame responses individually or in group settings by physically moving about a large diagram of the Compass of Shame laid out on the floor (T. Webb, personal communication, December 16, 2017). Webb suggests several steps that may be included in this exercise:

1. Place a paper marked "shame" in the center of the room.
2. Stand on shame, model its nonverbal display.
3. Ask how we typically respond to or defend against shame. Responses will usually fit the four Compass of Shame categories.
4. Label four sheets of paper with the Compass categories and lay them out in a compass configuration.
5. Model the categories and ask for participants' reactions. Discussion can include related emotions (anger, sadness) and correlates (isolation, depression, aggression).
6. Invite participants, one at a time (the model), to stand in the spot representing their most common response to shame. Ask the model what they notice about themselves and the reactions of others. Ask other participants what they notice about the model. Often, the model's expression will match the masking emotions in Fig. 26.1. Repeat these reflections as the participant moves to each of the points.

26.5.2 Visual Display and Empathy

Shame allows us to maintain positive relationships, but only when we address it. Others respond favorably to shame acknowledgment and nonverbal displays of shame, as opposed to avoidance or externalization. A variation of the Walking the Compass exercise is useful for illustrating empathic responses to shame (T. Webb, personal communication, December 16, 2017).

1. With others watching carefully, ask a participant (model) to stand in a spot representing their most common response to shame and to describe what they do there. Avoid long stories by asking others what they notice. They will typically report feeling uncomfortable due to the unaddressed shame, possibly noticing that words are being used to hide shame.
2. Ask the model how far they are willing to walk toward the center. Encourage a small, slow approach.

3. Ask others what they notice. Often this will be a true shame display.
4. Ask the model what they are feeling. Again, avoid long descriptions by asking others what they notice. They will typically notice that the model's words interrupt his or her shame display.
5. Ask the model if they can stay with shame, moving closer to the center.
6. If the model displays shame again, ask others how they feel about the model's shame. Focus on any empathic responses.
7. Ask the model how they feel about the empathic responses. They will often describe relief, the weight of shame being lifted.
8. Include all in a discussion of how shame is functional, allowing repair of relationships, but only when acknowledged.

26.5.3 Shame-Pain Analogy

The shame-pain analogy was described extensively above, so how can discussions personalize it? Specifically, when does shame help clients? Specifically, does their alarm system malfunction, either failing to go off or creating false alarms.

26.5.4 The Looking Glass

Similarly, the Looking Glass analogy was described extensively above, so how can discussions personalize it? Specifically, when do clients have unrealistic desires for what they will see there ("I want to be the best")? Do they create false alarms by seeing negative judgements where none exist? Who in their lives represent fun-house mirrors ("I can never please him")?

26.6 Conclusion

Taking an evolutionary perspective on shame, including the pain and Looking Glass analogies, directs our focus on shame's adaptive functions. This perspective also focuses attention on distinguishing adaptive from maladaptive instances of shame and shame-coping. Finally, the shame-pain analogy suggests a number of strategies for interventions designed to reduce maladaptive shame, replacing it with adaptive responses.

References

Campbell, J. S., & Elison, J. (2005). Shame coping styles and psychopathic personality traits. *Journal of Personality Assessment, 84,* 96–104.

Cooley, C. H. (1922). *Human nature and the social order.* New York: Charles Scribner's Sons.

Eisenberger, N. I. (2011). Why rejection hurts: What social neuroscience has revealed about the brain's response to social rejection. In J. Decety & J. Cacioppo (Eds.), *The handbook of social neuroscience* (pp. 586–598). New York: Oxford University Press.

Elison, J. (2005). Shame and guilt: A hundred years of apples and oranges. *New Ideas in Psychology, 23,* 5–32.

Elison, J., Garofalo, C., & Velotti, P. (2014). Shame and aggression: Theoretical considerations. *Aggression and Violent Behavior, 19*(4), 447–453.

Elison, J., Lennon, R., & Pulos, S. (2006). Investigating the compass of shame: The development of the compass of shame scale. *Social Behavior and Personality, 34,* 221–238.

MacDonald, G., & Leary, M. R. (2005). Why does social exclusion hurt? The relationship between social and physical pain. *Psychological Bulletin, 131*(2), 202–223.

Nathanson, D. L. (1992). *Shame and pride: affect, sex, and the birth of the self.* New York: Norton.

Scheff, T. J. (1988). Shame and conformity: The deference-emotion system. *American Sociological Review, 53,* 395–406.

Tangney, J. P., & Dearing, R. L. (2002). *Shame and guilt.* New York: Guilford Press.

Tomkins, S. S. (1963). *Affect/imagery/consciousness. The negative affect* (Vol. 2). New York: Springer.

Jeff Elison (Ph.D.) is a professor of psychology at Adams State University in Colorado, USA. He has published dozens of articles and conference presentations on shame, guilt, humiliation, and shame-regulation. He also authored the Compass of Shame Scale (CoSS), a self-report instrument to assess shame-regulation styles. The CoSS has been translated to 13 languages.

Chapter 27
Distinguishing Shame, Humiliation and Guilt: An Evolutionary Functional Analysis and Compassion Focused Interventions

Paul Gilbert

Abstract The self-conscious emotions of shame, humiliation and guilt are clearly related to our human capacity for self-awareness and sense of self as an 'object in the minds of others'. However, this chapter will highlight that the emotional and motivational processes that sit behind them are phylogenetically old and rooted in social competition for shame and humiliation, and care-giving for guilt. Insight into their phylogenetic origins and differences helps us to gain insight into the physiological processes that texture them and why they can have such profound effects not only on individual human behaviour but also whole societies and cultures. This chapter will explore the differences between these self-conscious emotions, how they are rooted in different motivational systems and how we can utilise care and compassion based motivational systems for the remediation and change.

Keywords Compassion · Guilt · Humiliation · Reputation · Shame

27.1 Introduction

Emotions evolved because they stimulate animals to behave in certain ways. For example, emotions such as anger, anxiety and disgust serve the function of detecting threats and creating physiological states for appropriate defences (fight, flight and avoid/expel). Positive and hedonic emotions stimulate resource seeking and acquiring. The physiological infrastructures supporting basic emotions are ancient and are often referred to as *primary emotions*. However, the evolution of a range of cognitive competencies over the last 2 million years including ones for self-monitoring, self-consciousness and self-identity, gave rise to *self-conscious emotions* (Gilbert, 1998a, 2007; Sedikides & Skowronski, 1997; Tracy, Robins, & Tangney, 2007).

P. Gilbert (✉)
Centre for Compassion Research and Training, College of Health and Social Care Research Centre, University of Derby, Kedleston Road, Derby DE22 1GB, UK
e-mail: p.gilbert@derby.ac.uk

University of Queensland, Brisbane, Australia

© Springer Nature Switzerland AG 2019
C.-H. Mayer and E. Vanderheiden (eds.), *The Bright Side of Shame*,
https://doi.org/10.1007/978-3-030-13409-9_27

There are a range of different self-conscious emotions that utilise primary emotions but blend them with self-conscious experience. The most common of these include shame, pride, embarrassment, humiliation, and guilt (Giner-Sorolla, 2015; Tracy et al., 2007). The central and peripheral nervous system did not evolve a different threat processing system for self-conscious emotions; the amygdala, hypothalamic-pituitary adrenal axis and autonomic nervous system remain the basic physiological mechanisms for all threats including to one's self-identity (Dickerson & Kemeny, 2004). Rather what evolved were new cognitive competencies that allow these threat systems to be triggered, textured and experienced in new ways (Tracy et al., 2007; Gilbert, 2009). Importantly, social threats linking to rejection, social loss and social devaluation, are core to our shame experience (Gilbert, 1998b; Sznycer, Tooby, Cosmedes et al., 2016), and are the most powerful activators of threat processing systems (Dickerson & Kemeny, 2004). Indeed, there is good evidence that rejection and experiences of shame operate through similar neurophysiological pathways as pain (Kross, Berman, Mischel, Smith, & Wager, 2011) although there may be physiological differences between acute and chronic rejection-shame experiences (Rohleder, Chen, Wolf, & Miller, 2008).

Importantly, there are different types of social threat that are linked to different types of self-conscious emotion. While shame and humiliation are both linked to the evolutionary salient problems of social competition, social reputation and social acceptance (Gilbert, 1992, 1998b; Sznycer et al., 2016), guilt is linked to a very different motivational process for caring and avoiding causing harm to others (Crook, 1980; Gilbert 1989/2016, 2009) (Elison and Malik, in this book). The next part of this chapter looks at some of the evolutionary origins of certain self-conscious emotion.

27.2   Intrasexual Competition

Shame and humiliation are rooted in various forms of social competition and operate through ancient, phylogenetic neurophysiological systems (Gilbert, 1989/2016, 1998b, 2007). There are two forms of social competition called 'scramble and contest'. In scramble competition individuals don't interact with each other whereas in contest competition they do. Contest competition can involve efforts of one individual(s) to prevent (an)other individual(s) access to resources or to accumulate more than others. While food or habitat can be a source of conflict the most common and intense forms of conflict are over sexual access. This is called *intrasexual competition* indicating competitiveness between same gender members. Intrasexual competition can be aggressive. In species where females come into uterus episodically and relatively short-term, the males can engage in intense aggressive competition for short periods of time. For example, the females of the Big Horn mountain goat secrete pheromones into the atmosphere as they come into uterus and this has an impact on the males who then start intense head-butting fights for dominance (Farke, 2008). Indeed, they have evolved highly thickened skulls that allow them to crash into each other at 35 km an hour! Although fights for dominance can occur at other times, outside periods of sexual competition, males live comparatively peacefully together.

Primates do not have any specific breeding seasons in competing for resources. Rather contest conflicts are regulated through the development of dominance and status hierarchies. These hierarchies are established partly through displays that are called *ritualistic agonistic display* behaviours. Such displays signal *resource holding power (RHP)*, sometimes seen as fighting ability, but also the alliances one can call on to help in a conflict (Caryl, 1988). These allow competitors to weigh each other up (utilise social comparison) and for those who assess themselves to be less powerful to back off or submit. Although typically associated with male competitive behaviour females also engage in agonistic behaviours that require submissive behaviours from subordinates. Looked at another way some individuals will escalate conflicts exhibiting more anger and aggression to a challenge or in a conflict, whereas others will show what has been called a fear-dove strategy of seeking to de-escalate the conflict using submissive and appeasing behaviour (Archer, 1988; Caryl, 1988). In many primate species females are as rank sensitive as males and dominant females can be very threatening to subordinate females and even their infants. In addition, they prefer courtships with more dominant males (Abbott et al., 2003). It is in these basic and ancient social dispositions we can see the human origins of shame and humiliation.

In humans, down rank competitive attacks are less physical (although they can be) and depend more on the symbolic representation of self and social presentation (reputation). Buss and Dreden (1990) found that the content of derogation and shaming differed for male-on-male and female-on-female shaming, with male-on-male shame focusing on notions of weakness and sexual incompetence and female-on-female shame focusing on appearance, promiscuous and sexual (un)attractiveness. Baumeister and Twenge (2002) suggest that female-on-female shaming for sexual activities and appearance can be a means of sexual competition to regulate female sexuality and that these become culturally shared values (e.g. women should not be promiscuous or use their sexuality to advance their careers). Shaming and reputation undermining are the means for controlling female sexual choice.

27.3 Submissiveness and Shame

Whether down rank attacks are physical or symbolic, understanding the origins and functions of submissive behaviour and signals, that try to limit the damage of such attacks, offer clues to the origins of shame responding and its behavioural profiles. Indeed, the submissive signal has long been linked to the phylogenetic origins of shame displays because they evolved to inhibit attacks by dominant, threatening others (Gilbert 1998b; Gilbert & McGuire, 1998; Keltner, 1995). It is the subordinate's ability to express a submissive display, that downgrades the hostile intent of the more dominant, which enables it to continue within a group where others are more powerful. Hence, submissive behaviours evolved as fundamental defensive social behaviours which facilitate control over aggression and enable social cohesion. As MacLean (1990) points out:

> ....Ethologists have made it popularly known..... that a passive response (a submissive display) to an aggressive display may make it possible under most circumstances to avoid unnecessary, and sometimes mortal, conflict. Hence it could be argued that the *submissive display is the most important of all displays* because without it numerous individuals might not survive. (italics added, p. 235)

There are a variety of submissive displays that depend on context, but as a general rule submissive displays involve eye gaze avoidance, curling the body to look smaller, social wariness, and inhibiting outputs (Gilbert, 2000a). These are also the basis of shame displays and have the same function as a submissive behaviour in an aggressive context, which is basically reducing aggressive or rejecting behaviour from more powerful others (Keltner, 1995). Martens, Tracy and Shariff (2012) review many studies showing that in contexts of potential conflict or transgression shame displays do indeed reduce hostility; although this can be relatively specific to in-groups. Submissive displays may not protect one from outgroup hostility. In self-report studies, shame proneness is also highly correlated with submissive behaviour (Gilbert, 2000b; Gilbert, Pehl, & Allan, 1994).

27.4   Intersexual Competition

Intersexual competition is related to the ability to attract or gain access to reproductive partners; members of the opposite sex. Whereas *intra*sexual competition can use the strategies of threat and inhibition *inter*sexual competition involves strategies of attraction, approach and positive affect. This is not to deny that males can be threatening towards females and even that some forms of copulation are not far short of rape; and of course, in humans' rape is tragically all too common. Nor should we overlook the fact that in some species males can kill off the young of other males in order to bring the female into oestrus. Nonetheless, for our purposes here we will focus on the most shame-relevant important dynamic of intersexual competition which pertains to the dimension of enticement and attraction and eliciting voluntary engaging and helpful behaviour from others (Gilbert, 1998b, 2007).

The desire to display positive characteristics of ourselves in order to stimulate positive emotions in others, and attract and elicit the positive intentions of others, is well established as a human motive. As the social anthropologist Barkow (1980, 1989) pointed out some years ago it is a strategy that now permeates nearly all forms of human social competition. Various forms of headdresses, cloths, make up and body shaping, athletic displays, displays of any skill or talent and of course displays of wealth such as fast cars, are forms of social display that invites positive audience judgement. It is believed that when metals were first discovered they were used as adornments rather than instruments or weapons. Rather than fighting or threatening aggression, competition by attraction is aimed to create positive evaluation in the minds of others so one is chosen as a partner in particular roles (Barkow, 1980). Gilbert (1989/2016, 1997; Gilbert, Price, & Allan 1995) suggested that whereas in the aggressive context, where the focus is on *resource holding potential* (Caryl, 1988) in the attracting competitive arenas it is on *social holding potential* (SAHP); that is the ability to influence the minds of others positively such that one is seen as a valued, desired and attractive agent and avoid being marginalised or rejected (Gilbert, 1997, 2007). To have positive SAHP is to be an individual who is liked and valued by others whereas negative SAHP would be an individual who is ignored, disliked and shunned; in other words the emotions created in the interpersonal field can be positive, indifferent or negative which will impact on the style of relating that individual can elicit from others. In her book *Survival of the Prettiest*, Etcoff (1999) highlights the benefits of being able to compete on various attraction dimensions. Individuals deemed to have physical attractiveness as well as attractive personalities have better outcomes in terms of choice of sexual partners, supportive social networks and job opportunities.

Using this concept, shame can be seen as an experience of having low or negative SAHP; that one is perceived to be unattractive in some way and worthy of marginalisation, exclusion, rejection or even persecution. Because the underlying dynamic is competitive then the defensive behaviour, to avoid exclusion, rejection or persecution remains, a submissive display rather than an overly confident, hubristic or aggressive display. Hence, many of the dimensions of shame are ones of social competitiveness. For example, the body and body appearance are major sources for people to experience a sense of inferiority, undesirability and shame (Andrews, 2002; Gilbert & Miles, 2002; Lamarche, Ozimok, Gammage, & Muir, 2017). But any display, be it of various athletic or intellectual talents and skills, that is rejected by an audience can be a source for shame because it indicates devaluation of self in the mind of others.

In his book *On The Expression of Emotions* in Man and Animals Darwin (1872) was clear that self-conscious emotions such as blushing, embarrassment and shame are all related to how we experience ourselves in the minds of others. Some years later Charles Horton Cooley, in 1902 coined the term *The Looking Glass Self* (Elison, in this book), highlighting the fact that we experience ourselves through the minds of others. Scheff (1988) articulated this theme in his approach to shame. One of the major shame theorist Michael Lewis (1992) highlights the social dynamic of shame by referring to shame as the *affect of exposure*. Mollon (1984) refers to the existential writings of Sartre to highlight the same theme:

> To see oneself blushing and to feel oneself sweating, etc., are inaccurate expressions which the shy person uses to describe his state; what he really means is that he is physically and constantly conscious of his body, not as it is for him but as it is for the Other….. We often say that the shy man is embarrassed by his own body. Actually, this is incorrect; I cannot be embarrassed by my own body as I exist in it. It is my body as it is for the Other which embarrasses me. (As quoted by Mollon 1984, p. 212)

Sznycer et al. (2016) also articulated an evolved model of shame rooted in competitive behaviour and reputation regulation. They investigated the relationship between social devaluation and shame in a number of different cultures including America, India (Bhawuk and Malik, in this book) and Israel. As expected shame was very highly correlated with experiences of social devaluation across cultures. What sits behind these concerns is social competition.

27.5 Shame and the Self

External shame then, focuses attention and cognitive processing on what's happening in the minds of others in relationship to the self. *Internal* shame focuses attention inwards, links to self-evaluation, often with forms of self-criticism (Gilbert 1992, 1998b, 2007; Giner-Sorolla, 2015). Competencies for self-awareness and judgement probably began to evolve around 2 million years ago. Early humans began to develop a form of social intelligence that allowed for new types of self-awareness, and self-insight (Gilbert, 2017b, 2018), Sedikides and Skowronski (1997) outline possible origins and precursors for a capacity to symbolise 'a self.'

Symbolic self-other awareness is the ability to imagine the self (or other) as an *object* and to judge and give value to self and other, to have self-esteem, pride or shame, or allocate positive or negative values to self and others (good and able, or worthless and useless). Our experience of ourselves, and our judgement of ourselves, is therefore partly linked to ourselves as a social agent and cannot be decontextualised from the social. The biblical myth of Adam and Eve is a story of shame. It conveys the ideas that shame is related to becoming self-aware, aware of another(s) security, and fear of transgression against authority with possible consequent punishment. It also attests to the antiquity of shame.

Although shame has been linked to failing to meet self-standards, the evidence does not support this view unless these 'failures' are seen to render one as an unattractive social agent in some way. Indeed, exploring the idea that shame was about failure to live up to ideals and using qualitative methods Lindsay-Hartz, de Rivera and Mascolo (1995) found that:

> To our surprise we found that most of the participants rejected this formulation. Rather, when ashamed, participants talked about being who they did *not* want to be. That is, they experienced themselves as embodying an anti-ideal, rather than simply not being who they wanted to be. The participants said things like. "I am fat and ugly," not "I failed to be pretty;" or "I am bad and evil," not "I am not as good as I want to be." This difference in emphasis is not simply semantic. Participants insisted that the distinction was important...... (p. 277).

Internal shame requires that there is some self-perception, evaluation or appraisal of self as actually "unattractive"—not just a failure to reach a standard (Gilbert, 1992, 1997, 1998b); that is to say it is closeness to an undesired and unattractive self rather than distance from a desired self that is at issue (Ogilive, 1987). The dynamic of an unattractive self, that's under scrutiny and seen as unworthy or incompetent in some way underpins many forms of mental health problems including depression (Gilbert, 2013) and social anxiety (Gilbert, 2014).

Although some authors regard shame as linked to a global self-evaluation, others have highlighted the fact that we can feel shame for specific aspects of ourselves. For example body shame (Andrews, 1995; Gilbert & Miles, 2002; Lamarche et al., 2017) and appearance (Kellett & Gilbert, 2001). Indeed, Andrews, Qian and Valentine, (2002) developed a self-report shame scale that measures characterological, behavioural and bodily shame as different dimensions of shame. Shame can be focused on specific characteristics of body function such as impotence, shape, size and appearance. Body focused shame underpins Body Dysmorphic Disorder (Gilbert & Miles, 2002). And shame can be a serious problem in how people seek out medical help for diseases that can be unattractive in appearance, secretions or deemed to be self-induced (Gilbert, 2017a). People can delay seeking help for bowel cancer or sexually transmitted diseases because of shame issues. Fear of shame can motivate concealment and non-sharing of personal information such as past trauma, behaviour or emotions or fantasies. Fear of shame can have very serious consequences on people's abilities to develop open trusting and affiliative relationships (Gilbert, 2009). Part of psychotherapy can be working with what people have 'shamefully' concealed and creates feelings of disconnection. In these contexts clients can monitor very carefully what they think the therapist might be thinking of them; their SAHP in the mind of the therapist.

While subordination, submissiveness and shame overlap, they are not the same. One can be submissive and recognise one's subordinate status without feeling shame. Indeed, in some contexts one may be willingly submissive to an adored leader. Another example that both Scott (1990) in his book, Domination and the Arts of Resistance and also Goffman's in his work on social stigma (1968), make clear is that there is a public and private face to acts of subordination. What is said and agreed in public may be very different in private. Compliance to authority, even public acts of (involuntary) subordination, do not suggest shame but social fear (Gilbert, 1992). It is also possible to have a sense of external shame but not to internalise that. For example, some people who have battled with sexual orientation may not experience internal shame but can be very hurt by experiencing stigma and external shame.

27.6 Humiliation

The term humiliation has many meanings. For example, a humiliating defeat can imply defeat in the face of an expectation of wining, perhaps where one had all the advantages. It can also be used to describe a large margin between the winner and loser. Figure 27.1 outlines some of these distinctions.

Although often seen as similar to shame, and with many overlapping features, humiliation differs from shame in important ways. Like shame, humiliation is rooted in the competitive dynamics and negotiating our social place in the world; status and social fit. Shame involves a sense of self as damaged as a social agent, and when internalised can be associated with negative judgements of the self even self-disgust and hatred. Although self-blame is not necessary for shame (we can be ashamed of a birth defect or deformity, for example, and we can feel a sense of shame through association with stigmatised or shamed others) for the most part there is some sense of personal identification with the shamed identity (Tracy et al. 2007). As noted elsewhere this is not the case for humiliation (Gilbert, 1998b). There is growing consensus that humiliation is associated with desires for vengeance in a way that shame may not be (Gilbert,1998b). Trumbull (2008) also highlights how humiliation generates aggressive, defensive responses directed at restoration of status, and to depose the humiliator and counter humiliate him or her.

In a major review of the literature on humiliation Elison (in this book) and Harter (2007) highlight the fact that the social devaluation is regarded as unjustified, as an injustice; individuals feel they have been ridiculed, taunted, bullied even tortured and devalued by others unfairly and unjustly; 'they have been wronged.' Whereas shame typically involves fear-based emotions, humiliation is one of anger and vengeance. Even if individuals feel they are in subordinate positions the desire for vengeance can be intense. Elison and Harter (2007) highlight examples of school shootings where individuals have often felt humiliated and ridiculed by others and their killing sprees were based on humiliated rage. This is true in groups, tribes and countries too where individuals who feel humiliated can have serious desires for vengeance. One of the drivers of the Second World War was the humiliation the allies heaped on the Germans for the First World War in the Treaty of Versailles (Mayer on shame in Germany, in this book). For the most part the humiliated person feels that the humiliator purposely and deliberately sought to create a sense of ridicule and inferiority in them. In torture for example, humiliating rituals even including being urinated and defecated on can be part of the process; it is a demonstration of power. Indeed, although we often think that torture and humiliation are to dehumanise people in fact it's the very awareness

SHAME   HUMILIATION

HAVE IN COMMON

Sensitivity to put down/injury
Desire to protect self
Increase in arousal
Complex emotions
Rumination

ARE DIFFERENT IN

Internal Attribution	External attribution
Self bad /flawed	Other bad
Inferiority	Not necessarily inferior
Heightened self conscientious	Attention focused on the other
Acceptance	Unjust
Not vengeful	Vengeful

Fig. 27.1 Similarities and distinctions between shame and humiliation (From Gilbert 1997, 2018)

of our human needs for connectedness and to be respected, valued and esteemed (to have positive SAHP) that the humiliator plays on. During the emergence of the Holocaust Jews were made to do humiliating acts such as scrubbing streets with toothbrushes and had symbols hung around their necks. While we could hurt and threaten animals, and they may well show submissive or fearful responses, we can't shame or humiliate them. We are humiliated and shamed not because we are like animals but because we are not and because we have human needs and sensibilities of self and social contextual awareness.

Another dimension to humiliation that is less acknowledged and requires research is that humiliation often crosses group boundaries. Individuals who feel humiliated can often feel excluded and marginalised as if they are an outgroup member. Many of Elison and Harter's (2007) examples that involved murderous vengeance suggest experiences of being an outcast, a ridiculed out-grouper, not just subordinated. This may explain partly why humiliated fury can often be taken out on a number of individuals who represent that groups identity. Humiliated fury can create the desire to 'do unto others as has been done to me' a sort of inversion of the golden rule. Another aspect of humiliation is it can create destructive envy and jealousy (Gilbert, 1992, 1998c). In a famous Beatles song *Run for Your Life*, (on the album Rubber Soul) are the words 'I'd rather see you dead little girl than to be with another man.' Sometimes jilted people refer to feeling humiliated rather than shamed by a rejection or infidelity, again with an intense desire for vengeance. Indeed, in some cultures it is a basis for honour killing. John Lennon later regretted writing the song and it was his least favourite, but it speaks to a dark theme of sexually, competitive driven humiliation. So in shame the focus is on the damaged reputation to oneself and as agent which is commonly internalised in negative self-evaluation whereas in humiliation the focus is on (what is seen as) unjustifiable devaluation harm and ridicule that's been done by another. In terms of competitive dynamics of humiliation, the experiencer seeks to dominate or injure the humiliator. These sentiments are not part of shame.

These distinctions can be depicted in Figs. 27.1 and 27.2.

Figure 27.2 depicts that in the first instance humans are born with extraordinarily sensitive needs to be cared for and looked after by others and be held in positive regard. From an early age they are constantly looking for approval of their displays and validation of their feelings. They are learning not only how they exist in the minds of others but how others are disposed towards them. They are particularly attentive to voice tones and facial expressions that indicate different emotions in the carer. Cold or rejecting facial expressions and voice tones can indicate that we are held negatively in the minds of others creating in the first instance an experience of external shame. We have a sense that we are not an attractive social agent, and this sensitises various threats systems, orientating attention and defensive manoeuvres (Gilbert, 1998b, 1998c). If on the other hand the individual perceives the environment is hostile, unfair and unjust then the experience is not rooted in self attribution's but in external attributions and humiliation.

Figure 27.2 also demonstrates that we can have reflected shame and a sense of humiliation whereby these can be brought to families or groups by its members

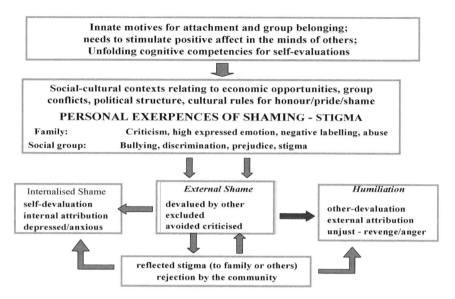

Fig. 27.2 An evolutionary and biopsychosocial model for shame and humiliation Adapted from Gilbert (2002)

or member. For example, in some cultures honour killing is for a family member, usually a young woman seeking their own sexuality who is deemed to have brought shame or humiliation to the family and tarnished the reputation and honour of the family (Gilbert, Gilbert, & Sanghera, 2004). Some cultures regard this as justified and indeed honourable whereas others as a crime and shameful.

Importantly, the self-conscious emotions can coexist. For example, it is very common in forensic services to find individuals who respond very aggressively to any threats upon them and who speak in the language of humiliation. However, as they engage in therapeutic explorations it becomes clear they also carry an intense sense of vulnerability, feelings of unworthiness and a sense of shame. Their aggressive humiliation-behaviour is actually a defence against experiencing this vulnerable, inferior sense of self. So aggressive behaviour itself is not a clear defining distinction between the two self-conscious emotions.

27.7   Guilt

Many authors tend to lump shame, humiliation and guilt together as part of the same family of self-conscious emotions, but an exploration of their evolutionary roots show them to be very different. The word guilt derives from the German word gelt which meant debt in the 8th century.

The evolutionary origins of guilt do not lie in the sexual and resource competitive dynamics of life but rather in caring motives and behaviour. With the evolution of parental investment and caring behaviour there was a focus on providing for infants such that they would be defended from harms and nurtured appropriately. Crook (1980) pointed out that for caring to evolve there had also to be a harm avoidance system such that carers are attentive to and avoid causing harm to the targets of their care and are motivated to take remedial action as soon as possible if they do. Indeed, MacLean (1990) highlighted the fact that some egg laying species such as some fish sometimes cannibalise their own young. So one of the first evolved processes for caring is kin recognition and 'don't eat the kids'! Second, harm avoidance will evolve with emotional consequences to having violated that general strategy and motivate reparations as quickly as possible. It follows therefore that the attentional focus of guilt will be different to that of shame and humiliation. For example, in guilt there is no aggressive desire for vengeance and no concern with social reputation. The focus is on having caused harm and desire for reparation. The emotions of guilt relate to sadness and remorse which partly motivate reparation and are very different to ones of anxiety and anger as in shame and humiliation. Guilt is linked to empathic and sympathy abilities (Tangney & Dearing 2002). Empathy is important for guilt but not necessary for shame or humiliation. Indeed, one can feel shamed and humiliated through projection.

Responses to having caused harm, even inadvertently can vary from shame to guilt. For example, imagine driving down the road and a dog runs out and you hit it. Externalising anger would focus on the damage the dog has done to your car (stupid dog); external shame would focus on fear of what others might say about your driving, internal shame on negative self-evaluation 'why am I not careful enough'. In such cases one might be tempted to drive on. Guilt focuses on sadness and sorrow and one is more likely to stop and help the injured animal. One's mind is not focused on what others might think or even judgements of one's driving but on the injured dog. Guilt is therefore a moral emotion in a way that shame often it is not (Tracy et al. 2007; Tangney & Dearing, 2002). Guilt supports prosocial behaviour, and builds interpersonal bonds (Baumeister, Stillwell, & Heatherton 1994). This suggests that the negative affect of guilt or the anticipation of guilt may nudge us towards care and compassion (Gilbert, 2009, 2017a). While shame may motivate individuals to try to repair the damage they caused, this is primarily to repair their own reputation and reduce external shame or sometimes to help themselves feel better about themselves.

Indeed, study after study has shown that guilt is significantly linked to moral behaviour and cooperation whereas shame is not (De Hooge, Zeelenberg, & Breugel-mans, 2007; Tangney & Dearing, 2002). Further guilt and it has low or no association with mental health problems (Gilbert, 2000c; Tangney & Dearing, 2002; SzentaÂgotai-Tătar, & Miu, 2016). In contrast, shame proneness, when rooted in a deep sense of an unattractive and an undesired self, is often associated with hostile forms of self-criticism and is linked to whole range of psychopathologies (Gilbert, 2009). Humiliation is seen as especially linked to the more aggressive, interpersonal difficulties. Approaches that over rely on cognitive explanations identify shame as linked to global self-evaluation whereas guilt is focused on behaviour. Although important these are not their defining features. Rather the underpinning motivational mechanisms that drive them are.

Another area where this distinction is very important is between restorative and retributive justice (Wenzel, Okimoto, Feather, & Platow, 2008). In retributive justice the focus is on shaming and humiliating, the idea is to cause suffering in some sense and for perpetrators to know their (lowered) social place. The desire is to induce fear, with a sense of subordination and defeat in perpetrators so they will not be tempted to do it again. In addition, retributive justice is a public demonstration that justice has been done and to act as a deterrent; hence it is designed to be callous (Gilbert, 2018). Restorative justice on the other hand, seeks to bring perpetrator and victim together in order to help the perpetrator empathise and understand the harm they have done. When this works well, rather than shaming and humiliating perpetrators, they are connected to a sense of guilt which allows them to begin to experience sadness and remorse. This internalised sense of responsibility taking, with a feeling of inner sadness for causing harm, is a more reliable source for subsequent prevention (Zehr, 2015). It should be noted, however, that clinically individuals who are blocked out on their ability to experience sadness can struggle with this approach and therapeutic work may be necessary to enable them to work on their own pain and suffering before they can appreciate the pain and suffering they have caused others (Gilbert, 2017b).

27.8 Compassion Focused Therapy

The evolution of social competition is ancient and often stressful. Indeed, there are many physiological markers linked to losing social status, and for humans being shamed, rejected or humiliated. In contrast, caring motivational systems evolved to 'look after, protect encourage and sooth (Gilbert, 1989/2016).' Caring motives organise our minds in very different ways and operate through different physiological processes to those of competitive motives. Caring, and its recent derivative compassion, are linked to hormones such as oxytocin and the myelinated vagas which is part of the parasympathetic system (Kirby et al., 2017; Thayer, Åhs, Fredrikson, Sollers, & Wager, 2012). Both have soothing functions. There is considerable evidence that access to caring others significantly attenuates stress. For example, if subordinate primates have access to support and soothing from kin they show less stress responses (Abbott et al., 2003). Many priming experiments show that attachment primes have a major impact on threatened stressed processing (e.g., Hornstein & Eisenberger, 2018)

Evolution based, compassion focused therapy suggests that one way to help people who are locked into problems of shame and humiliation is to switch them out of the competitive motivational systems into care and affiliative motivational systems (Gilbert, 2000c, 2010, 2017b). In this way the therapy seeks to change not only psychological processes but physiological ones too (Kirby et al., 2017). Hence there are a series of interventions and practices to help clients activate and stimulate caring motivational systems and their physiological mediators. These include:

- People are introduced to an evolutionary, psychoeducation formulation of how and why we can get caught up in different conflicting, motivational and emotion systems that can be unhelpful to us and others (called tricky brain). The focus is to help clients have an understanding that our minds are created by our genes and choreographed by our upbringing. It is not our fault the way we are but it is our responsibility to learn about our minds and utilise them cultivate mental processes and habits that can to maximise well-being and minimise causing harm to self; shifting from personalisation shame and blaming to compassionate responsibility taking.
- People are offered the definition of compassion as *sensitivity to suffering in self and others with a commitment to try to alleviate and prevent it* (Gilbert, 2009, 2017b) and is rooted in courage and wisdom. The next step is to help people to mindfully be aware of what emotion and motivation system they are operating from at any point in time and how to switch into motivational and emotional systems mediated through compassion processing that are physiologically and psychologically more conducive to well-being.
- People are helped to understand the link between motivation and physiological activation and provide people with a variety of postural and breathing practices, imagery and behavioral practices, that stimulate the vagus nerve and other physiological systems linked to caring motivation and affiliative emotion processing. In addition, clients are trained to use particular voice friendly and affiliative emotional textures to the thoughts, particularly self-referent thoughts. These build into a portfolio of practices to cultivate one's compassionate mind
- People are introduced to the nature of a compassionate self-identity that guides cultivating a compassionate mind and compassionate self. They are supported in exploring the benefits of practising, harnessing and living one's life from that orientation. This is accompanied by a range of guided meditation practices, ways of thinking and ways of engaging in compassionate behaviour.

By way of short case example consider Sally (not her real name and the details are changed here). Sally had experienced intense bullying as a young child about the weight. She came into therapy with low self-esteem, was highly self-critical, socially anxious and depressed. She also had a sense of shame not only around her appearance but also because she felt she hadn't really achieved very much in life even though she was intelligent. Her cognitive and motivational processes were highly linked to competitive motivational processing that included the typical competition motivational themes. These included: unfavourable social comparison, tendencies towards submissive behaviour, believing that other people saw her as inferior, wanting improve her standing/status in the eyes of others, to compete and achieve in the world, self-monitoring and self-critical thoughts that were internally self-downing and shaming with a hostile contemptuous tone to them.

The compassion focused therapist first provides a secure base and validating empathic connection to facilitate the client feeling validated and accepted. Talking about shame is itself painful and can be expressed as shameful in itself. Sally's transference was competitive in the sense that she believed that therapist would also judge negatively, compare her unfavourably with other clients, see her as less motivated or competent, and would expect her to achieve and do more. In CFT one would be very cautious about being pulled into that motivational system by focusing on doing and achieving. Instead CFT helped Sally to understand how our brains have evolved in such a way that we can become very focused on competitive social comparison, fears of what others think and feel about, us particularly if we've been bullied, and it's very easy to get caught in these loops.

We then explored 'what is the part of ourselves, may be linked to our inner strengths, that would really help us to face and work with the things that frighten and upset us.' The therapist then guides Sally to the core qualities of the compassionate mind, rooted as they are in courage and wisdom able to address pain and suffering. To help us with problems of shame we need a part of ourselves that can be supportive, validating and healing which we call the compassionate self. CFT spends time on discovering, recruiting and cultivating this aspect of self, including its physiological parameters.

Core to Sally's therapy was helping her to recognise the hostility and undermining nature of her and self-criticism. This is done in a series of steps using functional analysis and chair work. Sally was able to learn how to generate compassionate self-talk with friendly affiliative inner 'tones and textures' to her thoughts. As the internal compassionate competencies of Sally developed it became possible to help her use this aspect of her mind to address some of her shame and also engage compassionately in rescripting bullying trauma memories. So in brief Sally learnt to become more mindful and mind aware, recognise the value of refocusing on compassion motivation, activating the system and practising. Then, with the compassion focus, being able to move into and work with distressing areas.

CFT was specifically developed for people with high levels of shame and self-criticism often linked to complex or traumatic pasts. CFT suggest that if individuals do not have the inner physiological infrastructures (a form of inner secure base and safe haven to use attachment terms rooted in systems such as the vagus nerve) and psychological competencies for compassion and regulating threat processing, then working with shame and trauma can be very difficult for them.

27.9   Conclusion

This chapter explored some of the evolved differences between self-conscious emotions rooted in motivational systems and competencies for defence. Shame is linked to competitive dynamics which has an inhibitory function since it is linked to subordinate defensive strategies of inhibition. Humiliation is linked to competitive dynamics but is the opposite and generates aggression and desires for vengeance and retaliation. (Out) group identification is more common in humiliation. Guilt has a completely different evolutionary origin, rooted in caring behaviour with all of the competencies that go with it. In many studies, that other chapters to this volume explore, shame is associated with vulnerabilities to a range internalising type psychopathologies,

Table 27.1 Comparisons of external and internal shame humiliation guilt

	External shame	Internal shame	Humiliation	Guilt
Motivation	competitive rank	competitive rank	Competitive rank	Caring
Attention	Mind of the other	Own mind/self	Mind of the other	Mind of the other
Cognitive	They think badly of me	I think badly of me	How dare they think badly of me	I have hurt someone
Emotions	Threat-anxious	Threat-depressed	Threat-anger	Sorrow and remorse
Behaviours	Defensive submissive and avoidant	Defensive externally but offensive internally (self-attacking)	Offensive, vengeful	Reparative

such as depression and social anxiety while humiliation is associated more with vengeance and aggressive acting out. Shame is particularly toxic when it is rooted in a sense of self as bad, unworthy or even disgusting and where there is a high degrees of self-criticism through to self-hatred. In contrast guilt is associated with prosocial behaviour and is not linked to psychopathology or vengeance. This is partly because it's rooted in a completely different motivational system that its patterns, emotional dispositions and sense of self are quite differently to shame and humiliation (Giner-Sorolla 2015).

As a summary Table 27.1 gives a simplified overview of some of the differences between internal and external shame, humiliation and guilt.

These distinctions are important particularly in psychotherapy. For example, compassion focused therapy (Gilbert, 2010) helps individuals identify forms of shame-based self-criticism and how to switch into self-compassion. For humiliation it helps individuals work with their sense of anger, address potential underlying unprocessed emotions associated with humiliation and where appropriate develop forgiveness. If harm has been done then enabling people to process guilt is essential. For some individuals processing these emotions is very difficult because it takes them into their own emotional pain. Group relationships and cultural dynamics of what is and what is not shaming add new dimensions of experience that are lacquered into the sense of oneself as 'a confident desirable attractive person' or one 'vulnerable to criticism rejection and exclusion.' Seeing these experiences through the lens of evolved motivation systems offer new avenues for research and therapy.

References

Abbott, D. H., Keverne, E. B., Bercovitch, F. B., Shively, C. A., Mendoza, S. P., Saltzman, W., et al. (2003). Are subordinates always stressed? A comparative analysis of rank differences in cortisol levels among primates. *Hormones and Behavior, 43*(1), 67–82.

Andrews, B. (1995). Bodily shame as a mediator between abusive experiences and depression. *Journal of Abnormal Psychology, 104*, 277–285.

Andrews, B. (2002). Body shame and abuse in childhood. In P. Gilbert & J. N. V. Miles (Eds), *Body shame: Conceptualisation, research & treatment* (pp. 256–266). London. Brunner-Routledge.

Andrews, B., Qian, M., & Valentine, J. D. (2002). Predicting depressive symptoms with a new measure of shame: The experience of shame scale. *British Journal of Clinical Psychology, 41*(1), 29–42.

Archer, J. (1988). *The behavioural biology of aggression*. Cambridge: Cambridge University Press.

Barkow, J. H. (1980). Prestige and self-esteem: A bioscocial interpretation. In D. R. Omark., F. F. Strayer, & D. G. Freedman (Eds.), *Dominance relations: An ethological view of conflict and social interaction* (pp. 319–332). New York: Garland Press.

Barkow, J. H. (1989). *Darwin, sex and status: biological approaches to mind and culture*. Toronto: University of Toronto Press.

Baumeister, R. F., Stillwell, A. M., & Heatherton, T. F. (1994). Guilt: An interpersonal approach. *Psychological Bulletin, 115*(2), 243–267.

Baumeister, R. F., & Twenge, J. M. (2002). Cultural suppression of female sexuality. *Review of General Psychology, 6*, 166–203.

Buss, D. M., & Dreden, L. A. (1990). Derogation of competitors. *Journal of Social and Person Relationships, 7*, 395–422.

Caryl, P. G. (1988). Escalated fighting and the war of nerves: Games theory and animal combat. In P. H. Bateson, & P. H. Klopfer, (Eds.). *Perspectives in ethology. advantages of diversity* (Vol. 4, pp. 199–224). New York: Plenum Press.

Cooley, C. H. (1902). *Human nature and the social order*. New York: Scribner's.

Crook, J. H. (1980). *The evolution of human consciousness*. Oxford: Oxford University Press.

Darwin, C. (1872/2009). *On the expression of the emotions in man and animals*. Penguin Classics.

De Hooge, I. E., Zeelenberg, M., & Breugelmans, S. M. (2007). Moral sentiments and cooperation: Differential influences of shame and guilt. *Cognition and Emotion, 21*(5), 1025–1042.

Dickerson, S. S., & Kemeny, M. E. (2004). Acute stressors and cortisol responses: A theoretical integration and synthesis of laboratory research. *Psychological Bulletin, 130*(3), 355.

Etcoff, N. (1999). *Survival of the prettiest: The science of beauty*. New York: Doubleday.

Elison, J., & Harter, S. (2007). Humiliation: Causes, correlates, and consequences. In J. L. Tracy, R. W. Robins, & J. P. Tangney (Eds.), *The self-conscious emotions: Theory and research* (pp. 310–329). New York: Guilford.

Farke, A. A. (2008). Frontal sinuses and head-butting in goats: A finite element analysis. *Journal of Experimental Biology, 211*(19), 3085–3094.

Gilbert, P. (1989/2016). *Human nature and suffering*. London: Lawrence Erlbaum Associates.

Gilbert, P. (1992). *Depression: The evolution of powerlessness*. London: Lawrence Erlbaum Associates.

Gilbert, P. (1997). The evolution of social attractiveness and its role in shame, humiliation, guilt and therapy. *British Journal of Medical Psychology, 70*, 113–147.

Gilbert, P. (1998a). Evolutionary psychopathology: Why isn't the mind better designed than it is? *British Journal of Medical Psychology, 71*, 353–373.

Gilbert, P. (1998b). What is shame? Some core issues and controversies. In P. Gilbert & B. Andrews (Eds.), *Shame: Interpersonal behavior, psychopathology and culture* (pp. 3–36). New York: Oxford University Press.

Gilbert, P. (1998c). Shame & humiliation in complex cases: In N. Tarrier., G. Haddock, & A. Wells (Eds.), *Treating complex cases: The cognitive behavioural approach* (pp. 241–271). Wiley.

Gilbert, P. (2000a). Varieties of submissive behaviour: Their evolution and role in depression. In L. Sloman & P. Gilbert (Eds.) *Subordination and defeat. An evolutionary approach to mood disorders* (3–46). Hillsdale: N.J. Lawrence Erlbaum.

Gilbert, P. (2000b). The relationship of shame, social anxiety and depression: The role of the evaluation of social rank. *Clinical Psychology and Psychotherapy, 7*, 174–189.

Gilbert, P. (2000c). Social mentalities: Internal 'social' conflicts and the role of inner warmth and compassion in cognitive therapy. In P. Gilbert & K. G. Bailey (Eds.), *Genes on the couch: Explorations in evolutionary psychotherapy* (pp. 118–150). Hove: Psychology Press.

Gilbert, P. (2002). Body shame: A biopsychosocial conceptualisation and overview, with treatment implications. In P. Gilbert & J. Miles (Eds.), *Body shame: Conceptualisation, research & treatment* (pp. 3–54). London: Routledge.

Gilbert, P. (2007). The evolution of shame as a marker for relationship security. In J. L. Tracy, R. W. Robins, & J. P Tangney (Eds.), *The self-conscious emotions: Theory and research* (pp. 283–309). New York: Guilford.

Gilbert, P. (2009). *The compassionate mind: A new approach to the challenge of life.* London: Constable & Robinson.

Gilbert, P. (2010). *Compassion focused therapy: The CBT distinctive features series.* London: Routledge.

Gilbert, P. (2013). Depression: The challenges of an integrated biopsychosocial evolutionary approach. In M. Power (Ed.), *The Wiley Blackwell handbook of mood disorders*: Second edition (pp. 229–288.). Chichester, Wiley.

Gilbert, P. (2014). Evolutionary models. Practical and conceptual utility for the treatment and study of social anxiety disorder. In J. W. Weeks (ed.). *The Wiley Blackwell handbook of social anxiety disorder* (p. 24–52). Chichester: Wiley.

Gilbert, P. (2017a). Shame and the vulnerable self in medical contexts: the compassionate solution. *Medical humanities*, medhum-2016.

Gilbert, P. (2017b). Compassion as a social mentality: An evolutionary approach. In P. Gilbert (Ed.), *Compassion: Concepts, research and applications* (pp. 31–68). London: Routledge.

Gilbert, P. (2018). *Living like crazy* (2nd ed.). York: Annwyn House.

Gilbert, P., Clarke, M., Kempel, S., Miles, J. N. V., & Irons, C. (2004a). Criticizing and reassuring oneself: An exploration of forms style and reasons in female students. *British Journal of Clinical Psychology, 43,* 31–50.

Gilbert, P., Gilbert, J., & Sanghera, J. (2004b). A focus group exploration of the impact of izzat, shame, subordination and entrapment on mental health and service use in South Asian women living in Derby. *Mental Health, Religion & Culture, 7,* 109–130.

Gilbert, P., & McGuire, M. (1998). Shame, status and social roles: The psychobiological continuum from monkeys to humans. In P. Gilbert & B. Andrews (Eds.), *Shame: interpersonal behavior, psychopathology and culture* (pp. 99–125). New York: Oxford University Press.

Gilbert, P., & Miles, J. (2002). *Body shame: Conceptualisations, research & treatment.* London: Brunner-Routledge.

Gilbert, P., Pehl, J., & Allan, S. (1994). The phenomenology of shame and guilt: An empirical investigation. *British Journal of Medical Psychology, 67,* 23–36.

Gilbert, P., Price, J. S., & Allan, S. (1995). Social comparison, social attractiveness and evolution: How might they be related? *New Ideas in Psychology, 13,* 149–165.

Giner-Sorolla, R. (2015). *Judging passions: Moral emotions in persons and groups.* London: Routledge.

Goffman, E. (1968). *Stigma: Notes on the management of a spoiled identity.* Harmondsworth: Penguin.

Hornstein, E. A., & Eisenberger, N. I. (2018). A social safety net: Developing a model of social-support figures as prepared safety stimuli. *Current Directions in Psychological Science, 27,* 25–31.

Kellett, S., & Gilbert, P. (2001). Acne: A biopsychosocial and evolutionary perspective with a focus on shame. *British Journal of Health Psychology, 6*(1), 1–24.

Keltner, D. (1995). Signs of appeasement: Evidence for the distinct displays of embarrassment, amusement and shame. *Journal of Personality and Social Psychology, 68,* 441–454.

Kirby, J. N., Doty, J., Petrocchi, N., & Gilbert. P. (2017). The current and future role of heart rate variability for assessing and training compassion. Frontiers. *Public Health, 5,* 40. Retrieved from https://doi.org/10.3389/fpubh.2017.00040.

Kross, E., Berman, M. G., Mischel, W., Smith, E. E., & Wager, T. D. (2011). Social rejection shares somatosensory representations with physical pain. *Proceedings of the National Academy of Sciences, 108*(15), 6270–6275.

Lamarche, L., Ozimok, B., Gammage, K. L., & Muir, C. (2017). Men respond too: The effects of a social-evaluative body image threat on shame and cortisol in university Men. *American Journal Of Men's Health, 11*(6), 1791–1803.

Lewis, M. (1992). *Shame: The exposed self*. New York: The Free Press.

Lindsay-Hartz, J., de Rivera, J., & Mascolo, M.F. (1995). Differentiating guilt and shame and their effects on motivations. In Tangney, J. P. & Fischer, K. W. (Eds). *Self-conscious emotions. The psychology of shame, guilt, embarrassment and pride.* (pp. 274–300). New York: Guilford.

MacLean, P. D. (1990). *The triune brian in evolution.* New York: Plenum Press.

Martens, J. P., Tracy, J. L., & Shariff, A. F. (2012). Status signals: Adaptive benefits of displaying and observing the nonverbal expressions of pride and shame. *Cognition and Emotion, 26*(3), 390–406.

Mollon, P. (1984). Shame in relation to narcissistic disturbance. *British Journal of Medical Psychology, 57,* 207–214.

Ogilive, D. M. (1987). The undesired self: A neglected variable in personality research. *Journal of Personality and Social Psychology, 52,* 379–388.

Rohleder, N., Chen, E., Wolf, J. M., & Miller, G. E. (2008). The Psychobiology of trait shame in young women: Extending the social self preservation theory. *Health Psychology,* 27(5), 523–532. Retrieved from http://doi.org/10.1037/0278-6133.27.5.52.

Scheff, T. J. (1988). Shame and conformity: The deference-emotion system. *American Review of Sociology, 53,* 395–406.

Scott, J. C. (1990). *Domination and the arts of resistance*. New Haven: Yale University Press.

Sedikides, C., & Skowronski, J. J. (1997). The symbolic self in evolutionary context. *Personality and Social Psychology Review, 1,* 80–102.

SzentaÂgotai-Tătar, A., & Miu, A. C. (2016). Individual differences in emotion regulation, childhood trauma and proneness to shame and guilt in adolescence. *PLoS ONE,* 11(11), e0167299. Retrieved from https://doi.org/10.1371/journal.pone.0167299.

Sznycer, D., Tooby, J., Cosmides, L., Porat, R., Shalvi, S., & Halperin, E. (2016). Shame closely tracks the threat of devaluation by others, even across cultures. *Proceedings of the National Academy of Sciences, 113*(10), 2625–2630.

Tangney, J. P., & Dearing, R. L. (2002). *Shame and guilt.* Guilford Press.

Thayer, J. F., Åhs, F., Fredrikson, M., Sollers, J. J., & Wager, T. D. (2012). A meta-analysis of heart rate variability and neuroimaging studies: Implications for heart rate variability as a marker of stress and health. *Neuroscience and Biobehavioral Reviews, 36*(2), 747–756.

Tracy, J. L., Robins, R. W., & Tangney, J. P. (Eds.). (2007). *The Self-conscious emotions: Theory and research.* (pp. 283–309). New York: Guilford.

Trumbull, D. (2008). Humiliation: The trauma of disrespect. *Journal of The American Academy of Psychoanalysis and Dynamic Psychiatry, 36,* 643–660.

Wenzel, M., Okimoto, T. G., Feather, N. T., & Platow, M. J. (2008). Retributive and restorative justice. *Law and Human Behavior, 32*(5), 375–389.

Zehr, H. (2015). *The little book of restorative justice: Revised and updated.* Skyhorse Publishing, Inc.

Paul Gilbert (Ph.D.), FBPsS, OBE is Professor of Clinical Psychology at the University of Derby and until his retirement from the NHS in 2016 was Consultant Clinical Psychologist at the Derbyshire Health Care Foundation Trust. He has researched evolutionary approaches to psychopathology for over 40 years with a special focus on the roles of mood, shame and self-criticism in various mental health difficulties for which Compassion Focused Therapy was developed. He was made a Fellow of the British Psychological Society in 1993. In 2003 he was president of the

British Association for Behavioural and Cognitive Psychotherapy. 2002–2004 he was a member of the first British Governments' NICE guidelines for depression. He has written/edited 21 books and over 200 papers. In 2006 he established the Compassionate Mind Foundation as an international charity with the mission statement To promote wellbeing through the scientific understanding and application of compassion (www.compassionatemind.co.uk). There are now a number of sister foundations in other countries. On leaving the health service in 2016 he established the Centre for compassion research and training at the University of Derby and has recently been awarded an honorary professorship at the University of Queensland Australia. He was awarded an OBE by the Queen in March 2011 for services to mental health. He is now in the Director of the Centre for Compassion Research and Training at Derby University UK. He has written and edited many books on compassion. His latest Book is Living Like Crazy.

Chapter 28
Working with Shame Experiences in Dreams: Therapeutical Interventions

Claude-Hélène Mayer

Abstract Shame is a deep-rooted emotion which is of particular interest to researchers studying dreams and dream analysis, and to practitioners who work with it. Psychologists and therapists such as Freud, Breuer and worked with dreams for therapeutical reasons and healing purposes. They interpreted dreams in different ways and provided various explanations of the meaning of shame and its functions in the individual, such as repression, anxiety and self-esteem. Working with dreams can support individuals to transform shame and to value shame experiences in dreams as a source of personal growth and self-development. This chapter provides insights into therapeutical work with shameful experiences in dreams, and selected cases of shame in dream scenarios are presented. Conclusions on how to constructively work with shame in therapeutical practice are presented and recommendations for future research and practice are given.

Keywords Shame · Dreams · Dream work · Transformation of shame · Personal growth

28.1 Introduction

> A dream which is not understood
> is like a letter that is not opened.
>
> Talmud

In many cultures, shame is a taboo topic which often seems to be forgotten (Scheff, 2013) and stored in the unconscious. Psychologists and researchers have pointed out that shame constitutes an important aspect of life (Jacoby, 1996; Schultz, 1996). It impacts on thoughts, feelings and behaviour, as well as on creativity (Skov, 2018).

C.-H. Mayer (✉)
Institut für Therapeutische Kommunikation und Sprachgebrauch, Europa Universität Viadrina, Logenstrasse 11, 15230 Frankfurt (Oder), Germany
e-mail: claudemayer@gmx.net

Department of Management, Rhodes University, Drosdy Road, Grahamstown 6139, South Africa

© Springer Nature Switzerland AG 2019
C.-H. Mayer and E. Vanderheiden (eds.), *The Bright Side of Shame*,
https://doi.org/10.1007/978-3-030-13409-9_28

Shame is also present in dreams and dream analysis (Wittman & de Dassel, 2015) and can be a source of healing and reconstruction of the personality (Skov, 2018).

Research and practical, therapeutical work with dreams to uncover, transform and heal shameful experiences have been highlighted early in psychotherapeutical history by various psychologists such as Freud (1900, 1924, 1991) and Breuer (Freud & Breuer, 1895/1966), as well as by Jung (2009). It is, however, also an important topic in different psychological and healing approaches in specific cultural contexts and across cultures (Mayer, 2017; Vanderheiden & Mayer, 2017).

Shame, according to Freud, is related to the need for repression, to a mode of action formation and also to narcissism and ego ideal; it is basically a superego anxiety which threatens the self-esteem and standing of a person (Lansky & Morrison, 1997). Jung (2009) observes that a lack of self-esteem is the root cause of susceptibility to shame. In dreams, the individual connects to the individual and the collective unconscious; dreaming about shame and shameful experiences relates to the shadow which contains repressed and/or unacceptable experiences, thoughts or feelings (Jung, 2009). Shame, as a shadow aspect, is often unconsciously repressed (Lewis, 1971). The shadow is viewed in the psychology of the unconscious as the part of the personality which includes the unpleasant qualities individuals hide, the unconscious contents of the personality, as well as the functions which are insufficiently developed (Wharton, 1990).

As archetypal (collective, universal) phenomena, shameful experiences often find their origin in childhood experiences and the sociocultural environment (Jacoby, 1996) and reoccur in dreams either directly or in a symbolised way (Jung, 1976). According to Jung, fantasies, symbols, defences, resistance and dreams are viewed as creative functions and can be seen in a positive light as psychic purposes which, for example, serve as warning signals, as well as "opportunities of the mind to reflect on its own processes" (Jung cited in Knox, 2005, 617).

This chapter deals with shame in the context of dreams and dream work, thereby defining dreams from the viewpoint of Jung, seeing them as opportunities of the mind to reflect. The chapter presents insights into therapeutical work with dreams to transform shame—an emotion which is often experienced as negative—into a valuable aspect of self-development, actualisation and individualisation. The reader is provided with examples of dreams in the context of shame, and with therapeutical interventions to explore the value of shame from a positive psychology perspective (Vanderheiden & Mayer, 2017) through working with dreams of clients.[1]

---

[1]The chapter does not provide answers or interpretations of the cases presented; rather, it suggests which questions might be asked/which methods might be used as examples in a therapeutical context when working with shame as part of therapy.

28.2   Theoretical Background: Dreams and Dream Work to Transform Shame

Dreams are human universals which have, through time and across cultural contexts, been the subject of analysis and interpretation by humans wanting to explore their deeper meaning (Skov, 2018). It has been emphasised that shame connects to certain cultural patterns which have in many societies been used to create acceptable social behaviour and control (Skov, 2018). In dreams, however, individually or socio-culturally repressed feelings, thoughts and behaviour express themselves through the unconscious (Freud, 1900).

Dreams are both meaningful and significant and have always been seen as an important expression of intra-psychological dynamics of an individual; they present an important access to communications with the self (Ullman & Zimmerman, 2017; Fromm, 2013). According to Fromm (2013), there are three major approaches to understanding dreams:

For **Freud**, who was the first to bring different perspectives on dreams together in his work. The Interpretation of Dreams (Freud, 1900), dreams are expressions of irrational and asocial aspects of humankind which often contain unfulfilled wishes and desires. Freud worked with dreams in psychoanalytic contexts to reveal unconscious content in therapy. In particular, he made use of free association while interpreting dreams (Freud, 1900).

Dreams were classified by Freud as places in which the forgotten and repressed aspects of the psyche were stored, and he assumed that dreams were strongly influenced by daily experiences (day residue) (Freud, 1900). His perception of dreams as being similar to neurotic symptoms, however, was later revised. Lansky (2004) emphasises that ego–ideal[2] conflict in the context of anticipation of professional status loss resonates with early and unconscious shame dynamics which are associated with conflicts around guilt, competition and hostility in four of Freud's major dreams.

Jung, who in his youth was a friend and promising student of Freud's, describes dreams as revelations of unconscious wisdom which transcend the individual. He rejected Freud's assumption that dreams intentionally disguise their meanings, and argued that dreams are instead a direct and neutral expression of the dreamer's current concerns (Jung, 1967). In this way, the unconsciousness is viewed as playing a major role in defining the personality and the mind, impacting strongly on thoughts, feelings and behaviour, being based on an objective level of a dream's meaning (external influences on the dream) and a subjective level (internal influences such as feelings and thoughts) (Jung, 1967). Becoming self-aware through, for example, the work with dreams, can contribute to realising one's own potential, developing the self, becoming aware of one's own identity and leading a more meaningful and holistic life. Understanding dreams helps to improve self-understanding and to better comprehend relationships, interactions, development phases, unconscious movements and personal or social conflict, thereby functioning to balance imbalances in the

---

[2]In Freudian psychology, the ego-ideal (German Ich-Ideal) is the image of the ideal self (Akhtar, 2009).

personality of the dreamer, and to provide dreamers with prospective images of the future (Jung, 1967). Understanding dream content can also lead to personal transformation and the transformation of thoughts, feelings and behaviour through the integration of the unconscious content into a person's life.

Third, there is an approach to dreams which assumes that dreams express any kind of mental activity that occurs during sleep (Hobson, 2002), including rational and irrational aspects and light and shadow aspects of the self. Dreams carry content which is often supposed to guide the dreamer and provide new information about unconscious aspects in order to promote psychological well-being, guide the dreamer and even solve problems which might help the dreamer to cope with and resolve concerns and problems in waking life (Barrett, 2007). Dreams are often triggered by events or experiences which are emotionally important to the dreamer. The dream aims to give a balanced view of the situation, and is ideal for working with emotional content in the context of a "safe place" and finding solutions for challenges and problems (Hartmann, 1996). Dreams can become useful resources in understanding the self, complementing conscious knowledge and resolving conflictual issues.

In this chapter, I will use Hobson's (2002) definition of dreams as mental activity, and will mainly refer to Jung's dream analysis and interpretation in exploring how to understand and work with dreams regarding the topic of shame. It may even be possible to transform "toxic shame" to "healthy shame" through understanding the meaning of shame and integrating disowned parts of the psyche (Bradshaw, 2005).

In the following sections, the theoretical approach of the chapter will be explained, examples of shame in dreams narrated in therapeutical practice will be presented, and ways of exploring dream content with regard to shame will be exemplified.

28.3 Contextual Descriptions of Working with Dreams in Therapeutical Practice

For more than a decade, I have been working in counselling, coaching and therapy in my own therapeutical practice as a systemic family therapist, coach and counsellor. In this context I have worked with individuals, couples and families mainly in Germany, but also in South Africa. During this time, I have often come across dream narrations associated with shameful situations, and with feelings of shame and/or embarrassment. The sharing of the shame (in this case, with the therapist) seems, in itself, to be a healing resource which begins a healing process (see also Brown, Hernandez, & Villarreal, 2011). However, while working with shame in therapy, therapists needs to be highly aware of their own shame and their reactions to shame narrations of the client, in order to minimise shame projection or introjection, transference or countertransference (Skov, 2018). Often it seems that talking about the shame experienced in dreams is easier for the client than to talk about shame experienced in real-life situations. Lansky (2003) stresses that shame is an important instigation of the dream, and that hidden shame conflicts may react to the dreamer's anticipation of danger and exposure. Dreams carrying shame often occur in the context of specific life experiences and life changes, and are connected to particular life topics which the client and therapist can work on during therapy or coaching through the initiation of dream narration in therapy.

In my therapeutical practice, I realised that there are two main appearances of shameful situations in dream narrations:

1. Possibly shameful experiences are transformed within the dream itself, and leave the individual in the aftermath feeling irritated, positive, astonished, surprised or even amused about the original feeling of shame or how the shameful situation was transformed within the content of the dream.
2. Individuals experience shameful situations which stay unresolved and/or untransformed. These remain in the memory of the dreamer as strong and shameful dream experiences which leave the dreamer with a negative impression or feeling of shame, anger, anxiety and deep emotional upheaval based on shame and embarrassment.

In both cases, one can work with shame and its occurrence in dreams during therapy and coaching.

In the following short case, I offer examples of dreams in which shame played a role based on the subjective experience of the dreamer. I will then provide the reader with excerpts of questions which therapists can work with in terms of exploring the deeper meaning of the dream and its content regarding shame. I will also introduce the "social dream drawing" method. The methods described here can support the dreamer to transform the experience of shame into a resource for self-understanding, actualisation and development.

There are different ways of working with dreams and dream analysis in therapy. One can work with dreams extensively by focusing on the exploration of the dream to deeply understand the meaning and the intra-psychological conversation of the conscious and the unconsciousness within the person. Alternatively, one can refer to dreams within the context of other therapeutical approaches. The examples given below are only excerpts of how to work with dreams in the context of shame and can be expanded and combined with other methods, depending on the focus of the therapy. I do not provide an analysis and interpretation of the dreams described, but instead present the reflective questions and methods which can be applied or possibly transferred to other contexts.

28.4 Applied Methods in Transforming Shame in Dreams

28.4.1 Case 1: Running for Presidency

The first case example is a dream narrated by a ten year old boy, here called A. The dream was narrated during a time in which A had been shamed in a school context based on his origin and his behaviour which other children found "strange". During one of our sessions, A remembered a dream he had dreamt some days before the session.

> I was naked in the CBD,[3] I was just naked and I walked around a bit. The first few seconds, I felt ashamed about it, just being naked in the CBD. I don't know why. Then, in the dream, I became a comedian. I started to make people laugh, I told jokes and I acted a bit funny. And then I ran for becoming a president and everyone accepted me as a president, because I was so funny. And then I woke up. First, I did not like the dream, but then it was actually quite cool when I thought about this dream.

28.4.2   Exploring Associations, Images and Dream Messages

During the conversation, we worked with the dream and I asked him the following questions after he had reported the dream:

1. What do you associate with the dream? (Just to go with the associations of the client)
2. What are the images the dream shows you? (Work with the clients' images and explore them in detail, and with regard to feelings and thoughts about these images)
3. Which archetypes play a role in this dream? (Explain archetypes and provide, if necessary, ideas of which archetypes are at play in this dream, such as the comedian (jester), or the president (leader/ruler) for example
4. What does the dream tell you? What do you think is its message with regard to your personality? With regard to shame experiences?
5. How does shame play a role in the dream—from beginning to end? Is the feeling of shame transformed? If yes, how? Does it change; if yes, how does it change?
6. How does the dream impact on your view of shame in general?
7. What do you do with the message regarding shame in your life? How do you transform, acknowledge and integrate this message into your life?
8. Focusing specifically on shame, you said, you are shamed at school often. What does the dream tell you in terms of how to deal with shame at school?

These questions need to be explored together with the client and adjusted according to the client's age, socio-cultural background, and understanding of dreams and of shame.

28.4.3   Case 2: Winning Naked

The following dream was told by a young, adolescent man (C) who was swimming in his university's swim club. Sport was one of the most important activities in his life,

---

[3]City Bowl District.

carrying him through challenging and difficult life situations, providing him with strength and energy. One day, he came to our session and said: "I've had a strange dream!"

> I was with some friends from varsity[4] at a swimming competition. You know, I swim for the club … so, we were there and suddenly I lost my swim pants. It just slipped down and before the others could realise, I jumped into the water. I jumped and I swam to the other side. I swam as fast as I could … and back again. And I won! I won the competition! Then I had to come out of the water and I quickly grabbed my trousers and held it, as if I had it on. So, nobody realised what had happened, but first I had a shock when I lost my pants. Then I woke up. I felt quite embarrassed and shamed about it and still I am when I am telling you that story now.

28.4.4 Associations Regarding the Dream

I worked with C particularly concerning his associations based on this dream, to explore the deeper meaning for him and with regard to the systemic contexts he was in at that time.

1. What are the key words in this dream for you?
2. Where did the dream take place? What does this place remind you of? What do you associate with the swimming pool, the competition?
3. Who appeared in the dream? What relationship do you have with the students appearing in your dream in your life? Who did not appear in your dream and who would you have expected to appear in such a situation?
4. Which images, metaphors (e.g. "to jump in at the deep end"; opposite of "wearing the breeches"), symbols ("a certain lifestyle", "leisure", "duality—a world above, a world below", "sport") and feelings occurred in this dream? At which stage did they occur? What do these metaphors and symbols mean to you? How do you feel about them?
5. How did you feel in the dream? What do the feelings remind you of?
6. What do you personally associate with the dream images? What are your personal associations?
7. Which archetypes (primordial images and symbols of collective consciousness) do you associate with your dream? Which play a role here? Which associations do you think are archetypal and which content do they carry?
8. When you focus on your life and the relationships which play a role in your life, who do you think would interpret the dream, and how? What would the message be to the friends who were in the pool with you? What would the message to yourself be?
9. How does the message help you to build contemporary and future relationships between you and your friends? What does the dream tell you about yourself, your strength, weaknesses, transformative potential?
10. What do you learn from this dream for future situations?

---

[4]Varsity means university.

We examined the associations he had with the dream, the relationships and the transformative potential for C with regard to his own thoughts, feelings and behaviour, his relationships with his friends and his swimming talent and explored how the shaming situation of "losing the pants" turned into success.

28.4.5   Case 3: The Men in My Life and the Knot in My Stomach

Here, I describe the dream of a woman (M) who felt stuck in her unhappy marriage, while struggling to separate from her husband over the years. She started therapy with the wish to leave her husband. A few years ago she had engaged in a short, "two-night" affair with one of her colleagues (B), which nobody except she and B knew about, until today.

One day she came to therapy, and told me about the following dream. She said she felt very embarrassed even telling me about the dream, but she thought it might provide her with some guidance to understand herself better, as well as her feelings of shame, embarrassment and guilt.

> I am somewhere with B, you know, this black colleague I had an affair with, I am somewhere with him, but it feels as if we are having a conflict and we split up and walk different ways. I find a very attractive man soon after and we start holding hands and we pass by B who looks at us. I am not sure how to interpret his looks. This guy and I, we are jumping and running – just out of pure joy and happiness and we move on. He is blonde with blue eyes, and being with him just feels light. But somehow I feel bad about the situation and embarrassed and my stomach feels knotted. I turn around to look at B, but then I wake up. I wake up with a deep feeling of shame and embarrassment.

During the session, M explained that she felt extremely ashamed about the "racial conflict" in her dream, about splitting up with this black colleague and running away with this blonde blue-eyed man. We therefore started to explore the characters represented in her dream.

28.4.6 *Exploring the Characters in the Dream*

1. How do you experience yourself in the dream? How do you present yourself? How does the image of yourself in the dream change? How do you experience yourself in relation to the other characters in the dream? Where does shame and embarrassment play a role with regard to the different characters? (observing yourself and the dream characters as part of your inner self)

2. What does the dream communicate to you personally in terms of yourself, your relationships and shame? Who do you most often associate the feeling of shame with? Feeling the knot in the stomach: who or what does this knot connect with in the dream? (working with the ego)

3. What are the shadow aspects in the dream? What represents the hidden aspects, your unacceptable emotions, behavioural patterns, wishes, denied aspects? When you look at the desires, the wishes and emotions which are present in the dream, which of these does the shame mostly connect with? How do the different experiences of feelings interact how do they relate to each other in the dream (irritation, joy, happiness, shame)? (working with the shadow and selected shadow aspects)

4. What do the male and the female characters represent in your dream? How does shame connect to the male and the female aspects in your dream? How does shame relate to the rational thinking function (male) and/or the irrational, the feeling function (female) in the dream? What do the male and female representations and images tell you with regard to shame? (working with the anima, the animus) How do you understand the feeling of shame in your socio-cultural living context? (historical/contemporary South Africa)

5. How do you understand the feeling of shame in your socio-cultural living context? (historical/contemporary South Africa, upper-middle class living area in a large urban center etc.)

6. Focusing on the end of your dream, whom are you with at the end? Which character are you most connected to? How does this feel? How did the connections change throughout the dream? How did this change impact on the feeling of shame?

7. What is the most important message of this dream, taking the strong feeling of shame at the end of the dream into account? What does it tell you for your life, your relationships, and your self-conduct?

8. If the feeling of shame at the end of your dream could speak for itself, what would it say?

9. What (actions, thoughts, movements) would help you to untangle the knot?

10. Which overall meaning does the dream have for you and what meaning does the shame in the dream represent with regard to your life?

11. How does the dream, and particularly the experience of shame in the dream, comment on the overall patterns of behaviour in your life and how does both comment on your immediate life situation? If you wanted to, how would you change this pattern?

12. What transformative potential does the dream carry? What will you change in your life regarding the message of your dream? How will this impact on the feeling of shame in your life in the long term? What will you do to remind yourself of the dream's message in your life when it is necessary or helpful? (anchoring of the message in life/in the unconscious)

During the session, M interpreted the two men as parts of herself: the shadow parts which she hides, splits off from, does not acknowledge—and the light parts, which she loves to run away with. During the following session, we worked with the dream images of two male characters as expressions of shadow and light aspects of herself and allocated the topic of shame within this context. The shame about "racialisation" of her dream content, the shame about the affair, and the shame of not being able to leave her husband could (partly) be transformed through the new perspectives on the characters, the re-interpretation of dream content and the taking of ownership for thoughts, feelings and actions by evaluating the socio-contextual influences.

28.4.7   Case 4: Presenting in Front of High Achievers

The next dream occurred to a woman (K) who came to a coaching session to work on her self-esteem and on her anxieties about presenting herself in front of others, particularly in the male-dominated professional context of high achievers she worked in. Two days before K was due to give a very important presentation in front of government representatives, she had the following dream.

> I am arriving at the venue. I get out of my taxi and go in. I wonder – I seem to wear the wrong clothes! I pull my suitcase behind me, but there is no time and place to change anymore and the people are already waiting for me to greet me at the reception. I feel embarrassed that I am not dressed appropriately. I hold my presentation, but I seem to stutter and to miss the words and the connection to the audience. I wished the ground would open and swallow me. After the presentation I just want to leave, but I have to hold small talk with people from the audience. One old man comes to me and says: "I wished you had said something meaningful." I have to keep my countenance! However, I want to cry, cry, cry. I am relieved when I can leave the scenario, but my throat feels constricted and I feel embarrassed and shamed. I never want to return again. After I woke up, I felt that I just wanted to cancel the presentation two days ahead and I cried!

28.5   Social Dream Drawing

In this instance, I first talked with K about her dream and asked her questions as presented in the previous cases. However, she felt as if she was unable to respond to the questions. She was emotionally involved in talking about the dream, re-experiencing the shame, the pressure of the presentation, a kind of powerlessness, doubt and meaninglessness. We worked with her feelings and their connections to the dream, the dream message and images in the dream. One important aspect was the message regarding meaningfulness.

At the end of the session I decided to work differently with K; I asked her to draw her dream and put the dream into an image/images, based on the assumption that creating an image or several images of a dream can evoke dream images that would otherwise not come to the dreamer's awareness (Fisher, 1957). Allowing herself time between the dream, her conversation with me in the session, and finally time spent dream drawing later at home, freed her from the immediate experience (as described in Mersky, 2008). She could now take a distanced perspective while expressing the dream's content in a creative way.

K drew five images from her dream. During the next session, she displayed her images in the room, explained the drawings and I asked questions to clarify aspects of the images. I then offered my personal associations with the picture while K listened. She was then asked to share her reflections on my associations.

Usually the method of social dream drawing is used in a group or an organisational context, which often brings many new insights by elucidating material which is out of the awareness or consciousness of the individual and/or group (Mersky, 2017). However, it can also be used in single therapeutical sessions between the client and the therapist or between coachee and coach. Already Freud (cited in Fisher, 1957) and later Bion (1961) confirmed that drawing dreams supports the awareness and experience of the latent content of dreams, and can bring unconscious aspects of the dream into consciousness. The choice of which underlying psychological perspective to use in analysing and interpreting the material (such as Jungian analytic art therapy, psychoanalysis or socio-analysis for example) is up to the therapist and must be within the professional scope of the coach or therapist (Mersky, 2008).

In the context of the deep shame experienced by K, I used the following process:

1. The client narrates the dream in a therapy session
2. We talk about the dream (e.g. associations, images, metaphors, relationships, relevance to life situations)
3. We explore the topic of shame in the dream and its connection to life by highlighting the transformational aspects (also focusing on the context of other feelings, thoughts, behaviours)
4. The client draws an image/images of the dream
5. The client explains the drawing in the next session.
6. The therapist asks questions to understand the drawing fully
7. The therapist offers own associations regarding the drawing
8. The client presents own reflections on the associations

The topic of shame can become a focus area of the dream drawing process if the client presents it as such. Social dream drawing can also be applied in group therapy contexts, as well as in organisational contexts when the work with shame becomes relevant.

28.6 Conclusion

Although this chapter provides insight into how to work with shame in therapy by using narration of the client's dreams, the insight can only be of a limited nature. The aim is to create awareness of the often tabooed and silenced topic of shame in therapy. The focus should be on the transformation of toxic shame into healthy shame through work with dreams and dream content.

Further research is still needed to explore the limited scope and knowledge of shame in dreams and its connection to shame in real-life situations, the short-term and long-term transformational effects of working with dreams and shame in therapy, as well as its meaning for the client and for the therapist. Culture-specific research is needed in terms of dreams and shame (personal, cultural and archetypal images) and their transformation towards becoming a health resource for the individual.

Acknowledgements I would kindly like to thank the Centre of Applied Jungian Studies (CAJS) in Johannesburg, South Africa, for training me in Applied Jungian Studies through their programmes and inspiring my therapeutical practice.

References

Akhtar, S. (2009). *Comprehensive dictionary of psychoanalysis*. London: Karnac.

Barrett, D. (2007). An evolutionary theory of dreams and problem-solving. In D. Barrett & P. McNamara (Eds.), *The new science of dreaming* (pp. 133–154). Praeger Publishers.

Bion, W. R. (1961). *Experiences in groups*. London: Routledge.

Bradshaw, J. (2005). *Healing the shame that binds you*. Deerfield Beach: Health Communications Inc.

Brown, B., Hernandez, V. R., & Villarreal, Y. (2011). *Connections: A 12-session psychoeducational shame resilience curriculum*. Washington, DC: American Psychological Association.

Fisher, C. (1957). A study of preliminary stages of the construction of dreams and images. *Journal of the American Psychoanalytic Association, 5*(5), 60.

Freud, S. (1900). *The interpretation of dreams*. The Standard Edition of the Complete Psychological Works of Sigmund Freud (Vols. IV and V). London: Hogarth Press, 1900.

Freud, S. (1924). *The dissolution of the Oedipus complex*. Standard Edition (Vol. 19, pp. 173–179). London: Hogarth Press.

Freud, S. (1991). *Shame and the self*. New York: Guilford Press.

Freud, S., & Breuer, J. (1895/1966). *Studies on Hysteria*. New York: Avon.

Fromm, E. (2013). *The forgotten language. An introduction to the understanding of dreams, fairy tales, and myth*. New York: Early Bird Books.

Hartmann, E. (1996). Outline for a theory on the nature and functions of dreaming. *Dreaming, 6*(2), 147–170.

Hobson, J. A. (2002). *Dreaming: An introduction to the science of sleep*. New York: Oxford University Press.

Jacoby, M. (1996). *Shame and the origins of self-esteem. A Jungian Approach*. Hove: Brunner Routledge.

Jung, C. G. (1967). *The Collected Works of C.G. Jung* (Vol. 8). Princeton: Princeton University Press.

Jung, C. G. (1976). *Symbols and the interpretation of dreams* (Vol. 18). CW Princeton: Princeton University Press.

Jung, C. G. (2009). *The Red Book*. Liber Novus: A reader's edition. Edited and with an introduction by Sonu Shamdasani. London: W.W. Norton.

Knox, J. (2005). Sex, shame and the transcendent function: the function of fantasies in self development. *Journal of Analytical Psychology, 50*(5), 617–639.

Lansky, M. R. (2003). Shame conflicts as dream instigators: wish fulfillment and the ego ideal in dream dynamics. *The American Journal of Psychoanalysis, 63*(4), 357–364.

Lansky, M. R. (2004). Trigger and Screen: Shame Dynamics and the Problem of Instigation in Freud's Dreams. *The Journal of the American Academy of Psychoanalysis and Dynamic Psychiatry, 32*(3), 441–468. https://doi.org/10.1521/jaap.32.3.441.44782.

Lansky, M. R., & Morrison, A. P. (1997). *The widening scope of shame*. New York: Psychology Press Taylor & Francis.

Lewis, B. (1971). Shame and guilt in neurosis. *Psychoanalytic Review, 58*(3), 419.

Mayer, C.-H. (2017). Shame—"A soul feeding emotion": Archetypal work and the transformation of the shadow of shame in a group development process. In E. Vanderheiden & C.-H. Mayer (2016). *The value of shame—Exploring a health resource in cultural contexts* (pp. 277-302). Cham: Springer.

Mersky, R. R. (2008). Social dream-drawing: a methodology in the making. *Socio-Analysis, 10,* 35–50.

Mersky, R. R. (2017). *Social dream-drawing (SDD). Praxis and Research*. Doctoral thesis, University of the West of England, Bristol, UK. Retrieved from http://eprints.uwe.ac.uk/28881/12/Mersky.SDD.Praxis%20and%20Research.final.2017.pdf.

Scheff, T. (2013). *The S-word: Shame as a key to modern societies*. Global summit on diagnostic alternatives. Retrieved from http://dxsummit.org/archives/1286.

Schultz, J. M. (1996). *Shame. Reflections on Psychology, Culture and Life*. The Jung Page. Retrieved from http://www.cgjungpage.org/learn/articles/analytical-psychology/776-shame.

Skov, V. (2018). *Shame and creativity. From affect towards individuation*. Oxon: Routeledge.

Ullman, M., & Zimmerman, N. (2017). *Working with dreams*. London: Routledge.

Vanderheiden, E., & Mayer, C.-H. (2017). *The value of shame—Exploring a health resource in cultural contexts*. Cham: Springer.

Wharton, B. (1990). The hidden face of shame: the shadow, shame and separation. *Journal of Analytical Psychology, 35,* 279–299.

Wittman, L., & de Dassel, T. (2015). Posttraumatic nightmares from scientific evidence to clinical significance. In M. Kramer & M. Glucksman (Eds.), *Dream research. Contributions to clinical practice* (pp. 135–148). New York: Taylor & Francis.

Claude-Hélène Mayer (Dr. habil., PhD, PhD) is a Professor in Industrial and Organisational Psychology at the Department of Industrial Psychology and People Management at the University of Johannesburg, an Adjunct Professor at the Europa Universität Viadrina in Frankfurt (Oder), Germany and a Senior Research Associate in the Department of Management at Rhodes University, Grahamstown, South Africa. She holds a Ph.D. in psychology (University of Pretoria, South Africa), a Ph.D. in management (Rhodes University, South Africa), a Doctorate in political sciences (Georg-August-Universität, Göttingen, Germany), and a Habilitation with a Venia Legendi (Europa Universität Viadrina, Germany) in psychology with focus on work, organizational, and cultural psychology. She has published numerous monographs, edited text books, accredited journal article, and special issues on transcultural mental health, salutogenesis and sense of coherence, shame, transcultural conflict management and mediation, women in leadership in culturally diverse work contexts, constellation work, coaching, and psychobiography.

Chapter 29
Shame-Death and Resurrection—The Phoenix-Dance to Our Authentic Self

Barbara Buch

Abstract From the salutogenic, as well as from the shamanic point of view, shame in its largest intensity can be considered an emotional death experience, potentially leading to depression, addiction and suicide. 'Felt' death experience, encompassing the whole person, as a large stressor, implies the potential for dying or 'rising from the ashes', as a more empowered being. This has been described in the typical path of a shaman, as well as within the model of Salutogenesis, where the successful and often miraculous overcoming of a death (-like) experience leads to an increased Sense of Coherence and to empowerment. Shame occurs in everyone's upbringing and life to different degrees. In this context, mainly intergenerational, unjustified and toxic shame is considered, especially in regards to female and racial shaming. In order to use the transformative power of shame, different cognitive steps are suggested. However, strong emotions and traumata, like shame, are stored in our body tissues. Therefore physical processes, like embodiment techniques, are essential for their transformation. The recreation of oneself after shame requires the seeing and feeling, which creates believing. Exemplary movement with rhythmic music and body awareness practices with their underlying mechanisms are described, which may be able to rebalance, reassemble and recreate one's sense of self. The rebalancing and restoring of body, mind, spiritual and group-connection, which had been disrupted through shaming, based on new grounds and embodiment practices, is essential for transformation towards a more authentic self.

Keywords Female · Racial shame · Embodiment · Conscious dance & sexuality · Empowerment · Authentic self · Matriarchy

B. Buch (✉)
Burns Lake, BC V0J 1E4, Canada
e-mail: barbara@salutogenesis-shamanism.com

© Springer Nature Switzerland AG 2019
C.-H. Mayer and E. Vanderheiden (eds.), *The Bright Side of Shame*,
https://doi.org/10.1007/978-3-030-13409-9_29

29.1   Introduction

The complex emotional shame response to humiliation in front of others is a bio-socio-cultural adaptive dissociative body-mind reaction, which is an integral part of being a social human, who tries to belong (Buch, 2017). Shame in its different intensities can be considered an emotional death-experience, potentially leading to depression, addiction and suicide: "It encompasses the whole of ourselves; it generates a wish to hide, to disappear, or even to die" (Lewis, 1995, 2). Its main behavioral stress reaction—'freeze' and hide, isolates and cuts off from connections. The loss of these ties as generalized resistance resources (GRR), which are needed for a strong Sense of Coherence and health (Salutogenesis), like body-mind, social and higher power connections, reduce stress coping abilities. Extreme cases of (e.g. public-media) shaming (character assassination and defamation) can even lead to the loss of further essential resistance resources, like career and finances etc.. Thus, the psychological shame stress is exponentiated.

The experience of shame implies the potential for dying *or* 'rising from the ashes' (Phoenix) as a more empowered being. This has been described in the typical path of a shaman, as well as within the model of Salutogenesis, where the successful and often miraculous overcoming of a death experience leads to an increased Sense of Coherence (Buch, 2012). How can we access the salutogenic potential of shame to create us and our resources anew?

29.2   Cognitive Steps

29.2.1   Becoming Aware of How Shame-Driven Our Life Is: The Monster of Shame Lurks Behind Every Corner

Shame, as the master emotion, is a normal part of everyone's life (Brown, 2007). Most of us are driven to look good, to function and perform, avoiding the exposure of our deeply hidden, secret, learned belief system, that 'we're not good enough'. It is a devil's cycle: To avoid the pain of anticipated humiliation, we continuously re-create a shame-based symptomatic narcissistic self and society, where our inner self and pain is covered up by superficial norms, based on looks, finances, perfect social media profiles etc., disconnected from traditional environmentally adapted and authentic values (Buch, 2017). The more we adapt to these socio-culturally acknowledged success expectations, the more we are prone to the 'lurking monster of shame'.

Since re-integration after shaming is *not* an intrinsic part of our modern 'pseudo-connected' worldwide society (Buch, 2017),—once shamed—we are shame-tagged forever, while often lacking close social connective support systems. How can we be surprised, that shame is not only the root of depression, but of all addictions (Bradshaw, 2005; Lancer, 2014)?

In order to cut the chain of shame, we need to develop the awareness, to search for the often overlooked presence, root-causes, and consequences of shame, found within society, previous generations, therapeutic settings and our personal life. A crucial premise is the willingness and courage to look honestly into hidden (shame from shame) shame-pain. Here, the realization, that we are not responsible for past learned trauma-based behavior patterns (Wolynn, 2017), might lift some shame-burden off us. Cognitive self-reflective questions about occurrence and justification of shame, including the distinction from guilt and related terms, potentially direct us to a more authentic self. However, this might be impossible for some people, e.g. within the (shame-based) narcissistic dis-order spectrum.

29.2.2 The Analysis of the Who, Why and Which of Shaming

Historical systematic toxic shaming, based on stigmatization as a political tool (e.g. race, gender) leads to intergenerational psychological effects, which are often overlooked (Buch, 2017). Previous, trauma-related intergenerational and childhood shame increases the vulnerability and likelihood for its re-occurrence in life (Van der Kolk, 1994).

Would the effects of shaming have increased the social and biological functioning for our own, social groups' and earths' benefits? Was shame used to keep a particular power structure in place? Which values and norms is my social group based on and are they authentic with my values? What are my values? Where do they originate from, whom do they serve?

While shame is undeniably gender-related (Elise, 2008; Vanderheiden & Mayer, 2017), also the word-gender itself in many European languages (Buch, 2017), as well as the social-cultural convention of **shame is female** (Vanderheiden & Mayer, 2017)—at least since the creation of the Adam and Eve story in our western world. Female shame (Silverio, in this book), much more than male shame, is entangled with body, nudity, as well as sexuality. Typical *feminine* traits are based on the image of the *nurturing* mother, including empathy. Naturally, the *mother* earth, as the foundation for the subsistence of humanity, was honored in many pre-Christian, pre-colonial, matriarchal traditions. However, Christianity with its patriarchal, misogynist and hegemonial ambitions, systematically blamed, stigmatized, shamed, oppressed, and even eradicated women, as well as nature-connected, matriarchal societies. Historical manifestations are the medieval witch burnings, as well as colonization methods, which "native […] societies were forced to endure", like "the reduction of the cultural validation of women" (Klein & Ackerman, 1995, vii). The deeply engrained disrespect of the feminine (Nel and Govender on battered women, in this book), as what sustains, nurtures and provides for us, symbolized in mother and earth, still continues today, as does racial shaming.

Racial, gender, body etc.-shaming are based on *visible* characteristics—as different to the oppressing others—there is no chance, to hide your suggested flaw (**'outside shaming'**). Victims are trapped in the worthless, isolated shame state, often with no other escape than e.g. depression, addiction etc.. On the other hand, hideable shamed 'flaws' ('**inside shaming**'), like emotions (e.g. negligence), can be concealed through adaptive behavior patterns: Ranging from workaholic etc. to the narcissistic personality disorder-behavior adaptation. The latter, as emotionally dissociated 'master' of hiding shame-based flaws—plays the role of the 'superior', being in power and control. This theoretical distinction between both overlapping forms, can help us understand how and with which consequences shame occured. The prevalence of narcissism in men compared to women in western societies (Foster, Campbell, & Twenge, 2003), seems to confirm the theory of mostly outside-shamed females, versus men, who arc usually not shamed because of their obvious gender.

Shame asks us to re-evaluate our own value and norms on a deep level for the potential of adapting, or changing them, guided by *nurturing* aspects for oneself, the groups' and the earth's thriving (e.g. 'wheel of choices' by Daniel, 2012). However, even if the mortifying feeling of shame is comprehended and acknowledged as *justified* socio-cultural construct in retrospective, behavior change and self-forgiveness, as a conscious exercise of self-compassion, are needed to transform and empower.

The formulation, internalization and embodiment of shames' opposite aspects are crucial: Instead of blame, judgement, and stigmatisation, it is forgiveness (Baumann & Handrock, in this book), self-acceptance, and self-compassion, which essentially equals love. Taking time to re–connect on *all* levels, as well as to physically enact our cognitive insights, e.g. through conscious, self-explorative, physical embodiment methods, can be an expression of such self-compassion (love), which in return can increase our feelings of love by releasing endorphins (Freeman, 1998).

Connecting with supportive group settings, e.g. aboriginal (common ancestry, traditions) or gender-based (women's) groups and the more general, non-judgemental conscious dance groups (below), is essential for empowerment (Bradshaw, 2005).

"Analysis—like sex, interestingly—entails risking exposure of a sense of shame in the hope that the interpersonal outcome will not deepen or confirm one's humiliation but ameliorate it. Optimally, the negative self-concept is disconfirmed; when that occurs, exposure is connecting. Exposure uncovers a vulnerability of the self that is attractive; the toxicity of shame has been triumphed over" (Elise, 2008, 95).

29.3   Body-Based Practices

29.3.1   Resurrection from the 'Freeze' of Shame

The rebalancing and restoring of body, mind, spiritual, social- and group-connection, which had been disrupted through shaming, is fundamental for transformation (Bradshaw, 2005; Buch, 2017). Strong shame emotions are not only stored in our brains, but in our body postures and tissues (e.g. Van der Kolk, 1994; Fogel, 2009; Levine, 2010; Reich in Almeida & Albertini, 2014; Ogden, Pain, & Fisher, 2006). Therefore, perceptual movement processes are essential for their transformation to increased empowerment, by (re)creating resources and resilience (e.g. Fogel 2009; Levine, 2010; Reich's 'body armor' in Almeida & Albertini, 2014; Ogden et al., 2006).

The redefinition of oneself after shame needs the seeing and feeling (body-mind-emotion-awareness) of (re-)connection, which creates believing (Ryan, in this book and Baharudin et al., in this book) and thus integrating authentic compassion based values in our life. The following suggested embodiment methods can be practiced within different kinds of autodidactic, and within therapeutic settings.

29.3.2 Conscious Dance as Embodiment and Perceptual-Intuitive Awareness Practice

Our life is based on movement: Frequency and rhythm from the atomic level to the universe.

The embryo is engulfed in the rhythm of the heartbeat of its mother: The continuous drum of life. Through this constant communication, it feels connected, safe and alive, effecting its inner body chemistry, brain and emotions. Dance to rhythmic music is an ancestral, biologically and culturally rooted tradition, based on complex multisensory, emotional, cognitive and somatic practice (Hanna, 1995; Bachner-Melman et al., 2005). Embedded in rituals and ceremonies, they served different purposes from social-, courtship- to spiritual- (re)connection, as regular "group psychotherapy to prevent community disorders" (Hanna, 1995, 328).

There are countless dance forms today (Dance with your shame; Vanderheiden, in this book). However, I am focussing on freestyle, improvisational, meditative dance forms under the umbrella 'conscious dance'. Within this term, I include a number of worldwide contemporary community events with similar intention and structure: Conscious dance, 5-rhythm dance, ecstatic dance, open floor, just dance, Biodanza and others (e.g. Roth, 2010). These dance events offer regular kinesthetic experiences to increase one's own body-mind-awareness, potentially beneficent to counter act and transform the distorted sense of the shamed self (Hanna, 1995), as well as further multilevel (re)connecting potentials.

They are free-style, non-judgemental, meditative movement platforms for *every* body. Typically, uplifting world music is arranged in a particular 'wave-like' sequence, based on different rhythms: Starting slow, increasing in rhythm and reaching an ecstatic peak and finally slowing down (relaxation) (Roth, 2004, 2010).

29.3.2.1 (Re-)Establishing Social Connection

One of the largest shame effects is isolation: The links to the social group are broken. Based on the cognitive steps above, non-judgmental conscious dance groups can offer social re-connection, because they provide a platform for "positive interpersonal dynamics that provide what may essentially be a support group" (Hanna, 1995, 325).

As the mothers' heartbeat and voice connect child and mother, music plays a neurobiological role (Geldenhuis, in this book) in social bonding and religiosity (Freeman, 1998; Demmrich, 2017). Dance with rhythmic music "co-evolved biologically and culturally to serve as a technology of social bonding", creating trust (Freeman, 1998, 1; Wiedenhofer & Koch, 2017). Specific connecting group practices within conscious dance, such as contact improvisation (Novack, 1990), or instructional 5-rhythm dancing classes, can create increased bonding effects.

Besides non-verbal communication with others, the connective power of conscious dancing is based on group recognition, acceptance and sharing the same non-judgemental intention. Furthermore, dance in communal settings often builds up an elated spirit, which is infectious and connects people (Hanna, 1995). The rhythm sequences in conscious dance are particularly aiming for this trance-like, altered or ecstatic state of consciousness, which increases social connection through "mutual trust among members of societies" (Freeman, 1998, 2). Thus, dance in general, but particular conscious dance events, have social integrative effects and reduce feelings of isolation (Koch & Eberhard-Kaechle, 2014). Empowerment can be further enhanced through the kind of music woven into the music set. Depending on the affiliation to a particular culture or group, certain related, uplifting lyrical, traditional, as well as religious music can cause positive emotions, which again can trigger religious-dissociative conditions (Demmrich, 2017). In this sense, the known empowering factor of reviving ancestral connections, through integration of traditions (e.g. music), as well as rituals (e.g. smudging) can be integrated (e.g. McCormick, 2000).

29.3.2.2   'Reset Button': Altered States of Consciousness (ASC), Spirit-Connection and the Change of Belief

Rhythmic music with correspondent movements can cause emotional changes, as well as altered states of consciousness (ASC), often referred to as trance or ecstatic states (Hanna, 1995; Freeman, 1998). Technologies to enter ASC for healing purposes have been traditionally used worldwide for millennia (Buch, 2012). Through what is known as the 'Frequency Following Response (FFR)', brainwaves follow stimuli (beats, rhythm) and change frequencies through hearing, seeing and other senses (Dhaka, Chouhan & Singh, 2013).

Shame can break the connection to the divine (Ryan and Baharudin et al., in this book), as Broucek (1991, p. 3 and 4) describes Adam's fall: "The link with the divine Source was broken and became invisible, the world became suddenly external to Adam, things became opaque and heavy, they became like unintelligible and hostile fragents". Music, known as one of the most important triggers, and ASC, have always been connected with religious-dissociative, spiritual experiences, potentially creating a new belief system. Dance has served as prayer, communication and connection to a higher power (Demmrich, 2017). ASC-based states enable the dissolution of the ego-sense: If there is no ego, there is no feeling of shame, thus a reconnective experience can be established.

In past and modern times, there always is and was, survival stress in different modifications, including the social shame-stress-based functioning and performing. Within proper setting, ASC, carried by the connective agent music (Demmrich, 2017)—as moments of loss of a sense of reality—not only serve as break, but can counteract the effects of continuous survival-stress-mode, as a brain 'reset button'. Stress release, relaxation and access to our 'inner healer' is enabled. Different trance (altered) states are associated with the release of the according neurohormones. Strong 'ecstatic', euphoric emotions release endorphins (Freeman, 1998), which potentially block pain (analgesia), thus providing an emotional and physical release and escape (Hanna, 1995; Geldenhuys, in this book). Synaptic connections in the brain can be affected to loosen and allow the *breakdown* of pre-existing habits (Freeman, 1998), like *internalized shame behavior patterns.* Simultaneously, some states and neurohormones associated with prolonged social dance, stomping, singing and chanting (sensory overload) can cause a "remarkable state of malleability and an opportunity for re-education" (Freeman, 1998, 8).

So potentially, ecstatic dance experience is able to create "a wholesale change in beliefs and attitudes" (Freeman, 1998, 8), based on feeling connected with oneself (body-mind), with others (social, nature), and with a higher power (spiritual). As Fishbane (2007, 411) confirms: "A truly multisystemic perspective is biopsychosocial. Our future success [..] depends, I believe, on updating our theories and approaches based on an understanding of the humanbeing at a truly multisystemic level." In conclusion, the more engaged, intense and surrendering the dance experiences, through particular rhythms, the more likely is the transformative, empowering "biology of brainwashing" (Freeman, 1998, 8).

29.3.2.3 Moving Through Emotions

Based on cognitively new found values, we practice *moving* through emotions, like shame-death-pain—as Phoenix Dance—freeing ourselves. Conscious playful movement carried by rhythms, which correspond to our main emotions, is described and practiced with 5-rhythm dance by Roth (2010).

Emotions themselves, as main driving force of our behavior and actions, are based on varied frequencies and rhythms (EEG). They reflect the interaffectivity resonating in our bodies, where every social encounter causes a feedback (Fuchs & Koch, 2014). Moving *through* these rhythms and emotions is an integral part of a health-balanced, empowered life: The heart rhythm (ECG) and body- (bio-), emotional- etc. rhythms, all are in adaption to universal, seasonal, daily rhythms, all involving duality. The permanent re-balancing on the continuums of physical and mental health corresponds to **a dance on this wave-pattern.**

However, shame can interrupt this danceand lead to stagnation. Its body image of a frozen body and muscles, is comparable to the playing-dead reaction as self-defence in the animal kingdom. Here, it usually lasts until the animal is feeling absolutely safe, after the threatening predator has left. Then, mammals usually shake the life threating experience off from their body tissue (Levine, 2010). While animals—according to Levine—automatically apply these innate mechanisms to re-balance traumatic experiences, the human analog instinctive mechanisms are often blocked, by our 'rational' brains. Consequently, strong shame emotions still resonate in our "body-feedback system", acting "as a *medium* of emotional perception" (e.g. "sensations, postures, movement", Fuchs & Koch, 2014, 9), but cannot be released and thus are stored in our tissues (Roth, 1989; Ogden et al., 2006; Fogel, 2009; Levine, 2010; Reich in Almeida & Albertini, 2014). Mostly at early age, shame is internalized and becomes part of interrupted internal and external communications, re-creating and increasing the shame-anxiety-cycle: "Bodily sensations and behavior strongly influences one's emotional reaction toward certain situations or objects" (Fuchs & Koch, 2014, 1). Reich called the resulting, protective, 'shielding' body with its muscle tensions 'body armor' (Almeida & Albertini, 2014). Unreleased, they can lead to further mental or physical disease.

All these authors agree, that body-stored emotions can only be set free through multisensory body-based approaches (Ogden et al., 2006; Fogel, 2009; Levine, 2010; Roth, 2010). They all involve re-learning awareness of body, emotions and motility. Ogden et al., (2006) state, that the more movement vocabulary we (re-)develop, the higher our resiliency. Therefore, spontaneous dance movements, including shaking of the body, can help to liberate body stored emotional body trauma (Levine, 2010).

Music, as based on frequency and rhythm, triggers emotions. Intuitive body movement, immersed in music and rhythm, becomes expression and release of suppressed shame emotions (Roth, 2010), which eventually will re-surface through regular practice. We can get out of our rational brain, access, liberate and free former restricted emotions, moving through them, melting our 'body armour' (Reich in Almeida & Albertini, 2014) away. "The fusion of the mind and body and the expressive and communicative primacy of nonverbal body movement in revealing aspects of a person's mental and emotional state and range of adaptive behaviors", leads to "acquiring insight, experiencing catharsis, and discarding personal misconceptions" (Hanna, 1995, 328, 329).

If we project our shame-related feelings in our dance, detaching by moving through the play of them, we gain a sense of manageability (Salutogenesis) (Hanna, 1995). Furthermore, conscious dance also encourages to move through imagined fantasy worlds, which not only presents an escape of stress (Hanna, 1995), but also permits to experience us in different, more powerful, related personifications (seeing is believing). Through all these effects, the disturbed processes of embodied interaffectivity, caused by internalised shame trauma (Fuchs & Koch, 2014), may be counterbalanced.

29.3.2.4   (Re-)Establishment of Body-Mind-Neuronal Connections

Our brains are wired for relation (Fishbane, 2007). The more connective structures—plasticity—the healthier is the brain and its owner. Internalized shame equals chronic stress experience, which reduces synaptic connections (Kang et al., 2012) and can cause dissociative states. Hence, shame-based multileveled disconnection—socially, body-mind-spirit level etc.—can lead to consequences on the brain. However, dance activity, as well as music, seems to have enhancing effects on brain plasticity, confirming dancing to music as effective functional method to re-train the brain (Thaut, 2008; Karpati et al., 2015). Simultaneously, brain cells are re-connected by moving through emotions and physically, increasing resiliency through movement vocabulary (Ogden et al., 2006). However, research of the neuroscience of dance is just beginning (Karpati et al., 2015).

29.3.2.5 Dance and Body Awareness: Freeing Body, Mind and Self

Shame shuts down our self-expression completely and can feel like imprisonment in normative, suppressive standards. In contrast, free form dancing as "multisensory experience of self-expression other than speech or writing" (Hanna, 1995, 324) can feel like freedom. It encourages inner authentic -movement, -self-expression and thus -selves to appear: "There is no dogma in dance. If we let our body dance, we instantly shed off the lies and dogmas, and what is left, is nothing else than the spirit of life" (transl., Roth, 2010, 42).

Performance in front of others and shame are often connected. Therefore, conscious dance can be initially practised at home. Dance and the mastery of (new) movement to music through the experience of joy can contribute "to a positive self-perception, body image, self-esteem, and self-confidence" (Hanna, 1995, 326) and resiliency (Ogden et al., 2006). All of these need to be re-established after shaming. Conscious sexuality has the same potential (below).

Goal-oriented structured dance usually has restrictive rules, standards and expectations of how to dance, which leaves us in our normative, functioning, performing, and rational brain of daily consciousness. Therefore, free movement based dance outweighs health benefits regarding stress reduction and empowerment compared to goal-oriented—group dance activities (Wiedenhofer & Koch, 2017). Dance can be the empowering language of liberation and revolution:

> "Why do I dance? *Dance is my medicine*. It's *the scream* which eases for a while the terrible frustration common to all human beings who because of race, creed, or color, are 'invisible'. Dance is the fist with which I fight the sickening ignorance of prejudice." (Pearl Primus)

And Hanna (1995, 328) writes:

> "More than letting off steam, dance is a venue to guard against the misuse of power and produce social change without violence. A political form of coercion in a *shame-oriented society*, unheeded *dance communication* led to the famous 1929 'women's war' […]".

Concluding, conscious dance may improve health through enhancing the sense of manageability, meaningfulness by "getting a sense of control" through"(1) possession by the spiritual manifested in dance, (2) mastery of movement, (3) escape or diversion from stress and pain, and (4) confronting stressors to work through ways of handling their effects" (Hanna, 1995, 326).

29.4 Dance and Sex

While some animals dance as mating ritual, humans always had courtship dances. Both, dance and sexuality intertwine (Hanna, 1988) with eroticism, gender roles, body image, femininity, culture, sin and shame, not only through the still present shaming of both to different degrees (Kraus, 2010).

- Both are forms of non-verbal communication,
- Both do not need music but music enhances,
- Both can enable intense body-mind (Wolf, 2012), and social connections,
- Both can cause ASC,
- Both release 'happy/love/bonding' neurohormones (Freeman, 1998),
- Both activities are good for your health in a variety of ways (circulation/heart rate, muscle strengthening, detoxification, relaxation, breathing etc.),
- Both—conscious dancing and sexuality within non-judgemental, safe settings, have a large potential for empowerment through the free expression of emotions and motility (Roth, 1989, Wolf, 2012).

The gender difference in shaming of free sexual expression in our society contributes to repressed emotions, sexual dysfunction and *general disempowerment* of women, with widespread consequences on relationships and health (Lancer, 2014; Castleman, 2014). The sense of shame in women regarding sexuality inhibits enjoyment of particular sexual (Elise, 2008; Lancer, 2014), and other activities.

"The lack of adequate information given to the girl about her sexual body often leads to anxiety, confusion, and shame regarding her sexuality" (Elsie, 2008).

Sexual health is about "identity and relationships" (Rohleder & Flowers, 2018, 143), therefore "the pervasiveness of [shame-based] inhibition in female personality [...] can center in sexuality and then extend to other areas of failure to actualize desire" (Elise, 2008, 5). Thus "sexual health psychology must question the social organisation of sex, bodies and gender" and look at socio- cultural structures (Rohleder & Flowers, 2018, 147). Internalized female shame behavior responses contribute to missing boundaries, courage to stand up for oneself (the 'me too' movement puts awareness to this), as well as to develop a 'pleaser' behavior pattern. While these effects potentially lead to overwhelmed workaholics, they also open the pathway for the widespread sexual harassment of women in a male dominated society (Silverio, in this book).

Sensing and thus developing awareness and knowing one's own intimate body sensations, leads to body mind connectedness, as in conscious dance. However, potential empowerment of shamed women also needs the explorative development of female authentic sexuality combined with consciousness, cognitively reflected within our cultural climate (Wolf, 2012).

Taking time for oneself (self-compassion, Gilbert, Oosthuizen, Merkin and Vanderheiden, in this book), becoming aware of emotions and needs (e.g. whole body massage as fundamental in lovemaking for women (Castleman, 2014)), learning to find self-pleasure and joy e.g. through explorative, non-restricted body touch, equals self-empowerment. Although e.g. masturbation still a sin in many Christian groups, the health benefits are described (Kay, 1992), as well as the importance of the brain-vaginal connection (Wolf, 2012). Increased sexual desire and function was found in women, who took time out from daily responsibilities and instead focussed on meditation, mindfulness activities, and their own desires (Castleman, 2014). According to Ventegodt et al., (2006, 2066) conscious touch and acupressure in the genital area can cause the release of shame and guilt-emotions, which were "held by the tissues of the pelvis and sexual organs". Healing and empowering is about re-discovering our pleasure centres, at least partly disentwined from dominant suppressing culture, without the shame (Ratele, 2005). "Women need to regain a sense of grandeur grounded in the female body" (Elise, 2008, 91). "To unlearn our names we have to cultivate cultural unruliness, as we have to rebel against scientism, having become aware what the culture wishes us to look and feel like and that some 'science' can be a cover for conservatism, and often violent patriarchy" (Ratele, 2005, 42). As in conscious dance, sexual exploration needs to take place in safe non-judgemental, loving set and setting: Initially alone within a safe space or only with a trusted, respectful, empathic other. The cognitive processes need to involve like-minded, safe, empowering support groups (Bradshaw, 2005).

The conscious non-goal-oriented self-exploring—as in dance—involves awareness of body sensations, emotions etc. Self-help books and other sources on female sexuality (Wolf, 2012, e.g. Mintz, 2009 in Castleman, 2014) and learning techniques, which aim at conscious connection on multiple levels, involving gazing, touch, breathing etc. are recommended (Lewis, 2007). A trustworthy therapy setting as Ventegodt et al. (2006) described, can be supportive, but is unlikely to be found within the public medical system.

Transforming shame into empowerment is about cognitively and physically overcoming shame and consequently re-learning embodiment through our innate body-mind-communication as e.g. within conscious dance and sexuality. Only then we become aware of our nature: Authentic values, norms, needs, boundaries and can develop a sense of pride, respect, honor and are able to communicate them. The conscious dance with ourselves, based on our body sense, then can extend to a healthy, proud communication-dance with another—vertically as well as horizontally: Respectfully communicating, asking, replying, giving, taking.

29.5 Conclusion

The increasing awareness of shame, including narcissism, gives us the opportunity to cognitively re-evaluate our "psychosocial, sociocultural and geopolitical contexts" (Rohleder & Flowers, 2018) in order to honestly 'dig' into our personal hidden shame subjects: Asking and understanding the when, why, who, what questions, including the purpose of shaming.

> "The capacity to do battle with shame-ridden aspects of the personality is a developmental accomplishment that benefits one's entire personality, not to mention one's sex life." (Elise, 2008, 95)

Traditionally, shame involved the communal rehabilitation process: To learn to move through, adapt and potentially being empowered (pride) (Buch, 2017). Today, this process—in lack of coherent nurture-based restoring culture with authentic guides—has to be accomplished by individuals themselves.

As in nature conservation, if we want to enable an ecosystem to rebuild itself, it needs to be (re-)exposed to natural, nurturing rhythms (biotic and abiotic: Earth, water, light, wind, migration of organisms etc.), based on the removal of inhibiting artificial structures (e.g. agriculture with pesticides, drainages, dykes, straightened watercourses, highways, covered surfaces etc.). The analogy of re-creating and re-balancing nature within nature conservation applies to our personal human 'landscape' within health promotion.

The foundational human 'ground' must be prepared through cognitive replacement of value and norm-structures: Removal of what does not serve us, nor is based on compassion and authenticity. In order to release stuck shame-emotions and their physical consequences, our inner and outer human body-mind-'ecosystem' needs to have regular access to free unstructured (by outside norms, values) flow, involving explorative playfulness of nature's 'nurture' rhythms (movement, emotions and sexuality). Then, safe settings aiming at essential diverse bio-social, spiritual, body-mind-connections, allow equalizing and relational interactions (Fishbane, 2007). The rhythm of sound, closely interwoven with movement has the deeply—phylogenetically as well as ontogenetically repeated— rooted human potential, as ancient 'healing code'. Conscious dancing through musical sequences in the style of 5-rhythm dance in a wave pattern (Roth, 2010), as traditionally rooted ritual, can offer this 'empowering playground'.

While we cannot end shame experiences, nor our modern lifestyle, we can create regular times to allow intuitive, explorative mindful movement and body-touch awareness, as creative playfulness, within safe set and settings for non-goal oriented conscious dance, as well as sexuality. Both can lead to more authenticity and empowerment after shame and serve as health promotional tools. The embodiment of shame-emotions transforms them by reestablishing previous disrupted connections (body-mind etc.), based on a new cognitive understanding of values and norms (see above).

Thus, the cognitive and physical detoxification of shame, plus "a playfully transgressive freedom to internal experience" might enable to "access a transformative integration" of male and female "gendered experiences of shame" (Elise, 2008, 95). This 'Phoenix dance' after 'shame-death' can increase generalized resistance resources, resilience and the Sense of Coherence (SOC).

I hope, this article encourages to explore authentic embodiment practices and contributes to a wider acceptance of conscious dance as powerful health promoting and empowerment tool, leading to more and regular dance spaces also outside of urban areas.

References

Almeida, B. P., & Albertini, P. (2014). The notion of armor in the work of Wilhelm Reich. Publications from 1920 to 1933. *Psicologia USP, 25*(2), 134–143.

Bachner-Melman, R., Dina, C., Zohar, A. H., Constantini, N., Lerer, E., Hoch, S., Ebstein, R. P. (2005). AVPR1a and SLC6A4 gene polymorphisms are associated with creative dance performance. *PloS Genetics 1*(3), 394–403.

Bradshaw, J. (2005). *Healing the Shame That Binds You*. Deerfield Beach: Health Communications Inc.

Broucek, F. J. (1991). *Shame and the Self*. New York: The Guilford Press.

Brown, B. (2007). *I Thought it Was Just me (But It Isn't)*. New York: Penguin Random House.

Buch, B. (2012). Shamanism as applied salutogenesis? In C.-H. Mayer & C. Krause (Eds.), *Exploring Mental Health: Theoretical and Empirical Discourses on Salutogenesis* (pp. 99–117). Lengerich: Pabst Science Publishers.

Buch, B. (2017). Canada/North America: shame between indigenous nature-connectedness, colonialism and cultural disconnection. In E. Vanderheiden & C. H. Mayer (Eds.), *The Value of Shame* (pp. 157–185). Cham: Springer International Publishing.

Castleman, M. (2014). *Effective Self-Help for Women with Low or No Sexual Desire*. Retrieved from 19 Jan 2018 https://www.psychologytoday.com/blog/all-about-sex/201410/effective-self-help-women-low-or-no-sexual-desir.

Daniel, B. (2012). How effective is the inquiry based wheel of choices as a decision making tool for youth? Thesis, Vancouver Island University, Faculty of Education.

Demmrich, S. (2017). Musik, Religiosität und Dissoziation: Der Einfluß von Musik auf religiös-dissoziative Erfahrungen. In U. Wolfradt, P. Fielder, & G. Heim (Eds.), *Schlüsselthemen der Psychotherapie* (pp. 1–13). Lengerich: Pabst Publisher.

Dhaka, P., Chouhan, V. L., & Singh, D. (2013). The impact of light-sound stimulation on intelligence in teenagers. *Journal of Scientific & Industrial Research, 72,* 366–372.

Elise, D. (2008). Sex and shame: the inhibition of female desires. *Journal of the American Psychoanalytic Association, 56,* 73–98.

Fishbane, M. (2007). Wired to connect: neuroscience, relationships, and therapy. *Family Process, 46,* 395–421.

Fogel, A. (2009). *The psychophysiology of Self-Awareness: Rediscovering the Lost Art of Body Sense. The Norton Series on Interpersonal Neurobiology*. New York: Norton & Co.

Foster, J. D., Campbell, K. W., & Twenge, J. M. (2003). Individual differences in narcissism: inflated self-views across the lifespan and around the world. *Journal of Research in Personality, 37*(6), 469–486.

Freeman, W. (1998). A neurobiological role of music in social bonding. In N. Wallin, B. Merkure, & S. Brown (Eds.), *The Origins of Music*. Cambridge MA: MIT Press. Proceedings of a Conference in Florence, Italy, 31 May 1997, Chap. 22, pp. 411–424 (2000).

Fuchs, T., & Koch, S. (2014). Embodied affectivity: on moving and being moved. *Frontiers in Psychology, 5*(508), 1–12.

Hanna, J. L. (1988). *Dance, Sex, and Gender: Signs of Identity, Dominance, Defiance, and Desire*. Chicago: The University of Chicago Press.

Hanna, J. L. (1995). The power of dance: health and healing. *The Journal of Alternative and Complementary Medicine, 1*(4), 323–331.

Kang, H. J., Voleti B., Hajszan T., Rajkowska G., Stockmeier C. A., Liczerski P., … Duman R. S. (2012). Decreased expression of synapse-related genes and loss of synapses in major depressive disorder. *Nature Medicine 18*, 1413–1417.

Karpati, F. J., Giacosa, C., Foster, N. E. V., Penhune, V. B., & Hyde, K. L. (2015). Dance and the brain: a review. *Annals of the New York Academy of Sciences, 1337,* 140–146.

Kay, D. S. G. (1992). Masturbation and mental health—uses and abuses. *Journal Sexual and Marital Therapy, 7*(1), 97–107.

Klein, L. F., & Ackerman, L. A. (1995). *Women and Power in Native North America.* Norman: University of Oklahoma Press.

Koch, S., & Eberhard-Kaechele, M. (2014). *Wirkfaktoren der Tanztherapie.* Retrieved from https://www.researchgate.net/publication/272892640.

Kraus, R. (2010). "We are not strippers": how belly dancers manage a (soft) stigmatized serious leisure activity. *Symbolic Interaction TOC, 33*(3), 435–455.

Lancer, D. (2014). *Conquering Shame and Codependency. 8 Steps to Freeing the True You.* Minnesota: Hazelden Publishing.

Levine, P. A. (2010). *In an Unspoken Voice: How the Body Releases Trauma and Restores Goodness.* Berkeley: North Atlantic Books.

Lewis, L. (2007). Tantric Transformations, a Non-Dual Journey from Sexual Trauma to Wholeness: A phenomenological Hermeneutics Approach. Thesis MSc, Faculty of Health Sciences, University of Lethbridge, Canada.

Lewis, M. (1995). *Shame: The exposed Self.* New York City: Simon & Schuster.

McCormick, R. M. (2000). Aboriginal traditions in the treatment of substance abuse. *Canadian Journal of Counselling and Psychotherapy, 34*(1), 25–32.

Mintz, L. B. (2009). *A Tired Woman's Guide to Passionate Sex. Reclaim Your Desire and Reignite Your Relationship.* Avon, MA, US: Adams Media.

Novack, C. J. (1990). *Sharing the Dance. Contact Improvisation and American Culture.* Madison: The University of Wisconsin Press.

Ogden, P., Pain, C., & Fisher, J. (2006). A Sensorimotor approach to the treatment of trauma and dissociation. *Psychiatric Clinics of North America, 29*(1), 263–279. xi–xii.

Primus, P. Retrieved from 15 Feb. 2018 http://www.azquotes.com/quote/929470.

Ratele, K. (2005). Proper sex bodies, culture and objectification. *Agenda: Empowering Women For Gender Equity, 19*(63), 32–42.

Rohleder, P., & Flowers, P. (2018). Towards a psychology of sexual health. *Journal of Health Psychology, 23*(2), 143–147.

Roth, G. (1989). *Maps to Ecstasy: a Healing Journey for the Untamed Spirit.* Novato: New World Library.

Roth, G. (2004). The Wave. DVD, Audiobook, Sound True, Incorporated.

Roth, G. (2010). *Leben ist Bewegung. Tanz als Weg der Selbstbefreiung.* München: Wilhelm Heyne Verlag.

Thaut, M. H. (2008). *Rhythm, Music, and the Brain. Scientific Foundations and Clinical Applications.* New York: Routledge.

Vanderheiden, E., & Mayer, C.-H. (2017). An introduction to the value of shame exploring a health resource in cultural contexts. In E. Vanderheiden & C.-H. Mayer (Eds.), *The Value of Shame* (pp. 1–39). Cham: Springer International Publishing.

Van der Kolk, B. A. (1994). The body keeps the score. Memory and the evolving psychobiology of post traumatic stress. *Harvard Review of Psychiatry, 1*(5), 253–265.

Ventegodt, S., Clausen, B., Omar, H. A., & Merrick, J. (2006). Clinical holistic medicine: holistic sexology and acupressure through the vagina (hippocratic pelvis massage). *The Scientific World Journal, 6,* 2066–2079.

Wiedenhofer, S., & Koch, S. (2017). Active factors in dance/movement therapy: specifying health effects of non-goal-orientation in movement. *The Arts in Psychotherapy, 52,* 10–23.

Wolf, N. (2012). *Vagina: A New Biography*. New York: HarperCollins Publishers.

Wolynn, M. (2017). *It Didn't Start with You: How Inherited Family Trauma Shapes Who We Are and How to End the Cycle*. London: Penguin Random House.

Barbara Buch holds a Master's degree in Health Education (Faculty of Psychology, University Flensburg, Germany) and a Master's degree in Biology (Georg-August-University Göttingen, Germany). She offers workshops and courses on health-related subjects. Prior to her dedication to Health Promotion, she worked for years as a biologist, primarily in nature conservation. For many years, she lived with her family in a remote wilderness setting, where she managed an organic, permaculture farm. She focuses on further research about health, nature and traditional ways.

Chapter 30
Unemployed and High Achiever?
Working with Active Imagination
and Symbols to Transform Shame

Claude-Hélène Mayer

Abstract Work and employment are very important identity-building aspects in post-modern societies. Individuals who experience unemployment often face shame and humiliation. Particularly for high achievers, unemployment is experienced as being traumatic and the feeling of shame is multiplied. This chapter deals with the question of how the shame of unemployment can be overcome by high achievers. First, the theoretical background is described and the context of working with high achievers and unemployment with regard to a specific case is presented. Two intervention methods of self-management in therapeutic and coaching contexts are discussed: active imagination and symbol work. Both methods have been used to transform shame in unemployed high achievers successfully. They can be used as auto-didactical approaches or in therapeutical or counselling contexts.

Keywords High achiever · Unemployment · Shame · Symbol work · Active imagination

30.1 Introduction

Work and employment are very important identity-building aspects in post-modern societies. Research has shown that people who are unemployed in these socio-cultural postmodern and particularly Western societies experience shame and humiliation (Leahy, 2010).

It has been argued that employment is not supposed to be a privilege for human beings, but is rather a human right (CV Tips 2016). Individuals who are unemployed are deprived of the right to be employed and work. This often leads to reduced health and well-being and experiences of shame (Reneflot & Evensen, 2014).

C.-H. Mayer (✉)
Institut für Therapeutische Kommunikation und Sprachgebrauch, Europa Universität Viadrina,
Logenstrasse 11, 15230 Frankfurt (Oder), Germany
e-mail: claudemayer@gmx.net

Department of Management, Rhodes University, Drosdy Road, Grahamstown 6139, South Africa

© Springer Nature Switzerland AG 2019
C.-H. Mayer and E. Vanderheiden (eds.), *The Bright Side of Shame*,
https://doi.org/10.1007/978-3-030-13409-9_30

Research has shown that, particularly for high achievers,[1] unemployment is experienced as traumatic and the experience of shame is multiplied (Menkes, 2012). Men, particularly those who have been long-term unemployed, seem to be more ashamed of their unemployment than women and the short-term unemployed. Further, shame is not only caused by unemployment, but also by the financial hardships that unemployed individuals often experience (Rantakeisu, Starrin, & Hagquist, 1999). The more shaming the reaction of the environment to unemployment, the more mental disorders, deteriorating health conditions, and changes in living habits, activities and social relations are created in the unemployed individual (Rantakeisu, Starrin, & Hagquist, 1997). Shame experienced in these contexts generally supports the increase of psychological distress in situations of unemployment and confrontation with unemployment and poor social support (Reneflot & Evensen, 2014).

This chapter deals with the question of how the shame of unemployment can be overcome by high achievers. First, the theoretical background will be described, as well as possible contexts in which the methods can be effective. Second, two methods of how to work with the shame of unemployment in high achievers are described, using the specific case of a high achieving business manager who faced unemployment, shame and distress at a certain point in his life.

The first method to be described is active imagination, which was primarily invented by Carl Gustav Jung during the years 1913 to 1916 and counts as one of his major contributions to psychological science. Because active imagination often uses symbols, this chapter not only presents a specific way of conducting active imagination (there are various approaches and possibilities), but also a method of working with a symbol.

Both methods have been used to transform shame in unemployed high achievers successfully. They can be used as auto-didactical approaches or in therapeutical or counselling contexts, in combination or alone.

30.2   The Context

I have experience in working with unemployed individuals in coaching, as well as in therapy. Two typical cases are high achieving students who are long-term unemployed after having finished their university degrees, and high achieving male individuals who have dropped out of high-level management positions in business.

In this chapter, I describe working with a male unemployed high achiever (M) in a coaching context. First, I coached M when he was in a top managerial position in a German engineering organisation, preparing for expatriation work in a foreign country for three years. He contacted me again for coaching a few years later, when he had been retrenched by his organisation owing to restructuring processes. In the second part of our coaching process, M was 42 years old, a previously high achieving

---

[1] High achievers are here defined as achievers who achieve more in their work than the average person (Cambridge Dictionary, 2018).

mechanical engineer. He had worked for several years in middle and top management positions, was single and had a son of nine years from a previous partnership. The son lived mainly with the mother and visited him occasionally.

M was very frustrated when he was retrenched by his organisation; his life had changed completely. In this second phase of coaching, life appeared meaningless to him and he did not know what to do. He experienced high levels of shame at having "lost his job", and was anxious to re-establish social contacts, because he did not know what to say or talk about, since all his previous friends talked mainly about their work. We worked on overcoming the shame of unemployment and demotivation to enable him to reapply in the job market. At this point, the coaching aim was to regain inner strength and courage to return to being a high achiever in future in a new organisational position.

In this Chap. 1 describe two methods which I used for dealing with shame in the context of unemployment with M. They can be used as auto-didactical methods, but also as methods used by therapists, counsellors and coaches to conduct them with their clients. The methods can be combined or used as single intervention methods. I describe briefly the methods of active imagination and symbol work, to then provide insights into the work with the client using these methods.

30.3   Active Imagination

According to Jung, most fundamental ideas and views in life are based on experiences (Chodorow, 2006). According to Jung (1928), active imagination is a natural process for self-healing rather than a technique. It can be done through creative acts such as dancing, painting, crafts or writing, but it can also be used in relaxed states of mind and to analyse dreams. There are various forms of active imagination. Through active imagination and its different approaches, the gap between the conscious and the unconscious, between fantasy and a conscious viewpoint can be bridged.

Independent of the approach used, active imagination works with the images that arrive in the mind through the unconscious and without choosing them actively. However, the active part in active imagination starts when the individual engages with fantasies, moods and/or dreams through, for example, dialogue (Chodorow, 1997). In this manner, the individual does not work with passive fantasies, but is rather actively involved to engage with them.

By using active imagination, the focus of the individual shifts to the inner world to express the (unconscious) inner world symbolically. Through the active imagination exercise and application, the individual explores the unconsciousness and thereby gains a deeper insight into the inner world and new information about the self. Active imagination can further provide new ideas on how to address certain (life) topics, problems or how to develop oneself further. Active imagination uses different creative forms, such as visions and auditory images, relaxed state imagination, visualisation, dialogue with inner voices and/or figures, the expression of emotion through ritual and it is an inherent psychic function (Jung, 1928). The images appearing in front of the inner eye of the individual usually contain symbols and symbolic meaning. But what are symbols?

30.4 Working with Symbols to Overcome Shame in Unemployed High Achievers

Symbols are part of culture and are therefore part of historically derived and socially transmitted ideas (Wong & Tsai, 2007). In his major works, Jung (2009) defined personality and identifying symbols which are used on individual and collective levels to transform pathological practices, self-destructive attitudes, personal problems and emotions—such as shame—by recovering the general meaning in life and by reconnecting the individual with their soul. Jung's approach to healing is used by therapists and counsellors in various cultural contexts (Mayer, 2017) and can be used when working with and transforming shame in therapy, counselling and coaching with unemployed high achievers.

The advantage of working with symbols is that symbols carry unconscious content. When individuals struggle to find solutions or implement change on cognitive, affective or behavioural levels, unconscious knowledge can help them to find new options and solutions and to see beyond the immediate situation.

Shame is defined by Jung (1989) as a "soul eating emotion" (see Mayer, 2017) which is connected to other emotions often experienced and judged as negative (e.g. embarrassment or humiliation). Shame can lead to disempowerment of a person, victimisation and low self-esteem (Gamber, 2014), particularly in unemployed high achievers. To empower a person who experiences shame or has been shamed, different methods can be used to reactivate individual or collective resources to overcome and to deal with shame and the trauma of shameful experiences constructively on conscious and unconscious levels.

This chapter is concerned with Jung's work with active imaginations and symbols to overcome shame, and to self-reconcile and heal. The article presents selected applied approaches to use symbol work to constructively work with shame within a coaching context. By using active imagination and symbol work, clients are invited to create and re-create their world and their experiences by observing unconscious processes, and by engaging with meanings of symbols with which they actively identify. They thereby re-create a visual representation of the psyche's contents and widen their self-awareness, their self-actualisation and knowledge. In this process, unconscious material may reveal that which has previously been inaccessible, providing new ideas for change or movement. Through the work with symbols, clients gain new perspectives, explore deeper psychological content and relax through sensory stimulation as the healing process begins.

In the next section, I describe instances of active imagination and symbol work with M as a shamed and unemployed high achiever.

30.5 The Practical Application of Active Imagination and Symbol Work for Transforming Shame in High Achievers

When M came to his third session to work on his situation of shame and unemployment, we worked with active imagination.

For some days before the session, M had been extremely frustrated and depressed about his life situation. During an incident in which he had been questioned by a sports club friend about his unemployment, M had felt very embarrassed and ashamed of his state of being in the world without paid work and had been "swallowed up by meaninglessness and unhappiness". Since then, his reluctance to attend sports sessions—to avoid more situations like this—made him feel even worse, because his daily sports session provided his only joy during the day and with his only means of social contact.

M was still searching for a way to escape from the situation of unemployment and shame, which blocked his life energy and activities; however, he had no idea what to do in the conscious realm. I suggested doing something different during this session, and explained the process of active imagination to him. M was open to try something new. I made sure that he would stop the process actively, if something was not working positively for him during the process. He defined the aim of the process as trying to find new ideas on how to overcome his shame of the unemployment so that he could become more active again and return to his sports club sessions. The process took place in the following way.

1. In preparation for the active imagination process, I asked M to try "something new", a process I would guide him through. We defined the aim of this active imagination, regarding the topic he needed support and new information about from his unconscious.
2. M got into a conscious and aware state while relaxing in his chair.
3. I used a brief relaxation technique to prepare for the active imagination. We focused on the breathing, while relaxing the muscles, letting the body "sink" into the chair.
4. Then I asked M to stay in this state of relaxation and to wait for an image to appear in front of his inner eye, without forcing it to appear. If he wanted to, he could describe his observations out loud, or else keep them to himself, just observing in silence what was happening.
5. After a while, I asked him if he was seeing any image; he affirmed that he was. I then told him to continuing observing the image for a while. "Look at the image, explore what the image is doing, what is changing, how it unfolds in front of you, without controlling or leading it."
6. A few minutes later, I asked him to establish an active contact with the image. He could either talk to the image, ask the image questions, comment on the image or get actively involved in a dialogue. I recommended that he should wait for the image to respond without rushing forward. He should then signal me when he had finalised his interaction by lifting his left arm briefly.

7. Then I suggested he ask the image to show him a way forward, a visionary way to resolve whatever needs to be resolved and to respond to his defined aim of the session. He signalled to me again when this process was finished.
8. When the entire process of active imagination was over, we talked about the image and what had unfolded.
9. M described his interpretation of the image with regard to the session's introductory aim.

M said afterwards that he had enjoyed the process and that he felt free to just wait for any image to arrive for him. He felt safe. The image that appeared to him was a diamond which was yellow-orange in colour. He looked at it from all sides. It was shiny and bright and somehow a source of light.

He explained that his active interaction with the diamond was about telling the diamond that it was just beautiful as it was. He had felt that the diamond was just "smiling" at him. Neither M nor the diamond had something to say, M explained; it was just a "wonderful state of being".

With regard to the visionary way forward, M described how the diamond had started to jump and to turn, to move forward and to even increase its brightness.

Then, we worked on the transfer of this image and its message for M's situation and real life scenario. M interpreted the diamond as being his inner core, his soul, his inner being that had such a strong brightness within itself that nothing else counted as much as to trust his core, his inner strength and "diamond". Focusing on building his self-esteem in his inner being rather than on his work was the core message for M in this session, because he could recognise its beauty within himself. Holding such a strong and positive view of his inner being, M highlighted, was to prepare him with increased strength for any further attacks of shaming. In future, he said, he would focus more upon his inner being and his inner beauty than on employment as the main contributer to building self esteem.

30.6   The Symbol of the Diamond

During the next session, I decided to explore the symbol of the diamond with M further and its (un-)conscious meaning for him. We worked on the following questions:

1. Last week the image of the diamond appeared during our session and we have started to exploring it. What does the diamond symbolise in your opinion for you personally and with regard to the collective unconscious? Did the meaning change for you during the last week? Could you explore the symbol even more or was it not important anymore after you left the session?
2. What is the transformational power of the symbol for you when you think of your daily life? How do you use the power of the diamond? How could you expand the positive and constructive influence?
3. How does the diamond speak to you as a high achiever? What does it tell you?

4. How do you anchor this transformational power of the diamond in the context of unemployment and shame? How do you make sure that you can access this power in challenging situations?
5. How exactly can you use the diamond to transform shame and other negatively experienced emotions, such as anxiety (e.g. fear of failure, of unsupportive social contact), depression and frustration?
6. How does the diamond guide you in terms of your future?

During this session, M particularly worked with the meaning of the diamond, his personal meanings (e.g. beauty, elegance, exclusiveness) and the collective meanings (purity, undestructability, faithfulness, love, richness of self) with regard to his situation. Between the previous session and this session, M had explored the meaning of the diamond for himself—mainly through the internet—in the context of where this kind of diamond originates (worldwide only in South Africa and Australia). He was surprised about this diamond's origin, since he had lived and worked successfully and happily in South Africa for three years as an expat, and had always dreamed of living and working in Australia. The symbol of this specific yellow-orange diamond gave him faith and hope and a vision to start anew in another country (preferably Australia). He had in the meantime bought himself a stone (looking like a diamond) in the intense yellow-orange colour to remind him of the image of the bright diamond and the energy he associated with it. He showed me the "diamond" which he was now carrying in his purse and he told me that he wanted to sit down and reflect on a daily basis for five minutes, diving into the energy of this diamond. He said he still wanted to further explore the colours of yellow and orange and their resonance with his energy body (aura). M appeared to be lively, with regained energy and a new vision for himself. He did not feel ashamed of himself and his unemployment any longer and managed to look ahead.

After this session, we worked another five sessions together, often referring back to the symbol of the yellow-orange diamond. He had in the meanwhile found pictures of diamonds on the internet, and printed them to hang in his living room, while working on managing depression and frustration. These emotions reoccurred at times during the process of inner healing. M started to apply for positions internationally and eventually started to work for a French-Canadian company, again as a high achiever.

30.7 Conclusion

High achieving individuals who experience unemployment situations often experience shame and a loss of mental health and well-being. The method of active imagination and the work with symbols can help individuals to overcome toxic emotions such as shame, and turn them into healthy emotions which become integrated parts of the self, through acknowledging and reconciling with them.

References

Cambridge Dictionary (2018). *High Achievers. Definition.* Retrieved from https://dictionary. cambridge.org/dictionary/english/high-achiever.
Chodorow, J. (1997). *Jung on active imagination.* Princeton, NJ: Princeton University Press.
Chodorow, J. (2006). Active imagination. In R. K. Papadopouluos (Ed.), *The handbook of Jungian psychology. Theory, practice and applications* (pp. 215–240). London: Routledge.
CV Tips (2016). *The so-called shame of unemployment.* Retrieved from http://www.cvtips.com/ leaving-a-job/the-so-called-shame-of-unemployment.html.
Gamber, P. (2014). *Familientherapie für Dummies.* Weinheim: WILEY-VCH Verlag Gmbh.
Jung, C. G. (1928). The technique of differentiation between the ego and the figures of the unconscious. In *Collective works*, vol. 7, pp. 341–373. Princeton, NJ: Princeton University Press.
Jung, C. G. (1989). *Nietzsches Zarathustra:* Notes of the Seminar given in 1934–1939 by C. G. Jung. London: Routledge.
Jung, C. G. (2009). *The Red Book.* Liber Novus: A reader's edition. Edited and with an introduction by Sonu Shamdasani. London: W.W. Norton.
Leahly, R. L. (2010). The shame of unemployment. *Psychology Today.* https://www. psychologytoday.com/blog/anxiety-files/201007/the-shame-unemployment.
Mayer, C.-H. (2017). Shame - "A soul feeding emotion": Archetypal work and the transformation of the shadow of shame in a group development process. In E. Vanderheiden & C.-H. Mayer (Eds.), *The value of shame - Exploring a health resource in cultural contexts* (pp. 277–302). Cham: Springer.
Menkes, J. (2012). Tackling the trauma of unemployment. *Harvard Business Review*, March 27, 2012. https://hbr.org/2012/03/tackling-the-trauma-of-unemplo.
Rantakeisu, U., Starrin, B., & Hagquist, C. (1997). Unemployment, shame and ill-health - an exploratory study. *International Journal of Social Welfare, 6*(1), 13–23.
Rantakeisu, U., Starrin, B., & Hagquist, C. (1999). Financial hardship and shame: A tentative model.
Reneflot, A., & Evensen, M. (2014). Unemployment and psychological distress among young adults in the Nordic countries: A review of the literature. *International Journal of Social Welfare, 23,* 3–13.
Wong, Y., & Tsai, J. L. (2007). Cultural models of shame and guilt. In J. Tracy, R. Robins, & J. Tangney (Eds.), *Handbook of self-conscious emotions.* New York: Guildford.

Claude-Hélène Mayer (Dr. habil., PhD, PhD) is a Professor in Industrial and Organisational Psychology at the Department of Industrial Psychology and People Management at the University of Johannesburg, an Adjunct Professor at the Europa Universität Viadrina in Frankfurt (Oder), Germany and a Senior Research Associate in the Department of Management at Rhodes University, Grahamstown, South Africa. She holds a Ph.D. in psychology (University of Pretoria, South Africa), a Ph.D. in management (Rhodes University, South Africa), a Doctorate in political sciences (Georg-August-Universität, Göttingen, Germany), and a Habilitation with a Venia Legendi (Europa Universität Viadrina, Germany) in psychology with focus on work, organizational, and cultural psychology. She has published numerous monographs, edited text books, accredited journal article, and special issues on transcultural mental health, salutogenesis and sense of coherence, shame, transcultural conflict management and mediation, women in leadership in culturally diverse work contexts, constellation work, coaching, and psychobiography.

Chapter 31
Shame and Forgiveness in Therapy and Coaching

Maike Baumann and Anke Handrock

Abstract Shame and guilt are two emotions most people find very hard to endure. In order to avoid the feeling of shame, behaviors such as aggressive attacks or withdrawal from social relationships are common strategies. Such reactions can be socially impairing when they are shown on a regular basis or when they persist over a long period of time. They may even lead to antisocial behavior, social isolation or mental illness. In the secure environment of coaching sessions, counseling or therapy, it is possible to enable the client to find ways to disclose feelings of shame and guilt and to guide the client through a process of forgiving themselves or their offenders. Hence, it is possible to help the client to modify their perception of reality from focused upon past offenses to a hopeful, goal-oriented and meaningful future perspective. This chapter highlights the general process of a non-religious approach to forgiveness and offers practical exercises drawing on scientific results from, e.g., Schema Therapy, Positive Psychology and Imaginative Therapy.

Keywords Forgiveness · Shame · Coaching · Functional self · Therapy

31.1 Introduction

This chapter concentrates on the application of a non-religious approach to forgiveness and self-forgiveness in coaching and therapy, adapted to scenarios in which the experience of a shameful situation has led a client to repeated or continuous feelings of severe shame. The experience of shame may lead to unwanted psychological consequences, even to mental illness (for a detailed overview see Sinha, 2017).

M. Baumann (✉)
Institut für Lebensgestaltung-Ethik-Religionskunde, University of Potsdam, Am Neuen Palais 10, 14469 Potsdam, Germany
e-mail: mbaumann@uni-potsdam.de

A. Handrock
Steinbeis-Transfer-Institut Positive Psychologie und Prävention, at the Steinbeis Hochschule, 13467 Berlin, Germany
e-mail: info@handrock.de

© Springer Nature Switzerland AG 2019
C.-H. Mayer and E. Vanderheiden (eds.), *The Bright Side of Shame*,
https://doi.org/10.1007/978-3-030-13409-9_31

In the course of this chapter, we will briefly discuss the conditions under which forgiveness after experiences of shame might be a promising intervention in coaching or therapeutic contexts. We offer some distinguishing features between coaching and therapy. Furthermore, we provide directions for a practical implementation of our approach and present general constraints.

In this chapter, we use the term "client" to indicate a person wanting assistance from a coach to achieve a certain outcome. The term "patient" is used, when a client's psychological condition is too severe to be assisted by a coach only. For better readability, we use the term "client" unless the differentiation is of importance to the case. Note also that wc use the male singular pronoun throughout. This is for readability only and is of course intended to include all other genders as well.

31.1.1 Shame in the Context of Forgiveness

Self-critical emotions such as shame are experienced as dysphoric and aversive mental states and are therefore, if possible, avoided altogether.

Seen from an evolutionary perspective (Elison, 2019), self-critical emotions help to ensure the stability of social groups and to prevent group-internal conflicts and loss of resources due to, e.g., injuries resulting from fights for dominance. Well-structured social groups induce well-defined liabilities that are stable across time. Such groups show lower levels of social conflict and more success under selective pressure than heterogeneous groups without a reliable internal structure. The internalization of group-internal rules and values occurs during the process of socialization and is thus culture-specific and dependent on the individual's social role and position. Social rules and values that are consequently applied by attachment figures are integrated into the child's developing self-concept and persist on to adult-age (Coelho, Castilho, & Pinto-Gouveia, 2010). This kind of social information adds to a person's value structure in later life and may be seen as a constituent part of a person's identity (Berkman, Livingston, & Kahn, 2017; Goff & Goddard, 1999; Hitlin, 2003; Pinto-Gouveia & Matos, 2010). Furthermore, the internalized rules and values contribute to implicit basic beliefs and do feel ego-syntonic. This concerns a person's basic assumptions about themselves, the world in general, human relationships and general interaction processes.

By continuous self-monitoring it becomes apparent that the crossing of ego-syntonic rules, produces a nominal-actual value difference that is emotionally answered by feelings of guilt, shame or embarrassment. In order to experience shame, the person in question needs to feel responsible and to perceive the nominal-actual value difference between his behavior and his internalized self-concept (Roos, 2000).

In social groups, the feeling of shame functions as self-punishment, this way saving cognitive resources of other group members: The existence of shame ensures that group members rarely need to actively enforce group-internal rules on other adults.

Self-defining Shame

For our current purpose we distinguish between two distinct types of severe shame: self-defining and self-threatening shame. We do not, however, claim that these two types cover the full range of all possible dynamics. Rather, we will focus on those aspects of the emotion of shame that are directly relevant to the forgiveness interventions presented in this chapter.

The first type of severe shame presented here is, in our opinion, to be handled by a therapist only. If a patient attributes the cause of his shame to stable and invariable personal qualities (such as sex, being born in a certain caste, having a certain color of skin, or carrying some handicap), he perceives himself as defective and inferior. In this case, the character of these qualities lies within his socialization when these qualities were defined for him by relevant attachment figures as a taint. The feelings of defectiveness/shame have become part of the person's self-concept (e.g. Carvalho, Dinis, Pinto-Gouveia, & Estanqueiro, 2013; Pinto-Gouveia & Matos, 2010; Young, 1994; Young, Klosko, & Weishaar, 2003). For affected individuals the resulting experience of general deficiency becomes omnipresent and seems to be inevitable. They usually do not attribute their uncomfortable feelings to an identifiable human originator, because their causation happened early during childhood-socialization, and the emotion therefore feels ego-syntonic. We call this first type of shame "self-defining shame", because the felt deficiency and the resulting shame is an integral part of the individual's basic assumptions on himself.

Self-threatening Shame and the Functional Self

The second type of shame we consider is "self-threatening shame." In order to better understand the notion of "self" that we assume, it is necessary to introduce a working definition of a so-called "functional self".

We characterize it as follows: A person has developed a functional self, if he

- has developed a mainly benevolent and realistic set of basic assumptions about himself, the world, other people and his interactive options in the world;
- maintains a benevolent inner monologue in most situations and executes appropriate self-compassion and self-care;
- feels coherent with himself across time and in quality, which is consciously accessible in a single, integrative story of his life;
- follows realistically set, achievable and meaningful goals in a self-determined manner and is able to shift his inner time perspective at will to past, present and future, as well as to the interlaced conceptional qualities of a reality-oriented view vs. a perspective of potentiality and the emotional/evaluative vs. cognitive/descriptive perspective;
- can stand existing differences between his functional self and his ideal self and has a realistic view of his developmental options enabling him to choose realistic and achievable goals;
- has developed a good psycho-social integration and stability, adequate emotional regulatory strategies, adequate emotional self-efficacy and a certain resilience,

enabling him to successfully handle stress and common discrepancies to his basic assumptions (i.e., failure, criticism or interpersonal assaults).

The emotional quality of a functional self can be regarded as a feeling of oneness, of comfort with oneself, a certain inner quiescence and a feeling of purpose, rightfulness and inner coherence as well as feelings of care and friendliness towards oneself. We propose the functional self as a realistically reachable mental and emotional condition, which enables personal growth and flourishing. We understand the functional self as a *holistic* set of relatively stable and mostly functional, value-oriented basic beliefs.

Therefor the concept of a functional self is different in quality to the concept of health, as well as to the concept of a "fully functioning person" (Rogers, 1963) and also from the schematherapeutic terminus of the healthy adult mode (Young et al., 2003).

When a person has been given the chance to build a functional self, self-critical emotions will occur only as a reaction to considerable threats to that functional self and are usually experienced over (limited) periods of time, starting with a clear onset and usually finishing with a clear ending. So there is no constant feeling of defectiveness or fundamental insufficiency.

In cases of such "self-threatening shame", the person has developed a functional self *before* the shame-provoking event. On this generally stable foundation, the functional self may get under pressure and may even get shattered by shameful events of traumatic quality (Lee, Scragg, & Turner, 2001; Wilson, Droždek, & Turkovic, 2006). Nevertheless, the former experience of a functional self can be used as an emotional reference point and as a process-goal in therapy and coaching.

The functional self as proposed here draws on a number of concepts from self-psychology, research on personality and well-being. Discussing these concepts unfortunately goes well beyond the scope of this chapter.

31.2   Contextual Descriptions—Coaching versus Therapy

In order to enable practitioners to differentiate a coaching context from a therapeutic context and to indicate the different mandates as well as the transition from one context to the other, we present our way of classification below.

We understand coaching as a professional context in which a client actively engages a coach to assist him to meet a well-defined challenge. A client is in general able to cope with his life's challenges without assistance. He has developed an adequate functional self and is able to access his resources. Consequently, he can handle normal degrees of failure, legitimate complaints, feedback and criticism as well as minor to moderate interpersonal assaults. The client may show minor to moderate noticeable psychological problems, but his condition does not qualify to be classified as mental illness. The coach serves as facilitator. He supports the client in his process and takes the role of a mentor or assistant.

In therapy, we meet patients who qualify as mentally ill. In contrast to a client, we cannot expect a patient to exactly know what he wants to achieve. More often than not, patients can only articulate what they do not want. Consequently, a therapist has a more active role than a coach, taking control of the patient's process if necessary. Under the condition of mental illness, it is part of the therapeutic work to uncover the functionality of the patient's self and possibly to assist the patient to build a functional self - anew, or even for the first time.

31.3   Applicability of Forgiveness to Experiences of Shame

Many definitions have been offered on forgiveness (cf. Fernández-Capo, Recoder Fernández, Gámiz Sanfeliu, Gómez Benito, & Worthington, 2017; McCullough, Pargament, & Thoresen, 2000; Worthington, 2003; Worthington & Scherer, 2004). For the purpose of this chapter, we understand forgiveness as an intrapersonal emotional and cognitive process that changes the motivation of the forgiving person towards the offender(s), reduces feelings of anger and grudge, enables well-being and releases the former victim and the former culprit from these particular social roles.

For use in therapy and coaching, we consider only non-religious forms of forgiveness as appropriate.

Forgiveness is a process usually applied to handle guilt. As this chapter deals with shame, we need to address the question of how forgiveness can be applied to problematic experiences of shame.

In forgiveness processes following shameful events, it is possible to convert experiences of shame into anger at the causal agent of the harm and, as an effect, to produce an ascription of guilt to the offender. During the act of forgiveness, the victim then releases the offender from the ascribed guilt, while at the same time releasing himself from the past-centered social role of being a victim. Via the cognitive and emotional rejection of being a victim, the personal narrative of the humiliated person changes and time that was previously spent on rumination is available to be used freely. In our experience, the building up of an attractive and meaningful goal to be approached after having freed oneself from the victim-role, facilitates the process. A well-defined goal that is relevant to the person's identity, leads to a kind of double-bind that can be used in favor of the process of forgiveness: preserving the anger would mean to keep the role of the victim and to further give up precious lifetime to rumination and grudge. In making this negative circle explicit, the offended party usually decides immediately to move on with their lives towards the attractive meaningful goal, even if this does require forgiving the offender.

The intensity of felt shame can vary considerably. Under certain circumstances, shameful situations are memorized with traumatic quality, especially when caused by attachment figures (Coelho et al., 2010; Matos & Pinto-Gouveia, 2010).

Table 31.1 Comparison of forgiveness processes according to Enright and Worthington (adapted from Handrock & Baumann, 2017)

Process model of Enright	REACH-model of Worthington
Uncovering phase: getting in touch with the pain and exploring experienced injustice	R = Recall the hurt (differently to feelings of victimization or indulging in blame)
Decision phase: exploring the idea of forgiveness, cognitively deciding to forgive	
Work phase: seeing the offender with new eyes, trying to understand the offender from his context (reframing)	E = Emotionally replace negative unforgiving emotions with positive other-oriented emotions towards the offender; develop an understanding of the offender
Outcome phase: giving the gift of forgiveness to the offender, experiencing healing	A = Altruistic giving; give the altruistic gift of forgiveness to the offender
Discover unexpected positive secondary effects, understand the own suffering differently	
	C = Commit to the forgiveness
	H = Hold on to forgiveness through a series of maintenance-enhancing exercises

We see it as part of a coach's responsibility to evaluate whether the client's experience of shame can be handled within the setting of a coaching or is to be seen as a pathological condition.

The approach we offer (cf. Handrock & Baumann, 2017) is partly based on the work on processes of forgiveness by Worthington (2005) and Enright (2006). For a practice-oriented comparison of the approaches of Worthington and Enright, see Table 31.1.

We expand the general process of forgiveness by including interventions based on concepts from schematherapy adapted to coaching contexts and for short term therapy (Handrock, Zahn, & Baumann, 2016). In addition, we include the activation and building-up of personal resources and offer trauma therapeutic interventions and grief counseling if necessary. Furthermore, we provide assistance with the reorientation of the client's time perspective towards a meaningful future perspective. For a flow chart-overview of our approach with a focus on shame see Fig. 31.1.

31.4   Applications

The steps we describe in this section are adapted to cases where a client feels continuously ashamed or feels limited due to periods of intense shame. Often such shame-eliciting situations can be characterized as strongly externally influenced, such as sexual assault, being unwillingly exposed, having been exploited in some way, but can also include instances such as failure to assist a person in danger.

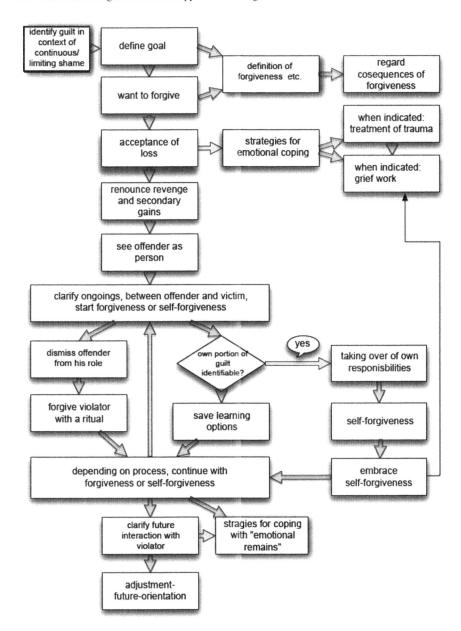

Fig. 31.1 Overview of an exemplary process of forgiveness/self-forgiveness (cf. Handrock & Baumann, 2017) adapted for intervention with clients who experience continuous/limiting severe shame

We confine ourselves in this chapter to present only some exemplary techniques we developed for our work with clients on forgiveness. For an in-depth discussion of the practical applications of our approach see Handrock and Baumann (2017).

At the beginning of the process, it is necessary to help the client to gain a general understanding of the situation(s) leading to his current feelings of shame. As shame feels extremely uncomfortable, clients have typically not retrospectively analyzed the situational parameters in depth as it feels much more comfortable to avoid the memories altogether. Whenever the memories are triggered, clients re-experience the shame and their attention is caught by the necessity to regulate the aversive emotion and usually again they are unable to analyze the situation. In order to enable clients to develop an understanding of the situational facts and to adequately assign responsibilities of action, we offer a set of basic questions.

In case the client feels too uncomfortable to talk directly about the incident, it is possible to offer a technique to keep an emotional distance. There are different ways to achieve such an emotional distance. Here we recommend the bystander-technique (see Box 31.1).

Box 31.1 Bystander-Technique: Keeping the Emotional Distance

Invite the client to imagine being a TV correspondent, witnessing the shameful incident and commenting on it. To better distinguish between the two different perceptual positions (the correspondent-client vs. the client's younger self in the action scene) it is advisable to mark different positions on the floor with colored pieces of paper for the "correspondent's space" and "the scene of action". This enables coach and client together to move to the correspondent's space and comment on the action scene from a safe distance. The physical distance, the boundaries of the pieces of paper on the floor and the different roles ascribed help the client to keep the emotional distance. The coach/therapist carefully monitors the client's speech and takes care that in the correspondent's space it is always spoken from an observer's point of view, detached from the action at the scene. This involves the client speaking about his younger self as a third party. Monitoring the client's use of third-party language is the coach's responsibility. Some clients also find holding a symbolic microphone or camera helpful. Once the defined space on the floor is left and the papers have been collected, props should be put aside and speech can be used normally.

Questions to offer to the client/correspondent include the following:

- Who is doing what to whom?
- Who has been hurt, either morally, or psychologically, or physically; or who has been killed?
- What consequences, defects or disabilities did result in the short and long term?
- What has been broken or ruined?
- Was the damage an irreplaceable loss, or was it reparable?

- What exactly did hurt emotionally or felt emotionally uncomfortable and what exact quality of feeling did this have?
- Which expectations and values were hurt?
- What was the offender's attitude (action, lack of action, acquiescence, intent or malice)?

> **Caution** We strongly appeal to coaches to stop the questioning immediately, if clients show signs of a trauma reaction during the questioning (e.g., signs of dissociation). In such case the client should be emotionally distracted to break dissociative tendencies (for instance, by a series of gymnastic exercises) and he should be redirected to a therapist.

These questions will be picked up again later during the process. The goal at this first stage is to elicit an ascription of guilt to different acting parties during the original shame-triggering situation. It is not advisable to explore the situation to its full extent. As soon as the client starts to realize responsible actions of different parties in the situation and starts to express anger and ascriptions of guilt, the questioning should cease. His answers will help him to understand and to differentiate his own and other's share in the incident. Usually this first round of questioning ends with the client's clear ascription of certain amounts of guilt accompanied by anger at an offender and possibly at himself.

In case the client starts to express anger at his younger self for having himself landed in the situation, the client's ascription of responsibility that causes the anger is in most cases based on different types of dysfunctional chains of thought. E.g., clients may apply the knowledge they gathered while answering the above questions to retrospectively ascribe stupidity or blindness to their younger selves for not anticipating what was in stall for them at a point of time when the younger self could still have fled the situation. In order to stop this verbal self-harm we recommend to guide the client through a reality check, gathering the facts accessible to the younger self at that time and to evaluate the decisions they (their younger selves) made based on these facts. In most cases, clients realize quickly that the behavior they chose at that time was indeed rational and understandable, considering the available facts.

If the client does bear part of the responsibility for the shameful experience, an additional process of self-forgiveness can be offered, following the same basic procedure as with interpersonal forgiveness.

Religious clients sometimes feel the urge to be spiritually forgiven before they feel able to actively forgive anyone. In such cases, the sessions on forgiveness should pause until the religious forgiveness has been reached, which happens solely in the responsibility of the religious denomination the patient belongs to. Once the client either feels forgiven, or realizes that he did not carry relevant responsibility for the shameful act at all, he often begins to feel sadness as well as compassion with his younger self. At the latest at that point, we experience that clients start to express anger towards the offender.

Sometimes no offender can be named as purely situational factors shaped the experience, in such cases forgiveness cannot be applied as a therapeutic tool. Instead, for most clients the analysis itself already works as reframing. They re-interpret the incident as an accident, In consequence the shame either vanishes or is replaced by a fading sense of embarrassment. Additionally, clients start to perceive the losses they suffered. Some clients start to feel sadness and begin to grieve (for example, over "lost" life-time, social relationships they could not stand being in, etc.). Elaborating further on therapeutic options to handle grief in a beneficial way unfortunately goes beyond the scope of this chapter.

The homework to write a "letter of rage" or a "bill of indictment" directed at the offender might be given to clients at this stage. The letter should be written in one go. The intention of this task is to externalize the rage (cf. Enright, 2006; Pennebaker, 1993, 1997). Clients should not give or send the letter to anyone, but keep it safe until a later stage during the process of forgiveness. In case writing the anger down intensifies the rage and infuriates the client, they should stop and not complete the writing task at that point in time.

Some clients are so intimidated by the offender that they do not dare to write down their anger. It can be a helpful suggestion for such clients to write down instead what their best friend would write in solidarity with them, if that friend was told the offender's deeds.

31.4.1 Deciding to Forgive

As a next step, the concept of forgiveness is introduced to the client. Sometimes clients refuse to consider forgiveness, especially when the ascription of guilt and the feeling of anger have only just been discovered "underneath" heavy shame. We find it helpful to introduce the concept of forgiveness anyway. Merely hearing about the option of a structured process of forgiveness seems to reduce the danger of clients feeling stuck in their feelings of anger and guilt. Here is a summary of the notion of forgiveness elaborated on above:

- No one can be forced to forgive, nor can anyone demand to be forgiven. Forgiveness is an act of a person's own free will.
- Forgiveness does not minimize the offending incident. It is neither forgetting, nor denying, nor the suppression of the offense. It is not meant to trivialize injuries or losses and inflicted pains. Forgiveness implies to be fully aware of all negative consequences of an offense, to acknowledge them and still to decide to forgive.
- Forgiveness is not forgetting: forgiveness is learning from the offense and discovering options of development and posttraumatic growth.
- Forgiveness is not making up with someone. This misconception corresponds to a common mix-up of forgiveness and reconciliation. A reconciliation process demands all parties to engage in a social exchange with the intention to re-establish a stable social bond after the previous social bond has been culpably shattered

(Schlenke, 2005). Hence, reconciliation necessarily needs the commitment and contribution of all parties involved in previously inflicted damage. This is different from forgiveness, which can be undertaken without the other party even knowing. Reconciliation and forgiveness can occur together, but this need not be the case.

- Forgiveness does not mean to abandon any rightful claims or to leave a legal position. Forgiving includes seeing the violator as a person again instead of reducing him to the offense. Giving up a rightful claim in consequence to the offense could do additional harm to the violated party and might consequently destabilize the system again.
- Forgiveness is not moral superiority. Regaining personal freedom and experiencing personal growth due to forgiveness is not an exceptional moral accomplishment. It also does not mean to use excuses for the violator ("he didn't learn it any better…"), as this would only result in feeling superior to the violator, but would not lift the social roles of offender and victim.

After getting to know the concept of forgiveness, the client might be curious to explore this emotional coping strategy further. Thus the phase of defining the client's goal for the possible process of forgiveness begins: First, the client reflects upon the question whether there is something to be forgiven at all. Once he answers this question in the affirmative, possible gains of forgiveness compared to the client's current situation are discussed. In order to provide the client with an emotional reference of how it would feel to have forgiven and of what to gain from the process, we make use of an adapted miracle question (cf. de Shazer, 1994; Daimler, Sparrer, & Varga von Kibéd, 2013). In addition, we utilize several reflexive future-oriented questions in order to have the client explore the connection between past orientation and rumination on the offense, anger and wishes of revenge in comparison to a concentration on future-oriented meaningful and therefore emotionally attractive goals (cf. Peterson, Park, & Seligman, 2005). Accompanying the development of a positive emotional attraction, the reflexive future-oriented questions enable the client to imagine himself having accomplished forgiveness already, thereby suggesting forgiveness as a realistic behavioral option. At this stage it is important to validate the client's doubts on his capability to forgive and to normalize such doubts as a typical step during forgiveness. This part of the process is completed by the client's explicit decision of wanting to forgive. In our opinion, the decision is best fixed in the form of a written and signed contract the client enters with himself (see Box 31.2).

Box 31.2 How to Formulate a Forgiveness-contract

A forgiveness-contract puts down the clients goals:
- to free himself from grudge and wishes to take revenge,
- to direct his life towards values he deems important,
- to experience more and more positive emotions in life, build good and stable relationships and
- to more and more take care of his health.

> Finally, the client writes down as a logical consequence of the above points to want to forgive and signs the contract.

Written and signed contracts, especially of self-chosen goals, add to the emotionally felt clarity of decisions, prompt the feeling of responsibility and lead to more consistent fulfillment. Additionally, forgiveness-contracts serve as an easily accessible resource during the following steps of the forgiveness process as well as for possible residual negative emotions.

31.4.2 Acceptance of Losses and Pain in its Entirety

During the following stage, clients work on understanding and accepting the full extent of their losses as a result of the original offense. The emotional-distance technique is used again and the questions from the beginning are asked again as well. However, this time all questions and lines of thought are followed on to the end in order to fully acknowledge the loss and all additional consequences. The full realization of the harm inspires in many clients a considerable aversion to "let the creep off the hook" by presenting the offender with the undeserved gift of the client's forgiveness. Here we validate the client's aversion by offering a systematic discussion of the costs and benefits of forgiving, compared to the costs and benefits of not-forgiving. We cover this in a semi-structured interview on possible consequences of forgiveness in the context of the client's momentary situation in life, their future hopes, the anticipated reactions of their friends, family members and others in their social circle as well as considering possible consequences for their own behavioral routines.

Schematherapeutic interventions

Next we introduce the concepts of the "fit adult" and the "sad/hurt inner child", which are adaptations from the schema mode model of Jeffrey Young (Young et al., 2003) that we adapted for use in coaching contexts (Handrock et al., 2016).

Using only these two slightly overgeneralized modes during a process of forgiveness, relieves the coach from introducing the entire schema-model while still enabling him to use the option of working with different "parts" of the client by using different spaces in the room (such as different chairs or with pieces of paper on the floor).

If the process of forgiveness succeeds a schematherapy it is possible to reduce the schema-mode model the patient already knows to the "fit adult" and the "sad/hurt inner child" to keep the process economical. The "fit adult" is introduced as the client's inner part being able to reason logically and wanting to reach forgiveness. The sad/hurt child (or "sad/hurt younger self") is introduced as the part feeling the emotions. This separation opens up a range of options, for example, to guide an imagination where the client takes the position of the fit adult and takes care of the hurt child. Such interventions may serve different purposes. For one, the client identifies himself with being (at least partly) someone capable to handle the emotional impact of the offense. Secondly, the emotions expressed by the "hurt child" are being validated adequately by the client himself without the danger of emotional flooding. The "hurt child" may be interpreted as a technique for emotional distance-keeping, as emotional externalization technique and as an intervention in self-compassion all in one.

At this stage it might become necessary to include grief work and it is to be expected that clients re-experience a want to revenge themselves. Here the forgiveness-contract can serve as a resource to keep the goal of an emotionally free life with a variety of positive developmental options. Furthermore, occasional wishes of revenge can be framed by the coach as expectable and usually only temporarily present. This part of the process is finished when the client reaches the definite decision to forgive in full cognitive and emotional knowledge of the harm done.

31.4.3   Forgiveness

The next step is to develop an understanding of the offender. We offer either a cognitive-based or an emotion-focussed approach to this task. We experience it most effective to begin with the cognitive process and then to add the emotion-focussed work. As the latter can be experienced as quite intense, the client should decide freely whether he feels confident to explore the emotional side any further.

During the cognitive work, the coach discusses with the client under which circumstances a person might behave in the way the offender did. It is helpful to have additional information on the offender's personal and social circumstances. Where such information is unavailable, the coach and the client together construct a logical, feasible and coherent narrative of the offender's behavior. If the client feels confident to explore the offender's behavior from an emotional perspective as well, we offer a technique working with different perceptual positions (see Box 31.3).

Box 31.3 Creating an Emotion-focussed Understanding of the Offender Using Perceptual Positions

The client is instructed to write on three differently colored pieces of paper the following terms: "victim", "offender", "camera". Then he positions the papers on the floor and the coach accompanies him to the camera position.

The client steps on the paper and imagines being a cameraman witnessing the scene. The coach asks him to describe the offender's and the victim's actions, while looking at the imaginary scene.

Next, the client is asked to take the offender's position on the floor and to describe the incident as fully and completely as possible from the offender's point of view.

The narrative from the cognitive work done previously should then be integrated in order to articulate the offender's thoughts consistent with the narrative. The coach is responsible for monitoring the client's use of language and to make sure he speaks from the first-person perspective of the offender. If necessary, the coach reformulates the client's sentences using an I-perspective of the offender. Additionally, the coach assists the client in his exploration with questions.

In most cases, it is not necessary to explore the victim's position any further. The client switches several times between the camera and offender's position until he understands the purpose and the line of action chosen by the offender. Note, however, that some clients feel uncomfortable when other persons touch or step on "their psycho-geography" on the floor. This should be kept in mind when switching between the different areas. In the end it is also advisable to let the client collect the pieces of paper from the floor.

After having reached a new understanding of the offender, the client formulates a bill of indictment. When this step has happened earlier, the client reviews his first version. Then he confronts the offender in an imaginary way with these complaints and tells him that he will forgive him now even though the offender never earned such a gift as the client's forgiveness and that the offender cannot do anything to stop the client in doing so. For this work, we again use papers on the floor to mark the client's and the offender's positions during the imaginary confrontation. Finally, the client destroys the bill of indictment and crosses out the term "offender" on the paper on the floor. The client then explores the imaginary reactions of the former offender, now called violator for better distinction. As a last step during this stage, the client gets the homework to write a certificate of forgiveness. He should design the certificate as beautifully and carefully as possible. The certificate serves as second resource to enforce the effectiveness of the process. These last steps of actually forgiving the offender can be very emotional and should be executed without time pressure. For details on questions to ask during these steps and on the exact process of confronting the offender, see Handrock and Baumann (2017). In case there have been several offenders or self-forgiveness is necessary in addition, the general process of forgiveness can be reentered and passed through again.

After finishing the entire process we add some interventions facilitating personal growth and improved coping with interpersonal stress such as the self-compassion mantra (Neff, 2012) and the meditation of loving kindness (Germer, 2012) (Gilbert, Oosthuizen and Vanderheiden, in this book). We then have the client decide on how he wants to arrange his future interaction with the violator, exploring together whether he sees an option for any contact at all, no contact at all, or even for a process of reconciliation. Here, the coach should carefully monitor the client's wishes for social harmony and point out possible dangers concerning the client's ideas of further interaction with the violator.

31.5   Conclusion and Recommendation

The process presented, requires the professional handling of intense feelings, possibly including trauma, intense grief and rage. We strongly recommend working with the approach, only when a coach/therapist is familiar and comfortable in handling such intense feelings of a client with high flexibility. The initial situation a client describes might be highly complex. In consequence it may be necessary to jump back and forth between parts of the process, depending on the client's needs. In order to gain this flexibility, we recommend to collect personal experience with the process in advance to working with clients. We find the success and the lastingness of the positive effects of the presented approach in clinical work and coaching very promising. In our experience this approach to therapeutic forgiveness is a powerful way of inducing posttraumatic growth in a structured way, helping clients to exit brooding-loops and to get free of inadequate feelings of shame.

References

Berkman, E., Livingston, J., & Kahn, L. E. (2017). Finding the "self" in self-regulation: the identity-value model. *Psychological Inquiry, 28*(2–3), 77–98. https://doi.org/10.1080/1047840X.2017.1323463.

Carvalho, S., Dinis, A., Pinto-Gouveia, J., & Estanqueiro, C. (2013). Memories of shame experiences with others and depression symptoms: The mediating role of experiential avoidance. *Clinical Psychology & Psychotherapy, 22*(1), 32–44. https://doi.org/10.1002/cpp.1862.

Coelho, S. A., Castilho, P., & Pinto-Gouveia, J. (2010). Recordação de experiências de ameaça e subordina-ção na infância, auto-criticismo, vergonha e submis-são: a sua contribuição para a depressão em estudan-tes universitários. *Psychologica, 52*(2), 449–474.

Daimler, R., Sparrer, I., & Varga von Kibéd, M. (2013). *Basics der systemischen Strukturaufstellungen. Eine Anleitung für Einsteiger und Fortgeschrittene.* München: Kösel Verlag.

de Shazer, S. (1994). Words were originally magic. New York: W W Norton & Co.

Elison, G. (2019). Interpreting instances of shame from an evolutionary perspective: The pain analogy. In E. Vanderheiden & C.-H. Mayer (Eds.), *The bright side of shame. Transforming and growing through practical applications in cultural contexts* (pp. 395–411). Springer International (Positive Psychology).

Enright, R. D. (2006). *Vergebung als Chance: Neuen Mut fürs Leben finden.* Bern: Verlag Hans Huber.

Fernández-Capo, M., Recoder Fernández, S., Gámiz Sanfeliu, M., Gómez Benito, J., & Worthington, E. L., Jr. (2017). Measuring forgiveness. A systematic review. *European Psychologist, 22*, 247–262. https://doi.org/10.1027/1016-9040/a000303.

Germer, C. (2012). *Der achtsame Weg zur Selbstliebe. Wie man sich von destruktiven Gedanken und Gefühlen befreit* (3.Aufl.). Freiburg: Arbor Verlag.

Goff, B. G., & Goddard, H. W. (1999). Terminal core values associated with adolescent problem behaviors. *Adolescence, 34*(33), 47–60.

Handrock, A., & Baumann, M. (2017). *Vergeben und Loslassen in Psychotherapie und Coaching.* Weinheim, Basel: Beltz PVU.

Handrock, A., Zahn, C., & Baumann, M. (2016). *Schemaberatung, Schemacoaching & Schemakurzzeittherapie.* Weinheim: Beltz PVU.

Hitlin, S. (2003). Values as the core of personal identity: Drawing links between two theories of self. *Social Psychology Quarterly, 66*(2), 118–137. https://doi.org/10.2307/1519843.

Lee, D. A., Scragg, P., & Turner, S. (2001). The role of shame and guilt in traumatic events: A clinical model of shame-based and guilt-based PTSD. *British Journal of Medical Psychology, 74*(4), 451–466. https://doi.org/10.1348/000711201161109.

Matos, M., & Pinto-Gouveia, J. (2010). Shame as a traumatic memory. *Clinical Psychology & Psychotherapy, 17,* 299–312. https://doi.org/10.1002/cpp.659.

McCullough, M. E., Pargament, K. I., & Thoresen, C. E. (2000). The psychology of forgiveness: History, conceptual issues, and overview. In M. E. McCullough, K. I. Pargament, & C. E. Thoresen (Eds.), *Forgiveness: Theory, research, and practice* (pp. 1–16). New York: Guilford Press.

Neff, K. D. (2012). *Selbstmitgefühl.* München: Random House.

Pennebaker, J. W. (1993). Putting stress into words: health linguistic and psychotherapeutic implications. *Behavioral Research and Therapy, 31*(6), 539–548.

Pennebaker, J. W. (1997). *Opening up: The healing power of expressing emotions.* London, New York: Guilford Press.

Peterson, C., Park, C., & Seligman, M. E. P. (2005). Orientation to happiness and life satisfaction: The full life versus the empty life. *Journal of Happiness Studies, 6*(1), 25–41.

Pinto-Gouveia, J., & Matos, M. (2010). Can shame memories become a key to identity? The centrality of shame memories predicts psychopathology. *Applied Cognitive Psychology, 25,* 281–290. https://doi.org/10.1002/acp.1689.

Rogers, C. R. (1963). The concept of the fully functioning person. *Psychotherapy: Theory, Research & Practice, 1*(1), 17–26. https://doi.org/10.1037/h0088567.

Roos, J. (2000). Peinlichkeit, Scham und Schuld. In J. H. Otto, H. A. Euler & H. Mandl (Hrsg.). *Emotionspsychologie. Ein Handbuch.* (pp. 264–271). Weinheim: PVU.

Schlenke, D. (2005). Versöhnung. In H. D. Betz, et al. (Hrsg.), *Religion in Geschichte und Gegenwart. Handwörterbuch für Theologie und Religionswissenschaften* (4.Aufl.). Tübingen: Mohr Siebeck Verlag.

Sinha, M. (2017). Shame and psychotherapy: Theory, method and practice. In E. Vanderheiden & C.-H. Meyer (Eds.), *The value of shame. Exploring a health resource in cultural contexts* (pp. 251–276). Cham: Springer.

Wilson, J. P., Droždek, B., & Turkovic, S. (2006). Posttraumatic shame and guilt. *Trauma, Violence and Abuse, 7*(2), 122–141. https://doi.org/10.1177/1524838005285914.

Worthington, E. L., Jr. (2003). *Forgiving and reconciling: Bridges to wholeness and hope.* Downers Grove: InterVarsity Press.

Worthington, E. L., Jr., & Scherer, M. (2004). Forgiveness is an emotion-focused coping strategy that can reduce health risks and promote health resilience: Theory, review, and hypotheses. *Psychology and Health, 19,* 385–405.

Worthington, E. L., Jr. (2005). *Handbook of forgiveness.* London: Routledge Chapman & Hall. https://doi.org/10.1177/1524838005285914.

Young, J. E. (1994). *Practitioner's resource series. Cognitive therapy for personality disorders: A schema-focused approach* (Rev ed.). Sarasota: Professional Resource Press/Professional Resource Exchange.

Young, J., Klosko, J. S., & Weishaar, M. E. (2003). *Schema therapy: A practitioner's guide.* New York, London: The Guilford Press.

Maike Baumann is a scientific associate at the University of Potsdam, Germany. She holds a diploma in psychology with specializations in clinical psychology/work-and organizational psychology and is curretly working as a therapist, coach and trainer. Beforehand she studied linguistics and philosophy with a special focus on the philosophy of religion (University of Potsdam, Germany). Extra-ocupationally she is doing a doctorate on the topic of cultural influences on social scripts at the Europa Universität Viadrina, Germany. Additionally she is internationally certified as a mediator with a special expertise in business mediation. She has published various articles and monographies on Schema Therapy, Forgiveness, psychology of Self, Positive Psychology and diverse topics in the field of work and organizational psychology.

Anke Handrock (Dr. med. dent.) is a pedagogue, holds a doctorate in dentistry, is a mediator, coach and head of the Steinbeis Transfer Institute of Positive Psychology and Prevention at the Steinbeis Hochschule Berlin. She has been training medical communication for over 20 years in different Universities, such as the Humboldt University zu Berlin (Campus Charité) as well as for private organizations and clinical staff. She developed trainings in systemic leadership and is an expert in human resource development, team coaching and on corporate cultures. Besides she provides trainings in therapeutic methods and communication for a wider audience, such as counselors, psychotherapists and for institutes of several christian dioceses in Germany. She has published several monographs and accredited journal articles on topics related to Schema Therapy, Forgivness, Neuro Linguistic Programming, Positive Psychology and medical communication.

Chapter 32
Somatically-Based Art Therapy
for Transforming Experiences of Shame

Patricia Sherwood

Abstract This somatically based model of therapy utilizes the nonverbal artistic languages of sensing, gesturing, breathing, visualizing and sounding to identify, explore and transform experiences of shame within individuals and groups. The three artistic exercises presented herein are particularly designed to promote healing from shame and include the shame to self-esteem healing sequence, the cutting negative voices sequence and the self-parenting sequence. These artistic exercises create images for new growth and healing of shame and are particularly suitable for children, adolescents and adults who prefer bodily sensate therapeutic experiences rather than verbal interventions alone. These art therapy exercises provide precise directions for diagnosis and interventions and are grounded in the socio-cultural soil of the individual's life. They are used to direct insight and awareness into the broader contextual factors that shape the individual's self-esteem and shame. They provide precise interventions for transforming these experiences from negative to positive self esteem enhancing experiences and opportunities. These nonverbal exercises have been effectively used in multicultural contexts to explore and transform shame experiences resulting from trauma and abuse within the family, community and society.

Keywords Shame · Art therapy · Psychotherapy · Somatic therapy · Dramatherapy

32.1   Shame and Guilt

Shame is best understood by also introducing its older brother guilt which lays the foundation for the shame relationship. Together they are like shadowy villains that carve into our connectedness with ourselves and others, leaving injuries that prevent our experience of wholeness as human beings. Just (2010) succinctly describes the shame guilt relationship as follows: shame is secondary to guilt in terms of morality and ethics because it is too entangled in the struggle for recognition, and too much

P. Sherwood (✉)
Notre Dame University, Broome Campus, PO Box 27, Boyanup, WA 6237, Australia
e-mail: cctrust111@hotmail.com

absorbed in self, rather than the other. They both leave us feeling less than who we are and undermine our sense of self-worth and self-esteem. Guilt is an experience of feeling inadequate because we have been judged by others to have violated social expectations, and the gesture is often an internal pressure of shielding oneself against the public humiliation of being judged by others for a particular behaviour. Shame is our self-judgment against ourselves. We buy into the judgment and often shore it up with our own self deprecation. The gesture is that of hanging one's head, slouching into the concave position, where the force of the gravity of one's own self-hatred and self-judgment weighs one down.

Keltner and Buswell's (1996) research had participants distinguish between shame and guilt. They coded events in which the actors failed to meet important personal standards as 'shame', and experiences in which they engaged in actions which harmed others or violated social rules as 'guilt'. In terms of gesture, participants accurately identified persons suffering from shame, but did not reliably label guilt. Tangney et al. (1996) also noted that participants distinguished between guilt and shame. Guilt's external gesture is having the finger of accusation and judgment pointed against one and shame is an internal gesture described as being invaded by and having internalised the negative judgments of others about one's self-worth. As Fromm (1944) so accurately notes; "there is nothing more effective in breaking any person than to give them a conviction of their own wickedness". Tangney and Dearing (2002) in their research demonstrated that while guilt was a judgment around a particular behaviour omitted or completed, shame was an internalised sense of moral pain about one's own self-failure. The interpersonal consequence was that persons suffering from guilt have higher levels of empathy than those suffering from shame who often defend themselves through anger or withdrawal into depression. You are unworthy, it is not just an unacceptable behaviour. You hold a litany of thoughts that are self-deprecating and pervasively negative about yourself. In the words of Gerard Manly Hopkins (2018):

> I am gall, I am heartburn God's most deep decree
> Bitter would have me taste and my taste was me.

There is the deprecating self-evaluatory and moral denigration directed towards self by those suffering from shame.

In this chapter, I will present three art therapy strategies that I use in the holistic counselling model that is somatically based and which tracks the experience of shame as primarily a bodily experience that is reinforced by negative mind-body feed back loops. In this somatic model, it is essential that the client completes exercises with their body so as to retrain the bodily memory and facilitate the transformation and release of the shame so as to create new biofeedback pathways for positive self-esteem. It is assumed in this somatic model that all experiences are stored in the bodily cell memory, transferred thought the senses and that traumatic experiences can be re-experienced through sites of bodily tension where they are stored. This is a common assumption of a number of somatic therapists including Lowen (1976), Pert (1999), Totton (2003), Rothschild (2011) and Van de Kolk (2015).

32.2   Shame in the Holistic Counselling Model

In holistic counselling elucidated in depth in Holistic Counselling: a new vision for mental health (Sherwood, 2010) the model is somatically and psychodynamically based as well as incorporating the art therapies such as colour, sound, gesture, clay and sand. Breathing is the most visible and immediately observable connection between mind and body as expressed through our gestures. In this model, distinctions are made between willful shame, inherited shame, and personal shame. These distinctions are etic descriptors that have been formed by a phenomenological investigation of clients experience in therapy. The material in this chapter is based upon clinical casework over a one year period working with the experience of shame and guilt and developing detailed profiles of these experiences from a sample of 20 adult female clients, all who could be described as white European Australians The age range was from 24 years to 65 years.

Three types of shame are expressed by these clients which in the holistic coun-selling model are deductively described as: inherited shame, willful shame and per-sonal shame. Each will now be briefly profiled but I will focus on interventions for inherited shame only.

32.2.1   Inherited Shame

Bedrick succinctly notes that the hallmark of shame is that there is something wrong with me which has too often been affirmed by the shaming witnesses, most often parents or authority figures. This is a typical description of what I call inherited shame. When I ask clients to sense where they feel the shame in their body by focusing on the tension there and then take a step forward imagining they are stepping into that part of the body, and draw how the stress is stored there, they will draw a scribble like a knot, a rock, a ball of string. All of these represent the tension in their body when they think of the shameful moment. When asked to make their whole body into the gesture of the drawing and then tell me what they feel they most often say fear and rejection. When asked the earliest memory underlying the fear and rejection of the shameful experience, most clients recall an experience under the age of 7 years when they recall being shamed by parents, teachers or friends. This process is known as the "enter-exit-behold" sequence as it involved the client in bodily movements based on drama-therapy and is the core method for finding out the underlying cause of the presenting shame. This method was developed by Tagar (2003) and modified by Sherwood. It is documented in precise detail in Sherwood (2007, reprint 2010). In other "enter-exit behold" sequences clients may also recall shame experiences later in their development, but it appears that in the majority of clients the foundation for intense feelings of shame is laid in the first 7 years of life. Thereafter upon this early shame foundation are built many stories of experience of shame.

I have thus posited that inherited shame comes about when an adult "I" or identity replaces the child's fragile "I" or identity with negative statements about the body, mind or capacities of the child especially during the under 7 year old developmental period. These value statements have such a pervasive effect on the early development of the child's "I" that they literally replace it with the toxic roots of the adult's "I" which condemn the child as dirty, stupid, unintelligent, ugly, lazy, hopeless, fat, or useless. These statements on the part of the adult can be seen as projections onto the child by the adult of their own wounded inner child. The child believes this is who they are as their identity formation is so strongly influenced by the adult in this early developmental period of their life. This adult negativity at the core of the emerging individuality is internalised by the child and results in low self-esteem in adolescence that often impairs adult life. Objective outsiders can see that the self-condemning shame judgments that the client makes, are inaccurate. The client may be physically beautiful but may believe that they are ugly. The client may have a fine intellect but insist they are stupid. They may have an attractive physique but describe themselves as fat and ugly. There is always a substantial gap between the client's perceptions and the observable reality in inherited shame. In my research on client experience of shame, the inherited shame client will experience and draw shame as distinct roots spread throughout the physical body and most often located in the bottom part of the body. Figure 32.1 below, is a typical drawing of inherited shame:

The client experiences inherited shame as though their very body is contaminated by these toxic roots which they experience bodily as well as mentally. The way through is difficult as the root of each shame based voice/thought or accusation must be removed from the body cell memory and a transplant of a positive self-valuing voice/thought/pattern be made in its place. Not all roots can be removed at once, so the process of restoring the self valuing voices/thoughts and reprogramming the cellular memory is gradual. Two art therapy based techniques for achieving this will be illustrated under interventions.

32.2.2   Willful Shame

Willful shame in essence, refers to decisions to cause willful injury to another person and having a conscience about the deed of shaming another person or persons. There are few mitigating circumstances for the deed, just a pure desire to acquire power or cause suffering to another being. Such willful shame arises through the inner awareness that this behaviour will cause suffering to another person but despite this awareness they will follow through on the action, deed or wrods. It is described by as necessary shame or healthy guilt, arising from one's consciousness of basic human rights and needs. This inner experience of willful shame is drawn by clients as brown blots over or near a golden yellow background. In holistic therapy, it is my observation in over more than 10,000 client cases that golden yellow in drawings of bodily experience usually represents the reflective or insightful self governed by frontal lobe which is the part of the brain where insight, reflective thought, emotional

Fig. 32.1 Inherited shame
(drawn by author)

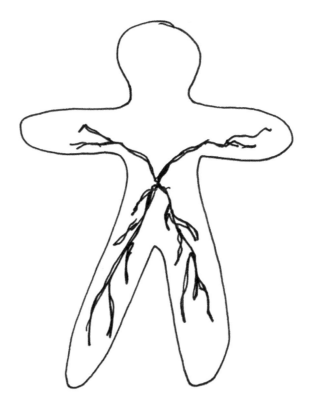

control and rationality are located (Filey, 2010) it stands in contrast to the reactive fight/flight responsive part of brain driven by fear. In willful shame, the collective moral conscience of a particular culture would agree with the client's judgment that the behaviour is a travesty of human rights, at the level of Kohlberg's stage 5 or 6 moral development. Willful shame may be experienced by youth and adults, mostly over the age of 12, when they have deliberately harmed or shamed another person and have regrets at a later time. Techniques for transforming this type of shame are documented in Sherwood (2012) Holistic counselling: through the shadow to compassion. An example is a mother who deliberately decides not to provide sufficient food for her children, knowing that they are hungry and finding satisfaction in this control she has in denying them food and spending the money on herself instead. Then when a child becomes ill through malnutrition, and a medical person confronts her she feels shame that her behaviour is now public and that she has deliberately created a situation of ill health for her child. Here, the initial technique to be used would be the "enter-exit-behold technique" outlined earlier in this chapter which engage the body in sensing the place of shame with it and literally using a drama therapy technique step into the body to identify the original cause of this behaviour. Once this has been identified a number of interventions are available to release the bodily memory driving the willful shame but these are too extensive to document herein.

32.2.3 Personal Shame

This occurs when the individual has extremely high personal awareness of the potential goodness within him or herself. In situations in which others would not judge them as inadequate, they judge themselves as inadequate and not manifesting the truth of their potential highest moral behaviour. They do not live up to their own inner potential and standards of what they know is good, desirable and right. An example is a client who came to counselling because she felt shame about leaving an injured kangaroo to die on the side of the road. Someone else had run over the kangaroo, and it was thrashing around on the road neither dead nor capable of jumping away from the scene. She was convinced however, that had she acted out of her highest and most moral self she would have had the strength to put the animal out of its misery by either killing it outright, or asking someone else to kill it, or by staying next to it and sending it love in its dying minutes. She had simply driven away and was ashamed that she had not followed the highest knowledge of compassion within herself. This type of shame is driven from within the individual, and like other types o shame does not have any influence in its formation from external persons. Techniques for transforming this type of shame are documented in Sherwood (2010). The basic technique would involve the clients completing an enter-exit-behold sequence followed by specific intervention sequences which are not the focus of this chapter.

32.3 Interventions: Inherited Shame

1. The shame tree

This chapter focuses upon interventions for inherited shame only, as this is the most common form of shame presenting in this sample of clients. The shame tree has been developed as a result of phenomenologically working with clients experiences of shame often experienced and drawn as roots in their body. From these drawings, I developed the shame tree intervention which begins as a diagnostic map drawn by the client which gives one a clear picture of the particular and precise nature of the client's shame thoughts. The client lists all the negative shame based devaluing thoughts that repeatedly go through their mind always beginning with "I". For example " I am stupid". The client is given an A4 sheet of paper and laid on the table in portrait position and asked to draw a tree with large roots. There is to be one root for each of the negative thoughts and most clients identify between 5 and 8 negative thoughts that are shame based and attack the very core of their self-esteem and integrity.

This is illustrated below (Fig. 32.2):

A self-esteem tree is then filled in which contains the same amount of roots as the toxic tree but with each root representing the positive alternative identity message. This self-esteem tree is illustrated below (Fig. 32.3):

Fig. 32.2 The shame tree (with permission by Tara Sherwood)

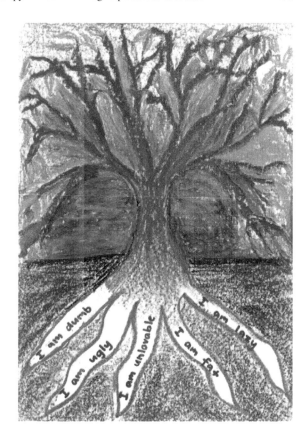

Common core messages in the self-esteem tree often include a selection from:

I am intelligent.
I am good.
I am attractive.
I am knowledgeable.
I am competent.
I am lovable.
I am hard working.
I am healthy.

The client and counsellor now have a diagnostic map of how the shame is expressed in their thinking and reflected in the shame roots that they experience in their body.

Fig. 32.3 The self esteem
tree with permission by Tara
Sherwood

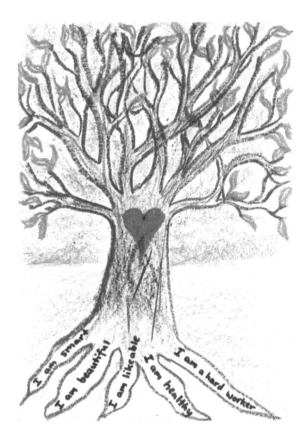

32.3.1 Active Abuse: Recovery Sequence

Each of the core messages in the self-esteem tree becomes the client's goal or intention
to transform in a therapy session.

32.3.2 Description of a Typical Therapeutic Process

Given for example the client's intention to believe that "I can accomplish things", the
counsellor begins by asking the client where in the body they feel the corresponding
shame root of "I am useless". The client does this by giving a real example of feeling
that voice in their life and then they place their hand on the part of the body where
they feel the most tension when they recount this incident. The client then literally
steps forward into that image of that part of their body, and draws the tension there.
Is it a knot? a lump? a ball? Once they have drawn this shape of how their breathing
is contracted by the tension they experience when they focus upon that part of their

body, they are literally asked to step into the shape they have drawn with their whole body. They must squeeze their whole body into the ball like shape or whatever they have drawn. When in this gesture, the counsellor first asks the client the feelings they have when their body is in this shape and which are always negative and often like, powerless, frustrated, scared, squashed, sad, lonely. Then, the counsellor will ask the client the earliest memory of feeling like that. The client's body will within a few minutes throw up an image from earlier life, usually childhood in which they first experienced this feeling. This technique is at the heart of holistic counselling's somatic foundations and this technique called "enter-exit-behold" is documented in Sherwood (2017, 104–106) Usually the client finds a younger inner child part of themselves from an earlier period in their life, being judged for some behaviour, shamed, scolded or beaten.

The counsellor then proceeds to work with the key feelings of the identified wounded little inner child that the client experiences within. There are usually two categories of interventions required, one that works to remove active abuse and one that works to overcome passive abuse.

Active abuse occurs when the client experiences in their bodily gesture the feeling of being attacked either physically, emotionally, mentally or psychologically. The clients experience these feelings of being attacked as leaving contamination within their bodies of some-one else's energy whether identified as someone else's judgment or physical force as in the case of hitting ore sexual abuse. Clients can clearly identify how they feel the force of the attack from the active abuse in their bodies. They will tell you that it feels like one of the following: being kicked, squeezed, suffocated, stabbed squashed, poked, shot at, or any other variation of a force that contract one's breathing. A empowerment/boundary sequence is used to remove the experience of the force attacking the body. This was developed by Tagar and is documented in Sherwood (2007; 141–144). It involves the following steps:

1. The client finds the shape of the force that the client experiences as attacking them e.g. stabbing.
2. finding a sound for the force.
3. preparing to face the sound of the force attacking them again by strengthening their bodily presence in the present moment by stamping their feet, clapping and repeating: "I am here, I am safe, I am protected".
4. pushing the sound of the attacking force away with a loud g, d, b, or "NO" and gesturing a blocking shield with their hands in the direction of the sound of the force. The sound of the attacking force is produced by the counsellor repeatedly directed towards the client until they no longer have any bodily aversion to the sound and tell the counsellor they now feel free of the attacking force.
5. using air or water sounds like whoosh the client now cleans out the energetic space within and around their body making the gesture of sweeping away.
6. establishing new boundaries using a strong earth sound like "dddd" successively repeated by the client while with their hands they actively create a safety dome around them made out of "d" while visualising a substance of choice such as steel, crystal, light that will be the material of the protective dome that they

are creating all around their body in a 360° circle using sound, gesture and visualisation. Further elucidation of this technique is documented in Sherwood (2000a, 2000b) and Tagar (2003).

32.4 Passive Abuse: Self-parenting Recovery Sequence

Clients in this model experience passive abuse when they describe feeling empty in their body, as though there are black holes and nobody is there for them. They also describe this experience as being abandoned and rejected, as being out in the cold, being alone and unloved. In the client sample above, all the clients had experiences of being abandoned by one of more of their parents, in at least one of the sessions and feeling empty holes in their body. They may have been verbally or physically attacked and afterwards experience often being rejected, abandoned and alone by the withdrawal of love, warmth, presence and/or affection from the significant adults. These attacks and ensuring experiences of abandonment are most commonly from the parents in the early childhood memories, that arise when they step into their bodily memories of shame.

32.5 Self-parenting Sequences

When the client's inner child, that is their earliest memory of shame from their childhood, experiences repeatedly debilitating and devaluing messages from a father or mother, which is the case in this sample of clients then self-parenting sequences are essential. The fatherhood sequence is used for experiences of abandonment or unavailability of the father, the motherhood sequence for rejection or abandonment by mothers. The mother archetype sequence will be required when the client's wish is to heal their inner child that was shamed and then experienced bodily as rejected or abandoned by the mother. The father archetype sequence is used when the client's wish is to heal the inner child that was shamed by the father and then rejected and abandoned by the father.

Shame work around rejection and or unavailability of the parent experienced bodily by the client as passive abuse or absence of the parental warmth, love and approval in his model requires the client to free their parents from the obligation to repair the client's experienced inner damage or to make the client feel loved unconditionally as an adult. Too many adults get caught up in negative spirals, demanding from their parents qualities that their parents do not have to give and possibly have never had to give. This self-parenting sequence, developed by Tagar is very liberating because the client becomes the parent to their own damaged and shamed inner child experience, and acts as the new guardian capable, with practice, of healing and protecting their own wounded inner child.

Tagar (1998, 56) describes this healing dynamic powerfully and poignantly in his profoundly moving poem titled *The motto of self-parenting:*

…But between me as the loving adult
And me as the child in need
There are traces of the unqualified adults
Who were my parents once.

They, incapable of the love and the protection
Which I was and I still am in need of
They are present there now as traces of unsafety
As traces of rejection and fear.

These traces are mine now
These things of darkness I must acknowledge as mine
Then I can confront them, tell them off, dissolve them,
And put in their place the best of my adulthood

My inner mother and my inner father
The best of the universe in me
With them, I now qualify
To care for my inner child…

The redemption from shame comes from our own endeavours at the anvil of our childhood experiences. I encourage the client to bring back to the rejected and abandoned child located in their bodily recall of the original feeling of being shamed, their our own capacity to heal and to consciously embrace that part of themselves that was shamed loving acceptance. The client gathers warm, present, caring, affirming supportive images of fatherhood or motherhood, that represent the qualities they did not have from their parents such as love, support, encouragement, affirmation, nurturing and protection. They resource their young inner child found within their bodily experience from the chosen images of positive parenthood. For each image they complete the following sequence:

- receiving one of those qualities from the selected image
- breathing in the quality
- giving it a colour
- giving it a gesture and making the gesture with one's body
- finding a sound or a song that represents the quality
- drawing the quality now flowing through the breath in our body.

Thus the client engages their highest resources to redeem their experience of their inner child found within their bodily cell recall when they completed the enter-exit-behold sequence, after describing their adult experience of shame. The body remembers the original cause of the adult shame that occurred in this sample of clients during experiences of shaming in childhood. In working with these original foundations for their adult shame, the shamed childhood experience, the client succeeds in removing the foundational memories for their adult shame. In so doing,

Fig. 32.4 I am ugly (drawn
by the author)

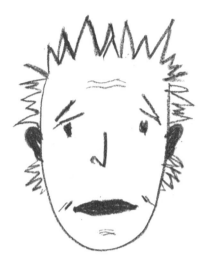

the client liberates themselves as adults from shame and fear and rebuilds their self-esteem. The client completes the above sequence for seven days as home care in their own environment with each of the five or six qualities identified as missing. These resourcing sequences for passive abuse are further documented in Sherwood and Tagar (2000a, 2000b).

32.6   Cutting the Chords of the Negative Voice

The aim of this sequence is to use a somatic process based on drama and sound therapy to engage the client in actively removing the negative thoughts within themselves that affirm their shame based messages and to replace them with positive self-esteem affirming voices. Here, in the pre-intervention phase, the clients draw a picture of the negative voice/thought that for example says; "I am ugly" (Fig. 32.4).

It is completed as a portrait with the eyes and mouth reflecting the negative message. Post intervention, that is after the enter exit behold sequence was completed and the sequences for active or passive abuse, every time the negative message comes to mind for example. "I am ugly" they imagine the negative portrait and cut it off and burn the image into ashes using the sounds of cutting and burning: kkk (cutting) and ffshh (burning). They then draw a portrait of the self-esteem voice that says "I am attractive" This is post intervention (Fig. 32.5).

They are encouraged to keep the positive images that they have drawn on their mobile phones. The negative thought/voice is drawn pre-intervention. The positive voice/thought is drawn post intervention following the burning off of the negative voice.

Fig. 32.5 I am attractive
(drawn by the author)

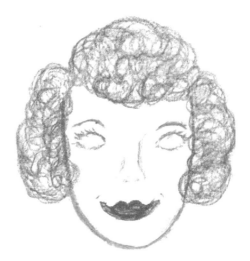

The counsellor also works with the client to identify changes they can make in their personal, social, work and community that will support this new perception of themselves following the completion of the session.

In summary, the following process comprises each counselling session

1. Identify which root or negative voice thought on the shame tree the client would like to transform in the session.
2. Draw a portrait of the negative voice.
3. Recount a current example in their lives of the negative thought.
4. Sense where they feel it in their bodies and complete an enter-exit behold sequence.
5. Identify the earliest memory of feeling like that "The shamed inner child".
6. Apply an empowerment/boundary sequence to remove the active abuse
7. Apply a resourcing sequence motherhood or fatherhood to remove the passive abuse.
8. Burn into ashes the negative voice and draw the new positive self-esteem voice.
9. Identify life changes to support the new positive self-esteem voice.

With this sample of clients, there was one counselling session for each root or voice of shame, drawn on their original shame tree. This sample completed between 5 and 8 sessions per person. The above process from 1 to 9 is undertaken for all the roots on the shame tree so that the client ends up with a gallery of negative portraits that are eventually torn up and burned literally as well as metaphorically and a gallery of positive portraits that are kept and placed in a significant place in their home to stand as a reminder of the positive self-esteem thoughts and associated actions that they are focusing upon in their lives post therapy.

32.7 Conclusion

Shame in this somatic model is a bodily experience resulting from shaming, and condemning statements about the person. In this sample, the origins arise from early childhood experiences of shaming from significant adults, most often parents. Hence the term "inherited shame" used to describe this type of shame. A pre-intervention diagnostic tool, the shame tree was used to capture the shame messages unique to each client while performing a map of the shame issues to be addressed in the ensuring therapy sessions. The structure of the intervention to release this shame and create positive self-esteem in this model includes the following interventions. An enter-exit behold bodily process to reveal the original shame experience underlying the current negative thought/voice. This is followed by empowerment/boundary sequence when the client experiences active abuse in the identified experience and a resourcing process to rebuild the clients positive self-esteem when the client experiences passive abuse in the identified experience. The interventions are completed by an art therapy process by which the negative voice/thought for each shame based message is drawn in the pre-intervention phase of the counselling process, then at the post intervention phase of the counselling process it is burned to ashes, and replaced by a drawing of a positive voice/thought. The therapy session is completed by reviewing behavioural changes that the client can make in their life socially, in their work life or personal life to implement the new positive voice/thought.

In essence, shame which is the parent of low self-esteem with all its self-sabotaging garments and messages that contaminate the client's life must be brought from shadows of the client's consciousness into the search light. Exposed to scrutiny, it will be revealed as a malnourished child that has developed on a poor diet of toxic parenting and self-deprecating nutrients. It is the role of the counsellor to reverse the parenting deficients through implementing positive self-parenting experiences as well as creating a fertile diet of positive messages, images and sensate creative activities that engage the client's body, soul and mind in carving out a new sense of self worth.

References

Bedrick, D. *The roots of shame: the shaming witness*. Retrieved from https://www.psychologytoday. com/blog/is-psychology-making-us-sick/201608/the-roots-shame. Accessed 15 Feb 2018.

Filey, C. (2010). The frontal lobes. *Handbook of Clinical Neurology, 95,* 557–570. https://doi.org/10.1016/s0072-9752(08)02135-0.

Fromm, E. (1944). *Individual and social origins of neurosis international psychoanalysis*. Retrieved from www.net/2013/06/19/erich-fromm. Accessed 24 Jan 2018.

Hopkins, G. M. *I wake and feel the fell of dark not day*. Retrieved from https://interestingliterature. com/2016/02/23/a-short-analysis-of-hopkinss-i-wake-and-feel-the-fell-of-dark-not-day/. Accessed 20 Jan 2018.

Just, D. (2010). From guilt to shame: Albert Camus and literature's ethical response to politics. *MLN, 125*(4), 895–912.

Keltner, D., & Buswell, B. (1996). Evidence for the distinctness of embarrassment, shame and guilt: A study of Recalled antecedents and Facial expressions of emotion. *Journal of Cognition and Emotion, 10*(2), 155–171.

Lowen, A. (1976). *Bioenergetics*. London: Penguin.

Pert, C. (1999). *Molecules of emotion*. New York: Simon and Schuster.

Rothschild, B. (2011). *The body remembers: The psychophysiology of trauma and trauma treatment*. New York: Norton and Co.

Sherwood, P. (2000a). Bridging the chasm: Philophonetics counselling and healing the trauma of sexual abuse. *Diversity, 2*(4), 18–25.

Sherwood, P. (2000b). Beholding: bridging the chasm between flooding and denial. Philophonetics counselling and sexual abuse survivors. *Journal of the Incest Survivors Association*, 23–32.

Sherwood, P., & Tagar, Y. (2000a). Experience awareness tools for preventing burnout in nurses. *Australian Journal of Holistic Nursing 7*(1), 15–20.

Sherwood, P., & Tagar, Y. (2000b). Self care tools for creating resistance to burnout: A case study in philophonetics counseling. Australian Journal of Holistic Nursing, 7(2), 45–46.

Sherwood, P. (2007). *Holistic counselling: A new vision for mental health*. Bunbury: Sophia Publications. Reprint 2010

Sherwood, P. (2012). *Holistic counselling: Through the shadow to compassion*. Bunbury: Sophia Publications.

Sherwood, P. (2017). *CBT and artistic therapies; an unlikely marriage*. Bunbury: Sophia Publications.

Tagar, Y. (1998). *Caring for the child within. Philophonetics love of sounds: Language for the inner life*. Melbourne: Persephone Publications.

Tagar, Y. (2003). Psychophonetics in South Africa: Psychophonetics (Philophonetics- Counselling) methodology, its application to recovery from sexual abuse and its initial introduction to South Africa. Pretoria: University of South Africa.

Tangney, J., & Dearing, R. (2002). *Shame and guilt*. New York: Guildford Press.

Tangney, J., Miller, R., Flicker, L., Hill, T., & Barlow, D. (1996). Are shame, guilt and embarrassment distinct emotions? *Journal of Personality and Social Psychology, 70*(6), 1256–1269.

Totton, N. (2003). *Body psychotherapy: An introduction*. Philadelphia: Open University Press.

Van der Kolk, B. (2015). *The body keeps the score: Brain, mind and body in the healing of trauma*. New York: Penguin.

Patricia Sherwood (Dr.) is an art therapist, mental health accredited social worker and has practiced as a somatically-based psychotherapist and counsellor for over 25 years, specialising in abuse and trauma recovery as well as panic and anxiety conditions. She is particularly interested in child and adolescent mental health issues. From 1984 onwards, Patricia held the position of Senior Lecturer at Edith Cowan University and in 2006 became an Adjunct Researcher until 2015. She now supervises doctoral students for Notre Dame University, writes books and continues private clinical practice. She has also served as the Director of Sophia College of Counselling from 2006–2015 during which time she designed and taught courses in holistic counselling, Buddhist psychotherapy and Artistic therapies specialising in developmental psychology, counselling skills and counselling models. Additionally, Trish also supervised practicums and casework throughout Australia and Singapore.

Chapter 33
"Nothing I Accept About Myself Can Be Used Against Me to Diminish Me"—Transforming Shame Through Mindfulness

Elisabeth Vanderheiden

Abstract In the context of positive psychology, shame is increasingly recognised as a potential resource of well-being, self-development and creativity in the sense of personal growth. Current studies on mindfulness have shown that mindfulness brings about various positive psychological effects such as the reduction of stress symptoms, depression, and shame-based trauma appraisals. It is also able to reduce negative reactions to emotionally charged situations and can reduce psychological symptoms and emotional reactivity, as well as improve behavioural regulation. This chapter combines those two approaches mindfulness and positive psychology and offers exercises to transform shame and explore shame as a resource.

Keywords Transforming shame · Mindfulness · Meditation · Positive psychology

33.1 Introduction

Vanderheiden and Mayer (2017, 3–8, 20–23) point out that shame can basically be regarded as a resource, for example with regard to one's own personal, social or creative development.

Numerous other authors have recently highlighted the positive implications of shame as a resource, as well as being a positive phenomenon (Tangney & Dearing, 2002; Brennan, Robertson & Cox in Vanderheiden & Mayer, 2017, 20) or shame as initiating self-reflection, individual learning and development processes (Hilgers, 2013, 20), or as a significant instrument in maintaining power, such as in group or mass humiliation (Briegleb, 2014, 10).

Lorde (2007). *Sister outsider* (p. 147). Berkeley, Calif.: Crossing Press.

E. Vanderheiden (✉)
Katholische Erwachsenenbildung Rheinland-Pfalz, Welschnonnengasse 2-4, 55116 Mainz, Germany
e-mail: ev@keb-rheinland-pfalz.de

C.-H. Mayer and E. Vanderheiden (eds.), *The Bright Side of Shame*,
https://doi.org/10.1007/978-3-030-13409-9_33

Since mindfulness originally has Buddhistic roots, it should also be referred to the corresponding Buddhist understanding of shame, which is also positively connoted:

> In any examination of behavior in relation to issues of ethics, the functions of shame and guilt need to be considered. In the Theravāda Buddhist perspective, shame or moral sensitivity (hiri-ottappa) is regarded as a sign of mental health. It is the emotional pain felt by a responsible person when they, for example, tell a lie or deliberately cause harm to another. It is regarded as a concomitant of physical pain that, similarly, usefully serves to protect the body. (Amaro, 2015, 69)

However, shame in general is regarded as deeply hurtful and toxic: "Shame is a powerful, painful feeling" (Krishnamurthy, 2018, 15, translated by the author or as "a soul eating emotion" (Carl Gustav Jung in Vanderheiden & Mayer, 2017, 277; see Mayer on dreams, in this book).

How can such potentially negative and painful shame experiences—which are in principle capable of profoundly injuring, disturbing and in extreme cases, destroying people—be transformed and become resources for growth and health? It is the concern of this chapter to thoroughly explore this question. Mindfulness can be considered as a meaningful way to shape such a transformation (Gilbert, Oosterhuizen, Merkin, in this book).

A number of studies have shown that mindfulness has a lasting positive impact on various indicators of psychological health, such as subjective well-being, reduced psychological symptoms and improved behavioural regulation (Keng et al., 2011, 1). During the last several decades, mindfulness has been more associated with psychological well-being and theoretical and empirical research in this area has been intensified. But what exactly is meant by mindfulness and which health effects can be scientifically proven? That is the focus of the next section of this chapter.

> Between stimulus and response there is a space.
> In that space is our power to choose our response.
> In our response lies our growth and our freedom.
> Viktor E. Frankl[1]

33.2 Mindfulness and Health—Insights into Relevant Research Results

Mindfulness finds its roots in ancient spiritual traditions, and is most systematically articulated and emphasised in Buddhism, a spiritual tradition that is at least 2550 years old. As the idea and practice of mindfulness has been introduced into Western psychology and medicine beginning in the 1970s, it is not surprising that differences emerge with regard to how mindfulness is conceptualised within Buddhist and Western perspectives.

---

[1]Pattakos (2010). *Prisoners of our thoughts: Viktor Frankl's Principles for Discovering Meaning in Life and Work* (p. Foreword). San Francisco, Calif.: Berrett-Koehler.

33.2.1 Definition of Mindfulness

All definitions of mindfulness are similar.

Jon Kabat-Zinn, who was one of the first to introduce mindfulness to the Western context of psychology research in 1979, defines mindfulness as

> being fully awake in our lives. It is about perceiving the exquisite vividness of each moment. We feel more alive. We also gain immediate access to our own powerful inner resources for insight, transformation, and healing. (Kabat-Zinn as cited in Amaro & Vallejo, 2008, 149)

Germer (in Germer et al., 2005 as cited in Keng et al., 2011, 2) describes mindfulness as a "psychological trait, a practice of cultivating mindfulness, a mode or state of awareness, or a psychological process".

Bishop (Bishop et al., 2004 as cited in Keng et al., 2011, 2) describes mindfulness as consisting of two components: "self-regulation of attention, directed to the present moment, together with an orientation component of curiosity, openness, and acceptance" (Keng et al., 2011, 2).

Keng sums up the central primary elements of mindfulness from a clinical psychology point of view as "awareness of one's moment-to-moment experience nonjudgmentally and with acceptance" (Keng et al., 2011, 1). Keng underlines the need to distinguish Western and Asian approach in regard to the context, the process and the content, noting that in the Western context, mindfulness is "generally independent of any specific circumscribed philosophy, ethical code, or system of practices" (Keng et al., 2011, 3).

33.2.1.1 Effects of Mindfulness Interventions on Health

Because of space limitations, only a few recent studies which have examined the relationships between mindfulness and well-being can be referred to in this chapter. A good overview of further studies is provided by Keng (see Keng et al., 2011).

Gilbert and Procter (2006, 353) found in their research that, after 12 two-hour sessions of compassionate mind training,

> results showed significant reductions in depression, anxiety, self-criticism, shame, inferiority and submissive behaviour. There was also a significant increase in the participants' ability to be self-soothing and focus on feelings of warmth and reassurance for the self. (Gilbert, in this book)

Based on two studies, Neff and Germer (2013) reported that their eight-week intervention programme of mindful self-compassion (MSC) resulted in increased happiness, life satisfaction, mindfulness, and self-compassion in addition to decreased depression, anxiety, and stress.

After a nine-week compassion cultivation training (CCT) programme, Jazaieri et al. (2013, 1113) reported more compassion for others, receiving compassion from others, and self-compassion experienced by the participants:

The amount of formal meditation practiced during CCT was associated with increased compassion for others. Specific domains of compassion can be intentionally cultivated in a training program. These findings may have important implications for mental health and well-being.

A meta-analysis of 39 studies mostly using mindfulness-based stress reduction (MBSR) and mindfulness-based cognitive therapy, demonstrated the efficacy of mindfulness-based therapy for reducing anxiety and depression symptoms (Hoffman et al., 2010). In 2016, Bartels-Velthuis and her colleagues found that by practising MBSR in two-and-a-half-hour weekly sessions over nine weeks, the levels of depression of patients reduced, and levels of mindfulness and self-compassion increased (Bartels-Velthuis et al., 2016, 809).

Pace et al. (2009) examined the effect of compassion meditation on innate immune, neuro-endocrine, and behavioural responses to psychosocial stress and evaluated the degree to which engagement in meditation practice influenced stress reactivity. These authors concluded that "engagement in compassion meditation may reduce stress-induced immune and behavioural responses" (Pace et al., 2009, 1) and, in another study, that in "individuals who actively engage in practicing the technique, compassion meditation may represent a viable strategy for reducing potentially deleterious physiological and behavioural responses to psychosocial stress" (Pace et al., 2010, 1).

Current studies even seem to suggest that programmes which are only offered via internet can have some success with trauma and stressor-related disorders, including post-traumatic stress disorder (PTSD) and related comorbid disorders such as anxiety, depression, and dissociative disorders in so far as participants report "improving self-regulation and well-being and reducing PTSD symptoms, anxiety, depressive, and dissociative experiences, as well as their experienced ease, helpfulness, and informational value" (Frewen et al., 2015, 1322). Stjernswärd and Hansson (2016, 751) also verify "significant positive improvements in mindfulness and self-compassion, and significant decreases in perceived stress and in certain dimensions of caregiver burden" in their research on a web-based mindfulness programme for families living with mental illness.

33.2.2 Introduction to Most Relevant Mindfulness Interventions on Health

Several mindfulness-orientated interventions seem to have proven particularly useful and have been carefully examined in research during the last decades (Oosthuizen, in this book).

Mindfulness-based stress reduction (MBSR)

MBSR is the oldest academic medical stress reduction programme in a Western context. Formulated in 1979 by Jon Kabat-Zinn (1990) at the University of Massachusetts Medical School, it teaches participants how to use their innate resources and abilities to respond more effectively to stress, pain and illness (Amaro & Vallejo, 2008, 2).

Compassionate mind training (CMT) and compassion-focused therapy (CFT)

Gilbert and Procter (2006) trialled CMT as an approach designed for people who experience chronic problems with high shame and self-criticism, in a pilot study with six participants who had severe and complex difficulties. There were significant reductions in shame, self-criticism, depression, and anxiety following 12 two-hour sessions. CMT was the basis for development of CFT (Gilbert et al., 2010), which includes mindful focus on breathing, compassion-focused imagery, compassionate chair work, directing compassionate feelings toward others, generation of experiences of receiving compassion from others, and compassionate letter writing. (Gilbert, in this book; Oosthuizen, in this book).

Mindful self-compassion (MSC)

While CFT is a therapy approach designed for use with clinical patients to enhance psychological resilience in both clinical and nonclinical populations, Neff and Germer developed the MSC programme specifically to enhance self-compassion. MSC focuses on both formal (sitting meditation) and informal (during daily life) self-compassion practices. The structure of MSC is based on MBSR, with participants meeting for two, or two and a half hours once a week over the course of eight weeks, and also meeting for a half-day meditation retreat (Germer and Neff, 2013, 3). The goal, according to Germer and Neff (2013, 4) is:

> to provide participants with a variety of tools to increase self-compassion, which they can integrate into their lives according to what works best for them. The program also teaches general skills of loving-kindness, which is a type of friendly benevolence given to oneself in everyday situations (compassion is mainly relevant for situations involving emotional distress).

All studies show that the intervention will be successful in the medium term. A certain continuity and regularity is therefore important for sustainable success. Most programmes assume a minimum period of one to three months, during which time interventions should be carried out on a regular basis.

Incidentally, Bartels-Velthuis et al. (2016, 810) mention a particularly interesting recent development, namely that some self-compassion training programmes have been developed and studied in non-clinical samples, with promising results (Fredrickson et al., 2008; Jazaieri et al., 2013; Neff & Germer, 2013; Pace et al., 2009, 2010) in which no preliminary experience with mindfulness is required.

33.2.3 Shame, Mindfulness and Health

Now that the relationship between mindfulness and health or well-being has been considered in more detail, and some of the better-known concepts and models have been introduced, the relationship between mindfulness, shame and health should be scrutinised.

Keng et al. (2011, 14) stress that mindfulness intervention maybe helpful in disorders where shame is involved:

> treatment of disorders that tend to involve excessive shame and guilt, such as eating disorders, may benefit from greater treatment emphasis on the acceptance and self-compassion aspects of mindfulness.

The research of Barbara Fredrickson and her colleagues (Fredrickson et al., 2008) demonstrates in several studies the positive impact of meditation practice, especially loving-kindness meditation (LKM, also called Mettā meditation). LKM is an intervention strategy which, over time, produces increased daily experiences of positive emotions, which, in turn, produce increases in a wide range of personal resources (such as increased mindfulness, purpose in life, social support, and decreased illness symptoms). In their studies, Fredrickson et al. (2008, 11) have also examined the impact of LKM on negative emotions, indexed by a composite of daily ratings for anger, shame, contempt, disgust, embarrassment, guilt, sadness, and fear.

In their research on the relationships of mindfulness, self-compassion, and meditation experience with shame-proneness, Woods and Proeve (2014) showed that mindfulness interventions were able to reduce shame in all participants of the study (Woods & Proeve, 2014, 21). Their findings indicated first, that self-compassion was a predictor of shame-proneness, but mindfulness was not, suggesting that self-compassion should be a particular focus of shame interventions. Second, they found that lower shame-proneness was associated with meditation (more than one session per month), compared to very infrequent meditation. The authors speculate:

> It is possible that the attitude of self-compassion which accompanies mindfulness meditation is the most effective aspect of meditation practice for influencing shame-proneness. Interventions that are intended to reduce shame experiences might effectively address self-compassion directly rather than indirectly through mindfulness. For example, mindfulness meditation may be supplemented by loving-kindness meditation (LKM), a technique for cultivating kindness toward all living things. (Woods & Proeve, 2014, 29)

> **Some reflections on being good, on not being good and on just being**
>
> You do not have to be good
>
> You do not have to walk on your knees for a hundred
>
> miles through the desert repenting
>
> You only have to let the soft animal of your body love
>
> what it loves
>
> Mary Oliver[2]

---

[2]Oliver (2004). Wild geese. Tarset: Bloodaxe.

33.3   Practising Mindfulness to Discover the Value of Shame

33.3.1   Practising Mindfulness—A Short Introduction

Mindfulness exercises can be set up in either single or group settings. Even if they lead to certain effects in the short term, they are particularly sustainable with long-term implementation as described above. For most people, it is certainly useful and helpful to book a course corresponding to one of the programmes mentioned above or similar offerings if they want to transform their toxic shame experiences through mindfulness. But for some people, it may make more sense to take their first steps towards transforming their toxic shame into a resource for more personal and social growth on their own. For these, the following comments can be helpful.

Usually mindfulness exercises begin with taking up a certain relaxed sitting or lying position, followed by a breathing exercise in preparation for deep relaxation. Breath awareness is a critical way to combine body, emotions and pirit. Conscious and mindful breathing is the "foundation of mindfulness" (Thích-Nhất-Hạnh, 2011, 43 translated by the author).

This is often followed by a so-called "body scan" exercise. Both are an important preparation for more demanding meditations such as Mettā meditations (LKM) with a special focus on the development of unconditional love for all beings. It makes sense to exercise 15 min daily for at least a few weeks, though evidence suggests that mindfulness increases the more it is practised. It is also useful and helpful to practise meditation in a group in order to strengthen and support one another, ideally under professional guidance.

33.3.1.1   Guided Breathing Exercise in Preparation for Deep Relaxation

Now that the relationship between mindfulness and health or well-being has been considered, you can follow the instructions below if you like to explore these technique.

1. "Find a relaxed, comfortable position. You could be seated on a chair or on the floor on a cushion. Keep your back upright, but not too tight. Or you could lie back on a sofa, on a bed or on a mat on the floor, hands resting wherever they are comfortable. Close your eyes. [*If you like, give yourself a smile and tell yourself that you are looking forward to the following meditation.*]"
2. Tune into your breath. Feel the natural flow of your breath—in, out. You don't need to do anything to your breath. Just breathe. There is no need to change your breath in any way. Just breathe, not long, not short, just natural.
3. Stay here for two to three minutes. Notice your breath, in silence. From time to time, you'll get lost in thought, then return to your breath."

33.3.2   Body Scan[3]

In the context of mindfulness, body, breath and emotions are closely linked. As Thích-Nhất-Hạnh points out, "If our body is in conflict, we are exposed to many violent emotions, our breath cannot be free… Mindful breathing not only brings our mind back to our breath, but also to our whole body" (Thích-Nhất-Hạnh, 2011, 45–46). In this deep relaxation exercise, you say "let" to yourself internally while inhaling; while exhaling you use the word "go". This choice of words helps you to enter into a deeper mental and physical relaxation.

1. "Now bring your awareness to your body. Smile to your body. Get in touch with your breath. Enjoy your breath. Watch as the breath enters through your nose, flows in and out again. Like waves that roll up to the sea and back into the ocean. Do not change your breath. Watch the quiet movements of your body as you come into contact with your breath. Take your breath away as it comes and goes without affecting it.
2. To get in touch with your present state of mind, inhale to yourself, smile at yourself and say, 'let', and exhale and use the word 'go'. This choice of words helps you to enter into a mental and physical relaxation.
3. Take a closer look at your body with every breath … let … go ….
4. Feel the different regions of your body. Give each part of your body a careful appreciation with a smile and a deep breath.
5. Smile to your right foot. Begin with the right heel: 'let go…', sole of the right foot: 'let go…', the toes of your right foot, big toe: 'let go…', second toe: 'let go…, third toe: 'let go…', fourth toe: 'let go…', little toe: 'let go…', right calf: 'let go…', the back of your right thigh: 'let go…', your right instep: 'let go…', the right shin: 'let go…', the right front of the thigh: 'let go…'.
6. Smile to your right leg: 'let go…'. Now go with your attention to your left heel: 'let go…', left sole: 'let go…', the toes of your left foot, big toe: 'let go…', second toe: 'let go…', third toe: 'let go…', fourth toe: 'let go…', little toe: 'let go…', left calf: 'let go…', the back of your left thigh: 'let go…', your left instep: 'let go…', the left tibia: 'let go…', the front of your left thigh: 'let go…'. Smile to your left leg: 'let go…'.
7. Both legs: 'let go…'.
8. Send a smile to your right buttock: 'let go…' and to your left buttock: 'let go…'. Both buttocks: 'let go…'. Your right back: 'let go…', your left back: 'let go…'. The whole back: 'let go…'.
9. Focus on your back and send a smile: 'let go…'. See how you sink more into your mat with each breath. Let all tension go to the ground. Relax deeper and deeper. Your breath flows calmly into your body, in and out.

---

[3]Some body scan excercises can be found for example in Amaro & Vallejo (2008) 89–97 or http://www.mbsr-kurs-koeln.de/achtsamkeitsuebungen/ or https://health.ucsd.edu/specialties/mindfulness/programs/mbsr/Pages/audio.aspx.

10. Send a smile to your right arm. The right back of your hand: 'let go…', the palm of your hand: 'let go…', your thumb: 'let go…', index finger: 'let go…', middle finger: 'let go…', ring finger: 'let go…', little finger: 'let go…'.

11. The right wrist: 'let go…'. The right forearm: 'let go…', the right upper arm: 'let go…'. The whole right arm: 'let go…'. Send a smile to your left arm. Your left back: 'let go…', the palm of your hand: 'let go…', your thumb: 'let go…', index finger: 'let go…', middle finger: 'let go…', ring finger: 'let go…', little finger: 'let go…'.

12. The left wrist: 'let go…'. The left forearm: 'let go…', the left upper arm: 'let go…'. Smile to your left arm: 'let go…'. Both arms: 'let go…'.

13. Focus on the front of the fuselage and send a smile. The lower abdomen: 'let go…', the upper abdomen: 'let go…', the chest: 'let go…'. The front of your neck: 'let go…'.

14. Send a smile to your face with your mouth: 'let go…', nose: 'let go…', tip of your nose: 'let go…', right cheek: 'let go…', left cheek: 'let go…'.

15. Both cheeks: 'let go…', right eyebrow: 'let go…', left eyebrow: 'let go…'. Both eyebrows: 'let go…', right eye: 'let go…', left eye: 'let go…', both eyes: 'let go…', forehead: 'let go…, the hairline down to the tips: 'let go…'. The back of the head: 'let go…'. The back of the neck: 'let go…'.

16. Focus on your whole body again. Watch how the whole body lies on the ground, smile and breath: 'Let go …'."

33.3.3   Transforming Shame Through Mindfulness

As the above remarks on mindfulness, health and shame have clearly shown, the regular practice of mindfulness exercises alone can lead to a transformation of potentially negative and distressing emotions such as toxic shame. But it is also conceivable that meditations can focus specifically on the transformation of shame. One such possibility is presented below. It would then follow a breathing and body scan exercise, so that a certain basic relaxation can be assumed.

Thích-Nhất-Hạnh (2011, 59) points out that there are three ways to transform suffering through mindfulness: one involves the possibility of "sowing and watering the seeds of happiness", the second is to practise constant mindfulness and so, the "seeds of the suffering are recognized as soon as they appear and to bathe them in the light of mindfulness, and

> the third way to deal with the suffering that has accompanied us since our childhood is to consciously invite these seeds into our mind consciousness. Forgetting, our regrets and longings, all the emotions that have touched us in the past have been very difficult for us, and we sit down and talk to them like old friends; but before we invite them, we need them safe so that the lamp of mindfulness burns brightly and continuously enough. (Thích-Nhất-Hạnh, 2011, 59)

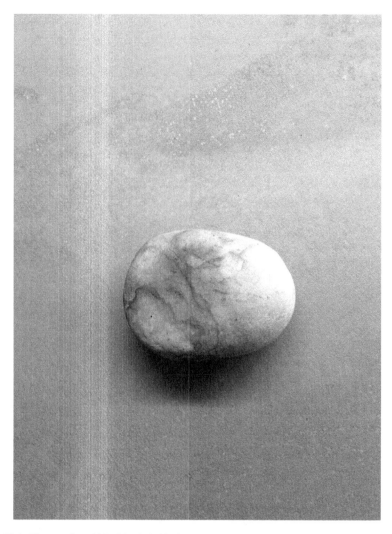

Fig. 33.1 Picture of a pebble (Vanderheiden)

Thích-Nhất-Hạnh points to a very central requirement, namely that this type of mindfulness exercise requires considerable prior experience!

It may be helpful for some people to look at the photo below before meditating, or to hold a real pebble in their hand and then let it drop before they begin to meditate (Fig. 1).

Exercise 1 Let (toxic) shame go

In addition to, and as a continuation of the body scan exercise, the feeling of shame can now be considered more closely. It is important to first perceive the shame, without evaluating it and, above all, without identifying with it. Recognise what thoughts and feelings are connected with shame, and just observe without rating them. And then, in a second step, let the shame go.

1. There is shame.
2. Watch the shame. What thoughts rise up in you? Just let the thoughts come and go like clouds in the sky. Do not try to rate them, just let them come and let go....
3. Is the shame particularly connected to a specific part of your body? Just observe, as if using a magnifying glass or a microscope. Do not rate.
4. Keep on breathing in and out ....
5. Observe and accept your thoughts and feelings about the shame as they are right now.
6. And let every single thought and every single emotion go as you are breathing out ... 'Let go...'.
7. If you find it difficult to let go of shame, imagine a pebble. Imagine you are standing by a lake. You raise your arm and throw the pebble, your shame, far into the water. Watch briefly as the pebble sinks. Breathing in and out ... As the pebble continues to sink into the depths of the water, what do you think, what do you feel?
8. Now the pebble has reached the bottom of the lake. What do you think or feel now? What has changed?
9. Stay for a while at 'your' lake, breathe calmly and feel relaxed. When the time is right for you, open your eyes again.

It may be useful to write down the thoughts and feelings that appeared during the meditation or to paint a picture. Another option could be to work on the pebble itself, painting it, or sculpting it (Mayer & Vanderheiden, 2016, 29–47).

Exercise 2 Acceptance of shame

A variation of this exercise could be to not only let the shame (with its negative emotional and mental implications) go, but to go one step further and actively accept it, for example by embracing shame, in the sense of the title of the book by Audre Lorde (2007): *Nothing I accept about myself can be used against me to diminish me* or inviting shame to dance. This can then be a real dance with shame that is incorporated into the meditation, or a dance as a purely mental thinking exercise.

Exercise 3 Reconciliation with shame and shamers

Handrock and Baumann (2017) justifiably point to the close connection between shame and forgiveness in their contribution to this book. Mindfulness can also make an important contribution in regard to this, for example through Mettā meditations. *Mettā* is a word from Pali, a language spoken during Buddha's lifetime; it means loving kindness and empathy. Mettā meditations have been practised in the Asian tradition for more than 2000 years and usually come into action in the established mindfulness programmes in the Western context at an advanced stage when a certain degree of self-compassion can be presupposed (Schuling et al., 2017, 2).

The intention of Mettā meditation is to create and maintain a stable field of loving kindness around oneself and gradually expand this field to others and all beings.

1. To practice Mettā, meditate on the following four sentences:

   May I be happy.
   May I feel safe and secure.
   May I be healthy.
   May I experience ease of well-being in my everyday life.

2. The extension takes place by sending these wishes also to humans or other organisms in your environment. Send your four sentences to someone you like, appreciate or love.

   May he/she/they be happy.
   May he/she/they feel safe and secure.
   May he/she/they be healthy.
   May he/she/they experience ease of well-being in their everyday life.

3. Afterwards you send the four wishes/blessings to a person with whom it is not easy for you to maintain a judgment-free relationship. You express your desires for those with whom you have had unpleasant experiences, for people who have hurt and shamed you, and for the entire environment, the entire world with all sentient beings.

   May he/she/they be happy.
   May he/she/they feel safe and secure.
   May he/she/they be healthy.
   May he/she/they experience ease of well-being in their everyday life.

4. The idea behind Mettā meditation is that you can liberate yourself from the person who hurt (and shamed) you. You do not have to deal so often with this person and their shaming. You accept him/her/them, wish him/her/them all the best and can liberate yourself mentally this way.
5. Mettā meditation is a sophisticated kind of meditation. But it can, like other forms of meditation—if regularly practised—provide a significant contribution to learning a different way of dealing with shame, transforming toxic into reinforcing shame, and generally being a crucial resource for resilience and well-being.

The Guest House

This being human is a guest house.
Every morning a new arrival.

A joy, a depression, a meanness,
some momentary awareness comes
as an unexpected visitor.

Welcome and entertain them all!
Even if they're a crowd of sorrows,
who violently sweep your house
empty of its furniture,
still, treat each guest honorably.
He may be clearing you out
for some new delight.

The dark thought, the shame,
the malice,
meet them at the door laughing,
and invite them in.

Be grateful for whoever comes,
because each has been sent
as a guide from beyond.

Jalāl al-Dīn Rūmī[4]

33.4   Conclusion

The health-promoting effect of a continuous mindfulness practice has been scientifically proven with regard to stress, burnout symptoms, nervousness, tension, pain, high blood pressure, heart problems, auto-immune and skin diseases and psychosomatic diseases, as well as depression, in view of usually negatively connoted emotions such as anxiety and shame, but also other mental stress disorders. A practice of mindfulness has a proven record of sustainable changes in attitudes about complaints and overall health awareness, as well as a new self-awareness and a new view of relationships with other people and the world. Various psychological research studies show that mindfulness leads to more sensitivity, concentration and openness to new experiences. It has been shown in this chapter that mindfulness can potentially turn shame into a resource for personal and social growth.

---

[4]Rumi and Barks (2004). *The essential Rumi*. San Francisco, CA: HarperSanFrancisco.

References

Amaro, A. (2015). A holistic mindfulness. *Mindfulness, 6*(1), 63–73.

Amaro, H., & Vallejo, Z. (2008). *Moment-by-moment in women's recovery: A mindfulness-based approach to relapse prevention.* Boston: SAMHSA & Northeastern University.

Bartels-Velthuis, A., Schroevers, M., van der Ploeg, K., Koster, F., Fleer, J., & van den Brink, E. (2016). A mindfulness-based compassionate living training in a heterogeneous sample of psychiatric outpatients: A feasibility study. *Mindfulness, 7*(4), 809–818.

Bishop, S. R., et al. (2004). Mindfulness: A proposed operational definition. *Clinical psychology: Science and practice, 11,* 230–241.

Briegleb, T. (2014). *Die diskrete scham.* Frankfurt: Insel Verlag.

Fredrickson, B. L., Cohn, M. A., Coffey, K. A., Pek, J., & Finkel, S. M. (2008). Open hearts build lives: Positive emotions, induced through loving-kindness meditation, build consequential personal resources. *Journal of Personality and Social Psychology, 95*(5), 1045–1062. https://doi.org/10.1037/a0013262.

Frewen, P., Rogers, N., Flodrowski, L., & Lanius, R. (2015). Mindfulness and metta-based trauma therapy (MMTT): Initial development and proof-of-concept of an internet resource. *Mindfulness, 6*(6), 1322–1334.

Germer, C., & Neff, K. (2013). Self-compassion in clinical practice. *Journal Of Clinical Psychology, 69*(8), 856–867. https://doi.org/10.1002/jclp.22021

Germer, C. K., Siegel, R. D., & Fulton, P. R. (2005). *Mindfulness and psychotherapy.* New York: Guilford Press.

Gilbert, P., & Procter, S. (2006). Compassionate mind training for people with high shame and self-criticism: Overview and pilot study of a group therapy approach. *Clinical Psychology and Psychotherapy, 13,* 353–379.

Gilbert, P., McEwan, K., Irons, C., Bhundia, R., Christie, R., Broomhead, C., et al. (2010). Self-harm in a mixed clinical population: The roles of self-criticism, shame, and social rank. *British Journal of Clinical Psychology, 49,* 563–576.

Handrock, A., & Baumann, M. (2017). *Vergeben und Loslassen in Psychotherapie und Coaching.* Weinheim, Basel: Beltz.

Hilgers, M. (2013). *Scham.* Göttingen: Vandenhoeck & Ruprecht.

Hoffman, S. G., Sawyer, A. T., Witt, A. A., & Oh, D. (2010). The effect of mindfulness-based therapy on anxiety and depression: A meta- analytic review. *Journal of Consulting and Clinical Psychology, 78,* 169–183. doi:https://doi.org/10.1037/a0018555.

Jazaieri, H., et al. (2013). Enhancing compassion: a randomized controlled trial of a compassion cultivation training program. *Journal of Happiness Studies, 14*(4), 1113–1126. doi:https://doi.org/10.1007/s10902-012-9373-z.

Kabat-Zinn, J. (1990). *Full catastrophe living.* London: Doubleday.

Keng, S., Smoski, M., & Robins, C. (2011). Effects of mindfulness on psychological health: A review of empirical studies. *Clinical Psychology Review, 31*(6), 1041–1056. doi:http://dx.doi.org/10.1016/j.cpr.2011.04.006.

Krishnamurthy, A. (2018). *Scham macht geschlecht* (p. 15). Opladen: Verlag Barbara Budrich.

Lorde, A. (2007). *Sister outsider* (p. 147). Berkeley: Crossing Press.

Mayer, C., & Vanderheiden, E. (2016). *Mediation in wandelzeiten* (pp. 29–47). Frankfurt: Peter Lang.

Neff, K. D., Germer, C. K. (2013). A pilot study and randomized controlled trial of the Mindful Self-Compassion Program. *Journal of Clinical Psychology, 69,* 28–44.

Oliver, M. (2004). *Wild geese.* Tarset: Bloodaxe.

Pace, T. W. W., et al. (2009). Effect of com- passion meditation on neuroendocrine, innate immune and behavioral responses to psychosocial stress. *Psychoneuroendocrinology, 34*(1), 87–98. doi:https://doi.org/10.1016/j.psyneuen.2008.08.011.

Pace, T., et al. (2010). Innate immune, neuroendocrine and behavioral responses to psychosocial stress do not predict subsequent compassion meditation practice time. *Psychoneuroendocrinology, 35*(2), 310–315. doi:http://dx.doi.org/10.1016/j.psyneuen.2009.06.008.

Pattakos, A. (2010). *Prisoners of our thoughts: Viktor Frankl's Principles for Discovering Meaning in Life and Work* (p. Foreword). San Francisco: Berrett-Koehler.

Rūmī, J. A. D., & Barks, C. (2004). *The essential Rumi*. San Francisco: HarperSanFrancisco.

Schuling, R., et al. (2017). The Co-creation and Feasibility of a Compassion Training as a Follow-up to Mindfulness-Based Cognitive Therapy in Patients with Recurrent Depression. *Mindfulness*.

Stjernswärd, S., & Hansson, L. (2016). Effectiveness and usability of a web-based mindfulness intervention for families living with mental illness. *Mindfulness, 8*(3), 751–764.

Tangney, J., & Dearing, R. (2002). *Shame and guilt*. New York: Guilford Press.

Hanh, T. N., & Richard, U. (2011). *Versöhnung mit dem inneren kind*. München: Barth.

Vanderheiden, E., & Mayer, C. (2017). *The value of shame*. Cham: Springer.

Woods, H., & Proeve, M. (2014). *Relationships of Mindfulness, Self-Compassion, and Meditation Experience With Shame-Proneness*. Retrieved from http://dx.doi.org/10.1891/0889-8391.28.1.20.

Elisabeth Vanderheiden (Second state examination) is a pedagogue, theologian, intercultural mediator, managing director of the Catholic Adult Education Rhineland-Palatinate, and the federal chairwoman of the Catholic Adult Education of Germany. She has published books and articles in the context of vocational qualifications, in particular qualification of teachers and trainers, as well as current topics of general, vocational, and civic education, and intercultural opening processes, mediation and shame. She lives in Germany and Florida.

Chapter 34
Healing Rituals to Transform Shame: An Example of Constellation Work

Claude-Hélène Mayer

Abstract Because shame is often a hidden and isolated experience, a mindful and conscious approach is needed in order to heal shame. This chapter deals with the healing ritual of constellation work to transform shame from a negative, challenging emotion into a health resource. The therapeutic method and ritual of constellation work allows for the identification of shame within its systemic context and its conscious exploration. Insight is offered into this powerful healing ritual and tool which explores and transforms shame, not only at an individual level, but also within a therapeutic group context.

Keywords Shame · Ritual · Healing · Transformation · Constellation work · Systemic therapy

34.1 Introduction

According to Nelson (2016), it is very natural for individuals to hide and isolate themselves when experiencing shame. However, shame requires a conscious and mindful approach in order to heal. Healing is thereby understood as a process which allows the building of positive qualities within an individual (Seligman & Csikszentmihalyi, 2000) to overcome disempowerment and the escape mechanisms which are often used by the person who feels ashamed (Masters, 2016).

Rituals are culturally defined practices (Wong & Tsai, 2007). They are socially and culturally transmitted, historically influenced and, according to Strickland (1997), are often based on community rather than on individual mores. Rituals are used in therapeutic practice (Imber-Black, 2002) and the power of rituals in various therapeutical contexts such as family therapy (Palazzoli, Boscolo, Cechin, & Prata, 1977)

C.-H. Mayer (✉)
Institut für Therapeutische Kommunikation und Sprachgebrauch, Europa Universität Viadrina, Logenstrasse 11, 15230 Frankfurt (Oder), Germany
e-mail: claudemayer@gmx.net

Department of Management, Rhodes University, Drosdy Road, Grahamstown 6139, South Africa

© Springer Nature Switzerland AG 2019
C.-H. Mayer and E. Vanderheiden (eds.), *The Bright Side of Shame*,
https://doi.org/10.1007/978-3-030-13409-9_34

521

or focused mind training (Gilbert & Irons, 2005) in different cultural contexts, has been widely emphasised and discussed.

This chapter presents the example of constellation work (CW) as a therapeutic tool and healing ritual for working with shame. CW has been successfully used within the family therapy context for clients to overcome and constructively work with shame. By applying the described ritual, healing processes are initiated which help to understand systemic influences on the experience of shame. Further, CW can help to transform self-criticism and the experience of the destructive emotion of shame in collective and socio-cultural contexts. CW, used in family therapy in a selected cultural context, will be described to show how shame can be addressed and transformed constructively.

34.2   Constellation Work as a Therapeutical Approach to Healing

CW is an experimental, psychotherapeutic approach which has been used in international therapeutic contexts since the 1980s (Anderson & Carnabucci, 2009; Mayer & Viviers, 2015a, 2015b). Payne (2005) describes CW as an intergenerational healing process and ritual work which uses a systemic approach to heal. In their book *Salutogene Aufstellungen*, Mayer and Hausner (2015) explain the ways in which CW can contribute to health through systemic intervention work, and how CW can affect the development of mental and physical health and well-being. This form of healing works with representations of the unconscious dynamics in systems such as family systems, systems of health and illness, or organisational systems.

CW has been described as a specific process (Cohen, 2008) which usually takes place in a group context. According to Cohen (2008), CW often involves from ten up to 30 individuals who participate voluntarily as clients, representatives or observers of the process. One group member (the client) then works on a specific issue which they would like to resolve within a systemic context.

In the beginning of the group CW process, the CW facilitator talks to a selected client, asking questions such as "What would you like to work on?" or "Who is involved in this situation?" The facilitator will explore more general questions with regard to the system and specific events in the system (e.g. sudden death, suicide, abortion, murder, causalities of war) which might influence the client and the current situation unconsciously. Group members are then used to represent individuals involved (e.g. mother, brother, husband) or as representatives of structural, abstract or otherwise materialised elements such as an illness, a symbol, a feeling, a burden, a pain, a place or location.

After the initial, usually brief talk with the facilitator, the client then selects representatives for the individuals or elements involved, and gives them a physical location within the room (Cohen, 2008). The individual representatives are then usually able to access feelings, thoughts, images or behavioural patterns within the context and system of the CW (Ulsamer, 2005; Schneider, 2007). The facilitator explores the emotions, thoughts, observations and impressions of the representatives by asking questions, or by asking for comments. Throughout the CW process, representatives are asked to take different positions. The aim at the end of the process, is to find a solution which is perceived by the system as a healing movement. This image of resolution at the end of a CW session needs to include a position for all representatives which is ideal for the individuals, as well as for the entire system. At the end of the process, the solution for the issue or problem is consciously acknowledged, while the issue/problem is released. The final images of the solution and ideal systemic situation is taken into account by the representatives, by the entire system and certainly by the client (Cohen, 2008).

CW makes use of ritual elements such as ritual gestures or ritual sentences, and can even be described as a group process ritual (Hunger, Weinhold, Bornhäuser, Link, & Schweitzer, 2010; Stiefel, Harris, & Zollmann, 2002), which includes strong individual and collective healing powers (Van Kampenhout, 2008).

Shame in CW can be recognised with regard to the constellation of shame within a person and within the constellation of the self[1] (Morrison, 1983). This might be the case when, for example in CW, individuals constellate parts of the self or identity or ego states (as described in Huyssen, 2015). However Anderson and Carnabucci (2009) also describe how shame in the context of family and suicide has led in one of their constellation cases to identification of the client with a family member who was shamed and committed suicide. This identification with the shame and the "victim" led to specific unconscious patterns of behaviour, emotions and thoughts in the client. The shame had been transferred over generations. Payne (2006) also describes how a client in CW managed to accept shame within his systemic context, and the consequences of shame in order to promote healing.

Shame has been recognised in descriptions of particular cases in CW practice. However, no research is available that specifically studies shame and its transformation in CW, nor does the chapter at hand study shame or how it is transformed in CW. Instead, this chapter provides insight into a detailed description of a CW case and how the constellation facilitator and the client worked with shame through CW.

34.3 My Context of Working with Constellation Work

Since 1998, I have attended several CW workshops internationally. My training as a CW facilitator took place in Germany over a period of two years and since then I have used CW in independent workshops, as well as in my systemic (family) therapy practice. I have found it to be a powerful ritual and tool in different therapeutical settings, working with individuals, but also working with couples and families. Further,

---

[1]I understand "the self" here as a person's essential being which distinguishes them from others and which includes personality characteristics, as well as ability, a person's attributes and an understanding and personal belief about who and what the self is (Baumeister, 1999).

I have led one- and two-day CW sessions with participants from various cultural contexts who aimed to resolve issues and problems through CW. Recently I have reflected upon the universality and/or culture-specifics of CW and have described the similarities and differences I have experienced in both German and South African CW settings (Mayer, 2018 in press).

As observed by Perry (2011), I too have witnessed that the topic of shame is often present in CW sessions and can be carried forward through generations. Shame is seldom mentioned by the clients themselves; rather, it occurs during the CW process and is named by the representatives. Shame is often not explicitly tackled within a CW process, but is treated as a side effect of other systemic dynamics. The following description, however, is of a CW case aiming specifically to transform shame.

34.4 Description of a Constellation Work Process Dealing with Shame

Here I describe the setting of the CW process, the client and the process of CW itself in this case which took place in Germany. My focus is on the interventions made with regard to resolving shame from a systemic perspective for the client and the family system. The topic of shame was mentioned as one of the core aspects the client wanted to resolve through family CW.

34.4.1 The Client

The client, U, was a male 43-year-old US citizen who had lived in Germany for the past 12 years. He was born in Miami, Florida, where, at the time of the workshop, his parents were still alive. He is the second-born of three children, with one elder sister and one younger brother.

At the age of 15, U realised that he was only interested in men – that he was homosexual. In the CW, he described this self-acknowledgement of "being gay" as a very difficult process, particularly since he was brought up in a "very traditional Christian mindset" in which homosexuality was taboo. In retrospect, he knew that he felt deeply ashamed of himself and did not see any way to deal with his homosexuality other than to "live far away from the family, so they could not find out". U left the US at the age of 18 without having told his parents about his sexual orientation. He had lived in various countries, searching for a place in which he could feel acknowledged, safe and accepted. However, in the workshop, 25 years later, he had to recognise that he had not found this "safe place", that he had lived in five different countries in the meantime, and that he was tired of searching without really knowing what to search for.

34.4.2 The Issue

In conversation with the facilitator, U said that through the CW, he wanted to "get rid of the feeling of shame for my sexual orientation" that he had carried since he was 15 years old. He had also left his job some weeks before to prepare to move back to the US, not particularly to Florida, but to California where a new job opportunity had opened up. He wanted to tell his parents about his homosexuality to find inner peace, and he hoped for acceptance from his parents.

34.4.3 The Constellation

The facilitator explored the topic of shame in the conversation upfront in more depth, asking questions, such as "Where do you find shame in your family of origin?", "What exactly are you ashamed about?", "When did the shame start?", "Who would it most matter to if you had transformed your shame in the family system?", "Could the shame also belong to anyone else in the family system?", "Who in the family does not care about your shame at all?", "Are there any extraordinary situations in your family of origin that happened in this or previous generations?" "Is there anything else notable you would like to add?".

After conversation about and exploration of the shame in the client's context, the facilitator decided to "constellate the index client", the father, the mother and the shame. The person representing shame was placed right in front of the client's representative, staring straight into his face, with about 20 cm between them (see CWI).[2] The father and mother stood next to each other, first looking at U's representative, then making a movement to turn around to look into another direction (see CWII). The representative of U also turned around and wanted to run away (taking a few steps out of the context of the family), closely followed by the shame representative. U's representative could not rest or stand in any particular place (Fig. 34.1).

The facilitator then worked with the individual representatives. Both mother and father said that they felt very ashamed of their son without knowing why. The shame representative had at this point in time put his arms around U's representative, holding him close (see CWII). U could hardly breathe and felt he had to move further away (Fig. 34.2).

In the following phase, the client, U, found a representative for the issue of homosexuality and placed the representative at his right side (CWIII). This made the shame representative move and turn around, staring at the father, moving a step in his direction. The mother said that she did not want to turn around, while the father said he felt suddenly very attracted to the shame representative. The shame representative also felt that he wanted to move closer towards the father, experiencing a feeling of belonging (Fig. 34.3).

---

[2] F = Father, M = Mother, U = Representative of client, Shame, Homosexuality. The arrow indicates the direction of the view and body of the representative. CWI = Constellation Work phase 1.

Fig. 34.1 Process Step 1
(Author's own construction)

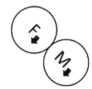

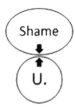

Fig. 34.2 Process Step 2
(Author's own construction)

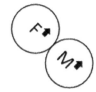

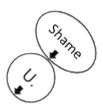

Fig. 34.3 Process Step 3
(Author's own construction)

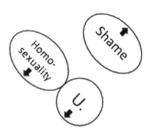

Fig. 34.4 Process Step 4
(Author's own construction)

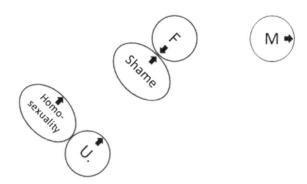

U's representative could breathe and felt much freer than before, but did not want to turn around to look at the situation behind him. He felt happy with the representative of homosexuality next to him, close.

The father and the shame representatives moved towards each other, holding hands soon after, while the mother turned in another direction, creating more distance from the father. At this point, U could turn around, holding onto the homosexuality representative who also turned around, both witnessing the situation (Fig. 34.4).

Through all stages of the process, the facilitator asked the representatives about their feelings, their thoughts, the changes in their bodies and physical perceptions and explored if the representatives felt better or worse after specific movements and dynamics within the system.

In the meantime, the facilitator always reconfirmed with U how he was feeling at the different stages, sometimes asking questions regarding of the transfer of information of the process. For example: "Were you aware that the shame seems to belong to your father originally?" or "Is there anything you know about your father's past which fits with this image?" U was very surprised at the movements and at the same time seemed to feel relieved, while the representative sat down, crying and staring at the shame and at the representative of the father.

The facilitator worked through several more interventions and exchanges of ritual. These were in the form of ritual sentences spoken out loud, such as "She is mine" (father), "Thank you for carrying the shame" (father), "Without you carrying it, I would have left long ago (mother), "I carried it for your marriage, but now I am free" (U), "I always belong to you—I am yours." (shame speaking to the father).

The final image was of U's representative standing in the middle of the room facing forward, the father to his left, and the mother behind them, on his right, looking at the two in acknowledgement. The shame found its place behind the father (CWV).

The facilitator ended the solution image at this stage and explained that she would not work further with the shame of the father since the father was not here and that she would respect the limits of this CW for U at this stage (Fig. 34.5).

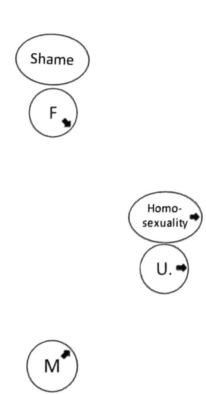

Fig. 34.5 Process Step 5 (Author's own construction)

U thanked all the representatives and released them from their representative roles. He reported that he felt very relieved, having seen that the shame did not actually belong to him and appeared to be unconnected to his homosexuality. Instead, he noted that the shame was a part of his father's history. However, he also felt sad that he had run away for many years without realising that he was carrying systemic content, the shame, of the previous generation (or even further back, since it might be possible that his father was also a carrier of shame from previous generations). U felt better about his homosexuality and emphasised that it was a good decision to "return home to the US." He felt confident about telling his parents about his sexual orientation after his return.

Since U was relieved of the burden of shame, he could see the shame (now at his father's side) as an acceptable aspect of his father and therefore could accept the shame he had experienced in the context of his homosexuality more easily. His father had become "more human" in his eyes and he now felt connected to his father. He also recognised that he had left home for his mother to be able to stay.[3]

U concluded that his future steps would probably be to accept his homosexuality at even deeper levels of his identity, accept himself the way he was, and forgive himself for having taken on the systemic shame with such consequences for his life and his movements in life. He expected that it would take some time for him to deeply reconcile with the shame and with his behaviour, based on the experience of shame, and then to turn this shame experience into a fruitful, acceptable and acknowledgeable experience and a health resource with growth and learning potential.

34.5   Conclusion

This example of CW with shame, as described, indicates that shame can be an issue that is passed down unconsciously by individuals through generations, if not resolved and acknowledged. When left in the unconscious, shame experiences in systems might strongly influence behaviour, thoughts and feelings of individuals. Often, clients who are at a distance (spatial, physical or in time) from those in whose context shame was first experienced, can explore shame consciously and on an in-depth level.

Shame, as a taboo topic in many cultures, needs to be understood and explored in terms of culture-specific knowledge by using an appropriate approach. CW, used as an intercultural intervention tool, might offer a practical way to transform shame in systemic contexts while working with unconscious content, turning it into a conscious health resource.

References

Anderson, R., & Carnabucci, K. (2009). *The challenge and promise for psychodrama of systemic constellation work*. Retrieved from http://www.awakening.com.au/download/diploma_library/SYS303%20Systemic%20Constellations/SystemicConstellationWorkand_Psychodrama.pdf.
Baumeister, R. F. (Ed.). (1999). *The self in social psychology*. Philadelphia: Psychology Press (Taylor & Francis).
Cohen, D. B. (2008). *Systemic family constellations and the use with prisoners serving long-term sentences for murder or rape*. Doctoral thesis, Unpublished. Saybrook Graduate School and Research Center, San Fransisco.
Gilbert, P., & Irons, C. (2005). Focussed therapies and compassionate mind training for shame and self-attacking. In P. Gilbert (Ed.), *Compassion. Conceptualisations, research and use in psychotherapy*. New York: Routledge.

[3]In CW we can see that often a family member leaves as a representative for another family member who would like/would have liked to leave (but could or did not due to different reasons).

Hunger, C., Weinhold, J., Bornhäuser, A., Link, L., & Schweitzer, J. (2010). Mid- and long-term effects of family constellation seminars in a general population sample: 8- and 12 month follow-up. *Family Process, 54*(2), 344–358.

Huyssen, K. (2015). Aufstellungen nach dem Modell der Ego-State-Therapie als salutogenetischer Integrationsprozess. In C.-H. Mayer & S. Hausner (Eds.), *Salutogene Aufstellungen. Beiträge zur Gesundheitsförderung aus der systemischen Arbeit* (pp. 173–188). Göttingen: Vandenhoeck and Ruprecht.

Imber-Black, E. (2002). Family rituals-from research to the consulting room and back again: Comment on the special section. *Journal of Family Psychology, 16*(4), 445–446. Retrieved from http://dx.doi.org/10.1037/0893-3200.16.4.445.

Masters, R. (2016). *Shame: From toxic collapse to healing exposure.* http://robertmasters.com/writings/shame-from-toxic-collapse-to-healing-exposure.

Mayer, C.-H., & Hausner, S. (2015). *Salutogene Aufstellungen. Beiträge zur Gesundheitsförderung aus der systemischen Arbeit.* Göttingen: Vandenhoeck and Ruprecht.

Mayer, C.-H., & Viviers, R. (2015a). Exploring cultural issues for constellation work in South Africa. Australian and New Zealand. *Journal of Family Therapy, 36,* 289–306.

Mayer, C.-H., & Viviers, R. (2015b). Constellation work principles, resonance phenomena and shamanism in South Africa. *South African Journal of Psychology, 46*(1), 130–145.

Mayer, C.-H. (2018). Reflektionen über universelle und kulturspezifische Aspekte der Aufstellungsarbeit. In K. Nazarkiewicz, & P. Boquin (Eds.), *Einflüsse der Welt—individuelles Schicksal im kollektiven Kontext. Praxis der Systemaufstellungen* (pp. 115–129). Göttingen: Vandenhoeck & Ruprecht.

Morrison, A. (1983). Shame, ideal self, and narcissism. *Contemporary Psychoanalysis, 19,* 295–318.

Nelson, H. D. (2016). *Unashamed: Healing our brokenness and finding freedom from shame.* Crossway: Wheaton.

Palazzoli, M. S., Boscolo, L., Cechin, G. F., & Prata, G. (1977). Family rituals a powerful tool in family therapy. *Family Process, 16*(4), 445–453.

Payne, J. L. (2005). *The healing of individuals, families and nations.* Findhorn: Findhorn Press.

Payne, J. L. (2006). *The language of the soul: Healing with words of truth.* Dyke Forres: Findhorn Press.

Perry, B. D. (2011). *Adoption and systemic constellation work. Doctoral dissertation.* Pro Quest Dissertations Publishing, Michigan, USA.

Schneider, J. (2007). *Family constellations basic principles.* Heidelberg: Carl-Auer-Systeme Verlag.

Seligman, M. E., & Csikszentmihalyi, M. (2000). Positive psychology: An introduction. *American Psychologist, 55*(1), 5–14. https://doi.org/10.1037//0003-066x.55.1.5.

Stiefel, I., Harris, P., & Zollmann, A. W. F. (2002). Family constellation–a therapy beyond words. *Australian & New Zealand Journal of Family Therapy.* https://www.newpathspsychology.com.au/wp-content/uploads/2015/10/Ingeborg-Stiefel_Australian_New-Zealand-Journal-of-Family-Therapy.pdf.

Strickland, R. (1997). Wolf warriors and turtle kings: Native American law before the blue coats. *Washington Law Review Association, 72,* 1043.

Ulsamer, B. (2005). *The Healing Power of the Past: The Systemic Therapy of Bert Hellinger.* Nevada City: Underwood.

Van Kampenhout, D. (2008). *Die Heilung kommt von außerhalb. Schamnismus und Familien-Stellen* (3rd ed.). Heidelberg: Carl Auer Verlag.

Wong, Y., & Tsai, J. L. (2007). Cultural models of shame and guilt. In J. Tracy, R. Robins, & J. Tangney (Eds.), *Handbook of self-conscious emotions* (pp. 209–223). New York: Guilford Press.

Claude-Hélène Mayer (Dr. habil., PhD, PhD) is a Professor in Industrial and Organisational Psychology at the Department of Industrial Psychology and People Management at the University of Johannesburg, an Adjunct Professor at the Europa Universität Viadrina in Frankfurt (Oder), Germany and a Senior Research Associate in the Department of Management at Rhodes University, Grahamstown, South Africa. She holds a Ph.D. in psychology (University of Pretoria, South Africa), a Ph.D. in management (Rhodes University, South Africa), a Doctorate in political sciences (Georg-August-Universität, Göttingen, Germany), and a Habilitation with a Venia Legendi (Europa Universität Viadrina, Germany) in psychology with focus on work, organizational, and cultural psychology. She has published numerous monographs, edited text books, accredited journal article, and special issues on transcultural mental health, salutogenesis and sense of coherence, shame, transcultural conflict management and mediation, women in leadership in culturally diverse work contexts, constellation work, coaching, and psychobiography.

Chapter 35
Discussion of HeartMath Techniques for the Transformation of Shame Experiences

Stephen D. Edwards

Abstract Shame may be generally defined as painful feelings and negative emotions, related to stressful experiences and psychological states such as anxiety, depression and aggression, which may impede ongoing positive experiences and feelings such as contentment, peacefulness and happiness. Shame experiences may also constitute source of resilience and health. The HeartMath system refers to scientific, evidence based self-regulation techniques that were specifically designed to be used in the moment to relieve stress, improve resilience and promote positive feelings, sense of coherence, health and performance. HeartMath techniques are informed by a large body of scientific research indicating that neural signals from the heart affect the brain centres involved in emotional self-regulation. Skill acquisition of HeartMath techniques is facilitated through heart rate variability (HRV) and heart rhythm coherence feedback training, heart focussed breathing and intentional generation of associated positive emotional feelings, emotional imagery, and remembered wellness. Perusal of the extensive HeartMath Research library indicates that the issue of shame has not been exclusively addressed. Various rigorous studies have indicated significant effectiveness of HeartMath practice in decreasing guilt as well other negative emotions as well as promoting positive feelings and resilience. The aim of the chapter is to explore the research hypothesis as to the effectiveness of HeartMath techniques to transform shame feelings. Specific techniques to address negative emotions, manage stress, promote positive feelings and build resilience will be discussed.

Keywords HeartMath · Shame · Stress · Feelings · Resilience

S. D. Edwards (✉)
Psychology Department, University of Zululand, 3 Antigua, 32 Chartwell Drive, Umhlanga
Rocks, KwaDlangezwa 4319, South Africa
e-mail: sdedward@telkomsa.net

© Springer Nature Switzerland AG 2019   533
C.-H. Mayer and E. Vanderheiden (eds.), *The Bright Side of Shame*,
https://doi.org/10.1007/978-3-030-13409-9_35

35.1   Introduction

Vanderheiden and Mayer (2017) have provided a comprehensive introduction to the value of shame as health resource in diverse cultural contexts. In keeping with the Institute of HeartMath (2014) model, the present discussion adopts a broad energetic approach to shame. It focusses on shame as a form of emotion (e-motion or energy in motion), immediately experienced subjectively as feelings and secondarily as emotions or relatively congealed feeling clusters. Feelings and emotions are never isolated but also associated with sensations, perceptions, cognitions and the full range of related experiences and behaviours of human beings in all their personal, social and wider worlds. Thus whether concerned with shameful feelings that are negative, positive, neutral, moral or mixed, an energetic approach implies opportunities for transformation and change, both in the moment as well as enduring over time. As negative emotion, shame experiences include major feeling clusters of anxiety, depression and anger, as well as their common variations, such as sadness, boredom, worry, frustration etc. As behavioural script, shame includes avoidance, withdrawal, attack self and attack other scripts as explicated by the Compass of Shame Scale (Elison, Lennon, & Pulos, 2006) (Elison, in this book). The HeartMath model is specifically concerned with the transformation of negative into positive energy patterns, in this case negative into neutral and positive feelings of shame. As energetic model it recognizes that each negatively perceived shameful feeling contains polarity seeds which present opportunities for transformation. Thus anxiety readily transforms into excitement, depression and loneliness into opportunities for connecting with greater Self and/or Being, anger into assertiveness, neutral into contented feelings. The following section is concerned with theoretical background and mechanisms for such transformations.

35.2   Theoretical Anchoring

The HeartMath Institute refers to an international scientific research and educational organization, with central vision and mission of promoting personal, social and global coherence (Institute of HeartMath, 2014). The HeartMath system refers to self-regulation techniques that can be used in the moment to relieve stress, improve resilience, health and well-being, as well as sport performance, while promoting what athletes describe as zone experiences. These techniques are informed by a large body of scientific research indicating that neural signals from the heart affect the brain centres involved in emotional self-regulation (McCraty & Shaffer, 2015). Skill acquisition of HeartMath techniques is facilitated through the use of heart rate variability (HRV) and heart rhythm coherence feedback training, heart focussed breathing and intentional generation of associated positive emotional feelings, emotional imagery, and remembered wellness (McCraty & Zayas, 2014). Based on Pribram's (2011) pattern recognition theory of emotion, it is hypothesized that HeartMath techniques use the heart as point of entry to facilitate neural identification of changes in the pattern of afferent cardiac signals sent to the brain and its associated cortical electrophysiological activity respectively.

Psychophysiological research continues to provide evidence that the vital role of the heart transcends physics and metaphor. The importance of bidirectional communication between the heart and the brain has been known for over 100 years (MacKinnon, Gevirtz, McCraty, & Brown, 2013). In addition to its sensory, organic functions, the heart has become recognized as a sophisticated information processing centre, with an intrinsic nervous system, capable of making autonomous, functional decisions (McCraty, Atkinson, Tomasino, & Bradley, 2009). Through its transmission of dynamic patterns of neurological, hormonal, pressure and electromagnetic information to the brain and throughout the body, the heart possesses a more extensive communication system with the brain than other organs (McCraty et al., 2009). Heart rate variability (HRV) performs a vital communicative function in this regard. A measure of naturally occurring beat-to-beat changes in heart rate, HRV is generated largely by interaction between the heart and brain via neural signals flowing through pathways of the sympathetic and parasympathetic (vagal) branches of the autonomic nervous system (ANS). These neural pathways, often respectively likened to the accelerator and break in a motor car, have different heart rhythm oscillatory patterns associated with their varying frequency bands, as discussed below in very simplified form.

Heart rate variability (HRV) is considered as a measure of neurocardiac function that reflects heart-brain interactions and ANS dynamics. It has great value as an index of adaptation, resilience and general health, owing to its resonant interconnections with psychophysiology in particular and the cosmos in general. HRV oscillations are typically dived into frequency bands, which include the high frequency (HF) from 0.15 to .4 Hz, low frequency (LF) between .04 and .15 Hz and very low frequency (VLF) band between .0033 and .04 Hz. The HF band reflects vagal parasympathetic activity. It is often referred to as the respiratory band because it corresponds to heart rate variations related to the respiratory cycle. The LF band has been called the baroreceptor band as it reflects resting blood pressure related stretch receptor activity. The heart produced VLF band, which relates to heat and hormone regulation, appears to be fundamental to health (Lehrer & Gevirtz, 2014).

The HeartMath psychophysiological coherence model postulates synchronization between positive emotions, cardiovascular, respiratory, and immune and nervous systems (McCraty et al., 2009). The model is based on research indicating that the heart's rhythm co-varies, not only with respiration, blood pressure and physical exercise, but also, independently, with positive emotions, which tend to naturally induce a rhythmic HRV sine wave pattern associated with increasing energy renewing hormone dehydroepiandrosterone production. Counteracting the energy depleting stress hormone of cortisol. (McCraty & Shaffer, 2015). The varying pattern of intervals between heart beats also produces a communicative Morse type signalling effect into the wider environment. This is the basic postulate of the Global Coherence Initiative (GCI) which will be discussed later.

35.3 There are Three Other HRV Related Psychophysiological Theories, Which All Offer Complementary Perspectives

Firstly, polyvagal theory is evolutionary and social in orientation, relating autonomic flexibility to experience in social interaction (Porges, 2011). The postulated
autonomic function hierarchy includes the ancient unmyelinated system, with a distribution to viscera below the diaphragm, and the evolutionarily recent "smart" vagus,
and distribution involving organs and muscles above the diaphragm, consisting of
myelinated nerve fibres, with a distinct central nucleus in the brainstem, the Nucleus
Ambiguus (NA). Porges (2011) postulates the "vagal brake" as a key functional mechanism during social engagement. This also implicates respiratory sinus arrhythmia
(RSA) a dynamic, naturally occurring, physiological mechanism, whereby heart rate
increases during inhalation and decreases during exhalation. Consequently Porges
advocates the measurement and enhancement of (RSA), as high amplitudes of HRV
have important implications for health and well-being.

Secondly, resonance theory is based on the physical principle that all oscillating
feedback systems with constant delay produce resonance characteristics. At rest,
phase relationships between respiration and heart rate (HR) are not synchronous,
possibly for reasons of organismic adaptability, as HR increases at about inhalation
mid-point and decreases at about exhalation mid-point. However, collaborative, respiration based, heart rate variability biofeedback (HRVB) research (Lehrer & Gevirtz,
2014). has indicated that maximal increases in amplitude of heart rate oscillation are
produced when the cardiovascular system (CVS) is rhythmically stimulated by paced
breathing at a frequency of about 0.1 Hz (about 5–7 breath cycles per minute). Substantial research evidence has confirmed that this resonant frequency, zero degree
phase relationship, is also associated with multiple other benefits, including most
efficient gas exchange in lung alveoli and optimal, baroreceptor related, blood pressure.

Thirdly, the Neurovisceral Integration Model (Thayer & Lane, 2000, 2009)
describes a central autonomic network (CAN) linking the brain stem NST (Nucleus of
the Solitary Tract) with forebrain anterior cingulate, insula, ventromedial prefrontal
cortex, amygdala and hypothalamus. The model postulates that vagally mediated
HRV is associated with higher executive regulation via a positive correlation; when
the CAN increases prefrontal cortical activation, HR decreases and HRV increases.
Alternatively, stress related, sympathetic autonomic overactivity is associated with
prefrontal cortical inactivity (Thayer, Ahs, Fredrikson, Sollers, & Wagner, 2012).
The model thus supports and extends the polyvagal theory of the importance of the
"vagal brake" operating in relation to higher level social, cognitive, affective, and
physiological regulation (Table 35.1).

All psychophysiological perspectives recognize the central role of heart in relation
to the ANS and emotional life. Derived from the Latin term, "movere"- "to move," the
word, emotion, literally means "energy in motion". In phenomenological terms, what
we think of as emotion is the experience of energy moving through our bodies that

Table 35.1 Heart rate variabilitiy mechanism, theories and models (Author's own construction)

Heart rate variability mechanis, theories and models
Respiratory Sinus Arrhythmia (RSA) is a naturally occurring physiological mechanism.
HeartMath Coherence Model indicates synchronization between physiological systems.
Neuroviscreral Integration Model postulates a Central Autonomic Network.
Polyvagal Theory is based on evolutionary and social communicative factors.
Resonance Theory describes oscillating feedback systems produce resonance.

generates ANS related physiological and mental reactions, as experienced in such strong feelings as love, joy, sorrow or anger. Feelings generally refer to a vast array of more subtle conscious experiences and sensations. In itself, emotional energy is neutral. Physiological reactions, feelings and thoughts give emotion meaning. Scientific research has repeatedly confirmed that reactive emotional energy manifests in brain activity before thought, that we live in a fundamentally pathic or feeling world, and tend to evaluate everything emotionally as we perceive it before thinking about it afterwards (Childre & Martin, 1999).

Coherence is a key concept in HeartMath research and praxis. The umbrella concept of coherence refers to a psychophysiological mode that encompasses entrainment, resonance, and synchronization—distinct but related phenomena, all of which emerge from the harmonious activity and interactions of the body's subsystems. The coherent mode is reflected by a smooth, sine wave-like pattern in the heart rhythms and a narrow-band, high-amplitude peak in the low frequency range of the heart rate variability power spectrum, at a frequency of about 0.1 Hz, which is also the resonant frequency of the planet via the earth's magnetic field. In practical healing terms, positive emotions and heart focussed breathing at about six breath cycles per minute facilitate vast interconnectivity (Childre, Martin, Rozman, & McCraty, 2016). In 2008, the GCI was launched to promote global health and well-being through heart-focused care. In pursuit of this mission a global network of ultrasensitive magnetic field detectors are being installed strategically around the planet to provide data on relationships involving physical, animal, human, planetary and cosmic ecologies. At present five sites are operational. Conceptual and practical implications of this initiative with special reference to global healing can be found on the websites: www.Heartmath.org and www.glcoherence.org.

35.4   Contextual Descriptions

Over the centuries, the heart has been recognized as a centre and source of spiritual, intellectual and emotional life in all cultures. For example, Yoga postulates that life-energy flows up and down the spine in terms of three main energetic pathways, called Ida, Pingala and Sushmna. Ida carries prana in the form of feminine lunar along the left side of the body, Pingala transmits masculine solar energy along the right side and Sushumna runs up the middle of the body connecting seven spinning energy wheels called chakras. The chakras are associated with particular anatomical locations of the spine and brain, plexuses of the nervous, endocrine and other human functional systems, as well as colours, sounds, patterns and symbols (Judith, 2004). For example, from perineum to crown, the chakras: muladhara, svadisthana, manipura, anahata, vishudda, ajna and sahasrara are respectively associated with systemic functions of elimination, reproduction, digestion, circulation, respiration, enervation and ultimate realisation through relation with the cosmos. As central, heart chakra for love and compassion, anahata expresses unconditional love for spirit, consciousness and all creation (Judith, 2004). Very similar healing patterns exist in traditional Chinese medicine, especially Taoist chi-gung, which emphasizes subtle consciousness/breath/energy work and/or exercises in relation to the lower, central and upper tan tien (Reid, 1998).

Similar recognition is given to the central, balancing, harmonising and subtle energetic function of the heart in other wisdom, spiritual and healing traditions. The Buddhist heart sutra extolls ultimate enlightenment through the union of emptiness and form, realized through loving kindness meditation and action. Judaic energy centres (sefirot) include the beauty, balance and harmony of the heart (tiffer et). In the Kabbalah, the heart is central sphere that touches all others (Childre & Martin, 2000). In Christian Heychastic traditions, the Prayer if the Heart involves differentiated focus on the human heart and the continuous repetition of a phrase, or the name of a Deity, with breath paced focus on the sense of self in the chest (Louchakova, 2007a, 2007b). A similar practice is found in Islamic Sufi traditions. For Bourgeault (2016, 5), the tripartite physical, emotional and spiritual organ of the human heart ultimately functions as "homing magnetic center" for a vital neurological shift in the mechanics of perception from the ordinary binary modes of dualistic consciousness to that nondual, holographic resonant heart, whereby one senses a single unified field, and is enabled to "see from wholeness". Although heart based practices such as Bhakti yoga and Prayer of the Heart have existed for millennia, it could be argued that never before have these been as scientifically grounded as is the case with HeartMath praxis and the GCI.

35.5 HeartMath Techniques and Tools to Transform Shameful Experiences

A practical energetics approach underlies HeartMath techniques and tools. Emphasis is on awareness of energy depletion, renewal and resilience in preparing for challenges, as well as shifting and resetting feelings after challenges, through sustained, regular HeartMath practice. HeartMath research has established that positive emotions are associated with psychophysiological coherence independently of respiration. However slower heart focussed breathing at about 10 s cardio-respiratory rhythm remains a practical, first step in most tools in order to modulate the heart's rhythmic activity and facilitate identification and focus on a particular positive emotion (McCraty & Zayas, 2014).

Depletion to Renewal Grid. The technique can be practised in relation to a visualized energy graph of the autonomic nervous system along the vertical axis and hormonal system along the horizontal axis. On the vertical axis, sympathetic activation yields high heart rates and parasympathetic relaxation rate yields low heart rates, while along the horizontal axis, depleting, negative emotions are associated with stress hormone, cortisol, and renewing positive emotions with growth hormone, dehydroepiandrosterone or DHEA (Childre & Martin, 1999; Institute of HeartMath, 2014; McCraty & Zayas, 2014). The technique can be used to assist with insight as to stressful effect of shame as emotion that could be given undue significance through cognitive appraisal as to threatening experiences and contexts as well as develop insight into the deleterious effect of stress hormones such a cortisol, the effect of which can last for eighteen hours in the body. On the other hand healthy hormones such as DHEA that increases significantly through the practice of such HeartMath techniques such as Cut-Thru and Heart Lock-In or tools such as emWave, emWave Pro and Inner Balance, practice of which can protect the body for up to 6 h.

Heart Focussed Breathing is valuable as immediate technique to improve consciousness and develop concentration. It is an immediate antidote to the evolutionary emotional default mode network expressed in the form of fight, flight and freeze reactions. Practised consciously heart focussed breathing slows the system down and facilitates the identification and focus on a particular positive emotion such as confidence, for example, as distinct from a morally shameful thought that could be associated with negative emotional valence.

Inner Ease refers to the conscious breathing in of a feeling of ease, for example to counteract expectation of an automatic or habitual social response such as blushing. Such a technique may constitute immediate relief felt in the moment of the blush being anticipated or in situations previously associated with such behavior.

Prep-Shift-Reset. Shameful thoughts, feelings, reactions and expectancies typical arise before challenging or stressful occasions. For example in organizational and business contexts, board room meetings provide a typical example. In such cases Prep-Shift-Reset is a specific practical application of resilience through preparing a calm feeling and/or using any HeartMath tool before any shameful, challenging or stressful situation, consciously shifting, resetting and restabilising the energy system when in the challenging event and practising sustaining coherence and resilience throughout the day.

Freeze-Frame. When practiced regularly Freeze-Frame has depth psychotherapeutic implications, for example in working through deep seated shame feelings that may be culturally occasioned, such as expectations of marriage and related experiences of intimate partner rejection, hesitation as to choice of marriage partner or confidence to make decisions as to engagement in any task. The same sequence of steps would be regularly practiced as when using Freeze-frame as one-minute technique that allows a major shift in perception. The technique can be described in five steps. Firstly, a shameful and/or stressful feeling is recognized and "freeze-framed" as one static image of a motion film. Secondly, heart focussed breathing is practised for at least 10 s. Thirdly, a positive, fun feeling or time in life is recalled and sincerely re-experienced. Fourthly, the heart is asked to provide a more efficient response to the shameful feeling and/or situation. Fifthly sincere listening to the deep, mature heart answer facilitates intuition, insight and action.

Heart Lock-In. This involves experiencing heart at a deeper level. Firstly there is heart focus, Secondly a positive feeling of love, care or appreciation for someone or context is cultivated. The feeling is maintained for at least five minutes. The feeling of love or appreciation is then sent to self and/or others to provide physical, mental and spiritual regeneration. It is suitable for example in contexts of shame and quilt associated with failure to perform certain tasks, engage in particular rituals or simply to deepen spirituality and improve health and performance. When regularly practised for longer time periods, this technique complemants all forms of meditation, prayer and contemplation and can be practiced regularly. By its very nature it forms an essential core of most wisdom, spiritual and healing practices.

Cut-Thru. Is valuable with shameful experiences associated with deeper, emotional issues. It is also designed to address the negative self-perceptions and emotional responses frequently triggered by novel situations. Thus, individuals are taught to alter their automatic responses to stress that are generated by old emotional programs involving hostility, shame, guilt and anxiety. Firstly an "inner weather report" identifies current emotional state. Secondly uncomfortable feelings are held in the heart area, to prevent attempts to analyse these negative feelings. Thirdly, a feeling of inner peace is generated. Fourthly there is reflection on when feelings of "overcare" about the negative emotional state developed. Fifthly a more efficient response or solution to the situation is generated and enacted.

All HeartMath techniques are taught in very specific sequences. For example, the following is an exact sequence of the Cut-Thru Technique that has been successfully used for shameful feelings in a client, who reported success in transforming shameful feelings with HeartMath techniques. The client emphasized the importance of staying in touch with heart focussed feelings as follows: The exact sequence of steps and a description of the client's personal experience follow:

Case Study

The following is a verbatim, reflexive, objective, experiential account offered by a client after he had confronted his shameful feelings.

Step 1: Be aware about how you feel about the issue at hand.

Questions to ask myself are: Am I in-touch with my feelings? Am I setting feelings aside that are draining me subconsciously and am I so caught up in it that I can't recognize it for what it is. Are they infiltrating other interactions at other points of my life? Am I carrying an emotional imbalance that is affecting the way I feel in other scenarios in my life? It is important to stay aware of how I feel at a particular moment? As I practice the technique I gradually become aware of events that may have affected my emotions and thus keep track of the shameful feeling. When an emotion begins to feel uncomfortable, it is important to recognize that worried feeling and then cut-through to balanced care on the spot. When any issue comes up, past or present, I observe my feelings more closely. If I am not feeling emotionally balanced, it is time to initiate a shift to a more beneficial emotional state.

*********FREEZE FRAME TECHNIQUE IS THE FIRST TO BE APPLIED**********

In freeze frame, an instant decision is made to remove one's self from being caught in a negative emotion or harmful pattern of thinking. The mind is cleared instantly and the acknowledgement of negative patterns of emotion damaging the physiology that are counter productive to health. The situation is confunded by emotions and that there is no actual harm in the present circumstances. It is time to overcome flight or flight reactions in the context where they are not necessary for healthy living. If step 1 which gives rise to freeze frame is not useful, then continue to implement CUT-THROUGH.

Step 2: Focus in the heart and in the solar plexus (that area above the diaphragm).

Breathe love and appreciation through the areas for ten seconds or more and help anchor your attention there. Breathe slowly from the CHEST into the STOMACH. Imagine that the breath is going in and out of this area. This will help create COHERENCE. This will help gain BALANCE AND STABILITY. You will stay grounded and focused. The solar plexus is connected to the lower brain through neurons and it is able to communicate with the brain. Strong emotions are felt in the solar plexus. The heart is used to ENTRAIN the oscillation of the heart with the solar plexus. This is the key to harmonizing the communication between the heart and the gut. You feel more centered after this process of entrainment. This entrainment can stop you from drifting on a sea of emotions and focus on a fixed secure and stable feeling. This entrainment can anchor you to a new reference point that can be the return point from negative emotional phases. With more anchoring to this entrainment, you feel bouyant and able to move beyond emotional distortion.

Step 3: Assume objectivity about the issue.

Think of the problem as if it belonged to someone else. When you are caught up in the emotions of the issue, it is hard to be objective. Don't make irrational or damaging decisions while so swamped with emotions that the bigger picture is completely lost.

Without objectivity, an issue can seem larger than it is, causing increased emotional reaction and overidentification with the issue. Many emotional decisions are due to overidentity where the head is thinking and reacting ahead of the heart. When you are more emotional, you are less objective. A cycle can occur where you can run out of emotional energy, end up in tears, break down or blow -up. You must break this cycle. The key to solving disputes is through compromise. You cannot compromise if you are always tring to win an argument or dispute. If you are determined to blame someone or something else at any cost, then there is no way to see things objectively. "Assuming Objectivity" is finding the integrity to disengage from the issue that is troubling you. This can be the most difficult step, especially if the issue is emotionally charged.

SEND A WHITE FLAG FROM YOUR HEART TO YOUR BRAIN

It is important to suspend feelings for a while so that you can address them in the midst of emotional turmoil. This can save the day. As in Gestalt Therapy, learn to disidentify with yourself and view yourself from an outside perspective. The next time you feel like you are about to appropriate an issue, ASSUME OBJECTIVITY. Disengage from it……Throw out the White Flag…..and pretend that you are watching another person deal with the issue……NOT YOU. How does the scene look from a distance? Ask yourself….Perception shifts can be amazing.

Assuming OBJECTIVITY allows you to be less identified with the issue and reduces the emotional energy that you invest in it.

REDUCE THE BURDEN OF SIGNIFICANCE PLACED ON A PROBLEM and EMOTIONAL COHERENCE will be regained.

Step 4: Rest in neutral in your rational mature heart.

Use heart intelligence to respond to the issue at hand. Neutral states allow for new possibilities to emerge. Find a neutral place to rest during your emotional storm which will change your attitudes and feelings. That will be an actual shift and not a perceived shift. You experience different attitudes and feelings when you surrender to your deep heart. The rational mature heart is more reasonable in its assessments. Perspectives and feelings occur that can help you consider what is best for your well-being. Understanding is gained that makes it easier to SHIFT YOUR ATTITUDE and find more BALANCED REGENERATIVE FEELINGS. New attitudes create a cognitive restructuring that is redirecting thoughts to interpret life's events in a more realistic and positive way. THIS IS NOT AN INTELLECTUAL EXERCISE>>>>>>THE HEART MUST BE ENGAGED for COGNITIVE SHIFTS TO TAKE PLACE. The rational mature heart offers a new direction that can help to retrain the MIND, encouraging it to let go of inflexible attitudes that confine your ability to make emotional shifts. From the deep heart, you can see what needs to change and why. Do not remain stuck in emotional dissonance.

Steps 5 and 6 clear out disturbed or dissonant feelings

Step 5: Soak and relax any disturbed or perblexed feelings in the compassion of the heart, dissolving their significance a little bit at a time.

There is no time limit for this. Remember, it is not the problem that causes energy drain as much as the significance that you assign to the problem. EMOTIONS ARE ENERGY IN MOTION. It is not the issue that is causing you discomfort but rather the significance that you assign the problem.

YOU INTERPRET ISSUES, and that is TOTALLY SUBJECTIVE. What you are releasing is not the truth but rather incoherent energy reinforced by a belief in its significance. That is what makes up disturbed feelings. You must use the coherent power of the heart to take out the weight or energy that you have invested in the issue and reduce the significance. The coherent power of the heart can do this. LET GO of IDENTIFYING with the EMOTIONS YOU ARE FEELING and soak in the coherent energy of the heart. FEEL COMPASSION. Soak out the stains on your heart and be sincere and sure that your heart is your own built in source of security and inner peace.

Step 6: From your deep heart, sincerely ask for guidance or insight.

If you dont get this, then APPRECIATE. Appreciation facilitates intuitive clarity on issues you are working on.

35.6 Conclusion

The HeartMath system, techniques and tools to assist persons transform shameful experiences as negative emotions, manage stress, promote positive feelings and build resilience have been discussed. There is great trust that the present chapter will contribute further towards personal, social and global heart based care and health. When practised sincerely with appropriate heart focussed care, HeartMath techniques and tools will transform negative shameful feelings into positive experiences and build presilience. These techniques and tools have been scientifically designed to as biofeedback devices to promote optimal heart rate variability, and psychophysiological coherence. They work by producing immediate cumulative entrainment effects on respiration, HRV, blood pressure rhythms and other physiological oscillatory systems. The HeartMath research library and numerous independent publications contain scientific documentary evidence of effectiveness of a may HeartMath programs, tools and techniques in a wide variety of contexts; psychophysiological, clinical, health, educational, organizational, intuition and energetics. This chapter has merely provided a taste of HeartMath theory and applications. For in depth study, readers are strongly encouraged to visit the user friendly HeartMath website at www. Heartmath.org. with its many facilitating illustrations and narratives. At present there are many thousands of GCI ambassadors from over 150 countries practicing heart focussed care, compassion and love towards improving global coherence (Childre et al., 2016). Many have become members after successfully transforming negative into positive feelings. Anyone motivated to promote planetary health and welfare can become GCI ambassadors at no financial cost. As more individuals, families, communities and nations transform negative into positive experiences, build resilience and raise coherence levels, this can lead to improved personal, social and global coherence, heart intelligence, and planetary consciousness. Finally, it seems appropriate to conclude this chapter with a brief description of the HeartMath technique of coherent communication that can be used to transform shame experiences that may arise in everyday dialogical and social contexts.

Shameful experiences typically arise in interpersonal and social contexts. In all cases coherent communication may improve relationships and focus discussion on meaningful specifics. The basic technique consists of three steps: (a) cultivating personal coherence before communicating, (b) listening to the essence of another person's communication without any prejudgements before the communication is complete, (c) confirming the essence of the communication heard from the other. When practised regularly, coherent communication facilitates such recognized therapeutic ingredients as empathy, respect and genuineness (Rogers, 1980).

Acknowledgements This work is based on research supported by the University of Zululand and the South African National Research Foundation (NRF). Any opinion, finding and conclusion or recommendation expressed in this material is that of the author(s) and the NRF does not accept any liability in regard thereto. Research collaboration with Dr. Rollin McCraty is appreciated.

References

Bourgeault, C. (2016). *The heart of centering prayer. Nondual Christianity in theory and practice.* Boulder: Shambala.

Childre, D. L., & Martin, H. (1999). *The HeartMath solution*. New York: Harper Collins.

Childre, D. L., & Martin, H. (2000). *The HeartMath solution*. New York: Harper Collins.

Childre, D. L, Martin, H., Rozman, D. & McCraty, R. (2016). Heart intelligence. In *Connecting with the intuitive guidance of the heart*. Maplewood: Waterfront Press, HeartMath.

Elison, J., Lennon, R., & Pulos, S. (2006). Investigating the compass of shame: The development of the compass of shame scale. *Social Behavior and Personality, 34,* 221–238.

Institute of HeartMath. (2014). *Building personal resilience. A handbook for Heartmath certified coachers and mentors*. Boulder Creek: HeartMath.

Judith, A. (2004). *Eastern body, western mind. Psychology and the chakra system as a path to the self*. Berkeley: Celestial Arts.

Lehrer, P., & Gevirtz, R. (2014). Heart rate variability biofeedback: How and why does it work? *Front Psychol, 5,* 756.

Louchakova, O. (2007a). Spiritual heart and direct knowing in the prayer of the heart. *Existent Anal, 18,* 81–102.

Louchakova, O. (2007b). The prayer of the heart, ego-transcendence and adult development. *Existent Anal, 18,* 261–287.

McCraty, R., Atkinson, M., Tomasino, D., & Bradley, R. J. (2009). The coherent heart. Heart–brain interaction, psychophysiological coherence and the emergence of a system wide order. *Integral Rev, 2,* 10–115.

MacKinnon, S., Gevirtz, R., McCraty, R., & Brown, M. (2013). Utilizing heartbeat evoked potentials to identify cardiac regulation of vagal afferents during emotion and resonant breathing. *Applied Physiology and Biofeedback, 38,* 241–255.

McCraty, R., & Shaffer, F. (2015). Heart rate variability: New perspectives on physiological mechanisms, assessment of self-regulatory capacity, and health risk. *Global Advances in Health and Medicine, 4*(1), 46–61.

McCraty, R. & Zayas, M. A. (2014). Cardiac coherence, self-regulation, autonomic stability and psychosocial well-being. *Frontiers in Psychology.* Retrieved from https://doi.org/10.3389/fpsyg.2014.01090.

Porges, S. W. (2011). *The polyvagal theory: Neurophysiological foundations of emotions, attachment, communication and self regulation.* New York: WW Norton & Co.

Pribram, K. H. (2011). *Brain and perception. Holonomy and structure in figural processing.* New York: Routledge.

Reid, D. (1998). *Chi-gung. Harnessing the power of the universe.* London: Simon and Schuster.

Rogers, C. (1980). *A way of being.* Boston: Houghton Mifflin.

Thayer, J. F., & Lane, R. D. (2000). A model of neurovisceral integration in emotion regulation and dysregulation. *Journal of Affective Disorders, 61,* 201–206.

Thayer, J. F., & Lane, R. D. (2009). Claude Bernard and the heart-brain connection: Further elaboration of neurovisceral integration. *Neuroscience and Biobehavioral Reviews, 33,* 81–88.

Thayer, J. F., Ahs, F., Fredrikson, M., Sollers, J. J., & Wagner, T. D. (2012). A meta-analysis of heart rate variability and neuroimaging studies: Implications for heart rate variability as a marker of stress and health. *Neuroscience and Biobehavioral Reviews, 36,* 747–756.

Vanderheiden, E., & Mayer, C.-H. (2017). An introduction to the value of shame—exploring a health resource in cultural contexts. In E. Vanderheiden & C.-H. Mayer (Eds.), *The value of shame—exploring a health resource in cultural contexts* (pp. 1–38). Cham: Springer.

Stephen D. Edwards discusses "HeartMath Techniques for the Transformation of Shame Experiences" which might then develop into a source of resilience and health. The HeartMath system is described as a scientific, evidence-based self-regulation technique which was designed to relieve stress, improve resilience and promote positive feelings, sense of coherence, health and performance. The aim of the chapter is to explore a research hypothesis concerning the effectiveness of HeartMath techniques to transform shame feelings. Specific techniques to address negative emotions, manage stress, promote positive feelings and build resilience are discussed.

Chapter 36
Dealing with Shame Using Appreciative Inquiry

Kathryn A. Nel and Sarawathie Govender

Abstract Although Appreciative Inquiry (AI) is often thought of as a framework used in Industrial/Organisational Psychology it has a much broader application. This chapter will focus on the applied use of AI in dealing with the 'shame' and 'guilt' experienced by individuals with HIV/AIDS in a sub-Saharan socio-economic context. The four key tenets of AI, namely: Discovery (the best of what is), Dream (what might be), Design (what should be) and Destiny (what will be) lend themselves to a reflexive approach for use in therapeutic settings. The appreciative interview, which is collaborative in nature, uses questions which are formulated so that a positive response is received. This gives clients a chance to discover positive things about themselves and their context (the client is not allowed to dwell on the negative). A second phase of discovery allows the client to reflect on satisfying moments in their lives which usually represents a strength that can be positively adapted to help them dream of a future which might be. The process continues in terms of the clients using different tools to design their provocative propositions which is their own positive statement and hope of what is or what might be. In recognizing that their destiny is not underpinned by 'shame' and/or guilt clients are able to deliver a positive approach (literally and metaphorically) to their lives which enables feelings of enhanced self-esteem.

Keywords HIV/AIDS · Discovery · Dream · Design · Destiny · Shame · Therapeutic tool

36.1 Introduction

This chapter demonstrates how Appreciative Inquiry (AI) can be used in an applied manner to help people deal with shame and guilt in a constructive way. For the purpose of this chapter shame is defined as a strong feeling or emotion which refers to a depreciation of self (Tangney & Dearing, 2002).

K. A. Nel (✉) · S. Govender
University of Limpopo, Private Bag X1106, Sovenga 0127, South Africa
e-mail: Kathryn.Nel@ul.ac.za

HIV and AIDS is arguably the most challenging pandemic in the 20th and 21st centuries (Nkosi & Rosenblatt, in this book). Global health systems, particularly in sub-Saharan Africa and countries such as Russia, face many challenges in coping with the disease. These include broad economic, health and social problems as well as issues that face individuals and families for instance, discrimination, stigmatisation, shame and guilt (Gutierrez, Albuquerque & Falzon, 2017; Tanser, Barnighausen, Grapsa, Zaida & Newell, 2013). Psychologists are well-placed to help People Living With HIV/AIDS (PLWHA) confront their life-challenges in a positive manner. Appreciative Inquiry (AI), in an applied format, helps people with HIV/AIDS find their own way forward in a way that emphasizes the positives in their lives. It helps them affirm their strengths and successes as well as recognizing their future potential which, in turn, allows them to enhance their self-esteem and self-determine their value to themselves, their families and their communities.

The theoretical approach for this chapter is AI which emphasises the positives in any situation either social, individual or organisational. The theory is underpinned by what Reed (2007) refers to the constructivist principle which is related to social constructionist theory. Essentially, constructivism is an individual's mental construct of their own experience which directly relates to principles within AI.

Theoretical models, used in a transformative manner can facilitate the release of shared goals and ambitions and help people problem solve by making decisions and taking action that they had previously not considered (Bushe, 2007). The chapter will give an overview of the approach. However, readers are urged to read further (a reading list is provided at the end of the chapter). This will help in understanding that AI has many applications and has been used in novel and transformative ways.

36.2 A Brief Overview of the Theory of Appreciative Inquiry (AI)

Historically, qualitative research approaches, theories and tools which have a positive influence stems from Lewin's (1946) introduction of *'Action Research'* into the Social Sciences. This led to various constructivist approaches and later the process of Affirmative or Appreciative Inquiry (AI) which was proposed in 1987 by David Cooperrider and Suresh Srivastva who were of the opinion that this type of research was problem oriented and did not encompass explorations which focused on feelings and perceptions (Fitzgerald, Muller & Miller, 2003). The approach was initially used in Industrial/Organisational Psychology as a way of helping workers identify their value, and that of their colleagues, to organisations. It was also used to identify positives and strengths in industrial contexts as before AI tools had looked at negatives thus workers tended to become disheartened as they felt they were not *'appreciated.'*

Nel and Govender (2018) report that AI looks at the potential within a system that reinforce the best *of what is; what might be; what should be* and the vision of *what will be*. It allows people within any system to appreciate themselves, as they identify the positives in the entity in which they exist and become aware of their inherent value and gain self-esteem. As a theory AI is flexible and integrates what Cooperrider and Srivastva (1987) named the four D's which are: Discovery (*the best of what is*), Dream (*what might be*), Design (*what should be*) and Destiny (*what will be*).

According to Nel and Govender (2018), in the *Define* stage the topic relating to the research or applied interview must be rigorously defined. The clinician must be properly grounded in AI which is ensured by extensive reading and consultation with experts in the method. This will guarantee that the focus of the applied AI interview (or research) is meticulously demarcated.

In the *Discovery* phase 1 interviews are undertaken so that people can narrate their stories. They are encouraged to tell these stories in a manner which focuses on the positive which helps them discover the positives, which they previously did not emphasise, exist. It is well known in psychology that people tend to remember and emphasise the negatives and forget anything good or positive (Williams, 2014). In this process people start to think about their lives and how they have been shaped by their own thoughts (often negative) and how these have focused their beliefs (in other words they engage in reflexivity). In phase 2 of the *Discovery* process people begin to *'see'* or have moments of clarity (*light bulb moments*) about events in their past and present which are positive and which help them in framing a desirable future.

This is followed by the *Dream* phase in which the positives they discovered are emphasized and which they use to help them frame an *ideal future*. When people *Design* their preferred futures they can narrate, draw or use any other method of developing a *Provocative Proposition* which is a written declaration of *what is* and the intent of *what might be* (Fitzgerald et al., 2003).

The last phase is *Destiny* or *Delivery* the person integrates his notions into every-day life in a positively framed manner. S/he reflects on this process, and with the enhanced self-esteem, built through the 4 D process is able to change and ensure that *Delivery* of the ideal future (with possible adaptations shaped through continuous reflexivity) takes place. During the entire process it must be emphasized that the researchers, individuals and/or clinicians ensure that the future *Dream* and *Destiny* is a sustainable and rational one (principles which shape AI are provided in Glossary 1 at the end of the chapter) (Fig. 36.1).

The Appreciative interview underpinned by the aforementioned theory was used as a therapeutic tool. In this regard the clinician helps the client create a picture of their existing reality which is generated using language, images, visions and beliefs (Tebele & Nel, 2011). This process is referred to as collaborative inquiry and helps people focus on the positives existing within their context (Cooperrider & Srivastva, 1987). The interviews take an hour with a ten to fifteen-minute period in the first session to build rapport with the client and a five to ten-minute de-briefing after every session. At the beginning of subsequent sessions, the clinician will summarise the client's narrative to verify it so that no misunderstandings occur (a generic questionnaire which can be adapted for different circumstances is provided in Glossary 2).

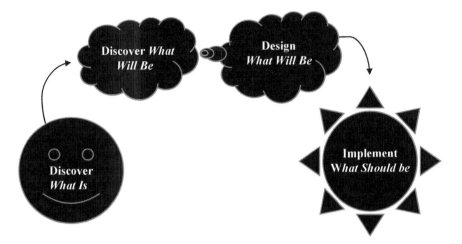

Fig. 36.1 Overview of the 4D process (Govender & Nel, 2018)

It is used to identify the best of *what is* and a client's future potential (*what will be*). This type of interview is dynamic and seeks to create an optimistic vision of the future which is both sustainable and positive. This type of interview mirrors the 4 D phase in AI theory.

Firstly, it seeks to help the clients describe and understand their past and existing day-to-day life challenges. As they engage in reflexion on their lives thus far they are able to understand how their own behaviour(s) could lead to feelings of negativity. At this stage questions such as: "Identify a time in your life when you felt most valued?" or "What do you most appreciate about your present life?" They have moments of clarity (*lightbulb moment*) and are able to appreciate that more positive thoughts and behaviours will have a very constructive impact on their lives, no matter what the context (*Discovery phases 1 and 2*).

In phase 2 a clinician could ask, "What are two or three things that are most important to your future life?" Secondly, in the *Dream* phase the clinician helps them conceive and plan their *ideal future* in manner that is realistic and can be maintained. The type of question in this phase could be, "What would you dream or envision as being a future life path?" or "Identify what your future could be?" Thirdly, the clients are requested to *Design* their ideal future in collaboration with the therapist. Questions here could be, "How would you go about getting to your ideal future?" or "Think of a plan that could help you get to your ideal future."

In the *Delivery* phase clients are expected to act upon their vision and put in place the positives they envisaged. In this phase the client could be asked, "In the past when you felt creative and decided to do something how did you feel and how did you implement that plan?" or "Tell me how you would implement your *ideal future*?" The interviews take place over a period of time usually 3–6 months but sometimes longer. During the process positives are emphasized and clients are encouraged in taking realistic steps to their *ideal futures*. They are encouraged, appreciated and challenged

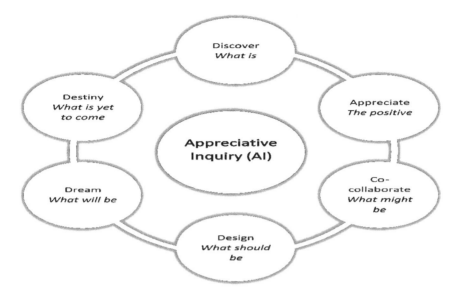

Fig. 36.2 Cyclical process of Appreciative Inquiry (Nel & Govender, 2018)

by the clinician to formulate and implement their plans (Nel & Govender, 2018) so that they can fulfil their true potential or *what should be.*

From data gleaned from the interviews key themes and provocative propositions were identified, from the data collected from the interviews, which illustrated the best of *what is,* the possibilities of *what should be* and the ideal *what will be* in Mrs M's experience of poverty (Fig. 36.2).

36.3 Background Descriptions

Dealing with shame and guilt constructively is difficult in any context but is even more challenging in the context of HIV/AIDS (Nkosi & Rosenblatt, in this book) where much stigmatisation and discrimination exist (Nqojane, Nel, Tebele, & Vezi, 2011). The use of AI as a therapeutic tool, and its effectiveness, is described and contextualized in this section.

Client 1: Ms M is a widow with two children whose husband died from an AIDS related illness. She initially met the clinician at a facility for grief counselling. At that time, she lived in informal housing, in a rural area, and her only income was a government stipend for her children. Her husband's family blamed her for his illness and her own family, who lived some distance away, did not support her for fear of discrimination and stigmatisation. She felt guilt and shame because the community 'knew' her husband had AIDS which is highly stigmatised and she was shunned by them.

Client 2: Ms G is a 33-year-old woman living with an HIV positive abusive husband who infected her with the retrovirus met the clinician at a clinic specializing in HIV/AIDS. When the counselling took place she had three children under the age of twelve. She was unemployed and had suffered physical, sexual and verbal abuse from her husband who she felt she could not leave because she needed money to care for her family. Her in-laws did not support her and, as lobola (bride-price) had been paid her own parents would not take her back into their home because they would be shamed. She reported that shame and guilt kept her from leaving her spouse.

Client 3: Mr S is 70-year-old widower whose wife died from Aids related complications. He is HIV infected and does not adhere to a strict medication regime. As a result, his overall health is poor and he also suffers from diabetes. Mr S has several girlfriends who do not know his positive status which makes him feel guilty and ashamed but he feels that he 'must keep up appearances.' However, this is stressful as he has diabetes as well and reported that he cannot '*satisfy*' his girlfriends (he did not have sex with them) which, in turn made him feel ashamed because he is a '*Man.*'

36.4 Appreciative Inquiry (AI) Used as a Therapeutic Tool for Dealing with Shame Constructively

Traditionally AI was used as a research method in Industrial/Organisational Psychology however, in recent years it has been use as both a method and a therapeutic tool in family and psychological counselling. An example of this is an investigation by Tebele and Nel (2011) which explored a rural woman woman's experience of poverty in a South African context using the appreciative interview.

Case Study 1

Mrs M stated that she was very unhappy and cried during the interview. She felt shame and guilt about being married to a man who was unfaithful and who had died of an AIDS related illness. It was apparent that she was feeling anger not grief. Her guilt and resentment spilled over to her mother and father (who refused to take her home) and her in-laws (who blamed her for their son's death). The shame and guilt that she felt because of the stigmatisation of HIV/AIDS in her community resulted in her feeling an overwhelming anger which made her depressed and suicidal. The clinician *Defined* the type of questions appropriate to the context and encouraged her to tell her story in *Discovery* phase 1.

It must be noted that South Africa is a traditional, patriarchal society in which women, particularly those in rural communities, have virtually no power in intimate relationships. According to Shivambu (2015), if lobola or bride price has been paid then it is even more problematic as many husbands feel that their wives have been bought and paid for thus belong to them. It is also true that the women's family experience 'shame' and 'guilt' if their daughter returns to them after lobola has been paid as a result, they do not allow them home even if they know of abuse that has taken place.

She was asked to identify how she felt she could improve the situation in her community where she felt she was shunned. After ruminating for some time she said:

"Well I can stop thinking about all the bad things and the shame I feel. I could just greet people and carry on with my life as I did before."

This made her feel better and started her *Discovery* process as she thought about the positive things she could do in order to lead a better (more fulfilled) life.

In the following interviews she was asked what else she had *Discovered* which was positive about her situation. She was able to state things such as she had a home and children who loved her. During this period, she noted that she was ashamed of 'wallowing' in her anger, shame and guilt and had come to the conclusion that she needed to look at her life differently (re-frame her story or narrative). Her quest was for a 'better' life and *Discovering* the *What might be*.

"I have started to think I could do something without my husband he is dead but I am not. My life was not happy but it could be."

She started to appreciate the *What is* and look at the *What might be* and then she began to think and speak about her *ideal future*. She often looked after children and felt she could start doing it for money as many people worked and needed this type of help. With the clinician's help she started to think of a realistic way of turning her *Dream* into the *What will and should be* and formulating her own *Provocative Propositions*. She devised a plan to implement her actions in a positive and sustainable way and began caring for children in an informal crèche for money. This occurred over a period of 6 months and, through the process of collaborative inquiry, Mrs M's ability to appreciate her situation and what she had was directly translated into a positive *ideal future*. She devised a plan to implement her actions in a positive and sustainable way and began caring for children in an informal crèche for money. This occurred over a period of 6 months and through the process of collaborative inquiry Mrs M's ability to appreciate her situation and what she had was directly translated into a positive *ideal future*. She informed the clinician that she really knew how to look for *"the good in my life."* It is apparent that in cases such as this a much lengthier period of therapy, using the appreciative interview as a tool, is required but it also indicates that mind-sets can shift and self-esteem enhances so individuals can see themselves as important and valuable. They are able to appreciate the positives in their lives and understand that feelings of shame and guilt are not constructive in this social context.

Case Study 2

Mrs H sought counselling because of her abusive husband. She had contracted HIV/AIDS from him as he had engaged in multiple affairs. Mrs H had stayed in the relationship because of pressures from both families (lobola had been paid) and because she had no source of income. She was severely beaten several times and had been in hospital because of this on more than one occasion. Mrs H was depressed and felt hopeless and could see no way out. She felt shame and guilt and even amongst her friends she did not discuss her predicament fundamentally, she suffered from 'Learned Helplessness.' According to Seligman (1975) this entails an individual believing that they deserve the abuse that is meted out to them. In this instance, Mrs H had learnt that she deserved the abuse and accepted the control of her male partner. On her first visit to the clinic she said:

"There is nothing I can do. You know when you are married you cannot move out, your families won't accept it. To do so would be shameful… anyway I have no money…my husband he doesn't mean it sometimes he corrects my behaviour…I feel bad about what I do [guilt]."

Mrs H reiterated this in different ways a number of times:

"We must stay together. If I left, I would be nobody and have nothing. I would have to face my family and be embarrassed [shame]. I have to think of my children having a father."

At the end of the first appreciative interview the clinician was able to *Define* the questions for future interviews which underpinned the *Discovery* phases. Mrs H did not defend her husband but felt her reality was not going to change because if she stood up to her husband he gave her a 'worse beating.' She was asked. "Tell me your present reality, I mean what happens to you on a day-to-day basis?" Mrs H then described her daily life and how she had to be *"very careful"* around her husband because she stated that, *"If I say or do the wrong thing according to him he hits me or throws things at me."* She stated she would *"take a beating because then he won't go to the children* [and beat them]." She was asked to think about the continual effects of these beatings on her children who witnessed many of them. Mrs H was also asked to identify any positives in her present reality and if she thought she could make any constructive change. In the second session she brought her thoughts which she had written down. Previously she had contacted the police and her husband was jailed but she had dropped the charges. She noted that for 6 months after this he had not beaten her. Mrs H said that this was a positive and she felt some pride (better self-esteem) that she had reported him. Furthermore, she thought that with support (from the clinician and the group she was attending) she would be able to follow through and go to court if it happened again (she was still *hoping* her husband would change at this stage). Mrs H came to the clinic and attended groups for around 3 months after this before she suffered another beating. This time her husband was jailed and she followed through with the charges. As the beating was particularly severe he was jailed for a substantial period. After this another 6 months passed with the clinician and Mrs H working on appreciating the *What is* and *What will be* in a collaborative endeavour. A breakthrough was made when Mrs H made the following comments:

"It is better now. You know before I didn't believe that it could be better. It took long but I see that life can be good. My family are proud of me and I are not ashamed that I left him. My children are my life and I have some money for them every month (from the State). You know my brother sells vegetables and I am helping him. We are even growing them."

Mrs H continued with therapy for another 6 months and during this period she made wonderful progress in *appreciating* her life. She had *Discovered* that she was indeed somebody in her own right and her *Dreams* were realistic. Mrs H wanted to look after her children and support them as best she could. She also became interested in helping other women who had been abused by telling her story to others at the clinic group.

Her *Dream* of looking after her family and providing for them might seem modest but after years of abuse she wanted her *ideal future* to be happy. She translated her *Dream* into the *What will and should be* and decided on a *Provocative Proposition.* Growing vegetables and selling them with her family and looking after her children meant those plans were implemented in a sustainable way. Her family allowed her to *come home* after the court case and at the end of the therapy sessions ($\pm$ 13 months) had decided to divorce him. She had gained self-esteem and appeared confident and in control.

Case Study 3

Mr S attended the HIV clinic a long way from his home village as he did not want anyone to know he was infected with the retrovirus. His wife, who had contracted the disease from him (owing to his having multiple affairs throughout their marriage) died the year before he met the clinician. His CD4 count was quite low (he did not always adhere to the medication regime) and he had diabetes. Problematically, he felt his standing in the community as a 'Man' was reflected by his liaisons with several younger women. This defined his own patriarchal definition of a man as "*being able to look after women and provide for the family*." He discussed missing his wife (who he stated he had really loved) and not really wanting his 'girlfriends' but felt that he had to have them otherwise the people (when pressed he said men) in his community would not respect him. He had not told his girlfriends about his HIV positive status which he stated that he knew was wrong however, he also noted that he did not have intimate relationships with them although '*others*' probably thought he did. He said this made him feel sad and it was something which he thought was shameful (he felt guilt). One of the issues he brought to therapy related to his diabetes. He reported that although he had girlfriends he was unable to '*service them,*' as he put it. He was depressed, spoke about "*joining his wife,*" and felt the situation was a hopeless one.

It must be noted that the clinician was aware that a rural African male of this generation was unlikely to have a 'sea change' in his beliefs about the roles of men, women and children. However, he had seven children the oldest of whom was 40 years and the youngest (from a girlfriend) 10 years old. He had helped them all in the past and professed to loving them dearly.

In *Discovery* phases 1 and 2 he was asked to first tell his story and then identify a time when he felt that he was effective and engaged with his life. When he narrated his story it was clear that his children and grandchildren made him proud and that he felt most useful and happy when engaging with them. The clinician asked him to identify the best in his life at that moment (*What is*). He was asked, "*Please identify what is the best thing in your life at present?*" His demeanor lightened when he spoke of his children and it was clear these were what he considered positives in his life.

"They are very good children and they love me and see me often."

It was also clear that he had been shocked and traumatized when he received his HIV positive diagnosis. He was asked:

"What one important thing you are going to achieve today?"

In this regard he said it was the ability to talk about the guilt in his life. He was ashamed and felt guilt that he 'gave' the disease to his wife. He spoke of some guilt about his girlfriends but as they had *"other boyfriends,"* did not appear to concerned which speaks to his mindset and patriarchal attitude towards women.

> "I did not want to go to the clinic but I was not well and my wife was sick…I suspected that I was HIV positive and got it from one of my girlfriends. I went to a clinic far away and it was not good, No, it was terrible when I found out – I had to tell my wife. She did live for a while but she was old and died. I couldn't tell my children it was my fault they just thought we were sick because we were old. I used to hide my treatment. I was ashamed as I am a respected man. I was worried that if people found out they would talk and I would be a no-one."

He was sent home to reflect on his life think about the positives and a potential *What will be.* When seen again he spoke of staying with his eldest son (who lived in another village) which would help on two counts (1) having people he cared for around him and (2) being able to say goodbye to his girlfriends. He told the clinician that his girlfriends had other (younger) boyfriends and while he was not going to tell them he was HIV positive he had told them to go and get tested. He said although he still felt guilty at least now they would know their status and, as he had not *'caused'* them to become infected through any sexual intimacy he did it so that they and their families would not have to go through what he did (loss of his wife). He identified his *ideal future* and created his own *Provocative Proposition* in order to fulfil his *Dream.* His *Dream was* to die in peace surrounded by his family who loved him. He did move to his son's home, which was closer to the clinic, and he seemed to gain from the experience of having someone listen to him in a non-judgmental manner. He eventually told his eldest son about his condition but no one else. At the last meeting he did say that he wished he had been able to just love (*appreciate*) what he had and not been so keen to see himself as a man as *"so many expect us to be men through having many girlfriends."* His depression had lifted and he had a positive outlook on what was left of his life.

36.5   Transforming Shame in the Cases Through AI

Appreciative Inquiry (AI) looks at the positives in life and allows people to reflect on their lives and appreciate what they have (What is) and what their lives can be (What will be). It does not allow them to focus on their guilt and shame and become immersed in misery that leads to mental health problems such as depression. They are able to recognize and reflect on what, in their past, caused their shame and guilt but are able to tell a new story going forward. Sometimes their shame is perceived shame (such as abuse by a husband, as in case study 2) and sometimes it is actual (such as not being truthful for instance, case study 3) and guilt because of anger that might be well founded (such as refusal of family to help as seen in case study 1). Appreciative Inquiry (AI) helps people formulate their futures without shame and guilt through self-reflexion and co-collaboration (with the therapist) in seeing a positive way forward. Consequences for the three clients in the case studies proved beneficial, they built self-esteem and worked towards positive sustainable futures.

36.6   Conclusion

The cultural context described in this chapter for using Appreciative Inquiry (AI) as a therapeutic tool may be foreign to many readers. Treating people from different cultures and backgrounds is not an easy task for any clinician. They have to try and understand the environment and the socio-cultural background that the client brings to the therapeutic setting. The clinician must be non-judgmental and do his or her best to empathize with the client in order to help them dispel any shame and guilt that they might have. This can be ethically challenging and requires diplomacy and above all the ability to understand that people do the best they can in their day-to-day lives. Respect is mutual and earned that is why when AI is used and the client and clinician work together (co-collaborate) they both appreciate the positives in working towards an *ideal future* which is sustainable and non-threatening to others.

Glossary 1—Key Terms in Appreciative Inquiry (AI)

4 D Cycle	This is the very essence of Appreciative Inquiry and can be captured as a 4D cycle which is the **discovery phasedream phase**, **design phase** and **destiny phase**. An appreciative enquiry emphasizes on an individual's positive aspects and potential rather than weaknesses.
Discovery Phase	This is a stage at which the direction of change is determined. This theme may be an opportunity for the individual to grow and thisis translated into an affirmative that invites formulations.
Dream Phase	In this stage of the 4D cycle people are expected to collectively assess their dreams versus their achievements in relation to their lifework and ambitions.
Design Phase	Drawing on the last two stagesvarious ideas and designs to implement the solutions are identified. These designs may be in the form of interventions to implement thoughts into practice and includes all steps need to make the dreams real

Destiny Phase	This is the last stage of the 4D cycle whereby participants are asked to fulfill different commitments and taskswhich may result in positive changes taking place.
Reflexivity	The researcher reflects on how their valuesbeliefs, experiences, interests and political orientation may affect their research.
Co-collaboration	Appreciative Inquiry is a collaborative process to engage people to discover the best in their context and is applied both from individual coaching and well as in a group context.

References

Bushe, G. R. (2007). Appreciative inquiry is not (just) about the positive. *OD Practitioner, 39*(4), 30–35.

Cooperrider, D. L., & Srivastva, S. (1987). Appreciative Inquiry in organisational life. In R. Woodman & W. Pasmore (Eds.), *Research in organisational change and development* (Vol. 1, pp. 129–169). Greenwich: JAI Press.

Fitzgerald, S. P., Murrell, K. I., & Miller, M. G. (2003). Appreciative inquiry: Accentuating the positive. *Business Strategy Review, 14*(1), 5–7.

Gutierrez, J., Albuquerque, A. A. A., & Falzon, L. (2017). *HIV Infection as vascular risk: a systematic review of the literature and meta-analysis. Plos One, 12(5)*, e0176686.

Lewin, K. (1946). Action research and minority problems. *Social Issues, 2*(4), 34–46.

Nel, K., & Govender, S. (2018). Transformative Research methods: Appreciative inquiry. In A. Fynn, S. Laher, & S. Kramer (Eds.). *Social Science Research in South Africa: theory and applications.* (In process) (DHET).

Nqojane, V., Nel, K. A., Tebele, C., & Vezi, M. (2011). Perceptions towards HIV and AIDS, condom use and voluntary counseling and testing (VCT) amongst students at a previously disadvantaged South African tertiary institution. *Journal of Human Ecology, 37*(1), 1–7.

Reed, J. (2007). *Appreciative Inquiry: research for change.* London: Sage.

Seligman, M. E. P. (1975). *Helplessness on depression, development and death.* San Francisco: Freeman.

Shivambu, D. (2015). *An investigation into psychological factors that compel battered women to remain in abusive relationships in Vhembe District, Limpopo Province.* Retrieved from http://ulspace.ul.ac.za/handle/10386/1311.

Tangney, J. P., & Dearing, R. L. (2002). *Shame and guilt.* New York: Guilford Press.

Tanser, F., Barnighausen, T., Grapsa, E., Zaida, J., & Newell, M. L. (2013). High coverage of ART associated with decline in risk of HIV aquistion in rural Kwa Zulu-Natal, South Africa. *Science, 339,* 966–971.

Tebele, C., & Nel, K. A. (2011). Appreciative inquiry: A case study of a woman's experience of poverty. *Journal of Psychology in Africa, 4,* 607–609.

Williams, R. (2014). *Are we hardwired to be positive or negative? On the capacity to emphasize the negative rather than the positive.* Retrieved from https://www.psychologytoday.com/blog/wired-success/201406/are-we-hardwired-be-positive-or-negative.

Kathryn A. Nel (Prof. Ph.D.) University of Limpopo (Turfloop Campus), Sovenga, Limpopo Province South Africa. She acted as HOD Industrial Psychology at the University of Zululand for a period of 3 years before moving to the University of Limpopo in 2009. She has a National

Research Foundation (South Africa) rating and broad research interests including gender issues, neuropsychology, social psychology, sport psychology and community psychology.

Associate Professor Saraswathie Govender University of Limpopo (Turfloop Campus), Sovenga, Limpopo Province, South Africa. She has acted as HOD Psychology in the Department of Psychology at the University of Limpopo (Turfloop Campus). She is Head of Research in the Department and serves on many of the institutions research committees. Her main areas of interest are neuropsychology, social psychology and Indigenous Knowledge Systems (IKS).

Chapter 37
Transforming Shame into Pride … and Vice Versa—A Meta-Model for Understanding the Transformations of Shame and Pride in Counselling, Mediation, Consulting and Therapy

Holger Lindemann

Abstract Whenever you are working with somebody who is ashamed of something or who is proud of something, you could ask how certain or doubtful he or she is about this feeling of shame or pride. Certainty and doubt do not exclusively refer to their self-evaluation but also to the evaluations of their social system, their community or to society in general. The dynamic of change and development may be clarified by visualising the antagonistic relationship between shame and pride in (self-)evaluation of their certainty or doubt. The transformations from shame into pride and vice versa are driven by the doubt about former evaluations and judgements. This short practical introduction will share a meta-model that can be helpful in counselling, mediation, consulting and therapy concerning shame or pride.

Keywords Transforming shame · Transforming pride · Certainty and doubt · Visualisation · Meta-model

37.1 Introduction

Literally, one can be ashamed of everything.[1] Heritage, living circumstances, knowledge, behaviour, appearance, sexuality, political conviction, incidents, job, financial situation and lots of other things. All of these aspects may refer to a person themself or may be linked to somebody else, such as someone from the family, neighbourhood, organisation, community or government (Salice & Montes Sánchez, 2016, p. 4). Of course, there is a qualitative difference. Shame about oneself can be considered

---

[1] Shame and guilt seem to be very similar emotions (Lindsay-Hartz, de Rivera & Mascolo, 1995, p. 298). For the purpose of this contribution, they are not differentiated here and I will only refer to shame. But the described dynamic can also apply to guilt.

H. Lindemann (✉)
Medical School Berlin, Calandrellistraße 1-9, 12247 Berlin, Germany
e-mail: holger.lindemann@medicalschool-berlin.de

© Springer Nature Switzerland AG 2019
C.-H. Mayer and E. Vanderheiden (eds.), *The Bright Side of Shame*,
https://doi.org/10.1007/978-3-030-13409-9_37

an emotion of self-assessment (Tangney, 1990; Lindsay-Hartz, De Rivera & Mascolo, 1995; Smith, Webster, Parrott & Eyre, 2002). These self-descriptions and self-evaluations depict what the person does not want to be (Lindsay-Hartz et al., 1995, p. 277). If the negative evaluation concerns other people, their behaviour, appearance, sexuality, political convictions or similar, shame can arise if a person thinks or feels that there is a relationship to themself. "We experience shame because that person is part of our self-definition" (Tangney, 2005, 541). Other people may draw a connection that links them to these other people. In this social sense, the self-devaluation of shame is reflected as a public reaction and social reputation (Kasabova, 2017, 110).

In contrast to the feeling and concept of shame, one can also be proud of everything: heritage, living circumstances, knowledge, behaviour, appearance, sexuality, political conviction, incidents, job, financial situation and more. References and links to a person or to somebody else also are possible. Pride also can be considered as an emotion of self-assessment, but a positive one (Tangney, 2005; Deonna, Rodogno, & Teroni, 2011).

An interesting fact seems to be that for every aspect about which someone is ashamed, someone else is proud, be it nationality, racism, drugs, overweight, underweight, habits and so on. "If, on the one hand, their phenomenological qualities are basically opposite (one being positive, the other negative), the way in which they relate to facts and objects, on the other hand, is almost parallel" (Salice & Montes Sánchez, 2016, 2). Shame and pride may be considered as counterparts or antagonists in negative and positive self-evaluation (Tangney, 2005, 541 ff.). Both feelings are also linked to antagonistic primary emotions: pride is based on anger and joy; shame is based on fear and sadness (TenHouten, 2017, 103).

In a social context of self-evaluation, it seems that whatever somebody is ashamed or proud of, they can find people, groups and the associated role models that confirm the self-evaluation, as well as for the exact opposite (Salice & Montes Sánchez, 2016, 4). While shame occurs with failure and lack of control, pride is likely to occur with the evaluation of something as a success and the experience of control (Turner & Husman, 2008, 138). Even here, shame and pride show an antagonistic dynamic: "This painful experience of shame results from the implicit self-comparison in the envious attack where the self is experienced as inferior, lacking or defective in the context of the other's success, creativity or good fortune in general" (May, 2017, 52).

37.2   A Transformational Meta-model

Building upon the introduced antagonistic dynamic, two assumptions can be made:

The *first* assumption is that transforming shame into pride needs success and the experience of control. This change of self-evaluation can be reached through direct action, and can be supported by focusing on people, groups, and associated role models, which show the possibility of being successful and gaining control (Kelly

& Lamia, 2018). Examples may be the self-acceptance of an overweight person or the coming-out of a gay person (Halpertine & Traub, 2009, 3 ff.).

The *second* assumption is that Transforming pride into shame needs failure and the loss of control.

> This change of self-evaluation can be reached by stopping actions, and through exposure to the evaluations of single people or groups who represent other values and evaluations. Helpful role models can show the possibility of being successful and gaining control. Examples may be the abandonment of (proud) drug abuse and drug dealing, the exit from a fascist group or from an religious sect. After a "phase of shame", the question may arise what it would be worth to be proud of instead. (Kelly & Lamia, 2018)

Whatever it is that leads to shame or pride, it is a complex interaction between cognitive, behavioural and affective aspects of the attitudes and beliefs someone has and shares with other people (Ajzen & Fishbein, 2005, 177; Louth, 2017, 186).

> "Shame and pride can be hetero-induced through a process of group identification. This shows that the evaluation of one's social self can be influenced by the evaluations deserved from other members of the group with which one identifies". (Salice & Montes Sánchez, 2016, p. 11)

However this identification is experienced, the evaluations and judgements of other people can stabilise or destabilise the feeling of shame as well as pride.

Every transformation of shame or pride contains a shift in group identification:

> "Seeing yourself as a member of a group, the actions and/or achievements of the other members acquire relevance when it comes to assessing your social self, and this is what triggers the emotive response". (Salice & Montes Sánchez, 2016, p. 7)

Transformational processes can be triggered by the experience of discrepancy between the different evaluations of whatever one could be ashamed or proud of (Salice & Montes Sánchez, 2016, 4; Buch, 2017, 160). These evaluations may be personal, social environmental (e.g. family, peers), communal, organisational or governmental. If somebody is ashamed of something, and experiences others who are also ashamed of it, or who are proud of the opposite, then they seem to be in good company.

With this in mind for every change and developmental process, it can be crucial to take a look at the referential groups and persons, and at their judgements (Kasabova, 2017, 103). Starting from this, the certainty/doubt of someone's shame or pride can be evaluated:

> *"Do you think it is justified/reasonable/legitimate to be ashamed about …?"*
>
> *"Do you think it is unjustified/unreasonable/illegitimate to be ashamed about …?"*
>
> *"Do you think it is justified/reasonable/legitimate to be proud of …?"*
>
> *"Do you think it is unjustified/unreasonable/illegitimate to be proud of …?"*

These self-evaluation questions can be completed with a social perspective by adding the evaluation of the social environment and community. The certainty and doubt about shame and pride in the different perspectives of oneself and the contextual social system can be visualised as a coordinate system in which the different judgements can be listed (Fig. 37.1).

An interesting point about this model is that doubtful judgements of pride or shame as unjustified, unreasonable and illegitimate are negatively connoted: "Don't be …" or "You don't have to …". From this negatively stated judgement of what not to be or do, no positive attraction can arise. Doubt, as an introductory step, can help to destabilise a state of shame or pride and seed questions about the former beliefs and judgements. If further development and change are in one's focus, it is crucial to answer the questions:

"What should I justified/reasonable/legitimate be ashamed of?"
"What should I justified/reasonable/legitimate be proud of?"

The first step of developmental transformation from shame or pride is doubt, a destabilisation of certainty. If someone is doubtful about a judgement, they may be open for other judgements and, what is more helpful, for the interaction with people who share other evaluations. The attraction to alter former judgements of shame or pride is higher when opposing observations and experiences can be made, involving other people who represent the new and different judgements. They are the best role models to construct an equivalent ego-state that is able to be ashamed or proud of something the person formerly was not ashamed or proud of.

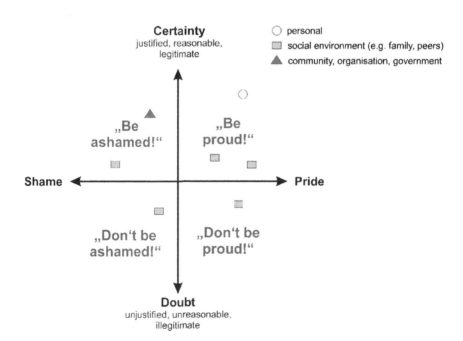

Fig. 37.1 Author's own construction: Coordinate system of shame and pride

There are some basic messages related to a change of judgements (vertical change) of either doubt (down) or certainty (up). Direct horizontal transformation from justified, reasonable and legitimate shame into justified, reasonable and legitimate pride is not very likely (Lindsay-Hartz et al., 1995, 296). Shame without doubt may more likely lead to helplessness and to passive and defensive behaviour (Lindsay-Hartz et al., 1995, 297). Doubt can directly refer to the feeling of shame, or to the insight that it does not include the whole personality but only a part of it.

Between shame and pride referring to the same aspect, the most likely dynamic will be a controversy. Understanding pride about something from a position of shame about the same thing is not likely. But the experience of this "gap" may inflict doubt. This dynamic may unfold in both directions. The same controversy can be assumed for the doubtful positions of unjustified, unreasonable and illegitimate shame versus unjustified, unreasonable and illegitimate pride. The main developmental (diagonal) directions of change are from a doubtful position of shame to pride, or from a doubtful position of pride to shame (Fig. 37.2).

For the clarification of this model, some examples may be helpful.

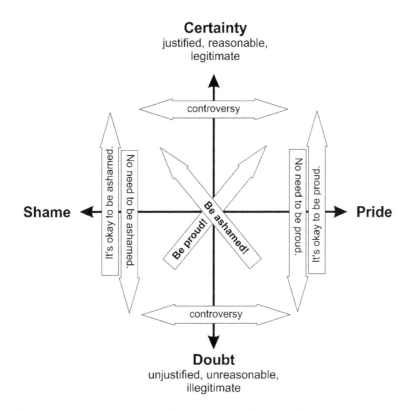

Fig. 37.2 Author's own construction: Messages and developmental directions in the coordinate system of shame and pride

1. There is a "rightfully proud, rich woman". She adores her possessions. From this state of mind, why should she be ashamed? Of what? She needs some doubt about her position of pride to open the door for shame. Receiving lots of negative input from media, friends, observations and experiences can lead her to a more unstable state of mind. So she can—as a first step—find some aspects of "rightful shame". From this point on, she can start a search for something (new) to be proud of and can even obtain a new group identification.
2. There is a "reasonably ashamed" gay husband who is married to a woman. They have two kids. After some reading, online conversation with peers and sleepless nights, he doubts that he should be ashamed. From there on, he can search for aspects of pride, and for the aligned group identification.

In this model and in these examples, doubt in pride and doubt in shame are the main pillars of development. The driving energy of transformation, of either shame or pride, is doubtfulness. Building on that, the search for new certainty through action, the experience of control and group identification can lead to being proud of something new (Turner & Husman, 2008, 138; Salice & Montes Sánchez, 2016, 11). Even if this transformation does not need people directly sharing the new value or evaluation, it is always the other people that someone will have in mind when they are undergoing self-evaluation (Salice & Montes Sánchez, 2016, 5 f.).

But what about the feeling of "rightful shame" that—in self-evaluation and in the evaluation of the social environment—stays justified, reasonable and legitimate with not the slightest seed of doubt? For example, someone who, while driving a car, completely drunk, feels ashamed after killing someone? Even here, the question may arise: what can this person be proud of? In the search for forgiveness, maybe they can do things to be proud of, even if the guilt and shame stay with them for the rest of their life.

This idea of using the dynamics of shame and pride is not meant to just change or replace one with the other. The direction and need for change should best be reflected towards the needs of clients and towards ethical considerations (Wurmser, 2015; Shweder, 2003):

Needs: What does the client seek? Freedom, peace, salvation, confidence, self-efficacy, participation, approval, control, take farewell etc.
Ethics: What does the client (and counsellor) think is ethically fair?

37.3 Application of the Meta-model to the Practice of Counselling, Mediation, Consulting and Therapy

At the end of this contribution I would like to offer some questions for use in counselling, mediation, consulting and therapy, that focus on the change from shame to pride and vice versa.

The presented meta-model for understanding the dynamics and transformation of shame and pride may help to identify what aspects of pride and shame can fuel a developmental process. With doubt as the starting point, changing pride or changing shame is best anchored by direct action and the experience of control (Smith, 2016, 112 ff.).

With the help of some systemic question techniques such as circular questions, scaling questions and hypothetical questions, it is possible to interview clients about their self-evaluation of shame, pride, doubt and certainty as well as about the evaluations of their social environment (Lindemann, Mayer & Osterfeld, 2018, 98–108). Some examples are given in the following table (Table 37.1). The questions focus on doubt, to take into account that a change of either shame or pride, needs doubt about the former evaluation. To stabilise a state of shame or pride, other questions may be helpful.

With an interview relating to the meta-model, the dynamics between shame and pride, certainty and doubt, can be explored. The "two sides of a coin" is a helpful metaphor to show clients and patients that a shift of perspective or "flipping the coin" may lead to a broader picture of their situation (Buch, 2017, 160).

37.4 Example in Practice

A young woman with an eating disorder has been to family counselling with her parents. In addition to her therapy, we have worked on family rules, school problems and how the family could organise their weekends. In one session, it became very clear that she was extremely proud of her self-discipline, as were her mother and father, both academics, equally proud of their own self-discipline. Her self-discipline led to weight control, while her parents' self-discipline, at first glance, led to professional success. They also showed great self-discipline in everything they did at home. Everything was functional and organised.

On recognising self-discipline as a driving value in the social context of the family, I had the hypothesis that the high esteem of self-discipline in the family system also contributed to the symptoms of the daughter. As a first step, I suggested that the family consider any doubts about their pride in being so self-disciplined. With some questions, I helped the family to explore the negative aspects of self-discipline in their lives, in their housekeeping and in their free-time activities. In this way, doubt could grow about whether self-discipline was something to be proud of in every aspect of their lives. While very functional in their professional context, it could be dysfunctional in their private context. In a reflection on what might be more serene, relaxed, spontaneous, delightful and unplanned in the family and parents' lives, the family defined some unplanned activities and spaces of imperfection, and took these on as experimental changes to bring into their everyday activities.

With the family's permission to reflect upon our work, the therapist and I exchanged our observations. In a following therapy session, the therapist helped the daughter to reflect on how she could help her parents to be more relaxed and undisciplined. I had a session with the parents, where they took their time to talk about the freedom and spontaneity they had lost while focusing on their careers.

Table 37.1 Questions regarding certainty and doubt about shame and pride

Self-reported certainty of shame	Self-reported certainty of pride
· What are you ashamed of?	· What are you proud of?
· If I asked your mother (father, brother, sister, boss, best friend …), what would she say you should be ashamed of?	· If I asked your mother (father, brother, sister, boss, best friend …), what would she say you should be proud of?
· How sure are you that it is justified (reasonable, legitimate) to be ashamed, using a scale from 1 "absolutely unsure I should be ashamed" to 10 "absolutely sure I should be ashamed"?	· How sure are you that it is justified (reasonable, legitimate) to be proud, using a scale from 1 "absolutely unsure I should be proud" to 10 "absolutely sure I should be proud"?
· If there is certainty about your shame, can you imagine something to do, as a compensation, so you can be proud of something else?	
Self-reported doubt of shame	Self-reported doubt of pride
· Can you tell something about your doubt that you should feel shame?	· Can you tell something about your doubt that you should feel pride?
· If I asked your mother (father, brother, sister, boss, best friend …), what would she say you should be doubtful about concerning your shame?	· If I asked your mother (father, brother, sister, boss, best friend …), what would she say you should be doubtful about concerning your pride?
· Which people you know, or have heard of, would agree with the idea that you should not feel shame?	· Which people you know, or have heard of, would agree with the idea that you should not feel pride?
· What social media or internet sites would support your doubt about your shame?	· What social media or internet sites would support your doubt about your pride?
· How does this doubt change the rating of your certainty, using a scale from 1 "absolutely unsure I should be ashamed" to 10 "absolutely sure I should be ashamed"?	· How does this doubt change the rating of your certainty, using a scale from 1 "absolutely unsure I should be proud" to 10 "absolutely sure I should be proud"?
· What could happen, or what could you do, to lower your rating by one more point?	· What could happen, or what could you do, to lower your rating by one more point?
· If there is doubt about your shame, can you imagine something to do that you can be proud of?	· If there is doubt about your pride, can you imagine something to be ashamed of?

They were ashamed about many opportunities which they had lost and activities had not done for years. They were particularly ashamed that their private life, and even their daughter, had to function in order to foster their careers.

My intervention was to help them regain some of these losses. I told them that this could indirectly help their daughter to let go of her very strict idea of control and discipline. Aside from reducing their working hours, they took more activities like "just driving and see where we get", sometimes using a directional roll of the dice, and cooking with a "surprise box of vegetables" an organic supermarket delivered to them every Friday.

The therapist and I helped to seed doubt about the family's pride in their self-discipline. Feeling ashamed about some aspects of their former life, the parents in particular were able to do other things to be proud of. In this example pride, shame and the social context of self-evaluation were used to reflect a consulting and therapeutic process and to define the starting point for coordinated interventions.

37.5 Conclusion

The purpose of this chapter was to link ideas of transforming shame to aspects of transforming pride and to give some hints how to combine both perspectives from a systemic point of view. Most publications reflect the qualitative aspects of shame (or pride). With the aspects of certainty and doubt, the meta-model that is presented here adds a quantitative level that allows questioning and identifying small steps up and down. This could help to add an "as well as" perspective to the "either or" perspective of shame and pride.

What could be interesting for further research and for practical interventions would be to explore the role of social media and online communication in the stabilisation and destabilisation of shame and pride.

References

Ajzen, I., & Fishbein, M. (2005). The influence of attitudes on behavior. In D. Albarracín, B. T. Johnson, & M. P. Zanna (Eds.), *The handbook of attitudes* (pp. 173–221). Mahwah: Erlbaum.
Buch, B. (2017). Indigenous nature-connectedness, colonialism and cultural disconnection. In C. H. Mayer & E. Vanderheiden (Eds.), *The value of shame. Exploring a health resource in cultural contexts* (pp. 157–185). Cham: Springer.
Deonna, J., Rodogno, R., & Teroni, F. (2011). *In Defense of Shame: The Faces of an Emotion*. New York: Oxford University Press.
Halpertine, D. M., & Traub, V. (2009). Beyond gay pride. In D. M. Halpertine & V. Traub (Eds.), *Gay shame* (pp. 3–40). Chicago: University of Chicago press.
Kasabova, A. (2017). From shame to shaming: Towards an analysis of shame narratives. *Open Cultural Studies, 1*, 99–112.
Kelly, V. C., & Lamia, M. C. (2018). *The upside of shame: Therapeutic interventions using the positive aspects of a "negative" emotion*. New York: Norton & Co.
Lindsay-Hartz, J., de Rivera, J., & Mascolo, M. F. (1995). Differenciating guilt and shame and their effects on motivation. In J. P. Tangney & K. W. Fischer (Eds.), *Self-conscious emotions: The psychology of shame, guilt, embarrassment and pride* (pp. 274–300). New York: Guilford Press.
Lindemann, H., Mayer, C. H., & Osterfeld, I. (2018). *Systemisch-lösungsorientierte Mediation und Konfliktklärung*. Göttingen: Vandenhoeck & Ruprecht.
Louth, S. (2017). Indigenous Australians: Shame and respect. In C.-H. Mayer & E. Vanderheiden (Eds.), *The value of shame. Exploring a health resource in cultural contexts* (pp. 186–200). Cham: Springer.
May, M. (2017). Shame! A system psychodynamic perspective. In C. H. Mayer & E. Vanderheiden (Eds.), *The value of shame. Exploring a health resource in cultural contexts* (pp. 43–60). Cham: Springer.

Salice, A., & Montes Sánchez, A. (2016). Pride, shame and group identification. *Frontiers in Psychology, 7*, 557.

Shweder, R. A. (2003). Toward a deep cultural psychology of shame. *Social Research, 70*(4), 1100–1129.

Smith, A. C. (2016). *Cognitive Mechanisms of Belief Change*. London: Pelgrane, Macmillan.

Smith, R. H., Webster, J. M., Parrott, W. G., & Eyre, H. L. (2002). The role of public exposure in moral and nonmoral shame and guilt. *Journal of Personality and Social Psychology, 83*(1), 138–159.

Tangney, J. P. (1990). Assessing individual differences in proneness to shame and guilt: Development of the self-conscious affect and attribution inventory. *Journal of Personality and Social Psychology, 59*(1), 102–111.

Tangney, J. P. (2005). The self-conscious emotions: shame, guilt, embarrassment and pride. In T. Dagleish & M. J. Power (Eds.), *Handbook of cognition and emotion* (pp. 541–568). Chichester: Wiley.

TenHouten, W. D. (2017). Social dominance hierarchy and the pride–shame system. *Journal of Political Power, 10*, 94–114.

Turner, J., & Husman, J. (2008). Emotional and cognitive self-regulation following academic shame. *Journal of Advanced Academics, 20*, 138–173.

Wurmser, L. (2015). Primary shame, mortal wound and tragic circularity: Some new reflections on shame and shame conflicts. *International Journal of Psychoanalysis, 96*, 1615–1634.

Holger Lindemann (Prof. Dr.) is full professor for developmental psychology and systemic counseling at the Department of Natural Sciences at the Medical School Berlin (MSB), Germany. He is private lecturer for special needs psycholo-gy at the Department of Special Needs Education & Rehabilitation at the University of Oldenburg, Germany. Director of HarbourCity Institute for Systemic Education and Training, Hamburg, Germany. He is qualified and works as a systemic supervisor (SG/DGSF), organizational consultant and certified mediator. He has published monographs, text collections, chapters and journal articles on school development, school inclusion, system theory and constructivism, solution focused mediation, systemic counseling and therapy, especially the use of metaphors counseling and therapeutic practice.

Chapter 38
A Cognitive Behavioral Approach Towards Bullying Remediation

Rebecca Merkin

Abstract This chapter updates literature on shame, guilt, and workplace bullying and introduces different possible cognitive behavioral approaches that could be used to help remediate the shame underlying bullying in the workplace. Differences between shame and guilt are distinguished in terms of their consequences. Given these consequences, a move towards guilt promotion (i.e., acceptance of responsibility) will be argued. Methods to move from shame to guilt will be explored using different cognitive behavioral approaches with an emphasis on strategies for overcoming shame and promoting pro-social work behaviors such as taking responsibility and experiencing empathy.

Keywords Shame · Guilt · Bullying · Cognitive behavioral approaches

38.1 Overview

Organizations (see Oosthuizen's chaptern with regard to organisations) are increasingly looking for effective ways to avoid the debilitating effects of workplace bullying (Bentley et al., 2017; Dollard et al., 2017). While cognitive behavioral approaches have characteristically been thought of as a treatment for depression, anxiety, and stress (Caplan et al., 2017), more generally, cognitive behavior therapy (CBT) has been aimed at improving emotion regulation (Barlow, Allen, & Choate, 2016). Merkin's (2017) research indicates that there is a need to examine the psychological states of bullies, who often are corporate psychopaths (Boddy, 2014). Bullies otherwise contribute effectively to organizations and are therefore retained (Boddy, 2014). Research shows that most bullies tend to be experiencing a state of shame from past experiences which diminish their ability to experience empathy for others (Merkin, 2017). Treating the bully at work with CBT could conceivably help to avoid the inevitable turnover of bullying targets by actually changing the bully's psychological state from maladaptive shame to the more pro-social state of guilt with

R. Merkin (✉)
Baruch College – CUNY, 1 Bernard Baruch Way VC 8-241, New York, NY 10010, USA
e-mail: Rebecca.Merkin@baruch.cuny.edu

© Springer Nature Switzerland AG 2019   571
C.-H. Mayer and E. Vanderheiden (eds.), *The Bright Side of Shame*,
https://doi.org/10.1007/978-3-030-13409-9_38

accompanying empathy and acceptance of responsibility for their behavior. Thus, an elaboration of possible CBT processes towards this end will be presented as possible remediation techniques for reducing bullying.

This chapter will begin by defining and describing both the distinctive states of shame and guilt and their relationship to workplace bullying. Then the consequences of shame versus guilt will be described based on the literature. Given these consequences, a move towards guilt promotion will be argued, followed by the introduction of cognitive behavioral approaches to remediate the shame behind bullying behaviors.

38.2   Distinctions Between Shame and Guilt

Shame and guilt can be seen as antecedents to conscience and moral behavior (Menesini & Camodeca, 2008). According to Berti and Bombi (2005), moral behavior develops from different mechanisms such as knowing the rules, internalizing them, being able to judge the difference between what is good and bad, and resisting temptation. Tangney (2015) points out that there are few differences in the kinds of occasions that produce shame or guilt. However, shame tends to be a more likely response to violations of social norms such as problematic drinking than guilt (Luoma et al., 2017). In fact, most anti-social events (e.g., lying, cheating, stealing) result in guilt for some people and shame for others (Tangney, 2015).

Because guilt is positively correlated with an acceptance of responsibility, guilt is more likely to be associated with moral adaptive productive relationships; while shame stimulates non-moral experiences that interfere with interpersonal relationships (Smith et al., 2002; Tangney, 2015). Thus, shame and guilt are termed self-conscious emotions induced by self-reflection and self-evaluation (Tangney, 2015). Although those in Western society tend to view shame and guilt interchangeably, there are important psychological, motivational, and interpersonal behavioral differences between these two emotions (Parker & Thomas, 2009; Pivetti, Camodeca, & Rapino, 2016; Tangney & Dearing, 2002).

> Shame is a silent emotion. People rarely announce that they feel shame – partly because shame is a deeply painful feeling of believing one is flawed and therefore unworthy of acceptance and belonging (Berti & Bombi, 2005; Brown, 2006; Lewis, 1971; Tangney, 2015). *Shame* is also characterized by a concern about feeling exposed and being judged negatively (Berti & Bombi, 2005; Lewis, 1971). It is typically accompanied by a sense of withdrawal and feeling one's exposed and lost face. (Lynd, 2013)

Shame is maladaptive (Roos, Hodges, & Salmivalli, 2014; Schlagintweit et al., 2017); partly because it has been shown to be related to problem gambling, maladaptive coping, bullying behaviors (Menesini et al., 2003; Merkin, 2017), bitterness, self-handicapping, hostility, social anxiety disorder (Hofseth et al., 2015; Levinson, Byrne, & Rodebaugh, 2016), disengagement (Menesini et al., 2003), greater impulsivity (Patock-Peckham, Canning, & Leeman, 2018), externalization of blame and detachment (Pivetti et al., 2016; Stuewig et al., 2010; Woodyatt & Wenzel, 2013), a lack of empathy (Menesini et al., 2003) and a decrease in pro-social behavior generally (Roos et al., 2014). A person's level of empathy determines whether or not he/she chooses to enact pro-social or antisocial communication (Sakurai et al., 2011). For example, delinquent adolescents tend to be less capable of identifying with others than non-delinquents (Schalkwijk et al., 2016). Finally, researchers have consistently reported a relationship between proneness to shame and a number of psychological symptoms; including depression, anxiety, eating disorder symptoms, subclinical sociopathy, and low self-esteem (Harder, Cutler, & Rockart, 1992; Tangney et al., 2007).

In contrast to shame, in guilt, the self is not the central object of negative evaluation, rather the specific behavior which tends to be less devastating (Lewis, 1971; Tangney, 2015). Feelings of guilt can be painful, nonetheless. People experiencing guilt often report a nagging focus on the specific transgression; ruminating and wishing they had behaved differently. Thus, whereas shame motivates avoidance, guilt tends to motivate reparative actions such as confessions or apologies (Aakvaag et al., 2016; Pivetti et al., 2016; Tangney, 2015). Tendencies associated with guilt are more apt to appease victims, resulting in greater empathy (Joireman, 2004; Stuewig et al., 2010; Tangney et al., 2007, 2015) and to handle anger constructively as opposed to shame which is linked to aggression (Stuewig et al., 2010). Since guilt is an understanding that one's own conduct is wrong because it caused harm to another who is now suffering (empathy); it is adaptive because it induces a deterrent to committing further transgressions (Pivetti et al., 2016; Tangney, 2015)—positively predicting self-forgiveness and negatively predicting excusing oneself (Griffin et al., 2016).

When bully's have negative feelings toward self, their shame can become particularly maladaptive resulting in unconstructive anger and hostility. This hostility may be redirected outward in a defensive attempt to protect the self by blaming others for their anger. In fact, research shows that shame leads to aggression via its influence on externalizing blame (Stuewig et al., 2010). While guilt orients people to be more constructive, proactive, and future-oriented, shame orients people toward separation, distance, and justification, (Lewis, 1971; Tangney, 2015), as in bullying (Menesini et al., 2003; Merkin, 2017).

38.3 Bullying

Griffin et al. (2016) assert that among perpetrators of interpersonal harm, shame is associated with wrongdoing. In particular, bullies, who are in a state of shame (Merkin, 2017), cope with offense-related emotion by expressing anger (Lewis, 1971; Scheff & Retzinger, 2001), detachment, lacking empathy, not taking responsibility for behavior, externalizing blame, (Cibich, Woodyatt, & Wenzel, 2016; Stuewig et al., 2010; Woodyatt & Wenzel, 2013), depression, substance abuse, and suicide (Hogh, Conway, & Mikkelsen, 2017; Roush et al., 2017). These coping attempts all act to alleviate emotional distress for the perpetrator. The extent to which these behaviors provoke negative interpersonal outcomes also needs to be addressed. Unfortunately, bullies tend to enact anti-social behavior such as manipulating and organizing people to inflict damages on others in subtle and destructive ways while avoiding detection themselves (Sutton, Smith & Swettenham, 1999).

It is important to understand more about the perpetrators of bullying because once they become part of the fabric of a work place, an intolerably toxic work environment results (Vega & Comer, 2005). In fact, bullying has been shown to diminish job performance, organizational productivity, and contribute to high rates of turnover (e.g. Hoel & Einarsen, 2008; Lutgen-Sandvik, 2006). While studies show that an increase of bullying is related to turnover outcomes in the workplace by targets, this does not appear to be the case with bullies (Bohle et al., 2017; Lutgen-Sandvik, 2006). What's more, a recent longitudinal study indicated that workplace bullies tend to remain intact in their jobs (Glambek, Skogstad, & Einarsen, 2016). They do not have an increased probability of intentions to leave, nor an increased probability of reporting illness. Actually, being a perpetrator of bullying is associated with a significantly lower probability of reporting sick days than non-perpetrators (Glambek et al., 2016).

Given the negative consequences of shame and bullying, it would be worthwhile to strategize how to move bullies towards guilt which has more pro-social consequences (Fisher & Exline, 2006; Roos et al., 2014). If increased feelings of guilt could be experienced by perpetrators of bullying upon hurting someone, it could help them to restore damaged relationships resulting in increased pride and self-esteem (Luciano & Orth, 2017). It is therefore warranted to examine how to convert shame into guilt. CBT has been shown to be successful in reducing shame associated with trauma in the veteran population (McKinney, Sirois, & Hirsch, 2017). Thus, it is likely to be relevant to expand this treatment to the shame associated with bullying.

38.4   Cognitive Behavior Therapy

Emotions contribute to the shaping of belief systems that support a person's actions (Svensson, Pauwels, & Weerman, 2017). Emotions also bond us to others (Scheff & Retzinger, 2001). Moral emotions guide people's choice of behavior (Svensson et al., 2017; Tangney & Dearing, 2002). Since emotions lead to action, to ultimately change feelings, it becomes necessary to attack the thoughts underlying shame-prone emotions. Thus, a person may feel shame but to change that feeling to guilt, therapists need to work with the shame-prone person's beliefs (e.g., "that was a really great put-down I made of Charlie in front of the guys") by eliciting their thoughts, discussing the thoughts' plausibility, and introducing more guilt-prone thoughts (e.g., how do you think that put down made Charlie feel? Why might it matter?).

CBT is one of the most extensively researched forms of psychotherapy (Butler et al., 2006). Hundreds of research studies have validated CBT's effectiveness (Beck, 2011; Clark & Beck, 2010). CBT has successfully treated multiple psychological conditions including depression, anxiety disorders, posttraumatic stress disorder, anger, somatic disorders, chronic pain, and obsessive-compulsive disorder (Butler et al., 2006). Research suggests that CBT can have a noticeable effect on building resilience and improving healthy cognitive processes (Grant, 2017). Theorists also suggest that CBT should be used to reduce feelings of shame (Gilbert & Woodyatt, 2017) (Gilbert, in this book). Therefore, it is proposed that CBT be attempted to help move those in a state of shame to one of guilt.

CBT is based on the notion that dysfunctional thinking (i.e., thoughts associated with shame) is common to all psychological disturbances which influence a person's behavior (Beck, 2011). Consequently, when people reevaluate their thinking more realistically, they experience an improvement in their emotional state and ensuing behavior (Beck, 2011). For example, three fundamental therapeutic components relevant to the treatment of emotional disorders have emerged (Barlow et al., 2016). They are (1) altering antecedent cognitive reappraisals; (2) preventing emotional avoidance; and (3) facilitating action tendencies not associated with an emotion that is deregulated. This CBT treatment method usually takes place in the context of provoking emotional exposure (Barlow et al., 2016). In the case of bullying, when exposed to the target, the bully needs to (1) alter his/her processing of the stimulus (e.g., this person is neutral) (2) accept responsibility for his/her anti-social responses, and consciously process his/her reaction responsibly (e.g., be civil, smile); (3) walk away.

Another process researchers suggest to move from maladaptive to adaptive thinking (Griffin et al., 2016) begins with a move away from the violated socio-moral values (i.e., bullying) then making a cognitive shift towards developing a conception of self as an accountable agent willing to accept responsibility for offenses, making amends when possible, and aligning behavior with adaptive values in the future (Griffin et al., 2016). It is likely that changing shame to guilt, which is theorized to bring about reparative feelings (Aakvaag et al., 2016; Tangney, 2015) will be positively associated with better interpersonal relationships and improved self-esteem for the bully (Smith et al., 2002; Tangney, 2015).

Leaders can have a strong impact on employee behavior through their influence on the context within which employees work. Managers in U.S. organizations often decide to keep maladaptive employees on board because they are productive in other ways; while the targets of their bullying activities tend to leave the organization due to their negative experiences such as stress (Pfeffer, 2007). To avoid the costs associated with high turnover rates, managers might consider mandating that bullying employees undergo in-house or out-sourced individual psychotherapy. Consequently, the context of private-practice therapy for applying CBT methods will be exhibited below.

38.5 Applied CBT Methods

38.5.1 Reflective Socratic Questioning

CBT therapists use reflective questions and Socratic questioning to identify their patients' underlying thoughts and assumptions (Beck, 2011; Bennett-Levy et al., 2009). The CBT example below will exemplify how reflective questioning could be employed to move bullies to reflect on their beliefs through acceptance of responsibility for their behavior.

In general, the following steps are suggested by therapists: revisit past experiences attributed to evoking shame, recognize the stimuli that triggered the shame, focus on how past behaviors had anti-social consequences, challenge the bully's thoughts, reframe perceptions to include taking responsibility for reactions to triggers and showing empathy, focus on moving from shame to guilt. False assumptions that are automatic thoughts are identified then, more constructive evaluations of these thoughts are created, and possible pro-social strategies are brainstormed. Finally, different strategies are practiced, past shame reinforcers are avoided, and positive behavior change is rewarded (Beck, 2011).

Research shows that shame leads to aggression via its influence on externalizing blame (Stuewig et al., 2010). Below is an example of a bully blaming someone else for making him/her feel angry. Redirecting the focus of the bully's thoughts to taking responsibility for the reaction is the goal of this Socratic questioning, based on Beck's (2011) method below:

Therapist: How were you feeling emotionally when you got upset at your coworker yesterday? Anxious? Frustrated? Angry?
Patient: Angry.
Therapist: What was going through your mind when you balled him out?
Patient: He was being a jerk. I was trying to concentrate and he was making noise talking and wouldn't shut up.
Therapist: What was going through your mind when you heard him making noise?
Patient: If he doesn't stop bothering me, I will have to explode.
Therapist: OK, you just identified what is called an automatic thought. These are the thoughts that pop into our minds. We all have them. We don't try to think this way. It's just what comes into our head. They're over quickly and we tend to just remember the emotions associated with the thoughts. Lots of times we have thoughts that are inaccurate but react as if they're true.
Patient: Hmmm.
Therapist: We're going to try to identify your automatic thoughts and then evaluate them to see if they are really true. For example, let's evaluate the thought, "if he doesn't stop bothering me, I am going to explode." What do you think would happen to your emotions if you discovered that your thought wasn't true—that the person would take your needs into account if he knew you couldn't concentrate with his noisiness?

Patient: I'd feel better.
Then an alternative scenario is suggested to illustrate the point…
Therapist: Suppose that you could speak reasonably to the person and the person would be quiet?
Patient: I hear…

The Socratic questioning process involves identifying the situation, the automatic thought, and the accompanying emotion. Once this is done, it becomes possible to deconstruct the faulty thinking process and redirect the patient to think more responsibly. For example, in this case the situation: hearing a coworker make noise → *automatic thought*: If he doesn't stop, I will have to explode → and *the emotion*: anger are used to redirect the bully's reactions. Reflecting on these elements helps to lead the patient to more rational thinking. (The automatic thought (anger) above is common thinking for those experiencing shame and for bullies. The idea is to use CBT to move from the anti-social thoughts common to shame and bullying to the more rational constructive thoughts associated with guilt).

38.6   Intellectual-Emotional Role Play

This technique is particularly useful when someone can intellectually see that a belief is dysfunctional but still feels the dysfunctional belief is true (Beck, 2011). This method can be executed by asking bullies to play the "emotional" part of their thoughts that strongly endorses the dysfunctional belief (e.g., the victim provoked me, which is a case of externalization of blame which is correlated with shame) while the therapist plays the intellectual part (moving the perpetrator towards the outcomes of guilt namely taking responsibility for one's actions). In the second segment the roles are switched, as elucidated by Beck (2011) and exemplified below:

Therapist: It sounds from what you're saying that you still believe that it's ok to tease strange people because you still seem to be having trouble leaving George alone.
Patient: Yeah
Therapist: I'd like to get a better sense of what evidence you still have that supports your belief.
Patient: Okay.
Therapist: Can we do a role play? I'll do the *intellectual* part of your mind that knows that when someone is odd, it doesn't mean it's okay to humiliate George. I'd like you to play the *emotional* part of your mind, that voice that still believes its fine to humiliate others. I want you to argue hard for your position so that I can really understand what's maintaining your belief. Okay, you start. Say "someone who is strange deserves to be teased".
Patient: Someone who is strange deserves to be teased.
Therapist: That's not true. I have a *belief* that someone who is strange deserves to be teased but every person actually deserves civility.

Patient: That's not true. Regular people don't get on other people's nerves and provoke people like "Weirdoes" do.

Therapist: That's not true. If people have idiosyncrasies, that doesn't mean that they are provoking others. All people have a right to be treated humanely.

Patient: Well I feel provoked, which is why I make fun of annoying people.

Therapist: That's not right, if you felt annoyed it is no reason to conflate that feeling with being provoked.

Patient: I guess that's true, I was just annoyed.

Therapist: Now let's trade roles. Now you be the *intellectual* part that disputes my *emotional* part and I'll use your same arguments.

Patient: Okay.

Therapist: I'll start. Someone who is strange deserves to be teased…

Once the patient and therapist switch roles, the patient has the opportunity to enact the intellectual voice, allowing him/her to practice the thinking that thwarts their faulty beliefs.

38.6.1 Mindfulness-Based Cognitive Therapy (MBCT)/Meditation

Mindfulness (based on meditation practices) (Gilbert, Oosterhuizen and Vanderheiden, in this book) could also possibly transform a bully's shame beliefs toward accepting responsibility. Mindfulness is a process of acquiring insight into one's mind and adopting a de-centered perspective (Safran & Segal, 1990) so that thoughts can be experienced in terms of their subjectivity (versus their necessary validity) and transient nature (versus their permanence).

The model of mindfulness for this illustration is based on Bishop et al. (2004) two-component model. The first component consists of self-regulating one's attention on immediate experiences. This allows individuals to increase their recognition of mental events in the present. The second component calls for an orientation toward present experience characterized by curiosity, openness, and acceptance regarding where the mind wonders.

Step one is maintaining *sustained attention* and *switching*. Sustained attention on ones' breath keeps attention affixed to the current experience; so that thoughts, feelings, and sensations can be detected as they arise in a stream of consciousness. Skills in switching allows one to bring attention back to one's breath once a thought or emotion has been acknowledged (Bishop et al., 2004). Finally, this process requires an *inhibition of elaborative processing,* so that cognitive processes are controlled and the stream of consciousness flows.

Mindfulness could move bullies towards a greater understanding of their unacknowledged shame state to achieve a more constructive perspective acknowledging greater responsibility. First, bullies receive mindfulness meditation training. Then meditate on experiences of shame while allowing thoughts to flow. The focus should be on the present, allowing the bully to begin to feel comfortable, bereft of dread. Mindfulness allows bullies to directly feel what they're going through and to notice thoughts about their experiences. It allows them to attend to their feelings of shame in the present without judging themselves and to consider alternative thoughts. For example, a bully may feel justified to leave a coworker out of social activities that others in their group are attending without remorse. Mindfulness could increase the bully's awareness of his/her own past experiences of shame (e.g., a mother raving about their *other* sibling). This might allow the bully to better understand that they are enacting the same behaviors that elicited their shame, perhaps arousing his/her conscience to possibly move the bully's perspective from blaming to feeling empathy for the target.

> **Mindfulness Checklist**
> Overview of the mindfulness approach
>
> 1. Bullies receive mindfulness meditation training.
> 2. Then sustained attention should be maintained. (Sustained attention on ones' breath keeps attention affixed to the current experience; thoughts, feelings, and sensations) should be allowed to flow—focusing is on the present.
> 3. Switching skills are applied to bring attention back to one's breath once a thought or emotion has been acknowledged (Bishop et al., 2004).
> 4. Finally, mindfulness processes requires an inhibition of elaborative processing, so that cognitive processes are controlled and the stream of consciousness flows.

38.6.2 Dialectical Behavior Therapy Technique

Rizvi and Linehan (2005) use an "opposite-to-emotion action" CBT technique termed dialectical behavior therapy (Neacsiu et al., 2010). They describe this process as a behavioral skill designed to regulate emotions. The premise behind this method is to focuses on opposite actions from the maladaptive ones. Thus, the patient changes an unwanted emotion (i.e., shame) by identifying the current emotional urges (e.g., hostile remarks) associated with it, determining the actions that are opposite to those urges (e.g., smiling), and then engaging in those actions.

This technique begins integrating opposite actions when the individual is faced with an emotion-eliciting cue—in our case, the presence of a bullying target. By thwarting maladaptive actions and generating new discordant response patterns, the initial emotional response is debilitated, and the incompatible response is fortified. Similar to Rizvi and Linehan's (2005) study of shame and bipolar disorder, two adjustments to the procedure are suggested. Namely, criteria for whether shame is considered justified should be expanded to include the following criteria: (a) that the action of the bully violated his/her own moral values, and/or (b) the action would cause others to reject him/her if they knew about it. If neither of those conditions are true, then the shame is considered to be unjustified. Second, given that bullying and shame are correlated with more than one maladaptive action tendency, opposite actions to each should be directed by response prevention and opposite actions (Rizvi & Linehan, 2005).

Some of the action tendencies associated with shame include a preoccupation with a negative action and with a negative evaluation of self (Dearing & Tangney, 2011; Tangney & Dearing, 2002). Bullies also tend to operate privately to avoid being detected (Aakvaag et al., 2016; Pivetti et al., 2016; Sutton et al., 1999; Tangney, 2015). Bullies have an action tendency to blame others for the event that elicited the emotion (Fischer & Tangney, 1995; Hofseth et al., 2015; Pivetti et al., 2016) and tend to express hostility toward themselves and others (Hogh, Conway, & Mikkelsen, 2017; Scheff & Retzinger, 2001; Stuewig et al., 2010). As Rizvi and Linehan (2005) pointed out in their pilot study, all shameful action urges would need to be altered if one would expect shame to be reduced (and not reinforced) using this method. Thus, various opposite actions would need to be identified on an individual basis.

In this process stress is placed in the beginning on familiarizing the client to a rationale for accepting responsibility and convincing the bully to commit to reducing shame. Moralistic information and basic research findings would be provided from the beginning during the rationale period. Then, homework and measures would have to be completed and consistently checked in a timely manner. The bullies should be reinforced for doing their work and for responsible behavior. Finally, and most significantly, owing to the particularly intimate nature of shame, an attachment to the therapist contributes to compliance. Consequently, effort expended by the therapist to be nonjudgmental and validating throughout the sessions is essential (Rizvi & Linehan, 2005).

More specifically, the dialectical behavior procedure for shame reduction aimed at shame transformation involves five steps (Rizvi & Linehan, 2005) (Table 38.1).

The last two steps are influenced by whether the shame is justified or unjustified. For example, if a participant described feeling justified shame over an event (e.g., the person hurt someone who was harming someone else) and an urge to hide that event from others for fear of losing face, the opposite action would not involve revealing that event to others. It would rather encompass disclosing that event to the

Table 38.1 Dialectical procedure for shame-transformation process

Identify cues that elicit shame
Assess if the shame cue is justified or unjustified based on the situation
The bully is exposed to the shame cue
Maladaptive emotion-linked action tendencies (e.g., avoidance, hostility) are blocked
Actions opposite to the emotion-linked action tendencies are elicited and reinforced

therapist only, working on making amends for the past behavior, and committing to not repeating that behavior again. In all cases this treatment involves a move from avoiding guilt to acknowledging responsibility for one's behavior and willingly accepting the rationalization for reducing shame.

38.7 Conclusion

Above are a number of possible options for employing CBT to help bullies move out of a shame orientation towards an acceptance of responsibility present in a guilt orientation. Future research is needed to test the actual viability of CBT in practice.

References

Aakvaag, H. F., Thoresen, S., Wentzel-Larsen, T., Dyb, G., Røysamb, E., & Olff, M. (2016). Broken and guilty since it happened: a population study of trauma-related shame and guilt after violence and sexual abuse. *Journal of Affective Disorders, 204,* 16–23.

Barlow, D. H., Allen, L. B., & Choate, M. L. (2016). Toward a unified treatment for emotional disorders-republished article. *Behavior Therapy, 47*(6), 838–853.

Beck, J. S. (2011). *Cognitive behavior therapy: basics and beyond*. New York: Guilford Press.

Bennett-Levy, J., Thwaites, R., Chaddock, A., & Davis, M. (2009). Reflective practice in cognitive behavioural therapy: the engine of lifelong learning. In J. Stedmon & R. Dallos (Eds.), *Reflective practice in psychotherapy and counselling* (pp. 115–135). New York: McGraw Hill.

Bentley, J. R., Treadway, D. C., Williams, L. V., Gazdag, B. A., & Yang, J. (2017). The moderating effect of employee political skill on the link between perceptions of a victimizing work environment and job performance. *Frontiers in Psychology, 8,* 1–14.

Berti, A. E., & Bombi, A. S. (2005). La media fanciullezza [Middle childhood]. In A. E. Berti & A. S. Bombi (a cura di), *Corso di Psicologia dello Sviluppo. Dalla nascita all'adolescenza* [Course of developmental psychology. From birth to adolescence] (pp. 231–322). Bologna: Il Mulino.

Bishop, S. R., Lau, M., Shapiro, S., Carlson, L., Anderson, N. D., Carmody, J., …, Devins, G. (2004). Mindfulness: a proposed operational definition. *Clinical Psychology: Science and Practice, 11*(3), 230–241.

Boddy, C. R. (2014). Corporate psychopaths, conflict, employee affective well-being and counterproductive work behaviour. *Journal of Business Ethics, 121*(1), 107–121.

Bohle, P., Bohle, P., Knox, A., Knox, A., Noone, J., Noone, J., …, Quinlan, M. (2017). Work organisation, bullying and intention to leave in the hospitality industry. Employee Relations, 39(4), 446–458.

Brown, B. (2006). Shame resilience theory: a grounded theory study on women and shame. Families in Society. *The Journal of Contemporary Social Services, 87*(1), 43–52.

Butler, A. C., Chapman, J. E., Forman, E. M., & Beck, A. T. (2006). The empirical status of cognitive-behavioral therapy: a review of meta-analyses. *Clinical Psychology Review, 26*(1), 17–31.

Caplan, R., Doss, J., Plioplys, S., & Jones, J. E. (2017). Cognitive behavioral therapy (CBT) treatment of anxiety disorders and depression in pediatric PNES. In *Pediatric psychogenic non-epileptic seizures* (pp. 147–160). Springer International Publishing.

Cibich, M., Woodyatt, L., & Wenzel, M. (2016). Moving beyond "shame is bad": how a functional emotion can become problematic. *Social and Personality Psychology Compass, 10*(9), 471–483.

Clark, D. A., & Beck, A. T. (2010). Cognitive theory and therapy of anxiety and depression: convergence with neurobiological findings. *Trends in Cognitive Sciences, 14*(9), 418–424.

Dearing, R. L., & Tangney, J. P. E. (2011). *Shame in the therapy hour*. Washington, D. C.: American Psychological Association.

Dollard, M. F., Dormann, C., Tuckey, M. R., & Escartín, J. (2017). Psychosocial safety climate (PSC) and enacted PSC for workplace bullying and psychological health problem reduction. *European Journal of Work and Organizational Psychology, 26*(6), 844–857.

Fischer, K. W., & Tangney, J. P. (Eds.). (1995). *Self-conscious emotions: the psychology of shame, guilt, embarrassment, and pride*. New York: Guilford Press.

Fisher, M. L., & Exline, J. J. (2006). Self-forgiveness versus excusing: the roles of remorse, effort, and acceptance of responsibility. *Self and Identity, 5*(02), 127–146.

Gilbert, P., & Woodyatt, L. (2017). An evolutionary approach to shame-based self-criticism, self-forgiveness, and compassion. In L. Woodyatt, E. L., Worthington, M., Wenzel, & B. J. Griffin (Eds.), *Handbook of the psychology of self-forgiveness* (pp. 29–41). Cham: Springer.

Glambek, M., Skogstad, A., & Einarsen, S. (2016). Do the bullies survive? A five-year, three-wave prospective study of indicators of expulsion in working life among perpetrators of workplace bullying. *Industrial Health, 54*(1), 68–73.

Grant, A. M. (2017). Solution-focused cognitive–behavioral coaching for sustainable high performance and circumventing stress, fatigue, and burnout. *Consulting Psychology Journal: Practice and Research, 69*(2), 98–111. https://doi.org/10.1037/cpb0000086.

Griffin, B. J., Moloney, J. M., Green, J. D., Worthington Jr, E. L., Cork, B., Tangney, J. P., …, Hook, J. N. (2016). Perpetrators' reactions to perceived interpersonal wrongdoing: the associations of guilt and shame with forgiving, punishing, and excusing oneself. *Self and Identity, 15*(6), 650–661.

Hogh, A., Conway, P. M., & Mikkelsen, E. G. (2017). *Prevalence and risk factors for workplace bullying. the wiley handbook of violence and aggression*. Chichester: Wiley.

Harder, D. W., Cutler, L., & Rockart, L. (1992). Assessment of shame and guilt and their relationships to psychopathology. *Journal of Personality Assessment, 59*(3), 584–604.

Hoel, H., & Einarsen, S. (2008). Bullying and mistreatment at work: how managers may prevent and manage such problems. In A. Kinder, R. Hughes, & C. L. Cooper (Eds.), *Employee well-being support. A workplace resource* (pp. 161–173). Chichester: Wiley.

Hofseth, E., Toering, T., & Jordet, G. (2015). Shame proneness, guilt proneness, behavioral self-handicapping, and skill level: a mediational analysis. *Journal of Applied Sport Psychology, 27*, 359–370.

Joireman, J. (2004). Empathy and the self-absorption paradox II: self-rumination and self-reflection as mediators between shame, guilt, and empathy. *Self and Identity, 3*(3), 225–238.

Levinson, C. A., Byrne, M., & Rodebaugh, T. L. (2016). Shame and guilt as shared vulnerability factors: Shame, but not guilt, prospectively predicts both social anxiety and bulimic symptoms. *Eating Behaviors, 22*, 188–193.

Lewis, H. B. (1971). *Shame and guilt in neurosis*. New York: International Universities Press.

Luciano, E. C., & Orth, U. (2017). Transitions in romantic relationships and development of self-esteem. *Journal of Personality and Social Psychology, 112*(2), 307–328. https://doi.org/10.1037/pspp0000109.

Luoma, J., Guinther, P., Potter, J., & Cheslock, M. (2017). Experienced-based versus scenario-based assessments of shame and guilt and their relationship to alcohol consumption and problems. *Substance Use and Misuse, 52*, 1692–1700.

Lutgen-Sandvik, P. (2006). Take this job and…: Quitting and other forms of resistance to workplace bullying. *Communication Monographs, 73*(4), 406–433.

Lynd, H. M. (2013). *On shame and the search for identity* (Vol. 145). New York: Routledge.

McKinney, J., Sirois, F. M., & Hirsch, J. K. (2017). *Posttraumatic Growth and Shame/Guilt in Veterans: Does Time (Perspective) Really Heal All Wounds?* Oral presentation. 32nd Annual Appalachian Student Research Forum, Johnson City, TN.

Menesini, E., & Camodeca, M. (2008). Shame and guilt as behaviour regulators: relationships with bullying, victimization and pro-social behaviour. *British Journal of Developmental Psychology, 26*(2), 183–196. https://doi.org/10.1348/026151007x205281.

Menesini, E., Sanchez, V., Fonzi, A., Ortega, R., Costabile, A., & Lo Feudo, G. (2003). Moral emotions and bullying: a cross-national comparison of differences between bullies, victims and outsiders. *Aggressive Behavior, 29*(6), 515–530.

Merkin, R. S. (2017). From shame to guilt: the remediation of bullying across cultures and the US. In E. Vanderheiden, C.-H. Mayer (Eds.), *The value of shame* (pp. 223–248). Cham: Springer International Publishing.

Neacsiu, A. D., Rizvi, S. L., Vitaliano, P. P., Lynch, T. R., & Linehan, M. M. (2010). The dialectical behavior therapy ways of coping checklist: development and psychometric properties. *Journal of Clinical Psychology, 66*(6), 563–582.

Parker, S., & Thomas, R. (2009). Psychological differences in shame vs. guilt: implications for mental health counselors. *Journal of Mental Health Counseling, 31*(3), 213–224.

Patock-Peckham, J. A., Canning, J. R., & Leeman, R. F. (2018). Shame is bad and guilt is good: an examination of the impaired control over drinking pathway to alcohol use and related problems. *Personality and Individual Differences, 121,* 62–66.

Pfeffer, J. (2007). Human resources from an organizational behavior perspective: Some paradoxes explained. *Journal of Economic Perspectives, 21*(4), 115–134.

Pivetti, M., Camodeca, M., & Rapino, M. (2016). Shame, guilt, and anger: their cognitive, physio-logical, and behavioral correlates. *Current Psychology, 35*(4), 690–699.

Rizvi, S. L., & Linehan, M. M. (2005). The treatment of maladaptive shame in borderline personality disorder: a pilot study of "opposite action". *Cognitive and Behavioral Practice, 12*(4), 437–447.

Roos, S., Hodges, E. V., & Salmivalli, C. (2014). Do guilt-and shame-proneness differentially predict pro-social, aggressive, and withdrawn behaviors during early adolescence? *Developmental Psychology, 50*(3), 941.

Roush, J. F., Brown, S. L., Mitchell, S. M., & Cukrowicz, K. C. (2017). Shame, guilt, and suicide ideation among bondage and discipline, dominance and submission, and sadomasochism practi-tioners: examining the role of the interpersonal theory of suicide. *Suicide and Life-Threatening Behavior, 47*(2), 129–141.

Safran, J. D., & Segal, Z. V. (1990). *Interpersonal process in cognitive therapy.* New York: Basic Books.

Sakurai, S., Hayama, D., Suzuki, T., Kurazumi, T., Hagiwara, T., Suzuki, M., …, Oikawa, C. (2011). The relationship of empathic-affective responses toward others' positive affect with pro-social behaviors and aggressive behaviors (English). *Japanese Journal of Psychology, 82*(2), 123–131. https://doi.org/10.4992/jjpsy.82.123.

Schalkwijk, F., Stams, G. J., Stegge, H., Dekker, J., & Peen, J. (2016). The conscience as a reg-ulatory function: empathy, shame, pride, guilt, and moral orientation in delinquent adolescents. *International Journal of Offender Therapy and Comparative Criminology, 60*(6), 675–693.

Scheff, T. J., & Retzinger, S. M. (2001). *Emotions and violence: Shame and rage in destructive conflicts.* Lincoln: Lexington Books.

Schlagintweit, H. E., Thompson, K., Goldstein, A. L., & Stewart, S. H. (2017). An Investigation of the association between shame and problem gambling: the mediating role of maladaptive coping motives. *Journal of Gambling Studies*, 1–13.

Smith, R. H., Webster, J. M., Parrott, W. G., & Eyre, H. L. (2002). The role of public exposure in moral and nonmoral shame and guilt. *Journal of Personality and Social Psychology, 83,* 138–159.

Stuewig, J., Tangney, J. P., Heigel, C., Harty, L., & McCloskey, L. (2010). Shaming, blaming, and maiming: functional links among the moral emotions, externalization of blame, and aggression. *Journal of Research in Personality, 44*(1), 91–102.

Sutton, J., Smith, P. K., & Swettenham, J. (1999). Bullying and 'theory of mind': a critique of the 'social skills deficit' view of anti-social behaviour. *Social Development, 8*(1), 117–127.

Svensson, R., Pauwels, L. J. R. & Weerman, F. M. (2017). The role of moral beliefs, shame, and guilt in criminal decision making. In W. Bernasco, J.-L. von Gelder, H. Elffers (Eds.), *The oxford handbook of offender decision making* (pp. 228–245). Oxford: Oxford University Press.

Tangney, J. P. (2015). Psychology of self-conscious emotions. In J. D. Wright (Ed.), *International encyclopedia of the social & behavioral sciences* (2nd ed., vol. 21, pp. 475–480).

Tangney, J. P., & Dearing, R. L. (2002). *Shame and guilt*. New York: Guilford Press.

Tangney, J. P., Stuewig, J., & Mashek, D. J. (2007). Moral emotions and moral behavior. *Annual Review of Psychology, 58,* 345–372.

Vega, G., & Comer, D. R. (2005). Sticks and stones may break your bones, but words can break your spirit: bullying in the workplace. *Journal of Business Ethics, 58*(1–3), 101–109.

Woodyatt, L., & Wenzel, M. (2013). The psychological immune response in the face of transgressions: pseudo self-forgiveness and threat to belonging. *Journal of Experimental Social Psychology, 49,* 951–958.

Rebecca S. Merkin (Ph.D., Kent State University) conducts research focused on communication in organizations; intercultural communication; sexual harass-ment in the workplace; job satisfaction; and social interaction processes such as impression management, identity, and facework communication. She has pub-lished articles in numerous journals including the Atlantic Journal of Communica-tion, International Journal of Intercultural Communication Research, Journal of Behavioral and Applied Management, Journal of Intercultural Communication, Journal of International Women's Studies, and International Journal of Intercul-tural Relations. Professor Merkin has also given presentations on communication at conferences of the Academy of Management, Eastern Communication Association, National Communication Association, International Communication Association, and the International Academy of Intercultural Research.

Chapter 39
Facing the Ambivalence of Shame Issues: Exploring the Use of Motivational Techniques to Enhance Shame Resilience and Provoke Behaviour Change

Len Andrieux

Abstract Shame is among the most intense and painful affects. It has been extensively defined from very different viewpoints: psychology, social sciences, clinical sociology and neurosciences. It has been looked at through the lenses of philosophy and drama from Ovid through Shakespeare, Jean Rhys, Jean Paul Sartre and numerous other authors. Nevertheless, there is no extensive literature about shame therapies and there are few established therapeutic approaches. Often studies related to shame are done with an accent on what causes shame rather than how to change one's behaviour from shame to shame resilient. This chapter examines the use of motivational interviewing techniques in coaching when faced with clearly identified shame issues, and the ambivalence resulting from the acknowledgment. Results of a qualitative and hermeneutic approach through coaching sessions, with three clients and self-observation show that this ambivalence can be alleviated by use of motivational techniques instead of or in concert with other therapeutic approaches. The key finding is that once a client has fully identified his shame issue, it is important to acknowledge it, without continuing to explore its causes but consider it as a starting point to enhance resilience and provoke behaviour change using motivational interviewing.

Keywords Shame · Resilience · Motivational interviews · Ambivalence · Behaviour change

39.1 Introduction

Shame is one of the most painful subjects to broach, it is the unspeakable, the secret memory of a narcissistic wound. The multiple faces of shame pervade all aspects of our existence, our body, our sexuality, morality, our social life, and our identity in its personal as well as its social aspects. Throughout cultures, and disciplines shame has been looked at through a great variety of lenses.

L. Andrieux (✉)
49 Promenade des Golfeurs, 77600 Bussy Saint Georges, France
e-mail: len@andrieux-consulting.com

© Springer Nature Switzerland AG 2019
C.-H. Mayer and E. Vanderheiden (eds.), *The Bright Side of Shame*,
https://doi.org/10.1007/978-3-030-13409-9_39

The purpose of this chapter is to examine Motivational Interviewing (MI) as an effective method to address the ambivalence, between the relative "comfort" of continuing to use one's shame defences and the desire to become the person freed of those defences and able to develop shame resilience thus allowing behaviour change. To do so I will start with definitions of shame by various authors and a brief overview of different therapeutic approaches which are not interrelated but illustrate how shame can be approached from different angles, from a psychodynamic approach to shame resilience without specifically addressing the ambivalence lingering with the client after having identified the shame issues. Motivational Interviewing addresses the residual ambivalence. The methodology will be illustrated through three coaching cases. Its impact and its effectiveness to spark change and develop shame resilience will be emphasised all along the coaching conversations. The Trans Theoretical Stages of Change model (Prochaska & DiClemente, 1984) will be used as a foundation to demonstrate the effectiveness of MI in the context of this study.

39.2   Shame Definitions and Established Therapeutic Approaches

According to Freud, the ego ideal is made up of ideal representations, grandiose fantasies, and parental representations. (see dream chapter in this book) Shame occurs when people perceive they have failed to approximate their ego ideal. (Freud, 1976) In social sciences shame is defined as a psycho-social-cultural construct, (Brown, 2006) an "intensely painful feeling or experience of believing we are flawed and therefore unworthy of acceptance and belonging".

Morrison defines shame as a feeling of intrinsic self-worthlessness, which underlies a range of psychological problems (1989, 1998): depression, addiction, sexual or eating disorders, and emotional problems linked to trauma, gender, illness, old age, infertility.

Shame is related to the belief that we cannot create positive images in the eyes of others: we will not be chosen, will be found lacking in talent, ability, appearance and so forth, we will be passed over, ignored or rejected (Gilbert, 1998) (see Gilbert's chapter in this book). The hallmarks of shame are fears of being weak, of losing control. The fear of shame is a compelling motivator, resulting in a challenge to achieve exceptional results, a drive leading to perfectionism, overcompensation, but also to a high sensitivity to criticism, poor listening skills, lack of empathy, and an intense desire to compete. Several of these shame related phenomena overlap with well-identified negative characteristics of "narcissistic personalities".

Most therapies focus on the root causes of shame. A psychodynamic approach will be centred on connections between the past and the present with a systemic view. The goals of psychodynamic therapy are a client's self-awareness and understanding of the influence of the past on present behaviour (Haggerty, 2006).

Gestalt therapy focuses on process (what is actually happening) as well as on content (what is being talked about). The emphasis is on what is being done, thought, and felt at the present moment (the phenomenality of both client and coach).

In Gestalt therapies (Merkin, in this book) clients will be supported to bear and explore shame feelings only to the extent that the therapists can be open to these difficult and isolating experiences (Wheeler, 1997).

Cognitive Behavioural Therapy (CBT) (Merkin, in this book) aims to solve problems concerning dysfunctional emotions, behaviours and cognitions through a goal-oriented, systematic procedure in the present. CBT focuses on the here and now and on alleviating the symptoms by questioning and testing cognition, assumptions, evaluations and beliefs and trying to find new ways of behaviour (Rachman, 1997).

Building on CBT and Dialectical Behavioural Therapies (DBT) (Lynch, Chapman, Rosenthal, Kuo, & Linehan, 2006), (Gilbert, in this book) Compassionate Mind Training (CMT) was developed for people with high shame and self-criticism, whose problems tend to be chronic and who find self-warmth and self-acceptance difficult and/or frightening (Gilbert, 2006).

By demonstrating the skills and attributes of compassion the therapist instils them in the client. Thus, the client is helped to develop an internal compassionate relationship with himself to replace the blaming, condemning and self-critical one, the "compassionate" approach continues to gain momentum in recent research.

Brené Brown from Houston University research faculty, approaches shame through the social worker's lens, she developed a Psycho-educational Shame Resilience Curriculum called "Connections" as a tool to help professionals and clients recognize shame and develop shame resilience in a group therapy (Brown, 2009). "Connections" is based on her Shame-Resilience theory (SRT) (Brown, 2006), offering a set of propositions about how shame affects men and women and how to build shame resilience.

In SRT, shame resilience is conceptualized as a continuum, with shame, fear, blame and disconnection anchoring at one end and empathy, courage, compassion and connection anchoring the other end. The sessions stretch from learning to recognize fear, towards practicing critical awareness, reaching out and speaking shame.

Brené Brown's definition and use of resilience is consistent with the original significance of the word. The etymology of resilience is the Latin resili, meaning, "to spring back." Resilience is the power or ability of a material to return to the original form, position, after being bent, compressed, or stretched.

The French neuropsychiatrist Boris Cyrulnik stresses the importance of the presence of "tutors of resilience" (Cyrulnik, 2010). The significance of tutor (tuteur) in French literally means a strong wooden or metal post with a point at one end, driven into the ground to support a tree or a plant's growth. Boris Cyrulnik's tutors are the people who actively support the person in the pangs of shame, reassuring and proposing a new project of existence.

Cyrulnik's resilience is a survival strategy, he argues that one has to "spring back" a little onwards, to move forward…and not to remain prisoner of one's shame. Resilience is then the capacity to resume life in spite of the wound (of shame), without settling on this wound.

This is a huge pace forward, covering a broad landscape of conceptualizations of shame, from psychodynamic research into the past and the root causes of shame through cognitive behavioural therapies, self-compassion and shame resilience, towards the capacity to change behaviours. This is where ambivalence comes into play and motivational techniques take all their significance as a method to alleviate shame.

39.3   The Ambivalence Lingering After Shame Issues Have Been Acknowledged

Each patient carries his own doctor inside him. They come to us not knowing this truth. We are at best when we give the doctor who resides within each patient a chance to go to work.

(Cousins, 1979)

The aim of this chapter is to share an approach of the particular ambivalence lingering when shame issues have been spoken and are acknowledged by the client and coach.

This ambivalence will be expressed verbally and non-verbally during coaching sessions aiming to resolve it and engage change, in an emergent process. I will be looking for a complex, detailed understanding of the ambivalence and the results of the use of Motivational Techniques to enhance resilience and provoke behaviour change. This can only be established by, talking to people, and studying their context.

I chose not to explore shame's root causes but rather to observe what happens once shame is named. My concern is with the journey towards relief; how to guide the coachee to grow into a happier person.

Data are collected from sessions with three coachees reporting shame issues. They agreed on the anonymous use of data from their sessions. I will first sketch the coachees' shame stories, to explore relevant exchanges during the sessions afterwards.

Case study 1: Nessa
Nessa is a successful business executive. She is an attractive woman and places high priority on decorum and manners.

She was accused of moral harassment, which she describes as being *"demanding"*. In answer to my probing she agreed that she is a very angry person, with violent outbursts because she wants *"things to be done the way they should be done"*.

She often feels *"stupid"*, stays late to rework *"afraid of being exposed*; *a nitwit without any academic education or any suitable family background"*. She is aware that "feeling stupid" fuels her anger and frenzies. She cannot manage her anger whenever she feels she is not *"good enough"*. She then uses shaming and blaming and *"hates"* herself *"even more."*

Case 2: Liam

Liam is co-CEO in a family business. His father sold 50% of the shares to Liam and insisted that he find a partner for the remaining 50%, because he didn't think Liam was solid enough to manage the company on his own.

The company grew beyond expectations, due to Liam's entrepreneurship and strong drive to prove his father wrong. His partner assures the stability and security in the company's functioning.

Liam does not feel recognised as a leader and feels trapped in the co-CEO arrangement, which in his opinion is the cause of his not being recognised as a leader.

Shame is a central theme in his childhood; Liam was born to the maid in his grandparents household and subsequently raised by the grandparents. His mother and father later had another child, which they raised themselves. Liam says he was *"ashamed of being alive"*, *"never good enough for his parents"*. This feeling of shame became persistent in his life.

Case 3: Einin

Einin is the only female partner in a Law firm; she came to me because she found it increasingly difficult to get on with her partners in a constructive professional relationship. The partners complain about her "numerous un-billable hours and her permanent quest for perfectionism which stifles her performance".

Einin's quest for perfection derives from a shaming event during elementary school; in order to "improve" her skills in dictation her teacher made her wear a cardboard on her back (for two years) with the following inscription: 0/10 in dictation! Whenever Einin cannot get her *"organisational ideas"* across to her partners she feels 0/10: *"Worthless"*. She then blames them and feels helpless and depressed.

39.3.1 Conceptual Framework for Observation

When shame is named, it can feel as a "aha" moment, it can bring relief and recognition of the underlying cause for behaviours, pain and discomfort. For some coachees this may be were they would like to go deep into the **why** of shame and linger with root causes and set up defences finding fault with the past or the present, blaming their shame on someone or something else. Others enter a **world of ambivalence**; "ok now I know why I behave that way, what hurts me, how it affects my life…where do I go from here? What can I change? …. Do I want to change? Can I deny this, get on with my life and forget now that I've come this far? Or… can I go further put these behaviours behind me, get out of the shame "spiel" and feel good?".

This is where the voyage starts. My hypothesis is that overcoming that ambivalence sets the coachee free: from the burden of shame affecting his/her behaviour, but also from denial and the pain intrinsic to the ambivalence. It is a process of change and of growing, connecting to one self in a healthy way.

The ambivalence is between:

- The "relative" comfort of the known territory; the defence mechanisms used to relieve shame and the resulting behaviour: the unwanted identity.
  AND
- The emergence of the ideal identity towards which reason commands to strive.

The figure below illustrates the ambivalence between status quo (defence mechanisms) and behaviour change with its ingredients necessary to attain the tipping point and change (Fig. 39.1).

39.4   Motivational Interviewing Sparking Change and Building Shame Resilience

Motivational Interviewing (MI) is a collaborative, goal-oriented method with particular attention to the language of change (Rollnick & Miller, 2002). MI is a style of interacting with the coachee intended to strengthen **personal motivation for and commitment to a target behaviour change** by eliciting and exploring an individual's own arguments for change (Rollnick & Miller, 2010).

It is designed to address the ambivalence when facing change within an atmosphere of acceptance. To address the ambivalence with the appropriate tool (Motivational Interviewing) enhances the desire for change and tips the balance.

Resilience, the first block on the behaviour change scale, is used with Boris Cyrulnik's acceptation: to spring back in a forward movement without settling on shame. In MI the coach is the tutor of resilience; a strong post to support growth, express empathy and accept ambivalence as a normal part of human experience.

Reason, the second block, represents the client's inherent reason(s) for and concerns about change; reasons are the basis for attitude and desire. Using MI as a tool the coach will develop discrepancy between the present state, the unwanted identity, and how the coachee wants it to be, the ideal identity. The goal is to override the inertia of status quo. The coach will roll with resistance and strive to understand the ambivalence from the coachee's point of view.

Desire for change, tipping the scale, happens when the coachee advocates for change. In MI spirit the coach supports the coachee's belief that he/she can carry out the necessary actions to commit to change and succeed in changing behaviour. The coachee remains the final arbiter of the change process.

39.5   Findings and Discussion

To reveal the ambivalence: the unwanted versus the ideal identity I use two questions adapted from the Connections curriculum (Brown, 2009) and give them to

Fig. 39.1 Ambivalence between status quo (defence mechanisms) and behaviour change

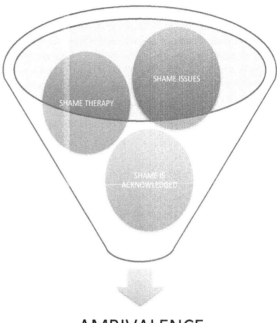

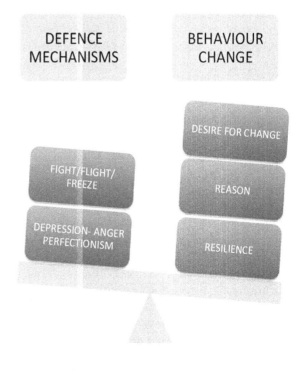

my coachees as homework. They list two or three ideal identities and two or three unwanted identities; it's a first description of their ambivalence.

MI focuses on exploring and resolving ambivalence as a key in eliciting change. MI works on intrinsic motivation for change, it centres on the motivational processes within the individual that facilitate change. MI is both, client centred and intentionally directive, directed towards the resolution of ambivalence in the service of change. The coach creates **an atmosphere in which the coachee rather than the coach becomes an advocate for change**.

39.5.1 Principles and Strategies

Miller and Rollnick (2000) described four basic principles of MI and identified two phases:

1. Building motivation for change.
2. Strengthening and Commitment.

To illustrate this I will briefly explore the use of the basic principles through extracts from the coaching sessions from the cases and subsequently go through the two phases to highlight my key findings.

Principle 1: Express Empathy
By practising empathy, the behaviours or decisions of the coachee become more comprehensible, the coach understands them **from the coachee's perspective**.

Why Nessa is lashing out, viewed from her perspective:

> "…, my parents both worked in the same factory… they both drank in the same pubs …ambition or achievement were dirty words. **I don't want to live like that; I want to be respected…**"

I can see where Nessa doesn't want to go; he aim to "be respected" makes special sense viewed from her perspective.

Asking open questions, listening reflectively, directly affirming and supporting, helps the coachee to verbalize her feelings. I will then **use summarizing** to link material together, to emphasise certain points, and to collect and elicit "change talk".

Principle 2: Develop Discrepancy
Change is motivated by a perceived discrepancy between present behaviour and personal goals and values. Awareness of this discrepancy can increase motivation to change. Particular attention is paid to the coachee's arguments for change, compared to those for not changing. The coach differentially **elicits and explores the coachee's own arguments for change as a path out of ambivalence.**

Liam's ideal identity: "*… a strong and very competent leader, standing straight on my own legs, … a visionary in my field*", versus his unwanted identities: "*… an outcast, a good for nothing, a second hand CEO, a mere salesman for the company*".

Discrepancy may be triggered by awareness of the cost of one's present course of behaviour. For instance in Liam's case when he develops arguments against change towards his ideal personality, I can start out with **simple reflections** (1), or increase the impact with a an **amplified reflecti**on (2) depending on the intensity of his argument, or give him a **double sided reflection** (3) to increase his awareness of the discrepancy.

Liam:

"I can't concentrate on improving my leadership right now, we're in the middle of high season I am too busy right now".

Coach:

(1) "You're really busy." (2) "You couldn't possibly concentrate on that now, given all that is on your plate" (3) "So at this point, it's hard to know where your work on leadership fits into these other competing demands, and on the other hand, you know you need it to attain what you desire."

The goal of developing discrepancy is to increase and amplify it till it overrides the inertia of status quo.

Principle 3: Roll with Resistance

Rolling with resistance is to **not** argue for change, but express an understanding of the coachee's point of view. It tends to diffuse rather than amplify the ambivalence and thereby diminishes resistance. It is **how** the coach responds to resistance that makes the difference, which distinguishes motivational interviewing from other approaches (Rollnick & Miller, 2002).

The goal is to decrease client resistance because this pattern is associated with long-term change. Using **reflecting skills** such as those evoked in Liam's example is one way to roll with resistance. More strategic elements can also alter the interaction pattern: shifting focus, reframing, emphasizing personal choice and control and coming along side.

To **shift the coachee's focus** away may be useful when we run into an area which doesn't seem productive; to diffuse the initial concern and direct attention to a workable issue. Another response is to **reframe**; the coachee's information is recast into a new form and viewed in a light more likely to be helpful and support change.

After Einin had written her ideal and unwanted identities, I felt she kept arguing quite strongly for status quo; this is called "sustain talk" in MI. Using **reflective responses** and **reframing** I discovered that her resistance was linked to anxiety of how she would be able to function once she left her old "habits" behind.

As if her knowledge and skills stayed in her known territory and the change process (the coaching sessions, ultimately me as her coach) was threatening her freedom of choice. I then used the emphasis on personal choice and control, and re-assured her that she was the only one who'd determine what she'd do, and that all along the process she had total freedom of choice.

I did express this reassurance earlier as an introduction of the process to come. It was ineffective then; at that stage Einin was still in the pre-contemplation phase of change (Prochaska & DiClemente, 1984) she had not yet fully engaged in the change process. Einin had not yet decided to operate a change; she was trying to imagine a change and toying with the possibility. During pre-contemplation the coachee may experience a feeling of being trapped and hindered in her freedom of choice and will react to this sensation.

Psychological reactance occurs in response to threats to perceived behavioural freedoms (Brehm, 1981). Einin's choice between status quo and behaviour change is a choice motivated by discomfort coherent with precedent behaviours, and a desire to cease those behaviours. The struggle goes on within her, there is no external threat; she did not react to the process or my coaching but expressed her anxiety linked to the ambivalence.

Another strategy to address resistance is **coming alongside**: when the coach defends the counter change side, it is a special case of amplified reflection.

MI is a dialogue about the coachee's ambivalence, the interviewer explores both sides. Coming alongside as the coachee argues against change is another way of defusing the argument and eliciting change talk. MI is the opposite of a confrontational approach in which the coach advocates for the change position and the coachee defends against it. It is nevertheless a conscious goal-directed approach and there is no reason why the coachee has to be kept in the dark about the dialogue.

With Nessa I set up a **direct debate** in which the coachee defends the need for change speaking in "you" language and the coach the counter argument speaking as "I". This kind of contrived dialogue is far from easy on the coachee. Even though it was awkward when we started out, the challenge appealed to Nessa and it elicited engaging change talk as she defended the need to change.

Principle 4: Support Self-efficacy

The support of self-efficacy is utilized when the coachee has sufficiently resolved ambivalence about change and begins to articulate **preparation-for-change** statements or begins to "dabble" with change, making small changes in behaviour, correcting attitudes and perceptions without full immersion in the process.

The approach seeks to elicit the coachee's ideas, experiences and perceptions consistent with her ability to change.

The coach and coachee **brainstorm** change-strategies, developing a change plan, and enhancing confidence, to stimulate creative, divergent thinking about how change might be accomplished. It is ok for the coach to suggest ideas but it is the coachee's creativity, which should generate possibilities; another format to elicit confidence talk.

The **elicit-provide-elicit style** recommended in MI consists in first asking for permission, offering the information, and then asking for the coachee's response.

The coachee remains the expert on what will and what won't work and is free to make choices about methods, timing and preferred strategies. Evocative questions such as: "Where would you start, if you decided to make a change to that particular behaviour?" "What other people or resources might help, if that's what you decided to do?" are very helpful.

Nessa had doubts about the perception of her ideal identity by others so I used the subjunctive syntax to query:

"Suppose that you succeeded in being perceived as … (the ideal persona) and you were looking back at it now: What most likely is it that worked? How did it happen?"

A common purpose that runs through all the techniques outlined here is for the coachee to talk about ways in which change can occur, about confidence and about how he or she can succeed. The coach's role is to stimulate further thought and specificity.

39.6   The Stages of Change

The five principles and the techniques and strategies developed above are used in two phases. In the paragraph "roll with resistance", I briefly evoked the Trans Theoretical Model (TTM) to illustrate Einin's anxiety (Prochaska & DiClemente, 1984). Identifying a coachee's status in terms of the stages of change is helpful in deciding which motivational strategies to use and in which phase. Considering TTM as a valid and very broadly applied model of change I will use it as foundation for my demonstration of the effectiveness of MI in the context of my study.

This figure schematises the Trans Theoretical Stages of Change (Fig. 39.2).

The departing point of my research is when a person has acknowledged and named his shame: in **pre-contemplation.** TTM has identified processes of change that have been implicated in movement from one stage to the next and in successful change (Prochaska & DiClemente, 1984). Cognitive and experimental processes of change appear to be more important in the earlier stages of change (phase 1 MI), and

Fig. 39.2 Determination Decision (Andrieux)

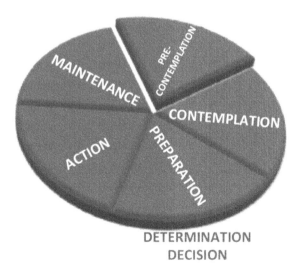

DETERMINATION
DECISION

behavioural processes appear to be more important in the later stages (phase 2 MI). MI approaches cognitive and experimental processes like consciousness raising, self-re-evaluation in the early stages of change (Rollnick & Miller, 2000). As coachees move forward in the process, MI influences efficacy and the behavioural processes of change.

The following development demonstrates that MI's two phases are aligned with this model. The philosophy in MI is appropriate for the participants facing ambivalence, as their change journey unfurls according to the TTM, the momentum of MI is clearly aligned albeit with the TTM model and with the feelings and abilities of the coachees. Thus guaranteeing the boosting of shame resilience and allowing behaviour change.

The coach's challenge is to understand where the coachee is in the change cycle and to offer the appropriate assistance.

PHASE 1: Building Motivation for Change—Enhancing Resilience

> "I have spread my dreams under your feet,
> tread softly because you tread on my dreams."
>
> W.B. Yeats

This first phase encompasses: the coachee's discovery of his/her ambivalence about the change of behaviour and the coach's first landmarks as a tutor of resilience supporting intrinsic motivation. In TTM this corresponds with the stages of **pre-contemplation and contemplation**, the cognitive and experimental processes of change.

In **pre-contemplation**, having named shame, identified the damages and pain shame causes in their life, recognised their recourse to defences impacting their behaviour the coachees are getting ready to envision a different future. During the ensuing coaching sessions I learn more about this vision by careful listening and providing feedback in an empathic manner. My focus is on the moment when tension starts building and the ambivalence emerges. By creating a safe space and insisting on the freedom for the coachees to make their own decisions the coach facilitates exploration of change in a nonthreatening manner. Motivational interviewing is effective because it avoids argumentation, allows the coachee to hear and assimilate her change statements in order to increase resilience and move towards the contemplation of a desire for change.

I materialise the transition to **contemplation** with the questionnaire on the ideal and the unwanted identity: the foundations of the coachees' ambivalence.

In **contemplation stage** the coach's goal is to help the client tip the balance in favour of change. When coachees experience their ambivalence most strongly, MI style and principles make it possible to alleviate the ambivalence tension and support the resilience. By helping the coachee to think through the risks of status quo and the potential benefits of change and by instilling hope that change is possible the coach accentuates the positive aspects. He listens for change statements: expressions of concern, problem recognition, optimism about change, or intent to change. Facilitators for change in this stage are: summarizing, feedback, double-sided reflections, and affirmations to boost the coachee's resilience.

Overcoming the ambivalence and shifting the decisional balance can take time and requires great patience and persistence on the part of the motivational interviewer.

PHASE 2: Strengthening and Commitment to Behaviour Change

The coachee shows signs of **readiness to change** (increased talk about change). The coach's focus then is on strengthening the commitment to change and help the client develop and implement a plan. The coachee is in the **preparation stage.**

All ambivalence is not resolved. The decision making process continues throughout the preparation stage.

Sometimes it is important to hold the ideal identity up to the light for scrutiny in order to transform the perfectionistic ideals into attainable self-accepting ideals translatable into goals and standards before preparing the plan. I worked through that with Nessa's professional ideal identity, which was tinted by her perfectionism and far removed from her present skills and capacities. I used summarizing and reframing with infinite care, threading softly because her lack of schooling was one of her causes of shame. It took time but Nessa developed a viable plan, and started moving into the action, implementing her plan.

Here the challenge is not to confound action with change; coachees in action might still have some conflicting feelings about change. They may miss their old defences and struggle to fit into new behaviours. Motivational interviewing helps coachees build resilience as they take action by focussing on their successes, reaffirming their decisions.

Maintenance is the final stage, the coachee works to consolidate the gains attained during the action stage and struggles to prevent relapse. Motivation to consolidate the change is needed.

Motivational techniques made it possible to alleviate Nessa's ambivalence and initiate a change of behaviour. Today Nessa is enrolled in a Masters program, acquiring the skills to live her ideal professional identity; she 's equally testing new behaviours, supported by the learning environment. She reports:

> "I often find myself believing I can do things without being afraid that they won't be good enough ...I discovered the world would not stop turning each time I'm wrong, nothing will happen I'll just learn something more from it. Of course it is not like that all the time but I'm getting there more and more."

Nessa has not yet consolidated her new behaviours and will continue coming to coaching sessions for a while, we have spaced out the sessions. She can now also rely on tutors of resilience in her environment (people who actively support her in her project—see §1).

MI is a process of shared decision making, of exploration and negotiation, in which the two partners bring aspirations. The relationship between the coachee and the coach is a major part of the therapeutic process; the coachee's thoughts about the coach (transference) and the coach's thoughts and fantasies about the client (countertransference) are part of the clinical effort. Coachees may become intensely dependent on their coach, and seek to hand over to them all responsibility for their health (Adshead, 2000). Motivational techniques lessen that dependence by restoring self-esteem, which is terribly important in the context of shame where the coachees have a very low self-esteem. MI techniques lay the foundations for durable change of behaviour because the coachee freely decides of every step. The coach is a tutor, in the French understanding, supporting the coachee's growth, not tutoring him/her about what should be done or deciding what would be the way to go about changing for the better!

Most established therapies for shame accompany the client to alleviate the pain provoked by shame, be it by self-soothing or mindfulness; they work on the symptoms. Nessa was too much versed in self-loathing to envision self-soothing or mindfulness, she needed to be in control of her change process.

Liam would view self-soothing as a weakness. MI gave him the possibility to vent all his reasons for not changing, all the "things" that made it impossible. But more importantly he was compelled to re-hear them when I rolled with resistance reframing and summarizing his argumentations against change. To me it was a real "aha" moment when he found faults with them! I was a very happy and proud of him when he counterattacked and started arguing for change! Liam is still a co-CEO he had positive conversations with his partner was able to express his expectations in a constructive way. He spent time with his parents, had long "tête-à-têtes" with his mother with whom he hadn't talked for ages. We have started working on his leadership style; he doesn't feel trapped in his co-direction of the company anymore. Today he knows that he can lean on his partner's steadiness and thus develop his own talents, this is a great "jump onward" from his main defence; blaming others (his father, his co-CEO…).

Einin has increased her talk of change; she is advancing in the preparation stage, phase two of MI. She has started sketching a plan, which could coincide with a new professional development in the firm. She also "experiments" with taking more time off in order to develop her talents as a painter thus leaving more space for her "*secret Me of my dreams*". My three coachees have tipped the scales!

39.7   Further Research

I have used Brown's (2006, 2008, 2009, 2010) approach in my coaching sessions first as the appropriate tool for my coachees to name shame, and then as a pivot to reveal the participants' ambivalence with the questionnaire on ideal and unwanted identities. Starting with MI techniques as a follow up of the partial use of the shame resilience curriculum, revealed MI's potential for enhancing the outcome of another approach. This clearly opens a scope for further research to evaluate the efficacy of the use of MI techniques in concert with other approaches.

Originally MI has been designed for the treatment of addictions, to address the ambivalence between status quo (remaining addicted) and behaviour change. Nowadays MI is also used in the treatment of psychological problems such as anxiety, depression, suicidality, and eating disorders (Arkowitz, Westra, Miller, & Rollnick, 2008). As well as with adolescents and young adults (Naar-King & Suarez, 2011). More than 100 randomized clinical trials of MI have been published (Burke, Arkowitz, & Menchola, 2003) and show significant greater behaviour change by people who received MI, relative to those not receiving MI. None of these trials concerned the use of MI in shame issues, it would be interesting to conduct an extensive research to identify those problems and types of people who respond best to MI and those for whom it might be less appropriate.

39.8   Conclusion

In this research panel all participants have initiated a change of behaviour; they are at different stages of their change process, all have travelled through ambivalence, tipped the balance and began designing their future behaviour.

The findings in these three coaching cases and the outcomes for the coachees illustrate the effectiveness of the Motivational Interviewing Techniques used are adapted to enhance resilience, trigger change behaviour and alleviate ambiguity. MI is about the present and has no à priori views about the why resistance and ambivalence occur. With the focus on the client's perspectives of the pros and cons of changing, motivational techniques augur a positive outcome in freeing the person of his ambivalence. MI is a directive technique, providing guidance to change with the coach and coachee in an equal partnership. The MI coach's objective is to perceive as much as possible the ambivalence from the coachee'sviewpoint, rolling with resistance and eliciting change talk so that the coachee voices the pros for change and is ultimately the expert of his change.

Shame is often the unspeakable as Boris Cyrulnik's title of his book, "Mourir de dire La Honte"—*Die to speak shame*—(Cyrulnik, 2010). The MI technique used is effective for it opens the way for the coachee to take charge, to build resilience and start changing behaviours induced by shame. It does so without probing into the causes of shame but concentrating on the behaviour changes the coachee herself wishes (as described in the ideal persona) and letting the coachee voice the steps required, initiate the change and take charge of it as a life project.

References

Adshead, G. (2000). Psychological therapies for post-traumatic stress disorder. *The British Journal of Psychiatry, 177,* 144–148. (G. A. MRCPsych (Ed.)).

Arkowitz, H., Westra, H. A., Miller, W. R., & Rollnick, S. (2008). *Motivational interviewing in the treatment of psychological problems* (1st ed.). In S. Rollnick & W. R. Miller (Eds.). New York: The Guilford Press.

Brehm, J. (1981). *Psychological reactance: A theory of freedom and control.* New York: Academic Press.

Brown, B. (2006). Shame-resilience theory: A grounded theory of women and shame. *Families in Society, 87,* 43.

Brown, B. (2008). *I thought it was just me (but it isn't)* (2nd ed.). In G. Books, (Ed.). New York: Penguin Group.

Brown, B. (2009). *Connections—a twelve session psychoeducational shame resilience curriculum.* Minnesota: Hazelden.

Brown, B. (2010). *The gifts of imperfection* (1st ed.). Minnesota: Hazelden.

Burke, B. L., Arkowitz, H., & Menchola, M. (2003). The efficacy of motivational interviewing: A meta analysis of controlled clinical trials. *Journal of Consulting & Clinical Psychology, 71,* 843–861.

Cousins, N. (1979). *Anatomy of an illness as perceived by the patient: Reflections on healing and regeneration* (1st ed.). New York City: W. W. Norton & Company.

Cyrulnik, B. (2010). *Mourir de dire la honte* (1st ed.). Paris: Odile Jacob.

Freud, S. (1976). *The complete psychological works of sigmund freud—on narcissism: an introduction* (1st ed., Vol. 14). In Hogarth, (Ed.). London, Britain: James Stratchey.

Gilbert, P. B. A. (1998). *Shame interpersonal behaviour, psychopathology and culture.* New York: Oxford University Press.

Gilbert, P. (2006). Compassionate mind training for people with high shame and self-criticism: Overview and pilot study of a group therapy approach. *Clinical Psychology and Psychotherapy, 13,* 353–379.

Haggarty, J. (2006). Psychodynamic therapy. Retrieved from https://psychcentral.com/lib/psychodynamic-therapy/.

Lynch, T., Chapman, A., Rosenthal, M., Kuo, J., & Linehan, M. (2006). Mechanisms of change in dialectical behavior therapy: Theoretical and empirical observations. *Journal of Clinical Psychology, 62*(4), 459–480. https://doi.org/10.1002/jclp.20243.

Morrison, A. P. (1989). *Shame the underside of narcissism.* New York: Routledge Taylor & Francis Group.

Morrison, A. P. (1998). *The culture of shame.* New York: Jason Aronson.

Naar-King, S., & Suarez, M. (2011). *Motivational interviewing with adolescents and young adults.* New York: The Guilford Press.

Prochaska, J., & DiClemente, C. (1984). *The transtheoretical approach: Towards a systematic eclectic framework.* Homewood: Irwin Dow Jones.

Rachman, S. (1997). *Science and practice of cognitive behavioural therapy—the evolution of cognitive behavioural therapy.* In D. M. Clark, C. G. Fairburn, & M. G. Gelder (Eds.). Oxford: Oxford University Press.

Rollnick, S., & Miller, W. (2000). *Motivational interviewing. Brief therapy for addictions video series.* San Francisco: psychotherapy.net.

Rollnick, S., & Miller, W. R. (2002). *Motivational interviewing—preparing people for change* (2nd ed.). New York: The Guilford Press.

Rollnick, S., & Miller, W. R. (2010). *What makes it motivational interviewing.* Stockholm: UniTryck.

Wheeler, G. (1997). Self and shame: A Gestalt approach. *Gestalt Review, 1,* 221–244.

Len Andrieux coaches international executives in global organizations. She is a member of EMCC and subscribes to their code of ethics. Her experience as an executive and as a consultant to senior executives convinced her of the need to develop one's awareness of how the "inner personality" affects the way one exercises leadership and manages others. Her aim is to allow her clients to envision a kaleidoscope of possibilities, to encourage them to reinforce their faith in their talents.

She has designed, organized and directed executive leadership programs and enables executives, to work on aspects of their leadership behaviours: improving self-awareness, honing their strengths, transitioning into new roles, developing resilience and self-esteem, refining their communication and relationship skills paving the way to enhanced performance and success. She has held various executive positions in areas of corporate development and strategy. She intervened as a keynote speaker in several conferences on varied subjects: Quality Management, Emotional Intelligence, Managing generation Y, Empowering Women in Business. She has a Diploma in Clinical Organizational Psychology and an Executive Masters in Coaching and Consulting for Change from INSEAD and attended HARVARD's Kennedy School of Government, training in The Art and Practice of Leadership Development. She's a certified practitioner in: HOGAN Leadership Inventory, LIMEF-E, ECP 360° Managerial Competences. She is actually perfecting her practice of Systemic Representations.

Chapter 40
PRACTICE REPORT—Transforming Shame Through Mediation and Nonviolent Communication

Liv Larsson

Abstract This chapter offers new perspectives on shame and mediation. It shows how we can reclaim power and choice through transforming shame. And as shame is present in almost all conflicts, this becomes central in order for reconciliation to happen. The tool called "The Compass of Needs" is a process based on the principles of Nonviolent Communication (NVC). When combined, they create a powerful foundation for anyone wanting to mediate or act as a third party and facilitate dialogue and connection. Shame is a life-serving signal that often is misinterpreted as if there is "something wrong with us" or "that we have done something wrong". In this chapter the aim of transforming shame is to create a certain quality of connection between parties in a conflict. When connection is established, the likelihood of reaching a solution increases.

Keywords Cultural shame · Natural shame · Nonviolent communication · Mediation

40.1 Introduction

This chapter discusses how we can embrace cultural (and often diminishing) shame and through that get back to a more life-serving or natural shame. To aid in this process, 'The Compass of Needs' will be introduced. This tool helps us recognize when shame is ruling us and to find freedom of choice. The assumption is that behind every human action, there is an attempt to meet a need. Even when people blame, withdraw, threaten or use violence, we can see this as attempts, albeit tragic ones, to meet needs.

Some points on the core of the chapter:

- How shame can be move from being a hindrance to become a tool to deepen empathy and openness.

L. Larsson (✉)
Mjösjölidvägen 477, 946 40 Svensbyn, Sweden
e-mail: liv@friareliv.se
URL: http://www.friareliv.se

© Springer Nature Switzerland AG 2019

603

C.-H. Mayer and E. Vanderheiden (eds.), *The Bright Side of Shame*,
https://doi.org/10.1007/978-3-030-13409-9_40

- How to listen to the life-serving signal in the shame attack and how to use these signals to gain connection.
- How to regain connection and inner balance after a shame attack and thus be of better service to others.
- How to become more effective as a mediator or therapist by transforming the cultural parts of shame to the more natural and need-connected shame.

40.2 Nonviolent Communication (NVC)

Some people say, "Shame is bad, let's get rid of it, it makes people unhappy and diminished." Others says, "shame is good, is shows us what is right and what is wrong so we know how to behave." Both opinions have a point, yet there is more to shame than that. Shame has both a cultural and a natural component and before we are clear about the difference, we cannot really say if shame serves us or not.

People who suggest that we get rid of shame are usually talking about what I call cultural shame. It is based on a certain way of thinking that tells us to do everything it takes to fit in. Cultural shame is based on what is "right and wrong" in the culture we are in and what our limits and possibilities are. It tells us how to behave to have others respect and acceptance and sometimes the price we pay is high. This is one of the reasons why people would like to get rid of shame rather than to embrace it to see if there is anything useful or supportive in it.

Most people with the opinion that "shame is good" are also referring to cultural shame. They have noticed that when, for example, a child shows shame and expresses regret it can be an opening to reconnection. They hear the expressing of the words "I'm sorry" as a sign that there will be some change in the child's actions in the future. And if the child learns to say those magic words, they will have what they need to fit in and to have the acceptance of others. What they don't see is that most of us have learned to say; "I'm sorry" in order to get out of the situation and that it doesn't necessarily lead to any transformation of behavior or compassion for the person that they might have caused harm to. The words becomes habitual and loose the capacity to heal a broken connection.

What I'm suggesting is that if we want shame to be useful, we need to know how to first transform cultural shame into natural shame. With natural shame I am referring to the reaction we have when we notice that, for example, something we are doing is harming another. It is not a matter of someone being "wrong" in any way as with cultural shame, but it is an inner regret and sadness over something we have done that was harmful for someone. When we connect to natural shame, it's easier to connect with the human needs behind it and from that point we can help people to connect, even in the fire of a conflict.

I'm suggesting that there is always a seed of natural shame in all cultural shame. That seed connects to the very human needs of acceptance, dignity and belonging. Therefore there is no need to get rid of cultural shame, what we need to learn is to transform it into natural shame.

40.3 Nonviolent Communication, Mediation and Shame

"Never do anything to avoid shame." I attended a training with Marshall Rosenberg, the man behind the process of Nonviolent Communication (NVC). He claimed that he was looking forward to the next time he would have a shame attack. He had to be joking I thought.

It took me a long time to understand what Rosenberg meant, even though I studied Nonviolent Communication intensively with him and through his books over several years. Nonviolent Communication (NVC) is sometimes described as a process language. With this process we use words and principles that help communication and connection between the parties to flow. The purpose of NVC is connection. Rosenberg based his work on the assumption that behind every action a human being takes there is a motivation to meet some need. If we can connect to those human needs in ourselves and others, empathy can happen.

Nonviolent Communication is an approach developed by Marshall Rosenberg starting in the 1960s. Based on the idea that all human beings have the capacity for compassion as long as basic needs are recognized (Rosenberg, 2003, 2015). Habits of thinking and speaking that lead to violent behaviour in a social, psychological and physical way are based on cultural learning. Rosenberg's theory supposes that conflict arises when strategies for meeting needs collide. NVC proposes that people identify needs they share and collaborate to develop strategies that meet them (Rosenberg, 2003, 2015).

NVC supports change on three levels: with the self, with other and with groups and social systems. NVC enables to do three things:

Increase our ability to live with choice, meaning, and connection.
Connect empathically with self and others to have more satisfying relationships.
Sharing of resources so everyone is able to benefit (Rosenberg, 2015).

The principles of the NVC are suitable for use in the context of mediation.

Studying NVC, I gradually learned that if we were willing to take a pause when we experience a shame attack, giving it space, and listening to what we need in these moments, we can gain access to valuable information about what we need. We also get the chance to connect to a sense of power and choice that is invaluable in our connection with others. Embracing shame in that way has given me easier access and more sensitivity in connecting to what I and others need. Being sensitive and human in this way opens a door to listening with empathy from a place within, rather than only through some technique or method. When I act as the third party or a mediator, being able to listen and be open is crucial for the results.

Mediation between conflicting parties is about helping them recreate connection. The aim is the same if we act as a third party (mediator) between our kids, when they have a fight, or when colleagues in a work place are struggling to find common ground for their work (Larsson, 2012b). The connection is about recognizing and honoring each other's feeling and needs, seeing the humanness in the other. Finding a solution to a conflict or a problem becomes so much easier when there is connection, so I operate under the suggestion; "Connect before correct". When I discovered how shame affected communication, one more piece of the puzzle fell into place.

Mediation can be described as a process in which a third party helps conflicting people to change their view of a conflict, to see behind it, to recognize its potential for development, and to reach an agreement on how to act in the future (Larsson, 2009, 19). Through meditation it is possible, through the intervention of the mediator, to help the two parties to get a more human picture of each other. The principles of the NVC can be used in mediation to help people find solutions to a particular problem or to reconcile themselves. The mediator is often concerned with helping to restore relationships—relationships that sufferers experience as painful and trusting each other as a challenge (Larsson, 2009, 20).

Talking about and reconnecting to things that have led to a need for mediation support—for example in a situation where we have done something that has not taken the needs of others into consideration - often triggers shame in us. This can happen even if we did not feel ashamed at the time, but only now, after taking in how the situation affected someone else, are we overcome with shame.

We may internally criticize ourselves for not having anticipated how our choices would affect others. Or we might judge ourselves for not standing up for ourselves and showing where our boundaries are.

For more than 20 years as a mediator, I have seen that one of the things that most gets in the way of connecting people in conflict, is when one or both of the parties are trying to avoid shame. When someone – either party, or even the mediator, – is trying to avoid shame, it becomes harder to create connection. If the situation does not feel safe, the sensitivity that shame can give us access to often gets pushed away when we avoid it, and it becomes harder to get to the core of the conflict. When someone tries to, at any price, escape the discomfort of the feelings of shame, this action lies in the way of both connection and the solution.

If we embrace feelings of shame, we can learn about mutuality and care, but only if we do not believe in the self-destructive thoughts that often accompany the feeling of shame. As a mutual willingness to talk with authenticity is one of the things that makes mediation work, the avoidance of shame, becomes an obstacle. For the mediation process to work, a small element of vulnerability and willingness to "sit with a feeling of discomfort" is needed (Larsson, 2011). Shame gives us that vulnerability, if it is received and allowed to exist. There is a lot a mediator can do that contributes to this.

Shame attacks are usually uncomfortable. When a person is feeling strong shame it is therefore often hard for them to pause and to connect with both their own and another person's needs. Many people try to handle shame by avoiding it in some way, at least until they get support in dealing with it in some more life- serving way. Empathy is far away when we are busy getting rid of the discomfort of shame.

As soon as someone is willing to embrace the shame she/he is feeling, a more open and vulnerable state arises which is a first step towards empathy.

To understand how we avoid shame is useful for all mediators (or anyone acting as a third party). Most of us experience feelings of shame as uncomfortable and therefore we try to immediately avoid or get rid of the shame.

The most common ways to try to avoid shame can be summarized into four categories (withdrawing, attacking, self-blaming and rebelling) as described below. How well mediators can recognize and deal with these strategies when used by the conflicting parties, will affect the outcome of all mediation processes.

Four strategies used to avoid shame:

1. Withdrawing physically, mentally or emotionally.
2. Becoming self-critical.
3. Rebelling against threats to freedom or lack of respect.
4. Criticizing others. We judge, demand, threaten and blame.

40.4 The Compass of Needs

The aim of the tool I call "The compass of needs" is to be able to reconnect with needs (Larsson, 2012a). As a mediator or therapist it is very useful to recognize these avoidance patterns. Recognizing them helps us to see that someone is experiencing shame and wants to avoid it. This is a sign to the mediator that a situation is sensitive or unsafe, but also potentially important to address. Usually slowing down and addressing the moment of shame creates more of a willingness to embrace and express the feeling. A mediator can use the moment to help the person return to their underlying needs. As shame is a "social feeling" (a feeling that is connected to being part of a community), most often the needs for belonging, acceptance and dignity are needs that are not being met, amongst other needs, when we are having a shame attack.

The compass points out four different types of behavior or thoughts we use to avoid shame. Let's take a closer look at them and the thought patterns that are usually connected to them.

1. Shame can be avoided with submitting, withdrawing, becoming quiet and in not expressing what we feel, need and want. Usual thoughts may be:

    I don't need anything; I can manage on my own.

    I might as well give up; it will not turn out as I was hoping anyhow.

2. This person criticizes him- or herself as soon as something that stimulates shame comes up. The inner critic has free reign to attack and judge. This person willingly shows they are losers, victims, not to be counted and so on. Self-critical thoughts are usually along these lines:

    If I could just learn to not be so…

    I'm not … enough.

    I am such a…

    Why do I always?

3. This strategy rebels against what is perceived as demands or threats to the person's freedom or a lack of respect. It is important for this person to show their independence and self-sufficiency. Thoughts associated with rebellion could be:

    I have come further than that—I do not care…

    I have no problems! If nothing happens soon I will leave.

    Look at me and I'll show you how things should go!

4. Attacking others is the fourth strategy to try to avoid shame. Blaming, attacking and criticizing others gives a sense of relief from the shame attack. Others are to blame and *they* should act differently. Thoughts that are a sign that one has moved in this direction of the compass may be:

    It is your own fault. You must start taking responsibility!

    They are cowards and too weak to be able to do this.

    She/he/they/you are too…

    She/he/they/you are not … enough.

Why we choose to use one or more of these strategies is simply explained by it being what we have previously learned as a method to avoid shame during a strong shame attack. After that we have used the same strategy over and over, but usually having to pay a high price for its usage. Now that the shame avoiding strategies have been clarified, let's take a look at how they influence a mediation or conflict situation and what the mediator can do about them.

Four strategies to avoid shame.

Strategy 1: Withdrawing from shame in a mediation process.

A person can be physically present in the mediation room, but at the same time not available emotionally or mentally. When a person moves in this direction to avoid shame, she or he can rarely listen deeply to others, even if she or he is silent, as it might increase the intensity of his or her shame. He or she can seem unaffected or cold, but is, in fact, overwhelmed by a deep sense of powerlessness. When someone does not know how to express this, information that would be useful for the solution of the conflict never comes up into the open.

If the mediator senses that this is going on, there are several ways to act. You can take a pause and talk to each party of the conflict in private. It can clarify your assumption that they feel strong shame and at the same time ease their internal pressure.

Slowing down the speed of the conversation and focusing on how what has happened is affecting the parties helps build connection. Give the person that seems to have withdrawn time to process what has been expressed and to find his or her own words. You want to avoid escalating the feelings of shame, as shame is involuntary is not supportive. At the same time you want to help the person to be fully present. Moving out of withdrawal and connecting with their own needs can stimulate strong feelings for someone, so give it time. This person needs confirmation that he or she is important as part of the conversation.

As a mediator some of the things I might *ask* in this situation are:

– Does this situation seem a bit hopeless to you, and you want to connect to what the purpose of this conversation is?
– Are you worried that whatever you say will make it even harder to connect?
– Are you nervous and want some confirmation that what you say will be taken seriously?
– Would you like to have more trust that it will make a difference to talk about these things, and that you will eventually have some peace around this matter?

As a mediator some of the things I might express in this situation are:

I want you to understand that it makes a difference that you are participating in this mediation. Even if you find it challenging to express what you feel, it is valuable for the outcome of this process that we also get to hear what you need and want. So I wonder if you can tell us what you need in order to take part?

The mediation may also be continued in two separate rooms—shuttle mediation—if it helps the person to manage their shame without withdrawing.

Strategy 2: Self- blame in a mediation process.

When someone attacks, blaming her- or himselfs for what has happened and repetitively asks for forgiveness, it is often difficult to come to a place of real reconciliation in a conflict. A person that is stuck in blame usually stops listening, as they believe that taking on all the guilt will resolve the situation as it takes away the feeling of shame. If the roles in their relationship are static and this person often gets the blame for conflicts or misunderstandings, the mediator can be of help if he or she makes sure both sides are listened to.

The situation becomes skewed if one party believes that everything will be fine only if she or he takes on the blame. It is skewed because in order to heal a hurt, action is often necessary. To heal from a conflict, openness to change is needed plus new agreements about how to act from now on. Trust might fully return if these actions can be kept for some time.

If someone attacks or blames him- or herself, this person often becomes the focus, instead of the focus being on how to establish connection and to find new agreements or solutions. Mediation à la NVC is based on the hypothesis that a conflict can be more easily resolved when the needs of both parties are heard. Having all needs "on the table" creates a quality of connection that is the base of coming to mutual agreements on how to act after the mediation.

The mediator is not there to judge who has done right or wrong, or to find a scapegoat, the mediator is there to establish connection. Remember that this idea of finding a scapegoat is a big part of how most societies manage conflict. It is a many-thousand-year-old habit that needs to be handled with care and clarity. I'm not saying here that both parties have hurt each other equally. I'm saying that if one person takes on the blame, the mediation is not as effective as it could be. Behind this idea of scapegoating, a need to deeply mourn and heal is usually found. Mourning usually means taking the time to really let every feeling and need come to the table and to find new ways to build trust.

As a mediator some of the things I might *ask* in this situation are:

> Do you want us to understand that knowing what you now know, you would have liked to have acted differently?
>
> Are you ashamed of what impact your actions have had on X and do you want to do everything in your power to make up for it?

After having connected with the needs the person wants to mourn, the mediator may express:

> I appreciate that you show that you want to take responsibility for what happened. I am also a bit worried, as mediation is not about finding out who is right or wrong, but about connection and in finding new agreements in how you can proceed from here. How is this for you to hear?

Strategy 3: Rebelling against shame and vulnerability in a mediation process.

When people rebel against shame, they push vulnerability away by showing that they are independent and free. They invade the sensitive parts of themselves; pushing every sign of dependency away. For a person that chooses this strategy to avoid shame it is usually very important to be self-sufficient and to be able to do "what they want" and not care so much about "what other people might think". They avoid showing vulnerability and shame, and as a consequence are often perceived as cold, superfluous or difficult to connect with at a deeper level.

In invading vulnerability or rebelling against shame they stop paying attention to the needs of others, and it becomes difficult to meet the needs for care, reciprocity, connection and love. Behind the tough exterior there is, of course, vulnerability still. For connection to be made between the parties, the rebelling person needs to feel safe enough to be vulnerable. This often happens by itself if they are seen and appreciated for their willingness to take responsibility for themselves.

A person, who is ready to invade and rebel against any sign of vulnerability, may choose not to participate in a mediation process. This "no", may be a way for the person to show that she or he does not need anyone else, and wants to prove that she or he has not done anything wrong.

If I as a mediator suspects that this is going on, I usually suggest separate meetings with the people involved. At this meeting I put my attention on the positive intention behind the chosen action, or on some positive result, rather than on the action itself. I do not need to approve of the action this person did, but it makes a difference in our connection if I'm able to acknowledge their intention in doing it. If you have the ability to see the "positive" in their motivations and express appreciation for that, it often lowers their guard. Beware, however, of giving appreciation in the form of "praise," that you think they are "good" or that they have done something "good." That kind of appreciation nourishes their rebellion and leads them to believe that you sympathize with their choices. Instead express the needs of yours that are met by them trying to act on the intention. Criticizing them usually does not lead to connection, but rather to more reactions where they want to prove their independence.

As a mediator you want to create connection, so you can eventually get to some "common ground." When you are connected, you can talk about what you are feeling distressed, angry or worried about. Connect your feelings to your needs. If they have difficulty hearing you, respond to their reaction with empathy and then go back to honesty again.

We try to meet them where they are, which could sound something like this:

> When you walked out during the mediation last time, after saying, 'I do not care about this anymore,' I wonder if it was because you yearn for more understanding of your choices?

An expression of honesty could sound something like this:

> When I hear what you said to X, I am worried because I do not understand what it is you want by expressing this. Are you willing to tell us what you need?

Often the connection with someone who has chosen to rebel needs to be built quite slowly step by step. The person might want to end the conversation if he or she experiences any attempt to limit their—highly valued – freedom and independence. Behind this reaction there is the fear of being confronted with the shame they have tried to run away from – maybe for a long time.

Strategy 4: Attacking—criticizing and judging others in a mediation process.

If someone gets angry, and attacks and criticizes the other party, it might result in the mediation talks breaking apart. Certainly we might want to separate the parties when the situation threatens to increase into physical violence. Sometimes it can continue with the often more time-consuming form of a shuttle mediation, with the parties in two different rooms and the mediators shuttling between the rooms.

It often helps me to connect if I remind myself that no one attacks anyone else, without having first experienced some form of violation or offense themselves. Often it is not conscious, but still has a strong influence on the person. Also in this direction, just as in the opposite direction of the compass of needs, the focus is on the issue of guilt. Who is to blame for the conflict? In this case, the person blames their opponents, instead of themselves.

To butt heads with someone who is choosing to move in this direction can be perceived as an invitation to compete about whom is the strongest. Since the argument is often a part of this strategy, it is constructive to choose another way to communicate, or the conflict will increase. Instead of attacking, connect to both parties with empathy, and help them to get in touch with which needs they are trying to meet with their relentless criticism.

When you do so, you become a role model, showing that there are other ways to handle a situation than by finding out who is right or to blame someone. When they have a sense of being understood, they become more open to listening to what we have to say.

I often remind myself that a person may feel cornered and does not know how she or he will have the capacity to feel even more shame. Either party may need a confirmation that you hear that the other person's behavior has affected him very much. He or she may struggle for quite a while to get his opponent to take on the blame.

40.5   When the Mediator or Third Party Feels Ashamed

It is valuable for a mediator to know how to deal with their own shame so that it does not become an obstacle in the mediation process. Knowing how to not spend energy in avoiding shame becomes an opportunity for in-depth vulnerability and connection. As a mediator, you may make mistakes, or say things you feel ashamed of. Or you might get embarrassed over something you hear the parties say. Maybe you feel ashamed "on their behalf" and get a secondary shame reaction. We can learn what situations often stimulate shame and thus learn to recognize when we need to be alert.

Shame attacks make us stupid in a certain way. It takes away our creativity when we are focused on surviving. When we feel shame, we often act in ways we later regret. At least if we try to pretend that we are not feeling shame or try to avoid it in some other way. When this happens, all the energy that would otherwise be used to create connection is used to conceal a natural reaction.

Shame can alert us in our interactions with other people. If we are not trying to avoid it, it can help us become more aware of our own and others' needs. When we embrace shame it becomes a door to a deeper capacity for empathy, so getting to know shame is really crucial for anyone wanting to support people dealing with a conflict.

First, learn to recognize shame by the physical symptoms. Some common symptoms are a warm wave running through your body, blushing or heat in your face, a dry mouth, your mind going into high gear, and if you meet a particular person's eyes, your mouth getting caught in a stiff smile.

Maybe you do not recognize these physical signs of shame before you've moved in either direction of the needs compass. In that case you need to learn those behaviors. When you start recognizing your favorite avoidance tactics you can start from there, and "go backwards" until you feel the physical shame impact again. The natural physical reaction provides information about what you need at that moment.

If you, in the role of a mediator, feel strong shame in the midst of mediation, you can, of course, take a break. Depending on what kind of mediation situation you are in, and if you think you can express yourself in a way that creates more connection, you can also ask the parties to listen to what is going on inside of you. Focusing on clearly expressing feelings and taking responsibility for them through connecting them to needs is crucial as it lessens the risk of the parties hearing what you say as blame.

The more you learn about shame, the more you can learn about needs and about empathy.

Reflection

Reflect on how you sometime try to numb or push out shame. Knowing what strategies you use to avoid shame and to embrace them will help you recognize them earlier in a mediation process. Therefore spend some time before a mediation where you guess there might be shame coming up, reflecting on your most usual avoidance strategies. Look for the signs in your body, face and words. Ask yourself what you usually need in that situation. Take some time to really connect with the need. Keeping the connection to your needs, rather than trying to avoid shame will keep you more attentive to your work as a mediator.

40.6 Four Steps to Regain Connection and Inner Balance After a Shame Attack

Dealing with shame in the manner proposed in the following four steps can be challenging, especially if you have a preconceived idea that a mediator is supposed to be perfect. Dealing with shame in this way thus is a path to more authenticity. It will give you easier access to empathy as it will connect you to how it is to be human, rather than to just be professional.

I believe that the more authentic the mediator can be, the greater role model for the parties in the mediation. When the mediator is willing to be vulnerable and open, it is inspirational for the parties to choose the same. Of course it is challenging to be in the middle of a conflict and to go for openness and authenticity, but knowing how to find your path can create enough safety to go for it.

Suggestions if you, as a mediator, have a shame attack:

- Allow yourself to feel how the shame affects your body and face. (Maybe you only notice this affect after having admitted to yourself that you are trying to avoid it).
- Get in touch with what you need. Start with asking if you have a need for acceptance, belonging or dignity, as they are part of the needs that are usually triggered.
- Take a deep breathe into that vulnerable need-connected place and allow for humanness and vulnerability.
- If you take a pause in the mediation, use it to connect with someone you know can listen with empathy.

References

Larsson, L. (2009). *Begegnung fördern*. Paderborn: Junfermann.
Larsson, L. (2011). *A helping hand*. Svensbyn: Friare LIV Konsult.
Larsson, L. (2012a). *Anger, guilt & shame*. Svensbyn: Friare Liv.
Larsson, L. (2012b). *Relationships, freedom without distance, connection without control*. Svensbyn: Friare liv.
Rosenberg, M. (2003). *Nonviolent communication* (2nd ed.). Encinitas: PuddleDancer Press.
Rosenberg, M. (2015). *Nonviolent communication* (3rd ed.). Encinitas: PuddleDancer Press.

Liv Larsson is a CNVC-certified trainer and passionate mediator. Based in Sweden, she has worked internationally sharing leadership, communication, and mediation skills for more than 20 years. Trained by Marshall Rosenberg, founder of Nonviolent-Violence Communication (NVC), her special interest is to see mediation in the context of social change towards more life-serving structures. One of her mediation contracts is as a mediator for FSC Sweden, mediating between the Sami, the indigenous people of Scandinavia, and the five biggest forest companies in the Sami region of Sweden. She is also contracted as a mediator between that same minority group and the biggest mining company in Sweden, LKAB. She regularly mediates conflict in families and organizations. Currently she is involved in a project with the Norwegian Red Cross and Danish Liv-Com on Domestic Violence. Giving trainings to police, social workers, health care workers etc. on the first response to a victim of violence. She has written 20 books on NVC, translated into many different languages for example English and German. Three of her books are especially useful for a mediator, as well as for anyone wanting to enhance their communication skills.

Epilogue

Elisabeth Vanderheiden & Claude-Hélène Mayer

In our previous book, *The Value of Shame. Exploring a Health Resource in Cultural Contexts* (Vanderheiden & Mayer, 2017), as well as in the work presented here, we have delved deeply into the subject of shame and the potentials associated with it. We have shaped our focus to provide a more detailed, multidisciplinary and transcultural perspective. We have moved a step further by incorporating additional views, illuminating new aspects, and extending practical applications. In this book, renowned experts have examined shame with regard to central fields of action and important areas of life, from different cultural perspectives, to develop concrete suggestions of ways to directly transform shame in context. This makes a decisive contribution to the fact that shame, in its non-toxic dimension, can actually lead to positive changes on an individual and a social level. Further, we have moved from a primarily positive psychology perspective PP1.0 towards a more integrated PP2.0 perspective.

Not only does this book generate new perspectives and responses to new, exciting research and theoretical discourses, but it also presents more questions which need to be addressed in future. For example, in his recently published book, the Swiss psychiatrist Hell (2018), points to specific sociocultural factors that contribute to the way in which shame currently "hides more and differently than it used to" (2018, 185, translated by the authors):

> Although shame is devalued as a blemish, it does not simply disappear but expresses itself for example in Fremdschämen or hides in political correctness. The shame goes more in the width today than in the depth. It expresses itself more in embarrassment than in deep terror

© Springer Nature Switzerland AG 2019
C.-H. Mayer and E. Vanderheiden (eds.), *The Bright Side of Shame*,
https://doi.org/10.1007/978-3-030-13409-9

about itself. Today's loss of tradition, however, does not erase shame, but increasingly binds feelings of shame and its defence to current trends. (185–186)[1]

Hell (2018) identifies the following as particularly significant trends in this context:

- forced individualisation
- religious loss of tradition and secularisation
- change of education or changed socialisation
- progressive mechanisation and "medicalisation" of life
- digitisation and communication change
- liberalisation and globalisation of the economy.

All of these affect body shame and sexual shame, but also social shame. It is worthwhile to explore further how those are reflected in different cultural contexts, and which strategies exist to (re)discover and further develop or transform shame as a resource. Some of the contributions in this book (see Silverio's and Gilbert's chapters) already illuminate this subject.

Another critically important aspect of shame as a resource is the socio-political context in which shame proves to be relevant. Important preliminary work on shame in this context has already been done by Lotter (as cited by Mayer, in this book), in connection with Nazism and the post-war period (see Mayer on shame in Germany, in this book), and lately f. e. by American author Jennifer Jacquet (2015), who suggests using shaming as a socialisation tactic to prevent and combat institutional abuse, such as corporate misconduct.

Shame could also be discussed as a possible resource when it comes to negotiating reparations in the context of colonisation, such as with Aboriginal people in Australia, First Nations in the United States and Canada in North America, and Hereros and Namas in Namibia. At the same time, however, shame or embarrassment can take on threatening forms in the political arena. One such example is a currently much-debated project of the Chinese government, which proposes to create a social credit profile for all citizens, recording their level of compliance with given social norms. These profiles are then intended to open or close access to certain resources such as education, loans, and jobs (FAZ.NET, 2018; Deutschlandfunk, 2018).

A particularly exciting field of research arises when considering the diverse dimensions of shame in an increasingly digitised world, especially when viewed in transcultural contexts. The Israeli philosopher Aaron Ben-Ze'ev (2003) observes:

> The relative anonymity of cyberspace and the ability to control which matters we wish to reveal allow us to safeguard our privacy while increasing emotional closeness and

---

[1] Hell (2018): "Scham wird zwar als Makel abgewertet, verschwindet aber nicht einfach, sondern äußert sich zum Beispiel im Fremdschämen oder versteckt sich in politischer Korrektheit. Die Scham geht heute mehr in die Breite als in die Tiefe. Sie äußert sich eher in Peinlichkeiten als im tiefem Erschrecken über sich selbst. Der heutige Traditionsverlust löscht aber Scham nicht aus, sondern bindet Schamgefühle und ihre Abwehr vermehrt an aktuelle Trends" (185–186). Translated by the authors.

openness. In fact, the nature of privacy itself has undergone a significant change in cyberspace since many matters that are usually kept private tend to be discussed in cyberspace. The greater tendency toward closeness and openness online has led to a redefinition of the nature of shame, which like privacy is connected to fundamental values that we want to safeguard. (Ben-Ze'ev, 2003, 1)

The following are suggestions of some potentially interesting and rewarding fields for further research:

- How does digitisation transform concepts and practices of relationships such as friendship, love and sexuality, through worldwide social media applications and dating platforms? What role might different, culturally-related concepts play? To what extent do these change through practices such as sexting (Ngo, Jaishankar, & Agustina, 2017; Anastassiou, 2017), and love or romance scamming (Whitty, 2018)?
- Although there are already studies that deal with cyber-bullying across cultures (see Craig et al., 2009, for example), a more intensive discussion of the issue of shame in this context is necessary, especially in the context of positive psychology. To consider how shame can be liberated and transformed from its toxic dimension in this highly dynamic context, and how this can be seen in different cultural contexts, would be another exciting research concern.
- In the context of digitalisation, there is also a dramatic increase in group-focused enmity. By way of example, the number of anti-Semitic comments on the internet seem to be increasing worldwide. A recent linguistic investigation undertaken by the Technical University of Berlin (Schwarz-Friesel, 2018) shows a dramatic increase in such internet statements from 7.51% in 2007 to more than 30% in 2017, for example for Germany. Several hundreds of thousands of texts and commentaries were examined in the Internet in Germany. At the same time, the language has become radicalised. Since 2009, Nazi comparisons, violent fantasies, and drastic doctrines that demonise Jews have doubled (Schwarz-Friesel, 2018). From our perspective, it would be worthwhile examining the question of which individual and collective ideas of shame and embarrassment reach or fail in this context, or which strategies could lead to more shame and developing its potential for individual and collective growth could help to reduce or, ideally, prevent group-focused enmity.
- Industry 4.0—as future trend of continuous automatisation and data exchange in manufacturing technologies, combined with the Internet of things, cloud computing etc.—will revolutionise the world of work globally, regionally and locally. It is already known that shame in connection with the workplace is a highly significant issue (Mayer, Viviers, & Tonelli, 2017), for example, in relation to bullying or other kinds of mistreatment by others, to poor work quality, exclusion and internalised failure in the workplace. How this will differ in relation to Industry 4.0, especially in various cultural contexts, may become a highly productive field of research.
- We also see need for extended research concerning the emergence of new forms of shame, which result from the physical and mental-optimisation pressure that many people feel today (Hell, 2018, 199). This is—almost inevitably—also connected with the danger of shameful failure.

Mistakes, errors or failure can, at the individual level, deeply shame and embarrass someone and cause severe personal, organisational and collective crises. However, it can also be viewed as a resource for self-development and organisational, collective and societal change. At the organisational level, mistakes, errors and failure can have serious consequences for individuals such as employees, leaders or clients in the field of transportation, or in the context of medicine or chemistry, for instance. They can also reveal inaccuracies in process chains, or weaknesses in a system. These concepts can, however, also trigger contingent and sustainable improvement processes on all levels. Even in the political context, actual or perceived wrong decisions can have massive and long-lasting consequences for individuals, societal groups and subcultures, and for society itself. Societal mistakes, errors and failures may then even be discussed in global contexts and in terms of their universal impact. Examining these aspects in terms of shame can also prove to be rewarding fields of research.

References

Anastassiou, A. (2017). Sexting and young people: A review of the qualitative literature. *The Qualitative Report, 22*(8), 2231–2239. Retrieved from http://nsuworks.nova.edu/tqr/vol22/iss8/9.

Ben-Ze'ev, A. (2003). Privacy, emotional closeness, and openness in cyberspace. *Computers In Human Behavior, 19*(4), 451–467. https://doi.org/10.1016/s0747-5632(02)00078-x.

Craig, W., Harel-Fisch, Y., Fogel-Grinvald, H., Dostaler, S., Hetland, J., & Simons-Morton, B., et al. (2009). A cross-national profile of bullying and victimization among adolescents in 40 countries. *International Journal Of Public Health, 54*(S2), 216–224. https://doi.org/10.1007/s00038-009-5413-9.

Deutschlandfunk. (2018). *Sozialkredit-System—China auf dem Weg in die IT-Diktatur.* [online]. Available at: https://www.deutschlandfunk.de/sozialkredit-system-china-auf-dem-weg-in-die-it-diktatur.724.de.html?dram:article_id=421115. Accessed July 17, 2018.

FAZ.NET. (2018). *Chinas Sozialkreditsystem: Die totale Kontrolle* [online]. Available at: http://www.faz.net/aktuell/feuilleton/debatten/chinas-sozialkreditsystem-die-totale-kontrolle-15575861.html. Accessed 17 July 17, 2018.

Hell, D. (2018). *Lob der Scham. Nur wer sich achtet, kann sich schämen.* Gießen: Psychosozial-Verlag.

Jacquet, J. (2015). *Scham. Die politische Kraft eines unterschätzten Gefühls.* Berlin: Fischer.

Mayer, C-H., Viviers, R., & Tonelli, L. (2017). 'The fact that she just looked at me...'—Narrations on shame in South African workplaces. *SA Journal of Industrial Psychology/SA Tydskrif vir Bedryfsielkunde, 43*(0), a1385. https://doi.org/10.4102/sajip.v43i0.1385.

Ngo, F., Jaishankar, K., & Jose R. Agustina, A. (2017, December). Sexting: Current research gaps and legislative issues. *International Journal of Cyber Criminology, 11*(2), 161–168. https://doi.org/10.5281/zenodo.1037369.

Schwarz-Friesel, M. (2018). Antisemitismus 2.0 und die Netzkultur des Hasses. Judenfeindschaft als kulturelle Konstante und kollektiver Gefühlswert im digitalen Zeitalter. Retrieved from https://www.linguistik.tu-berlin.de.

Vanderheiden, E., & Mayer, C. (2017). *The value of shame. Exploring a health resource in cultural contexts.* Cham: Springer International Publishing.

Whitty, M. (2018). Do you love me? Psychological characteristics of romance scam victims. *Cyberpsychology, Behavior, and Social Networking, 21*(2), 105–109. https://doi.org/10.1089/cyber.2016.0729.

Appendix

Page	Application	Context
15	Questionaire Random statements on collective shame in German therapeutical and counselling contexts	Opening the Black Box Part 1: On Collective Shame in the German Society Claude-Hélène Mayer
25	Questionaire Reflection on body shame	Opening the Black Box Part 2: Exploring Individual Shame in German Research Claude-Hélène Mayer
26	Questionaire Reflection Shame in the context of care	
46	ahiMsA in Speech: A Practice	lajjA: Learning, Unlearning, and Relearning dharma prakaza zarmA bhAwuk
57	Questionaiere Sharing experiences (of Japanese Returnees)	Shame as a Health Resource for the Repatriation Training of Japanese Returnees (kikokushijo) in Japan Kiyoko Sueda
73	Questionaire self-blame strategy functions	The Effect of Regulation on Shame in Adolescence in China Liusheng Wang & Biao Sang
98	Some applied recommendations to transform social shame through a social development initiative:	"The Group is That Who Protects You in the Face of Shame": Self-change and Community Theater Participation in an Argentine Agro-city Johana Kunin
110	Case study Shame and Trauma amongst refugees	A Sociocultural Exploration of Shame and Trauma Among Refugee Victims of Torture Gail Womersley
124	Questionaire Reflections on crime, criminal behaviour, and restorative justice within the context of shame and shaming	Crime and Shame: Reflections and Culture-Specific Insights Claude-Hélène Mayer

(continued)

© Springer Nature Switzerland AG 2019
C.-H. Mayer and E. Vanderheiden (eds.), *The Bright Side of Shame*,
https://doi.org/10.1007/978-3-030-13409-9

(continued)

Page	Application	Context
141	Practical application: possibility offered and reflection questions	Shame at the Bottom of the Pyramid: A Transformative Consumer Research Perspective Leona Ungerer
174	Case study 1 Shame and Guilt Experienced by Battered Women	Interventions for Shame and Guilt Experienced by Battered Women Kathryn A. Nel & Sarawathie Govender
176	Case study 2 Shame and Guilt Experienced by Battered Women	
177	Case study 3 Shame and Guilt Experienced by Battered Women	
180	Glossary 1: Questions for Person-Centered Therapy and Narrative Therapy	
181	Examples of questions for Narrative Therapy	
192	A Four-Step Strategy for transforming shame: Name—Claim—Tame—Aim	Transforming Shame: Strategies in Spirituality and Prayer Thomas Ryan
206	Muhasabah (Self-audit)	Shame Transformation Using an Islamic Psycho-Spiritual Approach for Malay Muslims Recovering from Substance Dependence Dini Farhana Baharudin, Melati Sumari, Suhailiza Md Hamdani
206	Tawbah (Repentance and forgiveness)	
	Constructing new narrative of the self	
208	Developing a stronger relationship with Allah (hablum min Allah) andother humans (hablum min annas)	
208	Case study	
223	Excercise Self-compassion in the organisational context	Managing Shame in Organisations: Don't let Shame become a Self-destructive Spiral Rudolf Oosthuizen
226	Exercise The Compassionate Image	
227	Exercise Gestalt Two-Chair	
238	Case study	Shame! Whose Shame, is it?
246	Practical application: possibility offered and reflection questions	A systems psychodynamic Perspective on Shame in Organisations: a Case Study Louise Tonelli
263	Case study to apply the theory of brainfitness	Transforming Shame in the Workplace: A Brainfit Approach Dirk Geldenhuys
271	Bicultural Management Development (BMD) Model which can be applied	Transforming Shame to Collective Pride and Social Equity in Bicultural Organizations in Japan Clifford Clark and Naomi Takashiro
291	"The highlight of the week"—Instructions	Building a Work Culture beyond Forgiveness—Shame as Barrier for Growth and Knowledge-management in Working Environments Maike Baumann and Anke Handrock
293	Meta structure of weekly team meetings	
294	Additional notes on the implementation	
304	SIBART-Model	Lecturers through a Stay-away Action Disowning Shame: Interventions from a system psychodynamic Michelle S. May

(continued)

(continued)

Page	Application	Context
342	Case Study of Li—a Chinese Student in a German School	Transforming Shame in the German Educational System Using the Team Ombuds Model Christian Martin Boness
358	Interventions for handling shame	Dealing with Shame in a Medical Context Iris Veit and Kay Spiekermann
370	Case Study Review Dialogue	From Shame to Pride—Initiation of De-Stigmatisation Processes in Review Dialogues Ottomar Bahrs & Karl-Heinz Henze
371	Review Dialogue I: Problem Dimensioning—Lack of Recognition and Lack of Energy in the Cycle of Excessive Demands	
373	Review Dialogue III: Problem-Solving —Stigma, Outburst Fantasies and the Need for Talking	
374	Review Dialogue IV: First Achievements and Future Planning— Being Recognised, Resources, Ownership	
385	Case Studies Who am I?	Working with Shame in Psychotherapy: An Eclectic Approach Aakriti Malik
399	Application: Before the Looking Glass: Desired Images	Interpreting Instances of Shame from an Evolutionary Perspective: The Pain Analogy Jeff Elison
403	The Compass of Shame	
437	Case 1: Running for presidency	Working with Shame Experiences in Dreams: Therapeutical Interventions Claude-Hélène Mayer
438	Case 2: Winning naked	
440	Case 3: The men in my life and the knot in my stomach	
442	Case 4: Presenting in front of high achievers	
455	Dance with Shame	Shame-Death and Resurrection—The Phoenix-Dance to our Authentic Self Barbara Buch
467	Case Study Active Imagination	Unemployed and High Achiever? Working with Active Imagination and Symbols to Transform Shame Claude-Hélène Mayer
478	Bystander-Technique: Keeping the Emotional Distance	Shame and Forgiving in Therapy and Coaching Maike Baumann & Anke Handrock
481	How to Formulate a Forgiveness-contract	
483	Creating an Emotion-focussed Understanding of the Offender Using Perceptual Positions	
494	The shame tree	Somatically-based Art Therapy for Transforming Experiences of Shame Patricia Sherwood
501	Counselling session (9 steps)	

(continued)

(continued)

Page	Application	Context
511	Guided breathing exercise in preparation for deep relaxation	"Nothing I accept about Myself can be Used Against me to Diminish me"— Transforming Shame Through Mindfulness Elisabeth Vanderheiden
512	Guided Exercise Body scan	
515	Exercise Let (toxic) shame go	
515	Exercise Acceptance of shame	
515	Exercise Reconciliation with shame and shamers	
524	Description of a constellation work process dealing with shame	Healing Rituals to Transform Shame: an Example of Constellation Work Claude-Hélène Mayer
540	Case Study Heart Math	Discussion of HeartMath Techniques for the Transformation of Shame Experiences Stephen D. Edwards
552	Case Study 1 Appreciative Inquiry	Dealing with Shame using Appreciative Inquiry Kathryn A. Nel and Sarawathie Govender
553	Case Study 2 Appreciative Inquiry	
555	Case Study 3 Appreciative Inquiry	
566	Application of the meta-model to the practice of counselling, mediation, consulting and therapy: Questions regarding certainty and doubt about shame and pride	Transforming Shame into Pride ... and Vice Versa—A Meta-model for Understanding the Transformations of Shame and Pride in Counselling, Mediation, Consulting and Therapy Holger Lindemann
567	Application of the meta-model to the practice of counselling, mediation, consulting and therapy: Example in practice	
576	Applied CBT Methods in the context of bullying: Reflective Socratic Questioning	A Cognitive Behavioral Approach Towards Bullying Remediation Rebecca Merkin
577	Applied CBT Methods in the context of bullying: Intellectual-Emotional Role Play	
579	Applied CBT Methods in the context of bullying: Mindfulness Checklist	
588	Case studies	Facing the Ambivalence of Shame Issues: Exploring the Use of Motivational Techniques to Enhance Shame Resilience and Provoke Behaviour Change Len Andrieux
607	The Compass of Needs	Practice Report—Transforming Shame Through Mediation and Nonviolent Communication Liv Larsson
613	Four steps to regain connection and inner balance after a shame attack	